UICC

International Union Against Cancer

Union Internationale Contre le Cancer

PR
IN

SEC

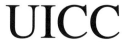

UICC International Union Against Cancer
Union Internationale Contre le Cancer

PROGNOSTIC FACTORS IN CANCER

SECOND EDITION

Edited by

M.K. Gospodarowicz
D.E. Henson
R.V.P. Hutter
B. O'Sullivan
L.H. Sobin
Ch. Wittekind

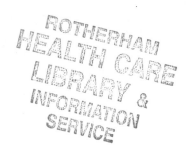

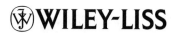**WILEY-LISS**

A JOHN WILEY & SONS, INC., PUBLICATION

New York • Chichester • Weinheim • Brisbane • Singapore • Toronto

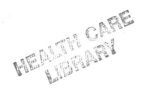

For ordering and customer service, call 1-800-CALL-WILEY.

Library of Congress Cataloging-in-Publication Data:

Prognostic factors in cancer / edited by M.K. Gospodarowicz. . .[et al.]. — 2nd ed.
    p.; cm.
  Includes bibliographical references and index.
  ISBN 0-471-40633-3 (pbk.: alk.paper)
  I. Cancer-Prognosis. I. Gospodarowicz, M.K. (Mary K.) II. International Union against Cancer.
  [DNLM: 1. Neoplasms — diagnosis. 2. Prognosis. 3. Neoplasm Staging. 4. Survival Rate. QZ 241 P964 2001]
  RC262 P688 2001
  616.99'4075 — dc21   2001017531

Printed in the United States of America.

10 9 8 7 6 5 4 3 2 1

CONTENTS

v

Medicine is a science of uncertainty and an art of probability

— *Sir William Osler, 1904*

This monograph is the result of an effort by the International Union Against Cancer (UICC) to study prognostic factors related to cancer. It is an extension of the long-term work on the TNM classification, and the follow-up to the first edition of *Prognostic Factors in Cancer*, published in 1995. Although anatomic extent of disease and histologic type are generally the most important indicators of prognosis for cancer patients and provide the main criteria for selecting therapy, they may not be sufficient to provide a powerful prognostic assessment. It has been recognized that other factors have a profound impact on prognosis of cancer patients.

The purpose of the second edition is to provide the framework for the consideration of prognosis and prognostic factors and for the application of prognostic factors to clinical practice for most tumor sites. The book has two parts. Part A, Principles of Prognostic Factors, deals with general issues surrounding prognosis and its measurement, the methodology of studying and classifying the prognostic factors, and the application of prognostic factors in clinical decision making. Part B, Prognostic Factors in specific Cancers, includes site- or tumor-specific chapters that provide a general overview of the relevant literature on prognostic factors. The authors have been asked to follow the template suggested in Chapter 1.2. Each site-specific chapter has a summary table that classifies the prognostic factors according to subject or topic and relevance. Since the anatomic disease extent is the main prognostic factor in most cancers, the current TNM classification is also provided in each chapter for reference. Finally, the last chapter aims to summarize common threads, explain the heterogeneity of Part B, and place the contents of the book in the context of the current research efforts in this area. To facilitate reading we have provided a glossary of selected terms used in this book.

We hope that this edition of *Prognostic Factors in Cancer* will be of value in (1) displaying the scope of this field; (2) stimulating the study of these and other prognostic factors; and (3) bringing some perspective to those working on specific factors.

ACKNOWLEDGMENTS

The Editors thank the International Union Against Cancer (UICC) for its support, and express appreciation to its secretariat for arranging meetings and facilitating communications.

This publication was made possible by grant number R13/CCR012626-01 from the United States Centers for Disease Control and Prevention (CDC). Its contents are the responsibility of the authors and do not necessarily represent the official views of the CDC.

M.K. GOSPODAROWICZ, *Toronto, Canada*
D.E. HENSON, *Bethesda, MD*
R.V.P. HUTTER, *Livingston, NJ*
B. O'SULLIVAN, *Toronto, Canada*
L.H. SOBIN, *Washington, DC*
Ch. WITTEKING, *Leipzig, Germany*

■■■■ CONTRIBUTORS

Jorge Albores-Saavedra Professor & Director, Division of Anatomic Pathology, UT Southwestern Medical Center, 5323 Harry Hines Blvd, Dallas, TX 75390-9073, USA

Sylvia L. Asa Professor of Laboratory Medicine and Pathobiology, University of Toronto, Faculty of Medicine, Department of Laboratory Medicine, Mt. Sinai Hospital, 600 University Avenue, Toronto, Ontario M5G 1X5, Canada

Luc Baert Professor and Chairman of Urology, KU Leuven, Herestraat 49, B-3000 Leuven, Belgium

Emma Bartfay Assistant Professor, Departments of Oncology, and Community Health and Epidemiology, Queen's University, Staff Scientist, Radiation Oncology Research Unit, Apps 4, Kingston General Hospital, Kingston, Ontario K7L 2V7, Canada

Pierfrancesco Bassi Assistant Professor, Department of Urology, University of Padova, Monoblocco Ospedaliero, Via Giustiniani, Padova 2, 35128 Italy

Richard J. Battafarano Division of Cardiothoracic Surgery, Assistant Professor of Surgery, Department of Surgery, Washington University School of Medicine, One Barnes-Jewish Hospital Plaza, Suite 3107, Queeny Tower, St. Louis, MO 63110-1013, USA

Goedele Beckers Resident in Urology, Division of Urology, KU Leuven, Herestraat 49, B-3000 Leuven, Belgium

Robert S. Bell Director, University Musculoskeletal Oncology Unit, Department of Surgery, Mount Sinai Hospital and the University of Toronto, Professor, Department of Surgery, University of Toronto, Mount Sinai Hospital, Suite 476, 600 University Avenue, Toronto M5G 1X5, Canada

J. Lou Benedet Professor, Department of Obstetrics & Gynecology, Division of Gynecologic Oncology, BC Cancer Agency & University of British Columbia, 600 West 10th Avenue, Vancouver, BC V5Z 4E6, Canada

Jeffrey M. Brandt President, Xaim, Inc., 6270 Lehman Drive, Suite 101, Colorado Springs, USA

James Brierley Associate Professor, Department of Radiation Oncology, University of Toronto, Department of Radiation Oncology, Princess Margaret Hospital, 610 University Avenue, Toronto, Ontario M5G 2M9, Canada

Robert G. Bristow Assistant Professor, Departments of Radiation Oncology & Medical Biophysics, University of Toronto, Associate Scientist, Division of Experimental Therapeutics, Ontario Cancer Institute, Department of Radiation Oncology, Princess Margaret Hospital/University Health Network, 610 University Avenue, Toronto, Ontario M5G 2M9, Canada

Michael D. Brundage Associate Professor, Departments of Oncology and Community Health and Epidemiology, Queen's University, Kingston Regional Cancer Clinic and Kingston General Hospital, Radiation Oncology Research Unit, Apps Level 4, Kingston General Hospital, Kingston, Ontario K7L 2V7, Canada

Joseph Califano Head and Neck Division, Department of Surgery, Memorial Sloan-Kettering Cancer Center, 1275 York Avenue, New York, New York 10021, USA

Vincent Chong Department of Diagnostic Radiology, Singapore General Hospital

Michael Crump Associate Professor, Department of Medicine, University of Toronto, Department of Medical Oncology and Hematology, Princess Margaret Hospital, 610 University Avenue, 5-110, Toronto, Ontario M5G 2M9, Canada

Bernard J. Cummings Chief, Department of Radiation Oncology, Professor, Faculty of Medicine, University of Toronto, Department of Radiation Oncology, Princess Margaret Hospital, Princess Margaret Hospital, 610 University Avenue, Toronto, Ontario M5G 2M9, Canada

Alastair J. Cunningham Professor, Department of Medical Biophysics, University of Toronto, Senior Scientist, Division of Epidemiology and Statistics and Behavioural Sciences, Ontario Cancer Institute, Princess Margaret Hospital/University Health Network, Director, The Healing Journey Program, Princess Margaret Hospital, 610 University Avenue, Toronto, Ontario M5G 2M9, Canada

Aileen M. Davis Director of Clinical Research, University Musculoskeletal Oncology Unit and the Division of Orthopaedic Surgery, Mount Sinai Hospital, Assistant Professor, Departments of Physical Therapy, Surgery and the Graduate Departments of Rehabilitation Science and Health Administration (Program in Clinical Epidemiology and Health Services Research), University of Toronto, Mount Sinai Hospital, Suite 476, 600 University Avenue, Toronto M5G IX5, Canada

Louis Denis Professor, Urology Vrije Universiteit Brussel, Director, Oncology Centre Antwerp, Lindenreef 1, B-2020 Antwerp, Belgium

Claire V. I. Edmonds Research Associate, Ontario Cancer Institute/Princess Margaret Hospital, The Healing Journey Program, 610 University Avenue, Toronto, Ontario M5G 2M9, Canada

Thomas G. Ehlen Assistant Professor, Department of Obstetrics & Gynecology Division of Gynecologic Oncology, BC Cancer Agency & University of British Columbia, 600 West 10th Avenue, Vancouver, BC V5Z 4E6, Canada

Dallas R. English Associate Professor, Department of Public Health, University of Western Australia, Queen Elizabeth II Medical Centre, 26 Leura St., Nedlands, Western Australia 6009

Charles Erlichman Professor of Oncology, Mayo Medical School, Director, Phase I Program and Associate Director for Translational Research, Mayo Clinic Cancer Center, Department of Oncology, 200 1st St. SW, Rochester MN 55905-0001, USA

Markus Feith Resident in General Surgery, Chirurgische Klinik und Poliklinik, Technische Universitat München, Klinikum rechts der Isar, Ismaningerstrabe 22, D-81675 München, Germany

Patrick L. Fitzgibbons Clinical Assistant Professor of Pathology, University of Southern California, School of Medicine, Director, Department of Pathology, Good Samaritan Hospital, 1225 Wilshire Blvd., Los Angeles, California 90017, USA

A. Fyles Associate Professor, Department of Radiation Oncology, Princess Margaret Hospital/University Health Network, 610 University Avenue, Toronto, Ontario M5G 2M9, Canada

Robert J. Ginsberg Chief, Thoracic Service, Department of Surgery, Memorial Sloan-Kettering Cancer Center, Professor of Surgery, Cornell University Medical College, 1275 York Avenue, New York, New York 10021, USA

Mary K. Gospodarowicz Professor, University of Toronto, Department of Radiation Oncology, Princess Margaret Hospital/University Health Network, 610 University Avenue, Toronto, Ontario M5G 2M9, Canada

Patti A. Groome Assistant Professor, Departments of Oncology and Community Health and Epidemiology, Queen's University, Scientist, Radiation Oncology Research Unit, Apps 4, Kingston General Hospital, Kingston, Ontario K7L 2V7, Canada

Peter J. Heenam Clinical Associate Professor, Department of Pathology, University of Western Australia, Queen Elizabeth II Medical Centre, 26 Leura St., Nedlands, Western Australia 6009

Donald Earl Henson Program Director, Cancer Biomarkers Research Group, Division of Cancer Prevention, National Cancer Institute, Executive Plaza North, Room 330, Bethesda, Maryland 20892, USA

Timothy J. Hobday Fellow in Hematology/Oncology, Mayo Graduate School of Medicine, Mayo Clinic, 200 1st St. SW, Rochester, MN 55905-0001, USA

David Hodgson Assistant Professor, Department of Radiation Oncology, University of Toronto, Institute for Clinical Evaluative Sciences, University of Toronto, Toronto, Canada, Department of Radiation Oncology, Princess Margaret Hospital, 610 University Avenue, Toronto, Ontario M5G 2M9, Canada

Simon Horenblas Chief, Dept. of Urology, Netherlands Cancer Institute/Antoni van Leeuwenhoek Hospital, Plesmanlaan 121, 1066 CX Amsterdam, The Netherlands

Philip J. Johnson Chairman, Department of Clinical Oncology, Chinese University of Hong Kong, Prince of Wales Hospital, Shatin, NT, Hong Kong

Ahmed Kara Department of Head and Neck, Centre Oscar Lambret, 3, Rue Frederic Combemale, B.P. 307-59020, Lille Cedex, France

Paul Kleihues Director, International Agency for, Research on Cancer (IARC), 150 Cours Albert-Thomas, 69372 Lyon, France

Heng-Nung Koong Fellow-Thoracic Service, Department of Surgery, Memorial Sloan-Kettering Cancer Center, 1275 York Avenue, New York, New York 10021, USA

Eric Lartigau Professor Radiation Oncology, Departments of Head and Neck and Radiotherapy, Centre Oscar Lambret, Rue Frederic Combemale, 59000 Lille, France

Jean-Louis Lefebvre Deputy Director Centre Oscar Lambret (Northern France Comprehensive Cancer Center), Chief, Head and Neck Department, Professor ENT, Head and Neck surgery, 3, Rue Frederic Combemale, B.P. 307-59020, Lille Cedex, France

William J. Mackillop Professor of Oncology, and Community Health and Epidemiology, Queen's University,, Head, Division of Radiation Oncology, Kingston Regional Cancer Centre, 25 King St. West, Kingston, Ontario K7L 5P9, Canada

Karen J. Marcus Assistant Professor of Radiation Oncology (Pediatrics), Division Chief of Radiation Oncology at Children's Hospital, Harvard Medical School, 300 Longwood Ave, Boston, MA 02115, USA

David G. McLeod Clinical Professor, Department of Surgery (Urology), Georgetown University Medical Center, Washington, DC, Professor of Surgery and Chief, Division of Urology, Uniformed Services University of the Health Sciences, Bethesda, Maryland, Chief, Urology Service, Walter Reed Army Medical Center, 6900 Georgia Avenue, NW, Washington, DC, USA

Lisa M. McShane Biometric Research Branch, National Cancer Institute, Bethesda, Maryland 20892, USA

Donna M. Miller Chair, Gynecologic Oncology Tumor Group, BC Cancer Agency, Assistant Professor, University of British Columbia, Vancouver Hospital & Health Sciences Centre, 855 12th Ave. W., Vancouver, B.C. V5Z 1M9, Canada

Mark Minden Professor, University of Toronto, Senior Scientist, Ontario Cancer Institute, Department of Medical Oncology and Hematology, Princess Margaret Hospital, University Health Network, 610 University Avenue, Toronto, Ontario M5G 2M9, Canada

Gerald P. Murphy Pacific Northwest Cancer Foundation

Hextan Y. S. Ngan Professor, University of Hong Kong, Dept. of Ob/Gynecology, Queen Mary Hospital, Room 605 6/F, Prof. Block, Pokfulham Rd., Hong Kong

Kazuhiro Nomura Deputy-Director, National Cancer Center, Tokyo, 5-1-1 Chuo-ku Tsukiji Tokyo, Japan

Franco E. Odicino Division of Obstetrics & Gynecology II, Gynecologic Oncology, Spedali Civili di Brescia, Piazzale Spedali Civili 1, 25123 Brescia, Italy

Hiroko Ohgaki Chief, Unit of Molecular Pathology, International Agency for Research on Cancer (IARC), 150 cours Albert Thomas, 69372 Lyon Cedex 08, France

Brian O'Sullivan Associate Professor of Radiation Oncology, University of Toronto, Department of Radiation Oncology, Princess Margaret Hospital/ University Health Network, 610 University Avenue, Toronto, Ontario M5G 2M9, Canada

Katja Ott Chirurgische Klinik und Poliklinik der Technischen Universitat Munchen, Klinikum rechts der Isar, Ismaninger Str 22, D-81675 München

Francesco Pagano Chairman, Department of Urology, University of Padova, Istituto di Urologia, Monoblocco Ospedaliero, Via Giustiniani, Padova 2, 35128 Italy

David G. Payne Associate Professor, Department of Radiation Oncology, University of Toronto, Department of Radiation Oncology, Princess Margaret Hospital, 610 University Avenue, Toronto, Ontario M5G 2M9, Canada

Sergio Pecorelli Director, Division of Obstetrics & Gynecology II, Gynecologic Oncology, Editor, FIGO Annual Report, European Institute of Oncology, via Ripamonti 435, 20141 Milano, Italy

Peter W. T. Pisters Associate Professor of Surgical Oncology, Department of Surgical Oncology, University of Texas M.D. Anderson Cancer Center, 1515 Holcombe Blvd., Houston, Texas, 77030-4009, USA

Graham Pitson Fellow, Department of Radiation Oncology, Princess Margaret Hospital/University Health Network, 610 University Avenue, Toronto, Ontario M5G 2M9, Canada

Raphael E. Pollock Head, Division of Surgery, Professor and Chairman, Department of Surgical Oncology, The University of Texas M.D. Anderson Cancer Center, Box 106, 1515 Holcombe Blvd., Houston, Texas, 77030-4095, USA

Michael Poulsen Clinical Associate Professor, University of Queensland, Department of Radiation Oncology, Mater Queensland Radium Institute, Raymond TCE, South Brisbane, Queensland, 4101 Australia

Guido Reifenberger Department of Neuropathology, University of Bonn Medical Center, Sigmund-Freud-Str. 25, D-53105 Bonn, Germany

Christoph Rie Klinik und Poliklinik, Martin-Luther-Universitat Halle-Wittenberg, Ernst-Grube-StraBe 40, Hem/Onk, Halle (Saale), 06120 Germany

Lynn G. Ries Health Statistician, National Cancer Institute, Cancer Statistics Branch, 6130 Executive Blvd. - MSC 7352, EPN 343J, Bethesda, MD 20892-7352, USA

Jürgen D. Roder Chirurgische Klinik und Poliklinik der Technischen Universitat Munchen, Klinikum rechts der Isar, Ismaninger Str 22, D-81675 München, Germany

David M. Rodvold Director of Technology Development, Xaim Inc., 6270 Lehman Dr., Ste 101, Colorado Springs, CO 80918, USA

Jérôme Sarini Head and Neck Surgeon, Head and Neck Department, Centre Oscar Lambret, 3, Rue Frederic Combemale, B.P. 307-59020 Lille Cedex, France

Mitsuru Sasako Professor of Surgery, Chief, Gastric Surgery Division, Department of Surgical Oncology, National Cancer Center Hospital, Tokyo, Japan, Department of Surgery, Leiden University Medical Centre, The Netherlands

Hans-Joachim Schmoll Director of the Institute of Hematology and Oncology, Internal Medicine IV, Martin-Luther-University, Ernst-Grube-Strasse 40, 06120 Halle, Germany

Carol L. Shields Associate Professor, Jefferson Medical College, Thomas Jefferson University, Philadelphia, Pennsylvania, Attending Surgeon, Oncology Service, 900 Walnut Street, Wills Eye Hospital, Philadelphia, Pennsylvania, PA 19107, USA

Jerry A. Shields Professor of Ophthalmology, Jefferson Medical College, Thomas Jefferson University, Philadelphia, Pennsylvania, Director, Ocular Oncology Service, Wills Eye Hospital, 900 Walnut Street, Philadelphia, Pennsylvania 19107, USA

Richard Simon Chief, Biometric Research Branch, National Cancer Institute, Bethesda, Maryland 20892, USA

Arun D. Singh Assistant Professor of Ophthalmology, Jefferson Medical School, Thomas Jefferson University, Philadelphia, Pennsylvania, Assistant Surgeon, Oncology Service, Wills Eye Hospital, 900 Walnut Street, Philadelphia, Pennsylvania 19107, USA

Peter B. Snow Vice President and Chief Technical Officer, Xaim, Inc., 6270 Lehman Drive, Suite 101, Colorado Springs, CO 80918, USA

Lena Specht Chief Oncologist, Herlev Hospital/University of Copenhagen, DK-2730 Herlev, Denmark

Ronald H. Spiro Professor of Clinical Surgery, Cornell Medical College, New York, Head and Neck Service, Department of Surgery, Memorial Sloan-Kettering Cancer Center, 1275 York Avenue, New York, New York 10021, USA

Hubert J. Stein General and Thoracic Surgeon, Oberarzt, Chirurgische Klinik und Poliklinik, Technische Universitat München, Klinikum rechts der Isar, Ismaningerstrable 22, D-81675 München, Germany

Cornelis J. H. van de Velde Professor of Surgery, Head of Department of Surgical Oncology, Endocrine and Head and Neck Surgery, and Gastro-intestinal Surgery, Leiden University Medical Center, P.O. Box 9600, 2300 RC LEIDEN, The Netherlands

J. Han J. M. van Krieken University Hospital Nijmegen, Department of Pathology, Professor of Tumorpathology, P.O. Box 9101, 6500 HB Nijmegen, The Netherlands

Hendrik Van Poppel Head, Uro-oncologic Clinic, Professor of Urology, KU Leuven, University of Hospitals Gasthuisberg, Herestraat 49, B-3000 Leuven, Belgium

J. N. Waldron Lecturer, Department of Radiation Oncology, Faculty of Medicine, University of Toronto, Staff Radiation Oncologist, Department of Radiation Oncology, Princess Margaret Hospital, 610 University Avenue, Toronto, Ontario M5G 2M9, Canada

Ian J. Witterick Department of Otolaryngology, Mt. Sinai Hospital and University of Toronto, 600 University Avenue, Suite 401, Toronto, Ontario M5G 1X5, Canada

Ling-chui Wong Professor, Division of Gynaecological Oncology, University of Hong Kong, Dept. of Obstetrics & Gynaecology, University of Hong Kong, Queen Mary Hospital, Hong Kong

Jay S. Wunder Associate Director, University Musculoskeletal Oncology Unit, Department of Surgery, Mount Sinai Hospital and the University of Toronto, Assistant Professor, Department of Surgery, University of Toronto, Mount Sinai Hospital, Suite 476, 600 University Avenue, Toronto M5G 1X5, Canada

Lawrence L. Yu Clinical Senior Lecturer, Department of Pathology, University of Western Australia, Queen Elizabeth II Medical Centre, 26 Leura St., Nedlands, Western Australia 6009

Lucia Zigliani European Institute of Oncology, via Ripamonti 435, 20141 Milano, Italy

PRINCIPLES OF PROGNOSTIC FACTORS

■■■■■■■ CHAPTER 1

The Importance of Prognosis in Cancer Medicine

WILLIAM J. MACKILLOP

THE ROLE OF PROGNOSIS IN THE PRACTICE OF MEDICINE

It is the best thing, in my opinion, for the physician to apply himself diligently to the art of foreknowing.

— Hippocrates

Prognosis: The Oldest of the Clinical Skills

Diagnosis, prognosis, and therapeutics are the three core elements of the art of medicine.[1,2] Today, diagnosis and treatment may seem to be of transcending importance, but prognosis has been part of the practice of medicine much longer than diagnosis. Sick people have always been preoccupied by their prospects for recovery, and physicians acquired genuine skill in prognosis long before therapeutics had anything real to offer.[3,4] *Mantic prognosis*, the foretelling of the outcome of an illness based on omens and magic, has been widely practiced since the beginning of recorded history,[5] but scientific approaches to prognosis also began long ago. *Semiotic prognosis*, the foretelling of the outcome of an illness based on clinical findings, can be traced as far back as the Sumerian civilization of 2000 B.C.[3] and reached a high level of sophistication in Greece in the era of Hippocrates about 400 B.C.[6] The Hippocratic school recognized complexes of symptoms and signs that predicted a good or bad outcome, and was also aware that environmental factors and characteristics of the patient could influence the prognosis. Hippocratic knowledge resembles modern medical knowledge in that it was based on clinical observation and applied by pattern recognition.[6] However,

Prognostic Factors in Cancer, 2nd edition, Edited by Mary K. Gospodarowicz
ISBN 0-471-40633-3   Copyright © 2001 Wiley-Liss, Inc.

Hippocratic prognostication differed significantly from modern prognostication in that the prognosis was inferred directly from the symptoms without passing through the process of diagnosis.[1,6] Although many of the symptom complexes described by Hippocrates are readily recognizable today as corresponding to specific diseases, Edelstein points out that "there is, in ancient medicine, no theory of disease per se."[6]

The Rise of Diagnosis

After Hippocrates, there were surprisingly few real advances in the science of medicine for almost 2000 years. Therapeutics flourished, but remedies were almost always directed by theories that had no empirical basis.[3,4] Modern medicine really began about 300 years ago when it was first clearly recognized that the right way to treat a patient could not be *deduced* from scientific theory, and that the effectiveness of treatment had to be *induced* by clinical observation.[7,8] Induction is the general process of inference that allows us to predict what will happen in a specific set of circumstances in the future, based on observations made in similar circumstances in the past.[7]

To apply inductive reasoning in medicine, it is essential to have a means of classifying clinical problems into groups of "similar" cases. In the seventeenth century, Sydenham provided the first "nosology," or classification of human diseases into diagnostic groups, based on the symptoms reported by the patient and the signs elicited by the clinicians.[3,4,8] Diagnosis from then on provided the link to past experience that permitted a rational choice of therapy. In the eighteenth century, postmortem studies began to reveal the pathological changes that were responsible for specific clinical syndromes, and this led to a more objective clinicopathological classification of diseases.[4,8] Successive advances in science and technology have since permitted many further refinements to this system of diagnostic classification, although our system today remains imperfect. The classification of neoplastic disease presents particular problems, and even modern diagnostic criteria do not create truly uniform groups of cases.[9]

The Ellipsis of Prognosis

In the modern era, the perceived importance of prognosis appears to have declined. In the late nineteenth century the standard textbooks of medicine all included extensive introductory sections dealing with this aspect of medical practice alongside diagnosis.[10–13] Modern textbooks of medicine, on the other hand, do not accord it any special status. Although there is some discussion of prognosis in sections dealing with specific diseases, here also the emphasis on prognosis has declined over the years. Christakis traced the decline in the emphasis in prognosis in the context of acute pneumonia through successive editions of Osler's textbook of medicine.[14] From being a dominant concern a hundred years ago, it almost disappeared altogether by the middle of the twentieth century. Christakis described this phenomenon as the "ellipsis" of prognosis, and attributed it to increasingly successful therapies that made the details of the natural history of the illness seem less relevant to the clinician. The theoretical basis of prognosis also receives scant attention in modern textbooks of clinical epidemiology, while diagnosis is discussed extensively and quantitative methods for measuring its accuracy are provided.[15,16] As we shall see, however, it is naive to believe that advances in diagnosis and therapy have made prognosis irrelevant; diagnosis and prognosis are complementary rather than competing aspects of medical practice.

The Relationship Between Diagnosis and Prognosis

Diagnosis means generalizing, transcending the particular; prognosis, however, means individualizing, allowing for the particular.

— Weissman, Theoretical Medicine and Bioethics

Prognosis differs from diagnosis in several ways. First, the goal of diagnosis is to discover a present fact, while the goal of prognosis is to predict the future. Second, the diagnosis may be static, but prognosis changes over time and may be modified by therapy. Third, the diagnosis is primarily a means to an end, providing a guide for therapy and prognosis; the prognosis, too, may guide therapy, but it is also an end in itself in that it directly addresses the patient's need for information about the future. Finally, and perhaps most importantly, the diagnosis is an abstract notion of the disease that is independent of the individual case, while the prognosis describes the probable course of the illness in a particular patient.[17-20]

THE BASIS OF PROGNOSIS

An expert prediction of outcome is based upon an accurate diagnosis, knowledge of the natural history of the disease, the disease's response to treatment, and the progression of the disease in the patient in question.

— Bailey, Concise Dictionary of Medical-Legal Terms

This definition, provided by a contemporary medical dictionary, makes it clear that two different frames of reference are used in predicting the outcome(s) of an illness. The first is an external frame of reference, provided by past experience in similar cases. The second is an internal frame of reference, provided by the previous course of the illness in the individual case. Both are important in oncology; the former is the dominant source of information at the time of diagnosis, and the latter assumes increasing importance during the course of the illness.

The External Frame of Reference: Past Experience in Similar Cases

There is a natural division of the subject into two parts. The first embraces prognosis as considered in its relation to diagnosis, and comprehends those general conclusions as to the future which are drawn from the known tendency of any given disease. The second comprehends those particular circumstances which belong to the individual case.

—Ash, The Cyclopaedia of Practical Medicine

Figure 1.1 illustrates how past experience in similar cases serves as the basis for prognosis in the individual case. Two different pathways lead to the prognosis. The first (α), starts with the assignment of a diagnosis based on clinical and pathological findings (α_1). The general prognosis associated with this diagnosis, which is sometimes referred to as the *ontologic prognosis*,[21] is then induced from past experience in patients with the same diagnosis (α_2). The prognosis is then attributed to the individual case (α_3). The second pathway, labeled β in Figure 1.1, involves the application of past experience relating to aspects of the case that are *not* included in the abstract notion of the diagnosis. These attributes were formerly referred to as "prognostics,"[10] but today they are usually known as "prognostic factors." In ancient Greek medicine, before diagnosis became established, the β pathway was obviously the only route to the prognosis. In modern medicine, the β pathway usually operates in conjunction with the α pathway and serves to modify the ontologic prognosis to provide the *individual prognosis*. In modern oncology the β pathway also functions alone in some circumstances, for example, in terminal illness, when the primary diagnosis ceases to be relevant and the classical Hippocratic signs become the best indicators of impending death.[22] Note that the distinction between "diagnosis" and "prognostic factor" is sometimes blurred. Measures of the severity of the disease, such as the

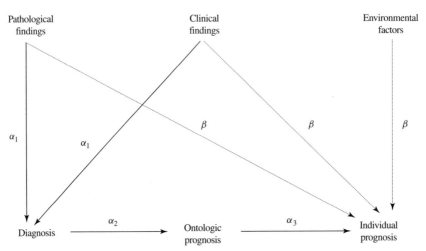

Figure 1.1   The basis of prognosis. The diagram illustrates the flow of information in establishing the prognosis in an individual case. The α pathway shows how diagnosis precedes and forms the basis for prognosis in modern medical practice. The β pathway shows how clinical findings were used to predict outcomes directly in the Hippocratic era. Today the β pathway serves to modify the ontologic prognosis established by the diagnosis.

grade or stage of a cancer, may be considered as prognostic factors by some, while others see them as inherent aspects of the diagnosis.

The Internal Frame of Reference: The Previous Course of the Illness

The prognosis may also be inferred from the trajectory of the illness observed in the individual case.[1,21] Tumor growth rates in individual cases have been observed to remain relatively constant over time.[23,24] If a cancer has been observed to grow slowly in the past, it is therefore reasonable to infer that it will continue to progress slowly in the future. Likewise, if the patient's functional status has declined rapidly, it will probably continue to deteriorate rapidly, and if the cancer has already failed to respond to several forms of systemic treatment, it will probably not respond to the next. Often, there is insufficient information available to use this form of reasoning at the time of diagnosis, but it becomes more and more important as the passage of time reveals the pace of the disease. Although the primary frame of reference here is internal, it does rely on the external frame to some extent; we would not be able to deduce the future behavior of an individual tumor from its previous behavior, if we did not know from past experience that the rate of tumor progression is generally fairly constant.

THE DIMENSIONS OF THE PROGNOSIS

The prognosis is multidimensional. Bailey defines it as "a reasoned forecast concerning the course, pattern, progression, duration, and end of the disease."[20] The prognosis is a dynamic quantity that changes as events unfold. The *natural prognosis* may be modifiable by therapeutic intervention(s), in which case, several *conditional prognoses* may be applicable to a given case at one point, depending on the choice of treatment. Furthermore, the patient's future may be affected by more than one illness, and a comprehensive prognosis must reflect the probable outcomes of all competing causes of morbidity.

The Prognosis is Multidimensional

The prognosis includes, but is not limited to, the issue of life and death. It may include any aspect of the future health or functional status of the patient. By the nineteenth century, the standard American and European medical textbooks all described the dimensions of prognosis. In that era, they were often referred to as the "objects of prognosis."[10-13,25,26] Today we would simply call them outcomes. In 1859, the following classic description of the types of questions that may have to be addressed in formulating the prognosis appeared in one of the standard textbooks of medicine:[12]

1) Will the disease end in death or recovery or will it continue indefinitely?
2) If it proves fatal will death come quickly or slowly and how will the patient die?

3) If the patient recovers, will some morbid condition remain either in the form of general ill health or some local problem?

4) How long will the illness last?

5) What events are likely to take place in its course, such as changes in symptoms, critical phenomena, the occurrence of complications?

6) Does having had the illness make the patient more or less susceptible to other illnesses?

This broad list of topics makes it clear that prognosis traditionally involved predicting not only survival, but many other outcomes as well. For a time in the 1960s and 1970s, when advances in chemotherapy made it seem that every cancer might soon be cured, the focus of prognosis in oncology seems to have narrowed to survival alone. Since the 1980s there has been a reawakening of interest in outcomes other than survival, and the broad classic definition of prognosis fits well with contemporary concerns about quality of life.

Before formulating the prognosis, Roberts recommended that the doctor should decide what outcomes are most important in the individual case.[24] This sensible approach remains valid today, except that the patient, rather than the doctor, now seems to us the right person to judge what is important. Empirical studies have demonstrated that many different aspects of the prognosis are important to cancer patients and to their doctors.[27-30] Table 1.1 shows some information provided by a survey of patients with ovarian cancer who were asked to score the importance of a number of questions about the illness that had been identified as possibly relevant in preliminary surveys of patients, doctors, and nurses.[27,28] It is interesting that each type of prognostic issue identified by Roberts more that 100 years ago is represented on this empirically derived list of contemporary concerns. This study revealed that questions concerning the prognosis were generally ranked much higher by patients than questions about the diagnosis or the treatment. The aspects of the illness that were most important varied widely from one patient to the next, and the concerns of the individual could not easily be predicted based on the characteristics of the patient. Thus, the only way to find out what prognostic information patients want is to ask them.

The Prognosis is a Dynamic Quantity

Perhaps the most important distinction between diagnosis and prognosis is to be made in terms of time. Diagnosis detemporalizes the disease process, and prognosis unrolls even a momentary state into a significant time sequence.

— Buchanan, The Doctrine of Signatures: A Defense of Theory in Medicine

The prognosis changes as events unfold over time, and new information becomes available. It obviously gets worse with the occurrence of any new event with adverse consequences; when a patient, treated initially with curative intent for an early cancer, develops evidence of distant metastases, the probability of long-term survival often drops to zero. On the other hand, if no adverse events occur, the prognosis may improve. If the patient survives without recurrence for five

TABLE 1.1   Questions Ranked Most Important by Cancer Patients Who are Faced with a Decision About Treatment

Questions	Rank	Median Score
Will the treatment cause the disease to go into complete remission?	1	9.29
Will the treatment cure me of the disease so that I may live a normal life span?	2	9.26
Will the disease lead to my death if left untreated?	3	9.21
How fast will the disease spread if left untreated?	4	9.16
How long will I live if the disease is left untreated?	5	9.10
What organs of my body will be affected by the disease if left untreated?	5	9.10
Will I have to be admitted to the hospital for treatment?	7	8.70
Will the disease be painful if left untreated?	8	9.07
Is the equipment at this hospital up-to-date for treating this disease?	9	9.06
How quickly does the treatment affect the disease?	10	9.04
Will the disease (if left untreated) affect my ability to care for myself?	10	9.04
Will the untreated disease cause me to be dependent on others?	12	9.02
If I refuse treatment, will my physician continue to care for me?	13	8.99
Will the disease spread to my brain if left untreated?	14	8.97
How many patients with this disease are ever cured by this treatment?	15	8.96

Source: Reference 28.

Note: Patients with ovarian cancer used a linear analogue scale to indicate the relative importance of 57 questions about the illness and its treatment. This table shows their top 15 responses.

years following radical treatment for an early cancer, the probability of long-term survival may be much higher than it was at the time of diagnosis.

The prognosis may also become more or less certain as new information becomes available. Consider the case of the patient treated radically for Stage IV cervical cancer. At the outset it is fairly certain she will die of the cancer, although there is a sufficient chance of cure to justify radical treatment. If she has a complete response to radiotherapy and no recurrence during the first few months, the outcome is much less certain. If she survives five years, it becomes fairly certain she will not die of her cancer. Thus, we go from near certainty about a bad outcome, through complete uncertainty, to near certainty about a good outcome, over a period of a few years.

Conditional Prognoses

The predictive inference depends on a dilemma between a prediction of the course of the trouble if left alone, and a prediction of the effect of the remedy if it is administered.

—Buchanan, The Doctrine of Signatures: A Defense of Theory in Medicine

In a short story entitled, *El jardin de los senderos que se bifurcan* ("The Garden of Branching Pathways"), Jorge Luis Borges used his title theme as a metaphor for life.[31] Whenever a person faced a decision that would affect the future, one part of him took each of the two paths available, and each went on through life in a parallel universe. In reality, for any individual there will only be one future, but there may be several possible futures from which to choose. The course of an illness may be dependent on external factors over which the patient or doctor has control, and present actions may modify the future. Whenever a choice of paths is available to the patient, each comes with its own prognosis. The prognosis, *if* the patient chooses the primary radiotherapy, may be quite different from the prognosis *if* the patient chooses surgery, or the prognosis *if* the patient chooses no active treatment, and each of these *conditional prognoses* requires to be considered before a rational decision about treatment can be made. Whether or not formal decision analysis is employed at the bedside, the comparison of conditional prognoses is at the heart of all rational therapeutic decisions.

The Comprehensive Prognosis

Most contemporary and historical definitions of the prognosis insist that it is a prediction of the outcome of a particular case *of a disease*.[17-20] However, the patient's future may be determined by the outcomes of several different diseases. The term, comprehensive prognosis, is used here to describe predictions of what will happen *to the patient*. A comprehensive prognosis must reflect the expected outcomes of all potential competing causes of death and morbidity, and not merely those associated with the dominant illness. Consider, for example, how the probability of death from competing causes sometimes dominates treatment decisions in early prostate cancer, where no active treatment may be indicated if it appears that other illnesses pose a greater risk to the patient's life and health than the cancer. It is always useful to consider causes of morbidity other than the cancer, even if this only leads to the conclusion that the chance of another illness becoming the dominant issue is so unlikely as to be irrelevant. Doctors may do this unconsciously, but it is better dealt with explicitly. Errors in decision making may result if comorbidity is ignored, or if its importance is overestimated. The comprehensive prognosis, which incorporates all competing risks, is the correct basis for medical decision making, and it is the quantity that has most meaning for the individual patient.

THE IMPORTANCE OF PROGNOSIS IN ONCOLOGY

The prognosis plays a central role in medical decision making, and is also valuable to patients in making decisions about aspects of their lives unrelated to their medical care. Providing prognostic information is a medico-legal responsibility. Good prognostication also contributes to the efficiency of medical care, and an understanding of prognostic factors facilitates our ability to learn from clinical experience.

Medical Decision Making

Whereas scientific knowledge is generalized and impersonal, medical practice takes place under conditions which are singular, individual, and irreversible.

— Weissman, Theoretical Medicine and Bioethics

Decision making in oncology is particularly difficult because the game is played for high stakes, and it is played for keeps. The potential benefits of cancer treatment are exceptional; unlike the situation in most other domains of medicine, cancer treatment can often eradicate the disease entirely. However, the morbidity associated with many forms of cancer treatment is also exceptional, and usually irreversible. Oncologists, therefore, rarely have the luxury of using a trial therapy to establish the correct course of action. The first treatment decision compromises all subsequent treatment decisions, and every effort has to be made to make the right choice the first time around.

The decision to treat is always based on the comparison of at least two conditional prognoses, the prognosis without treatment and the prognosis with treatment. The choice between two or more active treatment options is made by comparing the conditional prognoses associated with each course of action. This comparison may be made by formal decision analysis or more commonly, by some form of informal holistic judgment. In the past doctors often made these decisions on behalf of the patient. Today, modern medical ethics emphasizes the patient's right to self-determination, and patients are increasingly involved with what were formerly medical decisions.[32] It is clear that, under identical, external circumstances, different patients reach different decisions based on their personal values.[33,34] This is illustrated in Figure 1.2, which shows how different patients weigh gains in survival against increased toxicity, in choosing between more and less aggressive therapies for non-small-cell lung cancer. It illustrates how sensitive treatment decisions may be to prognostic information, and indicates that a fairly textured description of the probable outcomes of each alternative course of action may be required to permit the patients to make the best possible decision for themselves.

Personal Decision Making

Patients also need prognostic information to make decisions about other aspects of their lives. There are four distinct ways in which prognostic information can be useful in making personal decisions. First of all, knowing what the future may hold can provide an opportunity to take preemptive action to avoid a bad outcome. To use the weather as an analogy, the forecast may allow you to alter course to avoid a storm. In some instances, it may be possible for patients to modify their behaviors to decrease the risk of bad outcomes. Smoking cessation can decrease the risk of second primary cancers, and compliance with close follow-up, in some situations, can reduce the risk of death. Second, it may be useful to know what is coming in order to prepare for it; the forecast provides a chance to batten down the hatches and get ready for bad weather. Patients need to know their

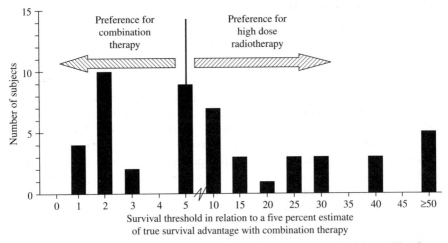

Figure 1.2 The effect of the prognosis on individual treatment decisions. The figure illustrates how much improvement in survival patients with Stage III non-small-cell lung cancer believe would be necessary for them to choose combined modality treatment as opposed to radiotherapy. The diagram shows a frequency distribution of the survival advantage at three years that made the combined approach seem superior to RT alone in a trade-off exercise from Brundage et al.[33]

prognosis in order to make decisions about their finances, their employment, and sometimes their accommodation in order to prepare to meet their future needs. Relatives may also need to make important personal decisions in order to prepare for a caregiving role, or for life without the support of the patient. The prognosis may also provide the opportunity for the patient to make spiritual preparations for the end of their lives. Third, knowing what is to come in the longer term is useful in planning one's short-term agenda; if it is going to rain tomorrow, you will want to do the outdoor things today. With the threat of deteriorating health down the road, patients may want to take the opportunity to do things that they promised themselves they always would, but have previously postponed. Finally, and sometimes most importantly, there is knowing for the sake of knowing. The argument here is not a consequentialist one; the knowledge itself simply meets the psychological need to know.

The Medico–Legal Perspective

He who is master of the art of prognosis, and shows himself such, will demonstrate such a superior knowledge, that the generality of men will commit themselves to the physician wholeheartedly.

—Hippocrates

In ancient Greek medicine, accurate prognosis was seen as a means of building patients' trust, of avoiding blame for bad outcomes, and of building a good reputation in the community.[6] These issues are still relevant in medical practice today, but potential liability for failure to provide prognostic information is an additional consideration. The physician is now expected to inform patients about the expected outcomes of any procedure or treatment before they are asked to give consent to it. Although practice varies around the world, this is an established principle under Anglo-American common law, and is also encoded as statute in some jurisdictions.[35,36] Failure to inform patients about the prognosis with respect to the potential benefits and material risks of treatment, and also about the risks associated with *not* undergoing treatment, may be deemed negligence.[35]

The Health Policy Perspective

On a societal level, skill in prognosis is useful as a means of optimizing the use of resources. Accurate prognosis is a precondition for good medical decisions, and good decisions lead to efficient care, whereas bad decisions waste money. The use of aggressive forms of active treatment in situations where the prognosis is hopeless can obviously be very expensive, but undertreatment can also have adverse financial consequences. Overlooking the chance for cure in a potentially curable patient is not only a lethal error, it is also an expensive one, because the cost of dying of cancer can greatly exceed the cost of effective treatment.

Prognostic information may also be useful in making allocational decisions. Some publicly funded health care systems have now begun to make decisions about which types of care they are willing to pay for, based on an economic appraisal of the benefits they achieve in the relationship to their cost. This type of decision making may be unfair unless the individual characteristics of the case can be factored into the equation. Consistently applying decisions at the level of the diagnostic group may seem sensible enough, but in circumstances in which individual characteristics of the case have a very large impact on outcome, it may prove too simplistic to be truly equitable. The principle of justice demands not only that like situations be treated alike, but also that situations that are unalike should not be treated as if they were the same.[32] Prognostic information is therefore essential for fair allocational decisions.

The Research Perspective

In cancer research, an understanding of prognostic factors is important in the design and analysis of clinical trials and retrospective reviews of clinical experience. Valid comparison of treatment and control groups requires that the expected outcome without treatment should be similar in both. Prognostic factors are used as eligibility criteria to ensure a relatively uniform study population, and they may also be used in the process of stratification that is undertaken to balance the case mix in each arm as far as possible. The more the variance in outcome due to prognostic factors other than the treatment can be controlled in the experiment, the more readily the effect of treatment itself can be determined. Identification of prognostic factors also allows identification of subgroups of cases that experience poor outcomes with standard treatment, in which experimental therapy should be tested. An understanding of prognostic factors is also important in cancer research because in some instances, prognostic factors may have a causal relationship to the outcome of the disease. When this is the case, strategies aimed at modifying the prognostic factor may also modify the outcome. For a more detailed discussion of these issues, see Chapter 10.

CONCLUSION

Thus, prognostic judgment remains an essential element of modern, medical practice. It meets patients' needs for information about the future that they can use to plan their lives, and it provides a basis for rational medical decisions. In the future, the importance of prognosis in oncology is likely to increase as new predictors of the prognosis permit increasingly accurate predictions of the outcomes of treatment. Over the last 30 years, advances in clinical epidemiology have greatly improved the practice of oncology; we understand much better today how to establish the *generalizability* of clinical observations. In future, however, the challenge will be to increase the *particularizability* of medical knowledge in such a way that the individual characteristics of the patient and the tumor are appropriately factored into treatment decisions. This will require characterizing patients, not only in terms of the diagnostic group to which they belong, but also in terms of all those individual characteristics that may influence the outcome of treatment. Hence, the importance of continuing to study prognostic factors in oncology, and of learning to use them correctly.

REFERENCES

1. Buchanan S: *The doctrine of signatures: a defense of theory in medicine*, Foreword by Edmund D. Pellegrino; Maycock PP, Jr. (ed.), 2d ed. Urbana and Chicago, University of Illinois Press, 1991.

2. Gibson AG: *The physician's art: an attempt to expand John Locke's fragment de arte medica*. Oxford, Clarendon Press, 1933.

3. Magner LN: *A history of medicine*. New York, Marcel Dekker, 1992.

4. McManus JFA: *The fundamentals of medicine: a brief history of medicine*. Springfield (IL), Charles C Thomas, 1963.

5. Sigerist HE: *History of medicine*, New York, Oxford University Press, 1951–61.

6. Temkin O, Temkin CL: (eds.): *Ancient medicine: selected papers Of Ludwig Edelstein*. Baltimore and London, Johns Hopkins University Press, 1967.

7. Howson C, Urbach P: *Scientific reasoning*. LaSalle (IL), Open Court Publishing Company, 1989.

8. Shryock RH: *The development of modern medicine: an interpretation of the social and scientific factors involved*. Madison, University of Wisconsin Press, 1979.

9. Mackillop WJ, O'Sullivan B, Gospodarowicz M: The role of cancer staging in evidence-based medicine. *Cancer Prev Control* 2:269–77, 1998.

10. Ash E: Prognosis in Forbes J, Tweedie A, Conolly J. (eds.): *The cyclopaedia of practical medicine* vol. III. Philadelphia, Blanchard and Lea, 1859, pp. 699–706.

11. Hartshorne H: *A system of medicine*, vol. 1, Reynolds JR, (ed.). Philadelphia, Henry C. Lea's Son, 1880, pp. 21–32.

12. Roberts FT: *A handbook of the theory and practice of medicine*, London, Lewis, 1885, pp. 10–21.

13. Flint A. *A treatise of the principles and practice of medicine*, 5th ed. Philadelphia, Henry C. Lea's Son, 98–109, 1881.

14. Christakis NA: The ellipsis of prognosis in modern medical thought. *Soc Sci Med* 44:301–15, 1997.

15. Sacket DI, Haynes RB, Guyatt GH, Tugwell P: *Clinical epidemiology. a basic science for clinical medicine*, 2d ed. Boston, Little, Brown, 1985.

16. Feinstein A: *Clinical epidemiology. the architecture of clinical research*. Philadelphia, W.B. Saunders, 1985.

17. *Encyclopaedia britannica*. Chicago, 1998.

18. *The Oxford english dictionary*, 2d ed., Simpson JA, Weiner ESC (eds.). Oxford, Clarendon Press, 1989.

19. *Dorland's illustrated medical dictionary*. Philadelphia, Saunders, 1988.

20. Bailey JA: *Concise dictionary of medical-legal terms*. New York, The Parthanon Publishing Group, 1998.

21. Wiesemann C. The significance of prognosis for a theory of medical practice. *Theor Med Bioethics* 19:253–61, 1998.

22. Mackillop WJ and Quirt CF: Measuring the accuracy of prognostic judgments in oncology. *J. Clin Epidemiol* 50:21–29, 1997.

23. Charbit A, Malaise EP, Tubiana M: Relation between pathological nature and growth rate of human tumours. *Eur J Cancer*, 7:307–25, 1971.

24. Mackillop WJ: The growth kinetics of human tumours. *Clin Phys Physiol Meas.* 11:121–3, 1990.

25. Trousseau A, Cormack JR: *Lectures on clinical medicine*, vol. 2, London, The New Sydenham Society, 1868, pp. 32–9 (translated from 2d ed.).

26. Holland H: *Medical notes and reflections*, 3rd ed. London, Longman, Brown, Green and Longmans, 1855.

27. Chammas S: MSc Thesis, Department of Community Health and Epidemiology, Queen's University, Kingston, Ontario, Canada 1991.

28. Feldman-Stewart D, Chammas S, Hayter C. Pater J, Mackillop WJ: An empirical approach to informed consent in ovarian cancer. *J Clin Epidemiol* 49:1259–69, 1996.

29. Feldman-Stewart D, Brundage MD, Hayter C, Davidson JR, Groome P, Nickel JC: What the prostate patient should know: variation in urologists' opinions. *Can J Urol* 4:438–44, 1997.

30. Feldman-Stewart D, Brundage MD, Hayter C, Groome P, Nickel JC, Downes H, Mackillop WJ: What prostate cancer patients should know: variations in professionals' opinions. *Radiother Oncol* 49:111–23, 1998.

31. Borges JL: *Ficciones*, Buenos Aires, Nuevo Mundo, 1946.

32. Applebaum PS, Lidz CW, Meisel A: *Informed consent. legal theory and clinical practice*. New York, Oxford University Press, 1987.

33. Brundage MD, Davidson J, Mackillop WJ: Trading treatment toxicity for survival in locally advanced non-small cell lung cancer. *J Clin Oncol*, 15:330–40, 1997.

34. Brundage MD, Davidson J, Mackillop WJ, Feldman-Stewart D, Groome P: Using a treatment trade-off method to elicit preferences for the treatment of locally advanced non-small cell lung cancer. *Med Decis Making*, 18:256–267, 1998.

35. Sneiderman B, Irvine JC, Osborne PH: *Canadian medical law*. Agincourt, Ont. Carswell, 1989.

36. The Consent to Treatment Act of Ontario, Ottawa, Ont. Canada.

CHAPTER 2

Prognostic Factors: Principles and Application

MARY K. GOSPODAROWICZ and BRIAN O'SULLIVAN

Since the beginning of time, man has wanted to prognosticate, or "know before." This desire explains the popularity of psychics and astrologers. After the birth of the idea of chance, prediction of the future has been largely handed over to statisticians. In studies of cancer and other diseases, identification of prognostic factors is the present-day equivalent of predicting the future. Nonetheless, it would be implausible to believe that we can predict precisely for the individual patient. In reality, all we can provide are statements of probability, and even these are more accurate for groups of patients, the study of whom provides us with our knowledge about prognosis. Furthermore, the practical management of cancer patients requires us to make predictions and decisions for individuals, and the challenge of prognostication is to link the individual patient to the collective population of patients with the same disease.

In this chapter we deal with the rationale for prognostic factors and describe classifications of these factors with attention to those used in this book. We also discuss potential endpoints relevant to oncology, the taxonomy of prognostic factors, and their applications in practice. Most importantly, we introduce a concept of a management scenario that forms the basis for defining prognosis at a given point in the course of disease.

RATIONALE FOR PROGNOSTIC FACTORS

The management of patients, or clinical practice, has four main components. Three comprise actions: namely diagnosis, treatment, and prophylaxis, and one is advisory, that of prognosis.[1] Appraisal of a patient's prognosis is part of everyday practice, and studies of prognostic factors are integral to cancer research.

Prognostic Factors in Cancer, 2nd edition, Edited by Mary K. Gospodarowicz
ISBN 0-471-40633-3   Copyright © 2001 Wiley-Liss, Inc.

However, the science of prognosis is rarely considered in a structured manner and, as in all areas of research, common definitions are required to allow communication of knowledge and new ideas.

Cancer is a heterogeneous group of diseases characterized by growth, invasion, and metastasis. The extent to which each of these occurs varies among apparently similar patients and cancers. To consider management of an individual cancer case, the fundamental pieces of information required include the site of origin (e.g., lung or breast), and morphologic type or histology (e.g., adenocarcinoma, or squamous cell carcinoma). In addition, the outcome in a cancer patient depends on a variety of variables referred to as *prognostic factors*. These factors are defined as *variables that can account for some of the heterogeneity associated with the expected course and outcome of a disease.*[2]

Knowledge of prognostic factors helps us to understand the progress of disease. However, we are seldom able to study the natural history of cancer, because some form of intervention is commonly applied in the hope that it will ameliorate the course of the disease. Treatment may have different goals, such as cure, avoidance or delay of symptoms, or prolongation of survival. Thus, the natural history of disease refers to the probable course of disease in a given patient, or

TABLE 2.1   Application of Prognostic Factors

Learning about the Natural History of Disease

Patient care
   Select appropriate diagnostic tests
   Select an appropriate treatment plan
   Predict the outcome for individual patient
   Establish informed consent
   Assess the outcome of therapeutic intervention
   Select appropriate follow-up monitoring
   Provide patient and caregiver education
Research
   Prognostic stratification
   • Improve the efficiency of research design and data analysis
   • Enhance the confidence of prediction
   • Demarcate phenomena for scientific explanation
   Design future studies
   • Identify subgroups with poor outcomes for experimental therapy
   • Identify groups with excellent outcomes for simplified therapy
   • Identify candidates for organ preservation trials
Cancer control programs
   Plan resource requirements
   Assess the impact of screening programs
   Introduce and monitor clinical-practice guidelines
   Monitor results
   Provide public education
   Explain variation in the observed outcome

groups of patients, defined by a set of prognostic factors and observed in the context of an intervention. Because prognostic factors affect disease outcome, they are an integral component of our ability to predict future disease-related events. Knowledge about prognostic factors is used in everyday patient care and in clinical research. To compare treatment outcomes among groups of patients, prognostic factors should be equally distributed, otherwise apparent differences in outcome could be explained entirely by a failure to compare "like with like," and not result from a putative effect of treatment. Therefore, knowledge of prognostic factors is essential for the interpretation of study results, and for the design of future studies. To answer a specific therapeutic question, it may be desirable to limit the patients studied to those characterized by selected prognostic variables.[3] In addition to clinical practice and research, knowledge of prognostic factors is essential to cancer control programs, because it permits inference to be applied broadly to other groups of individuals who may be at risk for cancer or benefit from educational or treatment-related programs (Table 2.1).

CLASSIFICATIONS OF PROGNOSTIC FACTORS

Even before anatomic extent of disease became the most widely adopted prognostic factor, it was appreciated that extent of disease was not the only factor affecting outcome in cancer patients. In recent years, with the availability of new cellular, molecular, and genetic factors, a renewed interest in prognostic factors in cancer has materialized. Both the American Joint Committee on Cancer (AJCC) and the International Union against Cancer (UICC) held meetings to discuss the optimal incorporation of prognostic factors, other than the anatomic disease extent, into a new prognostic system.[4] Following initial deliberations, the AJCC published criteria for interpretation of prognostic factors into an improved prognostic system that would enhance the existing TNM.[5] These criteria stipulated that to be included in a prognostic model, a putative prognostic factor had to be significant, independent, and clinically important. The AJCC proposal focused on the future use of molecular markers. In the early 1990s the UICC TNM-Prognostic Factor Project Committee embarked on a broad review of the state of the knowledge of all types of prognostic factors. This effort led to the publication of the first edition of the *Prognostic Factors in Cancer* book in 1995.[6,7] In this book, a topic- or subject-based classification was introduced and a statistical-significance-based rating proposed. Both the AJCC and the UICC encouraged that only statistically *significant and independent* prognostic factors be considered in clinical practice. In the previous edition, we suggested that the *significant prognostic factors* should be those found statistically significant in an analysis of at least one large data set. "Independence" implied the presence of new and additional prognostic information, with the implication that a new factor was not a surrogate for an already known factor. The establishment of independence required information from at least one multivariate analysis of prospectively collected data with adequate power to detect small but significant differences in outcome. However, few prospective studies exist that were designed with the primary objective of identifying prognostic factors, and secondary analysis forms the basis of recommendations about their use. Most databases and prospective therapeutic studies examine factors known to affect the outcome, or favor studies of new and fashionable molecular markers over *patient-related* or *environment-related* factors. Consequently, in this second edition of *Prognostic Factors in Cancer*, we propose an alternative approach for classifying the prognostic factors based on their relevance to clinical practice.

Subject-based Classification

Typically, most investigators regard prognostic factors to be those that directly relate to the given tumor. Examples include histologic type, grade, depth of invasion, or the presence of lymph-node metastasis. However, many factors not directly related to the tumor also affect the course of disease and the outcomes of interest. To comprehensively review these factors, three broad groupings are proposed: those that relate to disease or *tumor*, those that relate to the *host* or patient, and those that relate to the *environment* in which we find the patient[8] (see Chapter 6).

Tumor-related Prognostic Factors

Tumor-related prognostic factors include those directly related to the presence of the tumor or its effect on the host. Commonly used tumor-related prognostic factors comprise those that reflect tumor pathology, anatomic disease extent, or tumor biology. The most important disease-related prognostic factor is the anatomic extent of disease that is classified according to the UICC TNM classification.[9] In addition to the TNM categories and stage groupings, other factors describing disease extent, including tumor bulk, number of involved sites, or involvement of specific organs, may have an impact on prognosis.[10] Tumor histologic characteristics that influence the outcome include histologic type, e.g., follicular or papillary histology in thyroid carcinoma, and diffuse large-cell or follicular histology in lymphoma.[11,12] Tumor markers like PSA, AFP, and βHCG are used in everyday practice and strongly correlate with tumor bulk.[13,14] Hormone receptors, biochemical markers, expression of proliferation-related factors and, increasingly, molecular tumor characteristics have also been shown to affect outcomes for a variety of cancers.[15,16]

Host-related Prognostic Factors

Patient or host-related prognostic factors include inherent demographic characteristics such as age, gender, and ethnicity and other factors such as performance status, comorbid conditions, and immune status that may be acquired.[17-21] Although usually not related to the presence of the tumor, these factors may have a profound impact on the outcome.

Environment-related Prognostic Factors

Environment-related prognostic factors comprise those that operate external to the patient. In an ideal setting, these factors should lend themselves to modification to benefit an individual patient's outcome. This may also apply to groups of patients if specific health care policies are introduced to ensure the highest standards in a community. Unfortunately, the corollary also holds: failure to address these factors may well prejudice outcome for many patients. Interestingly, these factors are possibly the only ones that lend themselves to a realistic opportunity for immediate modification in the interest of improved outcomes. Environment-related prognostic factors could be specific to an individual patient (socioeconomic status, choice of treatment, quality of treatment), or more frequently, to groups of patients residing in the same geographic area (access to care, distance from medical facility, health care policy of the region, etc).[22-27] The impact of some of these factors may be profound (see chapter 6). Most studies dealing with prognostic factors deal exclusively with tumor-related attributes, with the exception of age and gender, which are easily available and therefore studied in many tumors.[28]

A combination of the subject-based and clinical-relevance-based classifications can be used to summarize in simple terms the prognostic factors for individual cancers for a selected management scenario. The template depicted in Table 2.2 illustrates a format, that has been used to summarize the salient information in Part B of this book. This table, which summarizes the prognostic factors relevant at diagnosis, is included in each chapter. Table 2.2 lists examples of prognostic factors in each category.

Prognostic Factor Groupings

While a classification within the three subject-based categories may be a useful working model, the distinction between these groupings of prognostic factors is not always clear and many prognostic factors overlap these categories. For example, performance status may be related to the tumor (which is causing debilitating symptoms), or, when compromised due to coexistent illness, could be a host-related prognostic factor. Similarly, the quality of treatment is a host-related factor if it relates to patient compliance, but is usually an environment-related factor relating to access to optimal medical care. An example of a prognostic factor that fits into all the subject-based categories is anemia and

TABLE 2.2 Summary Table: Examples of Prognostic Factors in Cancer

Prognostic Factors	Tumor Related	Host Related	Environment Related
Essential	Anatomic disease extent Histologic grade	Age	Availability of access to a radiotherapy facility
Additional	Tumor bulk Tumor marker level	Race Gender Cardiac function	Expertise of a surgeon
New and promising	p53 CD44	Germline p53	Access to information

all three could apply to the same patient. Anemia may be a direct result of the presence of tumor mass, as in superficial bladder cancer or cervix uteri cancer, because of persistent heavy bleeding. It may also be a host factor, as in a patient with thalassemia or anemia of chronic disease from an unrelated condition. However, in some parts of the world, as an *environment* prognostic factor, anemia also may be a result of malnutrition.

Several prognostic factors, each individually giving predictions with relatively low accuracy, can be combined to provide a single variable of high accuracy. Such a variable is called a *prognostic index*. When the T, N, and M categories in the TNM classification are combined, they form a stage grouping, which in reality is a specific prognostic index focusing mainly on anatomic disease extent. Another example of a prognostic index enjoying wide usage in clinical practice is the International Lymphoma Prognostic Index (IPI).[29-32] The IPI in lymphoma combines stage, age, performance status, lactate dehydrogenase (LDH), and number of extranodal sites, all previously shown to be independent prognostic factors in non-Hodgkin's lymphomas. Each factor is dichotomized as favorable, for example, stage I or II or unfavorable, for example, stage III or IV, or in performance status, favorable performance status (PS), Eastern Cooperative Oncology Group (ECOG) 1 or 2 versus unfavorable PS, ECOG 3 or 4. The patients with only one unfavorable factor have 70–80% 5-year survival, while those with all factors in an unfavorable category have only 25–30% 5-year survival (see Chapter 10).

Subject-based classification is discussed further in Chapter 6.

Clinical-relevance-based Classification

The assessment of prognostic factors allows for a prediction of a probable outcome and is a first step in a determination of a treatment plan. As noted earlier, the goals may include a variety of outcomes: cure, response with prospects of long-term disease control, or symptom relief only. To consider the relevance of prognostic factors in clinical practice, prognostic factors in this book are placed in the three distinct categories: *essential, additional*, and *new and promising factors*. Essential factors are those that are fundamental to decisions about the goals and choice treatment, including details of selection of treatment modality, and specific interventions. The essential prognostic factors are required to follow clinical practice guidelines. The additional factors allow finer prognostication, but do not add to the decision-making process. Their role is essentially to communicate prognosis, but do not influence treatment choice. Finally, new and promising factors are those that shed new light about the biology of disease, but for which currently there is, at best, incomplete evidence of an independent effect on outcome or prognosis. For some of these new factors, evidence may exist about their prognostic impact, but conflicting data may exist, or these factors are not currently in common usage for selecting treatment or communicating the prognosis. Factors included under the essential, additional, and new and promising categories are certain to change with time. With progress in understanding the biology of cancer, the ability to discriminate between localized and disseminated disease, and the introduction of new and more effective treatment methods, new factors may be required to select the optimal treatment. Furthermore, our ability to predict the outcome in the future may be enhanced by molecular tumor characteristics.

Essential Prognostic Factors

The most important essential factor is anatomic disease extent. The fundamental importance of disease extent was recognized more than 70 years ago with the first attempts at staging classifications. Steinthal initiated the development of an international language for the classification of cancer in the early twentieth century, following a proposal published in 1905 for the classification of the extent of breast cancer.[33] Subsequent work by Heyman, Lacassagne, and Voltz on cancer of the uterine cervix in 1928, and Portmann in 1937 on breast cancer, led to the publications on early staging systems.[34,35] The formal development of a systematic classification of the anatomic extent of disease using the TNM system is attributed to Pierre Denoix and the UICC through its TNM Project.[36] The TNM Classification has been translated into many languages and is accepted as the international standard for describing the anatomic extent of cancer. Today, the AJCC and the UICC TNM classifications are identical to facilitate worldwide communication about cancer.[37] However, factors other than anatomic extent of disease are also essential to the management of cancer. Tumor pathology also embraces domains beyond the diagnosis of malignancy, histologic type, or microscopic disease extent recognized in the staging classification. It includes the associated histologic features of cancer such as tumor grade and the presence of small-vessel invasion.[38] Newer imaging methods allow improved measurement of tumor bulk, an important addition to the description of anatomic disease extent. Tumor markers used in germ-cell testis tumors, prostate cancer, and ovarian cancer provide another dimension in measuring tumor burden.[10,13] Patient's age, a host-related factor, is integral to decision making in thyroid cancer and Hodgkin's disease, but does not appear to influence the choice of treatment in most other cancers.[39,40]

Additional Prognostic Factors

There are additional attributes that allow refinements in predicting outcome, although they are not currently used in the decision-making process. More detailed histologic features add to prognostic precision. These include patterns of invasion, phenotype, and surrogate indices for tumor proliferation such as percentage S-phase, expression of Ki-67 or MiB-1 antigens, and proliferative cell nuclear antigen (PCNA). However, they are usually not required for the generation of a treatment plan.[41-43] Most host-related factors, including performance status, comorbid conditions, and the function of vital organs, influence the suitability for surgery, chemotherapy, or radiotherapy. Therefore, they indirectly have an impact on outcome. Environment-related factors, although rarely considered in an individual case, have a profound impact on the outcome of groups of patients or on patient populations. The choice of an inferior treatment plan, poor quality of diagnostic tests, or treatment has potential to compromise the outcome.[23] Treatment of germ-cell testis cancer in a specialized unit, or breast cancer by a specialist surgeon resulted in an improved survival in population-based studies in Scotland.[25,26] Similar findings were observed in surgery for colorectal cancer.[44] As noted earlier, environment-related factors paradoxically lend themselves to modification with the opportunity for profound gain, in contrast to the other factors that are permanently set by the disease on the patient.

New and Promising Prognostic Factors

The explosion in biotechnology and an immense expansion of molecular biology has provided an abundance of new molecules, and more opportunities to study new biologic prognostic factors. These factors are not in general use at present, but are promising for future applications. Molecular factors may be used to predict response to a treatment modality, or they present a target for therapy. For example, the presence of Her-2/neu receptor predicts for response to chemotherapy as well as to trastuzumab (Herceptin®), and the presence of CD20 antigen is a prerequisite for response to rituximab (Rituxan®).[45,46] Another category includes factors that predict for the presence of occult distant metastases. Examples include polymerase chain reaction (PCR) for cells expressing prostatic-specific membrane antigen (PSMA), or the presence of high levels of cell-cycle-associated proteins, angiogenesis related factors, and so forth.[47] The numerous candidate prognostic factors allow prediction of the natural or treated history of a specific cancer. Most molecular factors fit into this *new and promising* category. Among them are the cell-cycle-associated proteins Rb, p53, p27, and so on, the cellular adhesion molecules CD44, *e*-cadherin, and so on, the proliferation antigens Ki-67, MiB-1, and the expression of protein products of translocations.[48−52] Further understanding of tumor biology may allow for greater accuracy and more specific prognostic ability, and in addition provide new and interesting targets for treatment.

MANAGEMENT SCENARIOS: FREEZING THE PROGNOSIS

Prognosis is not static. Prognosis will always change with time and will be affected by a large number of factors that may or may not be disease related. It is essential to be able to capture prognosis at a given time in order to formulate goals and plans for a specific intervention and to be able to discuss these issues with the patients and their support team. While prognosis changes with time, it also changes with the choices made. To determine the prognosis at a given time and in a given context, it is necessary to freeze the context in time. We consider this a *management scenario*. A management scenario comprises the prognostic attributes existing at the time, and is influenced by the choice of the planned intervention and the outcome of interest (Fig. 2.1). Intervention is axiomatic in cancer care, and in most instances it will affect the outcome. For example, in *scenario 1* during a normal physical examination prior to lumpectomy, a patient is found to have a 2-cm breast cancer. Considering the overall survival as the outcome of interest, her prognosis equates to that of reported survival for clinical stage I breast cancer in her peer group (age, race, socioeconomic status) and

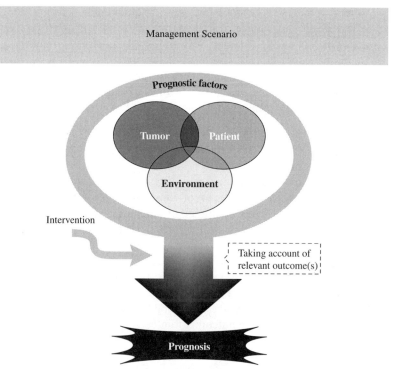

Figure 2.1   Representation of the interaction among the three domains of prognostic factors (tumor, host, and environment). The prognostic factors are expressed in the context of the proposed therapeutic intervention and for a given endpoint of interest (e.g., survival, response, local tumor control, organ preservation). In addition, the prognosis itself must be interpreted in the context of both the treatment (because it may change the prognosis) and the endpoint (which must be relevant to the prognosis).

in her geographic region. After the initial treatment is completed, the patient is in *scenario 2*. She has a pT1 pN0 tumor with pN0 status. Her prognosis is better than in scenario 1. She elects to be managed with partial mastectomy alone, her prognosis in scenario 2 is thus less favorable for local control than if she chose to have adjuvant radiation therapy. However, her prognosis for overall survival may not be affected by this decision. After some time, we can construct *scenario 3*. Thus some years later she develops local recurrence and distant metastasis (scenario 3). Her prognosis for survival is now much worse than in previous scenarios. The progress of time may also affect positively the probability of survival. A patient with stage IV Hodgkin's disease immediately following chemotherapy has a substantial probability of dying of Hodgkin's disease. However, after several years free of disease, the probability of dying of Hodgkin's disease is less.

Since the prognosis differs with a given scenario, prognostic factors should be considered within a given context or scenario. Most commonly, prognostic factors are considered at diagnosis before a definitive treatment plan is formulated. Prognostic factors differ with choice of intervention. Because treatment interventions have a major impact on the outcome, it is important to discuss prognostic factors in the context of a specific treatment plan or therapeutic intervention. Prognostic factors of value for survival prediction may not be of value for another outcome. Therefore, when considering prognostic factors, the endpoint or the outcome of interest must be a part of management scenario in determining the prognosis.

ENDPOINTS RELEVANT TO CONSIDER IN CANCER PATIENTS

It is important to focus again on the main purpose of prognostic factors, whether it is to facilitate the choice of treatment or communication about cancer. As noted earlier, prognostic factors allow prediction of outcomes. The relevant endpoints to consider in cancer include probability of cure, duration of survival, likelihood of response to treatment, probability of relapse, time to relapse, likelihood of local tumour control, likelihood of organ preservation, and possibility for symptom relief. Therefore, the outcomes may be very heterogeneous. Some prognostic factors facilitate prediction of more than one outcome, while others predict selected outcomes only. Consequently, prognostic factors always should be considered in the context of the outcome of interest. For example, the presence of bladder muscle wall invasion by a transitional cell carcinoma predicts for distant failure, while its absence virtually eliminates this probability. This knowledge permits clinicians to ignore the possibility of distant failure in patients with superficial bladder cancer both in diagnostic tests and therapeutic interventions. Another example is the number of involved nodal regions in stages I and II Hodgkin's disease that predict for risk of treatment failure, but not for survival. The number of tumours in superficial bladder cancer is predictive for recurrence, but has no impact on the overall survival.

Response to Treatment and Prognosis

Tumor response is an early endpoint in the assessment of treatment effectiveness. The formally agreed upon criteria for classification of tumor response were introduced in the late 1970s by the UICC and the World Health Organization (WHO).[53] The four categories of response (complete response, partial response, stable disease, and progressive disease) were originally proposed in the *WHO Handbook* and retained in the recently published United States National Cancer Institute (NCI) guidelines.[54] The preceding criteria were developed to assess the effects of drug therapy, but they may easily be applied to the outcomes of surgical or radiotherapy interventions. Response to treatment, whether to chemotherapy, radiotherapy, or surgery, has often been listed as an important prognostic factor. Indeed, as discussed below, complete tumor resection with negative margins could be considered as a complete response to surgical intervention, while positive resection margins could be considered as a partial response to surgical intervention. A response to treatment, however, is an early outcome in cancer. Knowledge of response can be incorporated into the next scenario in patient management. The extent of response is a surrogate for the anatomic extent of disease after the completion of therapy, and as such is a prognostic factor for further outcome. Positive response to treatment is almost always associated with a better outcome. Since the knowledge of response is not available until after treatment is completed, it should not be considered a prognostic factor for the scenario that preceded it. Therefore it may be used to predict outcome of the scenario, which follows the response assessment, and this is likely to be unfavorable for the nonresponders.

Surgical Resection Margins: Response to Treatment or Prognostic Factor?

For what has been discussed above, "incomplete response" defined as a positive surgical margin after attempted resection may be linked to different intentions and causes in the planned treatment strategy for a given *management scenario*. Incomplete excision, or residual disease, is most often characterized by the description of resection margins involved by tumor on pathologic assessment following attempted resection. The problem is made more complex by the fact that in organ conservation management of a given cancer, a close margin, or even a single focus of involved margin at a critical nonexpendable anatomic site, may be the intended strategy, with the intent of also delivering preoperative or postoperative adjuvant treatment. Such an approach would be unusual if adjuvant treatment were not included in the initial management plan. Clinical examples of these strategies to preserve function and/or cosmesis include breast conservation with lumpectomy combined with adjuvant irradiation in breast cancer,[55] and limb preservation strategies in soft tissue sarcoma of the extremity sites. For the latter adjuvant, preoperative or postoperative radiotherapy is very frequently used.[56]

The simple statement that the pathological margins "are involved" does not adequately explain the prognostic impact of this observation; nor can it attribute association or causality as to why residual disease was left. Thus for a given tumor, residual disease (positive resection margins defined as microscopic residuum or gross residuum) may result from a tumor that is indeed unresectable, or is only resectable with risk of disfigurement unacceptable to the patient. These probably have different prognostic expectations, although both are undesirable. This unsatisfactory situation has arisen because of "tumor-related" features, if caused by an extensive tumor. It would be "host related" if it resulted from a patient who could not tolerate the surgery for medical reasons or because of the wish to undergo function-preserving surgery. However, an "incomplete excision" could also arise as a consequence of inexperience or lack of skill on the part of the surgeon who attempted the resection, whereas a second surgeon might be able to achieve complete removal. In this instance, the adverse prognostic factor of incomplete resection is related to the "environment" in which the patient was first managed. Such an *environmental* cause could equally arise if the surgeon was highly skilled but lacked adequate access to oncologic staging procedures that would enable surgery to be planned in a manner that would minimize the chance of a positive margin.

Generally, a "positive margin" without further treatment has a far worse prognosis than if adjuvant radiotherapy is administered. Thus, the statement of residual disease following surgery has to be qualified by a statement about whether radiotherapy or other adjuvant treatment was or was not administered. Equally, it may be regarded as a response outcome following attempted surgical resection, or alternatively be prognostic for the ensuing management of the patient.

TAXONOMY: PROGNOSTIC FACTORS

In the English language, prediction, forecasting, and prognosis all indicate the probability of future events. In medical literature, however, the use of these terms has been highly variable.

In 1994 Burke proposed that the general heading of *predictive factors* describe three subtypes: *a risk, a diagnostic*, and *a prognostic factor*.[57] In his definition a risk factor was a factor where the main outcome of interest was incidence and the predictive accuracy was less than 100%; the diagnostic factor was where the outcome of interest was the incidence and the predictive accuracy was almost 100% of disease. A prognostic factor was where the outcome of interest was death and the predictive accuracy was variable.[57] This classification, however, has not been widely adopted. Burke's classification did not consider the temporal attributes of prediction and is associated with too narrow a view of relevant endpoint for patients with cancer (i.e., there is more than death at stake in contemporary oncology). In epidemiological literature, a *risk factor* is defined as "a clearly defined occurrence or characteristic that has been associated with the increased rate of a subsequently occurring disease"; thus, a risk factor is limited to patients who currently do not have a disease. In contrast, a *prognostic factor* refers to a probability of future event in patients who currently have a disease.

Henderson et al. and others have proposed an alternative use of the terms "predictive" and "prognostic".[58,59] Their proposal defines prediction as "prognosis for a measurable response" of overt tumor reduction following a treatment intervention and uses the term "predictive factor" as distinct from "prognostic" factor. The authors then consider a prognostic factor in the narrow context of a probability of cure or prolongation of survival. The initial description of the use of this model was in the area of breast cancer. An example of a prognostic factor that is not a predictive factor is the number of involved axillary lymph nodes in breast cancer. A high number of lymph nodes is associated with inferior survival, but the number of involved lymph nodes has no impact on response to treatment. An example of a factor that is both predictive and prognostic is the estrogen receptor status in breast cancer that predicts for response to hormonal therapy, but also prognosticates for a better survival. While this model fits the needs of breast cancer, it is questionable whether such a subtle distinction in terminology, which focuses on a single intermediate outcome (a measurable response to cytotoxic treatment) instead of defined endpoint relating to overall prognosis (e.g., local tumor control, survival), should be embraced. Indeed, to focus on the response to treatment alone may be misleading. Although a response to a particular treatment may be present, the treatment may not in itself benefit the patient. A response to treatment is not always predictive of a long-term survival. Examples of clinical situations where response is not an indication for the use of treatment include: chemotherapy in an asymptomatic patient with Stage III follicular small-cell lymphoma; androgen deprivation therapy in an asymptomatic patient with T1 prostate cancer; and radiation therapy in stage IV Hodgkin's disease. The informed reader will likely be aware of other examples. Effective treatment is always required to cure cancer. Surgery or radiation therapy is used, because they may lead to local tumor control, that is, a permanent complete response. Chemotherapy is used in germ-cell testis tumors because it leads to cure. In the final analysis, separation of these concepts may well be semantic. While the attempt to distinguish prognostic factors from predictive factors does bring attention to the importance of endpoint when considering any prognostic attributes, the danger of this proposal is that it narrows the concept of prognostic factors and may limit the scope of understanding the disease overall.

Generally, in the literature, the terms predictive, prognostic, and risk are being freely substituted for each other without much thought about consistent and accurate definitions.

Surrogate Diagnostic Factors versus Prognostic Factors

Prognosis implies prediction of an event that will occur in the future. The classic prognostic factors useful in forecasting cure, or long-term survival, clearly meet this objective. However, with better understanding of the mechanisms by which prognostic factors predict the future, new endpoints emerged. The common reason for failure to cure cancer is the presence of occult distant metastasis at the time of localized tumor presentation. In the absence of effective systemic treatment, patients with occult distant metastasis are destined to die. The forecasting of the probability of occult distant metastasis allows for a better understanding of the pattern of failure and targeting of treatment efforts. Where the probability of the presence of occult metastatic disease at the time of diagnosis is concerned, however, these factors predict for the current state and not for a future event. Two examples of such factors are the prostatic-specific antigen (PSA) level and the Gleason score in localized prostate cancer. These factors are considered as *prognostic* when survival or treatment failure probabilities are the endpoints of interest, but may be considered as *surrogate diagnostic factors* when they help discriminate different states at the present time. For example, they may help determine the probability of the presence of subclinical disease (e.g., disease lymph node involvement), as an endpoint of interest.

Time-dependent Prognostic Factors

Time dependent prognostic factors are variables that become available over the time course of the patient's disease. While they may be very predictive of outcome, they are also problematic because they risk disturbing the context of relevant disease outcome evaluation and decision making. This is because it may be impossible to separate real "causality" in the relationship between a time-dependent factor and an outcome of interest from a mere "association" caused by another factor common to them both. If the latter is the case, and it is not known whether there is causality, we are left uncertain whether influencing the time-dependent variable can have any effect on the course of the disease. Alternatively, we could incorrectly dismiss a causal association where one in fact exists because of a belief that the methodology for its evaluation was flawed.

Therefore, if not undertaken carefully, the clinical interpretation of time-dependent prognostic factors may be incorrect. In some cases, prognostic factors associated with a subsequent scenario have been considered together with prognostic factors at diagnosis. For example, the postradiotherapy PSA nadir level has been included in Cox models of prognostic factors in localized prostate cancer.[60] In truth, the PSA nadir is a surrogate for response to radiotherapy, and as such belongs to a different management scenario occurring subsequently. Another example of time-dependent covariates used in prognostic models is the use of hemoglobin level and patient weight in metastatic hormone refractory prostate cancer. The prognosis of patients with these features is worse than those with stable hemoglobin and weight.[61] These factors, when used as a prognostic factor in a later scenario, may be appropriate, but the problem arises when they masquerade as factors that were known at earlier times, such as when the disease is first diagnosed and staged.

Generally, time-dependent prognostic factors are entered into a Cox regression model in an attempt to adjust for the time bias in assessing the prognostic value of a specific covariate. Most often, these factors are a mathematical representation of disease progression or regression over time, but cannot be used to prognosticate about later outcomes at the time of an earlier scenario (e.g., time of diagnosis or initial treatment), since they have not had the opportunity to manifest yet. Gelman and Harris warned about using local recurrence in breast cancer as a time-dependent prognostic factor in a Cox model in an attempt to assess the impact of local recurrence on the overall survival.[62] In their view, no matter how well the mathematical formula of the Cox model performs in handling known prognostic factors, it is not able to eliminate potential bias between noncomparable groups such as those that respond to treatment initially and those that do not. Presumably, a prominent position in this matter of bias is occupied by unknown factors that are not accounted for in the model. Examples of such factors can include markers of biological aggressiveness, which contributed to the local recurrence in the first place and could also contribute to distant metastasis and therefore be a detriment to survival. As is shown throughout the remainder of this book, our knowledge of these markers remains quite preliminary for many tumors.

APPLICATION OF PROGNOSTIC FACTORS

Prognostic factors are used in daily clinical practice, in research (see Chapter 9), and in cancer control. In everyday clinical practice, the influence of prognostic factors dominates all the steps in decision making and the comprehensive management of patients with cancer, including selection of the primary goal of management, the most appropriate treatment modality, and the adjustment of treatment according to disease severity. Knowledge of prognostic factors allows clinicians to select treatment options that allow preservation of organs or function without compromising cure and survival. An example of such a situation is nonmetastatic soft tissue sarcoma of the extremities where the prognostic factors for local control, and hence limb-sparing approaches, differ from those for the risk of distant failure and disease-specific survival[63] (see Chapter 42). The availability of prognostic factor information is very helpful in population-based studies of the outcomes of treatment of cancer, especially if they focus on specific groups of patients. Measurement of the cost efficacy of cancer treatment has to include economic analysis of new treatment strategies and their impact on the health of the population. Cancer control efforts include population screening programs that require assessment of the prognostic factor in cancers detected by screening as an early endpoint of the effectiveness of such interventions. It is hoped that the implementation of clinical practice guidelines will improve the quality of decision making and in turn improve the outcomes in cancer patients. It is necessary to know the prognostic factors in order to evaluate compliance with practice guidelines before examining their impact.

Prognostic Factors and Milieu

The prognostic factors that are defined as essential for decision making depend on their relevance to the issues in cancer care in a particular milieu. What is important to cancer patient care in Toronto or Paris may not be relevant to a cancer patient in a small African village. The main issues in the developing countries are related to cancer prevention and early detection. Factors that predict for organ preservation and those that contribute to finesse in defining the prognosis may not be important in places with limited diagnostic equipment, and where funding for evaluation of assessment of response to treatment is not available. Therefore the list of *essential, additional*, and *new and promising factors* may vary depending on the milieu where the patient and health care professional are located. It is important to note that progress in such situations does not require new discovery, but merely economic development, education, and a process to ensure access.

FUTURE RESEARCH INTO PROGNOSTIC FACTORS

To be relevant to the clinical practice, prognostic factors must either have a significant impact on cancer outcome, or be used to select treatment methods. It is likely that with progress in treatment, and improved outcomes, prognostic factors will be more relevant for selection of treatment. An example is seen in the germ-cell testis tumors. The prognosis of patients with stage I is excellent, and knowledge of the individual patient or disease characteristics is not required to predict the cure. However, knowledge of prognostic factors is required to minimize the impact of treatment. Patients with favorable prognostic factors have a high probability of being cured with orchiectomy alone, while those with unfavorable factors such as small-vessel invasion are at a high risk of harboring occult metastatic disease and have an option of receiving adjuvant chemotherapy. Improved staging methods, and especially more accurate characterization of microscopic disease extent will allow a more homogeneous grouping of patients with similar disease characteristics, and the tumor-related prognostic factors for an individual disease may change. Knowledge of genetic factors will further add to the improved prediction of outcome and greater individualization of therapeutic interventions. However, grouping of patients into similar categories will continue to be required to assess the impact of new technology of patient assessment and new therapies on the outcome.

REFERENCES

1. Rizzi DA: Medical prognosis — some fundamentals. *Theor Med* 14:365–75, 1993.
2. Stockler M, Boyd N, Tannock I: Guide to studies of diagnostic tests, prognostic factors, and treatments, in Tannock I, Hill R (eds.): *The basic science of oncology*, 3d ed. Toronto, McGraw-Hill, 1998, pp. 466–92.
3. Byar DP: Identification of prognostic factors, in Buyse ME, Staquet MJ, Sylvester RJ (eds.): *Cancer clinical trials*. New York, Oxford University Press, 1984, pp. 423–43.
4. Yarbro JW, Page DL, Fielding LP, et al.: American Joint Committee on Cancer prognostic factors consensus conference. *Cancer* 86:2436–46, 1999.
5. Burke HB, Henson DE: Criteria for prognostic factors and for an enhanced prognostic system. *Cancer* 72:3131–5, 1993.
6. Hermanek P, Gospodarowicz M, Henson D, et al.: *Prognostic factors in cancer*, in UICC (ed.), (1st ed.): Heidelberg, Springer-Verlag, 1995.
7. Hermanek P: Prognostic factor research in oncology. *J Clin Epidemiol* 52:371–4, 1999.
8. Hermanek P, Hutter RVP, Sobin LH: Prognostic grouping: the next step in tumour classification. *J Cancer Res Clin Oncol* 116:513–16, 1990.
9. Sobin LH, Fleming ID: *TNM classification of malignant tumors*, (5th ed.) (1997). Union Internationale Contre le Cancer and the American Joint Committee on Cancer. *Cancer* 80:1803–4, 1997.
10. Sabbatini P, Larson SM, Kremer A, et al.: Prognostic significance of extent of disease in bone in patients with androgen-independent prostate cancer. *J Clin Oncol* 17:948–57, 1999.
11. Gelb AB: Renal cell carcinoma: current prognostic factors. Union Internationale Contre le Cancer (UICC) and the American Joint Committee on Cancer (AJCC). *Cancer* 80:981–6, 1997.
12. Shipp M: Prognostic factors in non-Hodgkin's lymphoma [published erratum appears in *Curr Opin Oncol* 5(1):251, 1993]. *Curr Opin Oncol* 4:856–62, 1992.
13. Mead GM, Stenning SP: The International Germ Cell Consensus Classification: a new prognostic factor-based staging classification for metastatic germ cell tumours. *Clin Oncol (R Coll Radiol)* 9:207–9, 1997.

14. Sassine AM, Schulman C: Clinical use of prostate-specific antigen in the staging of patients with prostatic carcinoma. *Eur Urol* 23:348–51, 1993.

15. Brien TP, Depowski PL, Sheehan CE, et al.: Prognostic factors in gastric cancer. *Mod Pathol* 11:870–7, 1998.

16. Kramer MH, Hermans J, Wijburg E, et al.: Clinical relevance of BCL2, BCL6, and MYC rearrangements in diffuse large B-cell lymphoma. *Blood* 92:3152–62, 1998.

17. Dolan R, Vaughan C, Fuleihan N: Metachronous cancer: prognostic factors including prior irradiation. *Otolaryngol Head Neck Surg* 119:619–23, 1998.

18. Aviles A, Yanez J, Lopez T, et al.: Malnutrition as an adverse prognostic factor in patients with diffuse large cell lymphoma. *Arch Med Res* 26:31–4, 1995.

19. Siu LL, Shepherd FA, Murray N, et al.: Influence of age on the treatment of limited-stage small-cell lung cancer. *J Clin Oncol* 14:821–8, 1996.

20. Moul JW, Douglas TH, McCarthy WF, et al.: Black race is an adverse prognostic factor for prostate cancer recurrence following radical prostatectomy in an equal access health care setting. *J Urol* 155:1667–73, 1996.

21. DeMario MD, Liebowitz DN: Lymphomas in the immunocompromised patient. *Semin Oncol* 25:492–502, 1998.

22. Feldman JG, Saunders M, Carter AC, et al.: The effects of patient delay and symptoms other than a lump on survival in breast cancer. *Cancer* 51:1226–9, 1983.

23. Selby P, Gillis C, Haward R: Benefits from specialised cancer care. *Lancet* 348:313–8, 1996.

24. Paszat LF, Mackillop WJ, Groome PA, et al.: Radiotherapy for breast cancer in Ontario: rate variation associated with region, age and income. *Clin Invest Med* 21:125–34, 1998.

25. Gillis CR, Hole DJ: Survival outcome of care by specialist surgeons in breast cancer: a study of 3786 patients in the west of Scotland. *BMJ* 312:145–8, 1996.

26. Harding MJ, Paul J, Gillis CR, et al.: Management of malignant teratoma: does referral to a specialist unit matter?. *Lancet* 341:999–1002, 1993.

27. Mackillop WJ, Zhang-Salomons J, Groome PA, et al.: Socioeconomic status and cancer survival in Ontario. *J Clin Oncol* 15:1680–9, 1997.

28. Fielding LP, Fenoglio-Preiser CM, Freedman LS: The future of prognostic factors in outcome prediction for patients with cancer. *Cancer* 70:2367–77, 1992.

29. Shipp MA: Can we improve upon the International Index? *Ann Oncol* 8 (Suppl 1):43–7, 1997.

30. A predictive model for aggressive non-Hodgkin's lymphoma. The International Non-Hodgkin's Lymphoma Prognostic Factors Project [see comments]. *N Engl J Med* 329:987–94, 1993.

31. Lopez-Guillermo A, Montserrat E, Bosch F, et al.: Applicability of the International Index for aggressive lymphomas to patients with low-grade lymphoma. *J Clin Oncol* 12:1343–8, 1994.

32. Hermans J, Krol AD, van Groningen K, et al.: International Prognostic Index for aggressive non-Hodgkin's lymphoma is valid for all malignancy grades. *Blood* 86:1460–3, 1995.

33. Steinthal PD: Zur Dauerheilung des Brustkrebses. *Beitr Klin Chir* 47:226–39, 1905.

34. Sellers A: *The classification of malignant tumours: Development of the TNM system.* Geneva, UICC, 1980.

35. Portmann U: Classification of mammary carcinomas to indicate preferable therapeutic procedures. *Radiology* 29:391–402, 1937.

36. Gospodarowicz M, Benedet L, Hutter R, et al.: History and international developments in cancer staging. *Cancer Prev Control* 2:262–8, 1998.

37. Fleming I, Cooper J, Henson D, et al.: *AJCC cancer staging manual*, 5th ed. Philadelphia, Lippincott, 1997.

38. Moul JW, Heidenreich A: Prognostic factors in low-stage nonseminomatous testicular cancer. *Oncology (Huntington)* 10:1359–68, 1374; discussion 1377–8, 1996.

39. Tsang RW, Brierley JD, Simpson WJ, et al.: The effects of surgery, radioiodine, and external radiation therapy on the clinical outcome of patients with differentiated thyroid carcinoma. *Cancer* 82:375–88, 1998.

40. Gospodarowicz MK, Sutcliffe SB, Clark RM, et al.: Analysis of supradiaphragmatic clinical stage I and II Hodgkin's disease treated with radiation alone. *Int J Radiat Oncol Biol Phys* 22:859–65, 1992.

41. Gisselbrecht C, Gaulard P, Lepage E, et al.: Prognostic significance of T-cell phenotype in aggressive non-Hodgkin's lymphomas. Groupe d'Etudes des Lymphomes de l'Adulte (GELA). *Blood* 92:76–82, 1998.

42. Sunderland MC, McGuire WL: Prognostic indicators in invasive breast cancer. *Surg Clin North Am* 70:989–1004, 1990.

43. Delahunt B: Histopathologic prognostic indicators for renal cell carcinoma. *Semin Diagn Pathol* 15:68–76, 1998.

44. McArdle CS, Hole D: Impact of variability among surgeons on postoperative morbidity and mortality and ultimate survival. *BMJ* 302:1501–5, 1991.

45. Goldenberg MM: Trastuzumab, a recombinant DNA-derived humanized monoclonal antibody, a novel agent for the treatment of metastatic breast cancer. *Clin Ther* 21:309–18, 1999.

46. McLaughlin P, White CA, Grillo-Lopez AJ, et al.: Clinical status and optimal use of rituximab for B-cell lymphomas. *Oncology (Huntington)* 12:1763–9; discussion 1769–70, 1775–7, 1998.

47. Olsson CA, de Vries GM, Buttyan R, et al.: Reverse transcriptase-polymerase chain reaction assays for prostate cancer. *Urol Clin North Am* 24:367–78, 1997.

48. Aaltomaa S, Lipponen P, Ala-Opas M, et al.: Alpha-catenin expression has prognostic value in local and locally advanced prostate cancer. *Br J Cancer* 80:477–82, 1999.

49. Gascoyne RD, Aoun P, Wu D, et al.: Prognostic significance of anaplastic lymphoma kinase (ALK) protein expression in adults with anaplastic large cell lymphoma. *Blood* 93:3913–21, 1999.

50. Gascoyne RD, Adomat SA, Krajewski S, et al.: Prognostic significance of Bcl-2 protein expression and Bcl-2 gene rearrangement in diffuse aggressive non-Hodgkin's lymphoma. *Blood* 90:244–51, 1997.

51. Grignon DJ, Caplan R, Sarkar FH, et al.: p53 status and prognosis of locally advanced prostatic adenocarcinoma: a study based on RTOG 8610. *J Natl Cancer Inst* 89:158–65, 1997.

52. Stauder R, Eisterer W, Thaler J, et al.: CD44 variant isoforms in non-Hodgkin's lymphoma: a new independent prognostic factor. *Blood* 85:2885–99, 1995.

53. WHO handbook for reporting results of cancer treatment. Geneva, World Health Organization Offset Publication, 1979.

54. Therasse P, Arbuck SG, Eisenhauer EA, et al.: New guidelines to evaluate the response to treatment in solid tumors. *J Natl Cancer Inst* 92:205–16, 2000.

55. Gage I, Harris JR: Radiation therapy and breast cancer. *Curr Opin Oncol* 9:527–31, 1997.

56. O'Sullivan B, Wylie J, Catton C, et al.: The local management of soft tissue sarcoma. *Semin Radiat Oncol* 9:328–48, 1999.

57. Burke HB: Increasing the power of surrogate endpoint biomarkers: the aggregation of predictive factors. *J Cell Biochem Suppl* 19:278–82, 1994.

58. Gasparini G, Pozza F, Harris AL: Evaluating the potential usefulness of new prognostic and predictive indicators in node-negative breast cancer patients [published erratum appears in *J Natl Cancer Inst* 85(19):1605, 1993]. *J Natl Cancer Inst* 85:1206–19, 1993.

59. Henderson IC, Patek AJ: The relationship between prognostic and predictive factors in the management of breast cancer. *Breast Cancer Res Treat* 52:261–88, 1998.

60. Preston DM, Bauer JJ, Connelly RR, et al.: Prostate-specific antigen to predict outcome of external beam radiation for prostate cancer: Walter Reed Army Medical Center experience, 1988–1995. *Urology* 53:131–8, 1999.

61. Vollmer RT, Kantoff PW, Dawson NA, et al.: A prognostic score for hormone-refractory prostate cancer: analysis of two cancer and leukemia group B studies. *Clin Cancer Res* 5:831–7, 1999.

62. Gelman R, Harris JR: Editorial comment on "The link between local recurrence and distant metastasis in human breast cancer" by Serge Koscielny and Maurice Tubiana. *Int J Radiat Oncol Biol Phys* 43:7–9, 1999.

63. Pisters PW, Leung DH, Woodruff J, et al.: Analysis of prognostic factors in 1,041 patients with localized soft tissue sarcomas of the extremities. *J Clin Oncol* 14:1679–89, 1996.

CHAPTER 3

Statistical Methods for the Analysis of Prognostic Factor Studies

LISA M. MCSHANE and RICHARD SIMON

Prognostic factor studies in cancer relate covariates describing clinical features and tumor characteristics to clinical endpoints such as therapy response, disease recurrence or progression, or survival. Examples of covariates in cancer prognostic factor studies include tumor size, nodal status, presence of metastases, and tumor-specific measurements such as expression levels of certain proteins, presence of chromosomal aberrations, or gene mutations. Typically, the relationship between the covariates and the clinical endpoints is examined by development and testing of a prognostic model. The modeling approaches discussed in this chapter include logistic regression for binary endpoints, Cox proportional hazards regression for survival outcomes, and neural networks and recursive partitioning for both binary and survival outcomes. In the final section, techniques for model validation are discussed.

LOGISTIC REGRESSION

If the clinical endpoint of interest in the prognostic factor study is a binary variable indicating some outcome such as response to therapy or disease recurrence within some fixed time window, then a commonly used modeling approach is logistic regression. Logistic regression bears similarities to the more familiar linear regression for normally distributed data, but it is specifically designed to handle binary dependent (outcome) variables. In classic linear regression, one models the expectation (mean) of a normally distributed dependent variable, Y, as a linear function of covariates (predictor variables) $x_1, x_2, \ldots, x_p$. For example, the model for the mean may be written as $E(Y) = \beta_0 + \beta_1 x_1 + \beta_2 x_2 + \cdots + \beta_p x_p$, where $E(Y)$ denotes the expected value of Y. The model coefficients

Prognostic Factors in Cancer, 2nd edition, Edited by Mary K. Gospodarowicz
ISBN 0-471-40633-3   Copyright © 2001 Wiley-Liss, Inc.

$\beta_0, \beta_1, \beta_2, \ldots, \beta_p$ measure the linear relationship between the variable Y and the covariates $x_1, x_2, \ldots, x_p$. There are several problems with using this standard regression model for a binary dependent variable. First, the assumption that Y is normally distributed is clearly inappropriate for a binary variable. Second, the mean of a binary variable is equal to the probability that it takes on the value 1, and this quantity must lie between 0 and 1 (inclusive). There is no guarantee that fitting the classic linear model will yield mean-value estimates between 0 and 1.

Logistic regression is a modeling technique applicable to binary outcome variables.[1] The expected value of a binary outcome variable associated with covariates $x_1, x_2, \ldots, x_p$ will be denoted by $p(x_1, x_2, \ldots, x_p)$, and it is equal to the probability that the binary variable takes on the value one, or equivalently the probability that the clinical event occurs. The logistic regression model is

$$\log[p(x_1, x_2, \ldots, x_p)/(1 - p(x_1, x_2, \ldots, x_p))] = \beta_0 + \beta_1 x_1 + \beta_2 x_2 + \cdots + \beta_p x_p.$$

The right-hand side of this equation is a linear function of the covariates. The left-hand side is the logarithm of the odds ratio, and is known as the *logit*. The logit can take any value between positive and negative infinity, and therefore using it as the basis for modeling rather than $p(x_1, x_2, \ldots, x_p)$ eliminates the difficulty associated with ensuring that the fitted regression function lies between 0 and 1. The mathematical methods for estimating the coefficients in the model assume the dependent variable has a binomial distribution rather than a normal distribution, as is assumed in classic linear regression.

An attractive feature of the logistic regression model is the interpretability of the β coefficient associated with a covariate x. For every unit increase in the variable x, the odds that the outcome event occurs increases by a factor $\exp(\beta)$. This interpretation of the β coefficients, excluding the intercept term β_0, remains valid even for a retrospective study in which events are oversampled. Also, it is critically important for proper interpretation of the model and its coefficients that the criteria for event occurrence are strictly adhered to. For example, the fitted model when the outcome event is recurrence within 1 year may look quite different than the fitted model when the outcome event is recurrence within 10 years. Different factors (covariates) may be responsible for early versus late recurrences. Survival analysis methods, discussed in the next section, provide a means of analyzing time-to-event data without requiring prespecification of a time window for event occurrence.

Example 1. Ravdin et al.[2] used logistic regression methods to develop a model to predict axillary lymph-node involvement in breast cancer patients using clinical information and characteristics of the primary tumors. They considered tumor size, patient age, quantitative estrogen (ER) and progesterone (PgR) receptor levels, DNA ploidy, and S-phase fraction to be potential predictors. Some of the predictor variables were transformed prior to modeling to reduce the impact of outlying values. Three possible binary "outcome" variables were considered: ≥ 1 positive node, ≥ 4 positive nodes, or ≥ 10 positive nodes. Model selection procedures were applied to identify the subset of independent predictors in

TABLE 3.1   Logistic Regression β Coefficients (SE)

	β Coefficients (SE)		
Variable	≥ 1 Positive Node	≥ 4 Positive Nodes	≥ 10 Positive Nodes
Log(tumor size + 1)	4.342 (0.216)	4.522 (0.270)	4.555 (0.383)
Log(S-phase + 1)	0.3992 (0.0918)	0.4241 (0.112)	0.8471 (0.161)
Age	−0.01343 (0.0021)	−0.00843 (0.0026)	—
Log(PgR + 1)	0.06919 (0.0259)	—	—
Constant	−2.201 (0.193)	−3.720 (0.239)	−5.625 (0.247)

Source: Reproduced from Table 2 in Ravdin et al.[2] with permission of the authors.

multivariate models for each of the three binary outcome variables. Table 3.1 presents the fitted logistic regression model parameters based on data from 5963 patients. Note that the set of predictors that was found to be independently prognostic varied with the definition of the binary outcome variable. For example, PgR (transformed as log(PgR + 1)) was a significant predictor for node positivity (≥ 1 positive node), but not for ≥ 4 or ≥ 10 positive nodes. To translate the regression coefficients into estimated risk probabilities, we can invert the regression model to obtain

$$p(x_1, x_2, \ldots, x_p) = \exp(\beta_0 + \beta_1 x_1 + \beta_2 x_2 + \cdots + \beta_p x_p)/$$
$$[1 + \exp(\beta_0 + \beta_1 x_1 + \beta_2 x_2 + \cdots + \beta_p x_p)]$$

and substitute in the estimated β coefficients. For example, the model-predicted risk of ≥ 1 positive node for a 60-year-old woman with a tumor size of 2.2 cm, S-phase 7.7, and PgR 181 is calculated to be

$$\exp(-2.201 + 4.342 \times \log(3.2) + 0.3992 \times \log(8.7) - 0.01343 \times 60 + 0.06919$$
$$\times \log(182))/[1 + \exp(-2.201 + 4.342 \times \log(3.2) + 0.3992 \times \log(8.7)$$
$$- 0.01343 \times 60 + 0.06919 \times \log(182)] = 0.43.$$

COX PROPORTIONAL HAZARDS REGRESSION

Frequently in prognostic factor studies, the primary outcome of interest is time to an event such as recurrence, progression, or death. In medicine, the analysis of time-to-event data is termed survival analysis. Here the term "survival time" will be used generically to refer to any time-to-event. In the discussion that follows, it will be assumed that the survival time is recorded on a continuous time scale. Survival analysis methods for discrete or grouped survival times are discussed elsewhere (Reference 3, sec. 4.6).

A survival-time distribution can be characterized by its survival function, $S(t)$, which is defined as the probability of survival until at least time t. An alternate characterization of a survival-time distribution is in terms of its hazard function, denoted by $\lambda(t)$, which is the instantaneous rate of failure immediately following time t, given survival up until time t. There is a one-to-one relationship between the survivor function and the hazard function. That is, one can be mathematically derived from the other, so that modeling one yields a model for the other. It is generally easier mathematically to model the hazard function than to model the survival function when one wishes to assess associations of covariates with survival.

Cox porportional hazards regression[4] is a widely used, flexible statistical method for the analysis of survival data. It specifies a model for the hazard function of the form

$$\lambda(t) = \lambda_0(t) \exp(\beta_1 x_1 + \beta_2 x_2 + \cdots + \beta_p x_p).$$

The function $\lambda_0(t)$ is called the baseline hazard function. It models the hazard as a function of time only, and it is equal to the overall hazard function when all covariate values are identically zero. The term "proportional hazards" derives from the fact that the hazard, $\lambda(t)$, is proportional to the baseline hazard, $\lambda_0(t)$, with the proportionality factor $\exp(\beta_1 x_1 + \beta_2 x_2 + \cdots + \beta_p x_p)$. This formulation lends itself to a convenient interpretation for each of the β coefficients. A unit increase in a covariate x corresponds to multiplication of the baseline hazard function by the factor $\exp(\beta)$, if all of the other covariates in the model are held fixed.

Proportional hazards regression is often cited as an example of a "semi-parametric" method. No assumptions are made about a parametric form for the baseline hazard, $\lambda_0(t)$, but a parametric form is specified for the proportionality factor, $\exp(\beta_1 x_1 + \beta_2 x_2 + \cdots + \beta_p x_p)$. However, the parametric form specified for the proportionality factor does not have to be a function of the linear combination of covariates, as was originally proposed. It may have very flexible forms, including replacing the linear form with spline[5] or neural network models.[6]

Parameter estimates and standard errors are obtained by maximum likelihood methods applied to a "partial likelihood," and confidence intervals for β or $\exp(\beta)$ are usually based on assumptions of approximate normality. Any proportional hazards regression analysis should be accompanied by an assessment of the appropriateness of the proportional hazards assumption. Several methods are available for making this assessment.[7]

Example 2. Brown et al.[8] used Cox proportional hazards regression modeling to assess the prognostic value of a cell proliferation marker, Ki-67, for predicting disease-free survival (DFS) in axillary node-negative breast cancer patients. The modeling was based on data from a nonrandomized retrospective series of patients. Using data from 314 cases for which complete data were available, the only independent predictors of DFS in a multivariate Cox model were tumor size (≤ 2 cm vs. >2 cm), S-phase fraction ($\leq 6.7\%$ vs. $>6.7\%$), and Ki-67 ($\leq 5\%$ vs. $>5\%$) when a larger set of variables that also included histologic type, age, hormone and hormone receptor status, ploidy, and treatment received, was considered. Thresholds for defining the dichotomous predictor variables were obtained using optimal cutpoint selection methods, and the impact of this

TABLE 3.2 Multivariate Analysis of DFS[a]

Covariate	High-risk Group	HR (95% CI)[b]	P value[c]
Tumor size	>2 cm	1.90 (1.1–3.2)	0.019
S-phase fraction	>6.7%	2.04 (1.2–3.4)	0.006
Ki-67	>5%	1.93 (1.1–3.2)	0.014

Source: Reproduced from a portion of Table 4 in Brown et al.[8] with permission of the authors and the American Association for Cancer Research.

[a]DFS truncated to 60 months (see Reference 8 for details).

[b]HR, hazard ratio; CI, confidence interval.

[c]P value from Wald χ^2 statistic.

selection on reported significance levels was discussed by the authors. Hilsenbeck and Clark[9] discuss the general problem of optimal cutpoint selection. Table 3.2 presents adjusted hazard ratios along with their associated 95% confidence intervals for the variables that were found to be independent predictors in multivariate Cox modeling. Because the marker values are represented as binary variables with a value of one indicating high-risk category, the hazard ratio associated with a particular marker can be computed as $\exp(\beta_{est})$, where β_{est} is the estimated regression coefficient for that marker variable. For example, the interpretation of the hazard ratio of 1.9 reported for Ki-67 is that high Ki-67 (>5%) is associated with a 1.9-fold increase in risk of recurrence ($P = 0.014$) after adjustment for tumor size and S-phase fraction.

Two particularly useful extensions of the proportional hazards regression model are models that incorporate strata and models that allow for time-dependent covariates. The stratified model specifies the hazard function in the form

$$\lambda_s(t) = \lambda_{0s}(t) \exp(\beta_1 x_1 + \beta_2 x_2 + \cdots + \beta_p x_p)$$

where s indexes the stratum. That is, subgroups (strata) are permitted to have distinct baseline hazard functions, but the relative effects of the covariates are assumed constant across strata. This approach can be useful in situations in which covariates do not follow the proportional hazards assumptions. Furthermore, the stratified model provides one means of graphically assessing proportional hazards assumptions (Reference 3, p. 88). Time-dependent covariate models allow for the value of a covariate to vary over time. For example, if the prognostic factor under investigation is some new measure of minimal residual disease, and patients are monitored at several timepoints, then minimal residual disease status should be incorporated into the prognostic model as a time-dependent covariate.

NEURAL NETWORKS

Neural networks ("neural nets") have become a popular tool, particularly among nonstatisticians, for addressing a variety of classification and prediction problems. Recently, several authors have adapted neural network algorithms for use with survival data. In this section, basic neural network methodology is described, followed by a limited discussion of some of the extensions to survival data.

Feedforward neural networks are the most commonly used type and are summarized briefly here. Typically, neural networks for prediction consist of three layers: an input layer, a hidden layer, and an output layer. Each node in the input layer corresponds to an input variable, or covariate. The form of the output layer depends on the type of prediction problem. In a simple, two-category (positive/negative) classification problem, there will be a single output node, and the output variable can be interpreted as a probability of positive response. In a K-category classification problem, there are K output values, with the ith output value representing the relative probability of membership in category i. For a regression problem, the output of a neural net is an estimate of the expected value of the response variable y, given covariates.

In the hidden layer between the input and output layers, nonlinear transformations are performed. Between each input node and all but one of the hidden nodes, there is a direct connection, and with each connection there is an associated connection weight. Transmission of the covariates $x_1, x_2, \ldots, x_p$ to the jth node in the hidden layer results in the value $w_{0j} + w_{1j}x_1 + w_{2j}x_2 + \cdots + w_{pj}x_p$, where w_{ij} denotes the weight of the connection between input node i and hidden node j, and w_{0j} is a constant shift term. Feedforward neural nets do not allow feedback loops or backward transmissions. In the case of a single output node, an "activation" or "squashing" function, f, is applied to the output of the hidden layers, and a weighted linear combination of the transformed outputs from the h hidden nodes, using weights $\alpha_1, \alpha_2, \ldots, \alpha_h$ and constant shift α_0, is transmitted to that output node. A common choice for the activation function f is the logistic function. Another activation function g can be applied at the output node, yielding the net value

$$g \left\{ \sum_{j=1}^{h} \alpha_j f \left(\sum_{i=1}^{p} w_{ij}x_i + w_{0j} \right) + \alpha_0 \right\}.$$

Generalizing to K output nodes, the value at the kth output node is

$$O_k(x, \theta) = g \left\{ \sum_{j=1}^{h} \alpha_{jk} f \left(\sum_{i=1}^{p} w_{ij}x_i + w_{0j} \right) + \alpha_{0k} \right\}$$

where x is a vector of covariates $(x_1, x_2, \ldots, x_p)$ and θ denotes the vector of unknown parameters $(w_{01}, \ldots, w_{ph}, \alpha_{01}, \ldots, \alpha_{hK})$. Additional generalizations are possible, such as allowing the activation function f to vary by hidden node or g to vary by output node. Figure 3.1 presents an example of a single hidden layer neural network with two hidden nodes and two output nodes.

Some noteworthy special cases include linear regression and logistic regression. By omitting the hidden layer and setting the activation function to the identity function, a linear regression model is obtained; setting the activation function to the logistic function results in a logistic regression model.

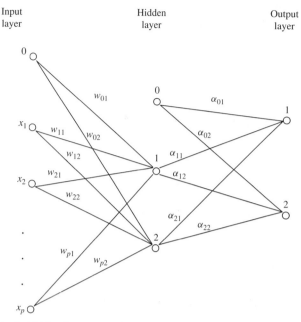

Input layer   Hidden layer   Output layer

Figure 3.1 Single hidden layer neural network with two hidden nodes and two outputs.

The process of estimating the parameters is known as training the neural net, and it requires the availability of a training data set consisting of sets of covariates and the observed outcome responses associated with them. Parameter estimates are chosen to minimize a cost function. The most commonly used cost function is the quadratic, or squared-error cost function:

$$\sum_{n=1}^{N} \sum_{k=1}^{K} \{O_k(\boldsymbol{x}_n, \theta) - y_{nk}\}^2$$

where $O_k(\boldsymbol{x}_n, \theta)$ is the net value at the kth output node for the nth observation with covariate vector $\boldsymbol{x}_n$, and observed response vector $(y_{n1}, y_{n2}, \ldots, y_{nK})$. The most common algorithm for minimizing this quadratic cost function is the back propagation algorithm, which is based on a gradient descent method. Faraggi and Simon[10] propose an alternative method, in which they estimate net parameters by maximum-likelihood techniques applied to a logistic likelihood function.

Recently, several authors have proposed adaptations of neural networks for use with survival outcomes. Liestol et al.[11] demonstrate how neural network methodology can be used to obtain maximum-likelihood estimates in survival regression models, based on partitioning the time axis into disjoint time intervals. Faraggi and Simon[6] present a neural network approach to nonlinear proportional hazards regression modeling of survival data. Also, Faraggi et al.[12] have considered a Bayesian neural network model for survival data.

Neural network models provide a means of modeling nonlinear effects of covariates on binary or survival outcomes that may be encountered in prognostic factor studies. They allow for modeling complicated functional relationships between covariates and outcomes, including complex interactions between covariates. With this flexibility comes some drawbacks. First, the model parameters lack a natural interpretation like the interpretation of the regression coefficients in logistic regression or proportional hazards models. Thus, while the neural network model may in some cases provide good predictions, it does not easily lend itself to increasing scientific understanding of relationships between the prognostic factors and outcome. Since there is no single regression coefficient that represents the effect of a covariate on response, statistical significance tests of the influence of specific covariates are not available. Second is the danger of overfitting the models, because the number of parameters increases rapidly as the number of hidden nodes increases. Hence, it is easy to obtain a model that fits the training data well but that has no predictive value for independent data. Consequently, the use of model validation procedures is especially critical for proper assessment of the usefulness of a neural net.

RECURSIVE PARTITIONING

Recursive partitioning methods, also known as tree-based models, which include classification and regression trees, are exploratory tools for elucidating nonlinear relationships between covariates and outcome. Presented with data sets of covariates and associated outcomes, the goal of these methods is to either predict membership in one of several possible classes (classification tree) or to predict some continuous outcome (regression tree). The basic algorithm consists of successively splitting the data into smaller subgroups to achieve homogeneity within each of the final subgroups while maintaining diversity across subgroups. Each split corresponds to a "node" of the tree and it separates the group of observations at that node into two (not necessarily equal-size) subgroups. Data splitting proceeds until the resulting collection of subgroups, or "terminal nodes," are sufficiently "pure" or satisfy some other optimality criterion.

Many different criteria can be applied to determine the "best" split at each node. For growing classification trees, one of the classic approaches is to base splitting decisions on the degree of purity achieved in the resultant nodes. At each node, one can examine the proportion of observations that fall into each of the possible classes. An absolutely pure node is one in which all of the outcome observations at that node belong to a single class. An example of a very impure node would be one in which the observations at that node are approximately equally divided among all possible classes. Other splitting criteria not based on node purity measures include the "twoing rule" (Reference 13, sec. 4.3) and likelihood ratio-based methods (Reference 14, chap. 9). For growing regression trees, splitting criteria include methods based on quantities such as within-node variance estimates or likelihood ratio-based methods. After no more optimal splits can be determined, each of the terminal nodes is assigned an output value. For classification trees, this value is typically the dominant class, that is, the class to which the greatest percentage of observations in that node belong. For regression trees, the assigned value may be the mean of the observed outcomes in that terminal node.

Usually trees that are grown by any of these methods are too large in the sense that they overfit to the data and are likely to have poor predictive power. To address this problem, various techniques such as tree pruning and tree shrinking (recombination of branches) are employed. Pruning often involves the use of sample reuse methods such as cross-validation or bootstrapping, which are described in general terms in the next section.

Advantages of recursive partitioning methods are that they can gracefully handle missing covariate values, they are good at modeling complex interactions, and they provide easily interpretable models. Recently, these methods have been generalized to the analysis of censored survival data (Reference 15, and references therein), which broadens their applicability in prognostic factor modeling. One of the major disadvantages of recursive partitioning methods is that the resulting tree structures are often unstable. That is, different trees are obtained if the data are slightly changed or a small subset of cases is omitted. Approaches for assessing the stability of tree models or other modeling techniques involving variable selection are discussed in the next section. The trees are also subject to misinterpretation due to "variable masking." This misinterpretation occurs if one erroneously concludes that a variable is unrelated to classification membership because the variable does not appear in the tree when, in fact, the variable's effect is explained by other variables in the tree. In addition, trees do not perform well in situations in which the data structure depends on combinations of variables rather than one variable at a time (Reference 13, chap. 2).

MODEL VALIDATION

When developing a prognostic model that depends on a large number of covariates, or has a very complicated structure involving a large number of parameters, there is a great tendency to "overfit" the model to the data. Overfitting means that some of the apparent structure in the model has actually been fit to random noise in the data. One way to determine if overfitting has occurred is to validate the model on an independent data set. Each set of covariates in the new data set is "plugged in" to the fitted model to predict an outcome. These predicted values, as they are called, are then compared to the outcomes actually observed in the new data set. If the prediction from the model is a continuous value, then the prediction error can be summarized as the average prediction error sum of squares. To compute the average prediction error sum of squares, the difference between each observed value in the new data set and its value predicted from the model is computed, each of these differences is squared, and then the squared differences are averaged. If the prediction from the model is a classification, then the misclassification rate can be used as a measure of prediction error. If these measures of prediction error are computed using the original data set that was used to build the prognostic model rather than using a new, independent data set, the true prediction error would be underestimated. This is because the data used to build the model has an inherent advantage in achieving a smaller prediction error because the model was chosen to provide a good fit to that data.

Rarely in practice is one so fortunate to have available an independent data set for validation purposes. In this situation, a popular alternative is to use "cross-validation" techniques. In cross-validation, one reuses the original data set by splitting it into parts in which one part is used to fit the model and the other part is used to validate the model. In its simplest form, cross-validation splits the data set into two equal parts. One half is used to fit the model ("modeling" or "estimation" set), while the remaining half ("test" or "validation" set) is used to assess the predictive value of the model and to calculate an estimate of prediction error. Then the roles of the test and validation sets are reversed to obtain a second estimate of prediction error, and the two estimates of prediction error can be averaged to obtain a single estimate of prediction error. If the original data set is not very large, then it may be difficult to fit a complex model with many covariates to only half of the data. In these circumstances, k-fold cross-validation is recommended. With k-fold cross-validation, the data are partitioned randomly into k subsets. The data for one of the subsets are omitted, and the model developed in the remaining $(k-1)/k \times 100\%$ of the data. The outcomes for the cases in the omitted subset are then predicted using the model developed without use of that subset. This is repeated k times, each time excluding a different one of the k subsets, developing a model on the remaining data and predicting outcomes for the cases in the excluded subset. This results in a prediction for all cases, and these can be used to estimate prediction error. Popular choices of k are 5 or 10, and sometimes k is equal to N, the number of observations in the complete original data set. This last option is referred to as "leave-one-out" cross-validation. For large data sets, the fitted model may be insensitive to deleting one observation, so leave-one-out cross-validation may not be very informative. Also, for large data sets and complex model-fitting algorithms, leave-one-out cross-validation may be computationally prohibitive.

The prediction error estimates obtained by cross-validation are particularly useful for comparing fits of two or more models. These comparisons may be between models of two different classes, for example, a logistic regression model versus a neural network model. The models need not even contain the same effective number of parameters for the comparison of the cross-validation prediction errors to be meaningful. Alternatively, the comparisons could be between models of the same class in which some additional restriction must be imposed on the model. Examples of such restrictions include the size of a classification or regression tree, or the maximum number of predictor covariates included in a regression model. For the classification and regression tree example, one might compute cross-validation prediction errors for each of several tree sizes, and choose the tree size that minimizes the prediction error. For regression modeling involving a large number of predictor covariates, variable selection procedures such as stepwise regression tend to overstate the significance of variables in the final selected model. Applying cross-validation techniques to this problem, one can compute cross-validation prediction errors for variable selection procedures that are forced to terminate when the number of variables included in the model reaches some limit, and then choose the limit (number of variables) that minimizes the prediction error.[16]

Bootstrapping is another technique involving sample reuse that can be used to assess the stability of parameters in a fitted model. An overview of bootstrapping and its theoretical justification can be found in Efron and Tibshirani.[17] Bootstrapping is performed by selecting one observation at a time, with replacement, from the original data set, until a sample the same size as the original data set has been created, and then repeating this procedure until many (often 100–200) "artificial" data sets have been generated. The idea is that each of these artificial data sets (called bootstrap samples) is generated from a process similar to the process that generated the original data set. Therefore, the degree of variability exhibited by an estimated parameter across the many bootstrap samples should provide an estimate of the stability of that parameter estimate computed from the original data set.

Bootstrapping is particularly useful in settings where the parameter of interest is estimated by some complex procedure. One example is the selection of optimal cutpoints to dichotomize continuous prognostic factors. If the cutpoint applied to a prognostic factor that is recorded as a continuous or multilevel variable is chosen from the data to maximize the significance of the resulting dichotomous variable, then it is well established that the test of significance of that dichotomous variable will be biased in the direction of overly optimistic. Bootstrapping can be applied in this situation by recording, for each bootstrap sample, the optimally determined cutpoint. Confidence intervals and standard error estimates could then be calculated for the estimated optimal cutpoint. Faraggi and Simon[18] discuss an alternative approach to the problem of cutpoint selection using cross-validation.

Boostrapping may also be used to assess that stability of the "selected" set of variables in a model selection problem. For example, one can record for each covariate the proportion of bootstrap samples in which that covariate was included in the subset of covariates resulting from application of a model selection procedure. Altman and Andersen[19] describe a bootstrap approach for evaluating the stability of a proportional hazards regression model built using variable selection. Their bootstrap approach assesses both the stability of the choice of variables included in the model and the predictive ability of the model. This approach can also be applied to examining the stability of tree models.

The sample reuse methods discussed here are valuable tools in the process of developing prognostic models, but they can never replace validation of the model on a completely independent data set. The final validation on an independent data set requires prespecification of all variables to be considered for inclusion in the prognostic model, as well as specification of any cutpoints that will be applied to continuous or multilevel variables. The validation data set also must be of sufficient size to provide acceptable power for detecting prognostic factor effects of clinically relevant magnitude. Probably the most common problem in prognostic modeling is misrepresentation of the significance of covariates and the predictiveness of the model by selecting covariates based on the same data used for testing their significance and estimating predictiveness.

REFERENCES

1. Hosmer DW, Lemeshow S: *Applied logistic regression.* New York, Wiley, 1989.
2. Ravdin PM, De Laurentiis M, Vendely T, Clark GM: Prediction of axillary lymph node status in breast cancer patients by use of prognostic indicators. *J Nat Cancer Inst* 86:1771–5, 1994.
3. Kalbfleisch JD, Prentice RL: *The statistical analysis of failure time data.* New York, Wiley, 1980.
4. Cox DR: Regression models and life tables (with discussion), *J R Stat Soc, Ser B* 34:187–220, 1972.
5. Durrleman S, Simon R: Flexible regression models with cubic splines. *Stat Med* 8:551–61, 1989.
6. Faraggi D, Simon R: A neural network model for survival data. *Sta Med* 14:73–82, 1995.
7. Grambsch P, Therneau TM: Proportional hazards tests and diagnostics based on weighted residuals. *Biometrika* 81:515–26, 1994.
8. Brown RW, Allred DC, Clark GM, Osborne CK, Hilsenbeck SG: Prognostic value of Ki-67 compared to S-phase fraction in axillary node-negative breast cancer. *Clin Cancer Res* 2:585–92, 1996.
9. Hilsenbeck SG, Clark GM: Practical p-value adjustment for optimally selected cutpoints. *Stat Med* 15:103–12, 1996.
10. Faraggi D, Simon R: The maximum likelihood neural network as a statistical classification model. *J Stat Plann Inference* 46:93–104, 1995.
11. Liestol K, Andersen PK, Andersen U: Survival analysis and neural nets. *Stat Med* 13:1189–1200, 1994.
12. Faraggi D, Simon R, Yaskil E, Kramar A: A Bayesian neural network model for censored survival data. *Biometrical J* 39:519–32, 1997.
13. Breiman L, Friedman JH, Olshen RA, Stone CJ: *Classification and regression trees.* Belmont, CA, Wadsworth, 1984.
14. Chambers JM, Hastie TJ: *Statistical Models in S.* Pacific Grove, CA, Wadsworth and Brooks Cole Advanced Books and Software, 1992.
15. LeBlanc M, Crowley J: Survival trees by goodness of split. *J Am Stat Assoc* 88:457–67, 1993.
16. Thall PF, Simon R, Grier DA: Test based variable selection via cross-validation. *J Comput Graphical Stat* 1:41–62, 1992.
17. Efron B, Tibshirani RJ: *An introduction to the bootstrap.* New York, Chapman & Hall, 1993.
18. Faraggi D, Simon R: A simulation study of cross-validation for selecting an optimal cutpoint in univariate survival analysis. *Stat Med* 15:2203–13, 1996.
19. Altman DG, Andersen PK: Bootstrap investigation of the stability of a Cox regression model. *Stat Med* 8:771–83, 1989.

CHAPTER 4

Evaluating Prognostic Factor Studies

RICHARD SIMON

Most types of human cancer are heterogeneous with regard to clinical features, natural course, histologic, and molecular characteristics. Better diagnostic classification systems would improve the ability to select an appropriate treatment and facilitate the development of more effective regimens. For example, accurate classification of small breast tumors with regard to metastatic potential would permit many patients to avoid systemic therapy.

The medical literature is filled with reports of prognostic factor discoveries. There are numerous inconsistencies among reports, and for many types of cancer the literature can at best be called confusing.[1,2] In contrast to clinical trials, there are no standards for prognostic factor studies, and hence it is easy to publish methodologically poor studies in reputable journals. Nearly all prognostic factor studies are "exploratory studies" rather than "confirmatory studies." Because of problems of multiple significance testing, most conclusions of exploratory analyses will not be correct. The phenomenon of "publication bias" assures that the most positive and erroneous of these studies will be published in reputable journals and receive attention.

Technological developments are likely to make the confusion in the literature of prognostic factor studies much worse. Genomics is providing huge numbers of DNA polymorphisms that can be used as prognostic factors in future studies. DNA microarrays currently permit the expression profiling of tens of thousands of genes for each tumor sample, and these expression levels are potential prognostic factors. It is therefore important for clinical investigators and clinicians to have a better understanding of the flaws of many prognostic factor studies and to establish standards for the type of evidence about a prognostic factor that we should have before accepting the factor in clinical practice. These are the objectives of this chapter.

Prognostic Factors in Cancer, 2nd edition, Edited by Mary K. Gospodarowicz
ISBN 0-471-40633-3   Copyright © 2001 Wiley-Liss, Inc.

TYPES OF PROGNOSTIC FACTOR STUDIES

Prognostic factor studies can be classified as exploratory or confirmatory. Most are exploratory. These latter are unfocused studies that may examine a variety of factors with regard to a variety of endpoints in a heterogeneous population of patients. Exploratory studies usually have no specific prespecified hypotheses. They generally involve numerous analyses of factors, endpoints, and subsets of patients. For example, the data may be heterogeneous with regard to stage and treatment, and no therapeutically relevant focused question about a prespecified set of patients is asked. They may involve multiple analyses with different cutpoints for prognostic factors.[3] Exploratory studies often do not report all of the analyses performed; only those that resulted in "statistically significant" differences are described. In contrast, a confirmatory prognostic factor study is based on a prespecified hypothesis involving one, or at most a few, prognostic factors for a defined therapeutically homogeneous set of patients. With a confirmatory study the endpoint is prespecified, the patient population is prespecified, and any cutpoints used are prespecified. This helps avoid the high error rates resulting from exploratory testing of multiple hypotheses, particularly data-derived hypotheses. A confirmatory study should either be a prospective study in which patients are accrued and samples taken after the study is defined, or should simulate a prospective study as much as possible. For example, a consecutive series of patients should be included in the study, not a selected set for which tissue was retrospectively available. Some of the important characteristics of a confirmatory prognostic factor study are listed in Table 4.1.[4]

Before a prognostic factor or new classification system is adopted into clinical practice and used for therapeutic decision making it is desirable that (1) at least

TABLE 4.1   Guidelines for Confirmatory Prognostic Factor Studies

1 Intra- and interlaboratory reproducibility of assays should be documented
2 Laboratory assays should be performed blinded to clinical data and outcome
3 An inception cohort of patients should be assembled with <15% of patients nonevaluable due to missing tissue or data. The referral pattern and eligibility criteria should be described
4 Treatment should be standardized or randomized and accounted for in the analysis
5 Hypotheses should be stated in advance, including specification of prognostic factors, coding of prognostic factors, endpoints, and subsets of patients and treatments
6 The sample size and number of events should be sufficiently large that statistically reliable results are obtained. Statistical power calculations that incorporate the number of hypotheses to be tested and appropriate subsets for each hypothesis should be described. There should be at least 10 events per prognostic factor examined per subset analyzed
7 Analyses should test whether new factors add predictiveness after adjustment for or within subsets determined by standard prognostic factors
8 Analyses should be adjusted for the number of hypotheses to be tested
9 Analyses should be based of prespecified cutoff values for prognostic factors or cutoffs should be avoided

one confirmatory study of the factor has been conducted; (2) any assays used have been determined to be reproducible between laboratories; (3) the factor has substantial predictive value beyond that of standard prognostic factors; and (4) the predictions have therapeutic implications.

STATISTICAL SIGNIFICANCE

Statistical significance refers to the test of a hypothesis specified in advance. For example, consider the regression model $\phi(y) = b_1x_1 + b_2x_2 + \cdots + b_px_p$, where the x's are prognostic factors, the b's are regression coefficients, and $\phi(y)$ is some specified function of the endpoint y. For linear regression $\phi(y)$ is the expected value of the variable y that is being predicted. For logistic regression, y can be thought of as a binary variable taking value 0 for nonresponse and 1 for response, and $\phi(y)$ is ratio of the probability that $y = 1$ to the probability that $y = 0$. For proportional hazards regression, $\phi(y)$, represents the probability that an individual with covariates $(x_1, x_2, \ldots, x_p)$ failed at any specified time relative to the probability that an individual with all covariate values equal to zero failed at that time. Statistical significance of the first prognostic factor, or "covariate," x_1 refers to a test of the null hypothesis that b_1 equals zero. Testing the null hypothesis that $b_1 = 0$ is not meaningful unless we specify the model in which b_1 is a regression coefficient. That requires that we specify what other covariates are in the model and that we specify how all covariates are represented in the model. Only if we specify all of the components of the model in advance can we validly assign a statistical significance level to x_1.

Many commonly used methods of prognostic factor analysis do not produce valid statistical significance values.[5,6] For example, if we screen covariates one at a time for those that seem correlated with response and then include them in a regression model, the significance levels for the covariates in the regression model are not valid. Similarly, none of the step-up, step-down, or stepwise variable selection procedures result in valid statistical significance levels for the variables in the model. If we have a continuous covariate (e.g., age) or a quantative covariate with many levels (e.g., number of lymph nodes involved), it is not valid to find an "optimal cutpoint" for dichotomizing the covariate and then test significance of the binary covariate using the optimal cutpoint. Similarly, it is not valid to group a categorical variable (e.g., histologic type) in a manner suggested by the outcome data and then test the significance of the grouped variable.

If one wishes to have valid statistical significance values, one must completely prespecify the regression model to be used. This specification will generally be based on the findings of previous exploratory studies that focused attention on one or a small number of candidate prognostic factors, suggested cutpoints for their representation, suggested the endpoint for which the factors appeared prognostic, and suggested a set of patients homogeneous with regard to the stage and therapy that should be addressed. If the investigators plunge into their data analyses without focusing their study and prespecifying their hypotheses, then their study will most likely not result in valid assessments of statistical significance and will represent only another exploratory study. There is generally no lack of exploratory prognostic factor studies, but confirmatory studies conducted in a manner that provide statistically valid assessments of significance and definitive answers to therapeutically relevant questions are rare.

WHICH PROGNOSTIC FACTOR IS MOST IMPORTANT?

Many prognostic factor studies claim that a new factor, call it x_1, is more important than a standard factor, call it x_2, because x_1 was selected before x_2 by a variable selection algorithm. As indicated earlier, the significance levels resulting from variable selection algorithms are not valid. The order of selection is also not an indicator of importance. The order of selection depends on a number of things other than the discriminatory values of the factors. The question of which factor is most important is generally the wrong question. It is usually more relevant to know whether the new factor is predictive after incorporating the standard factor. From a regression model viewpoint, this can be expressed by asking how useful is the model containing x_1 and x_2 relative to the model that contains only the standard factor x_2. Comparing the likelihood of the data for the model containing both x_1 and x_2 to the likelihood of the data for the model containing only x_2 provides a statistical significance test of the null hypothesis of interest. This approach is often better than assessing the significance of x_1 for the model containing x_1 and x_2, although for very large sample sizes the two approaches are equivalent.

Statistical significance is really just a test of a null hypothesis, not an assessment of whether a new factor is prognostically important. If the standard factor x_2 is categorical, for example, stage or grade, then one should evaluate whether x_1 is significant and whether it is prognostically important within the categories of x_2. For example, suppose that x_1 represents the presence or absence of a chromosomal abnormality or the overexpression of an oncogene (using a prespecified threshold for immunohistochemical assays). Then one should examine survival curves (if that is the endpoint) for the categories of x_1 within the categories of x_2. In some cases, x_2 will be categorical and will represent an entire classification system in common use. As can be appreciated, reliable assessment of the prognostic importance of the new factor x_1 within the categories of the standard classification requires a large sample size.

In some cases several new factors are of interest. If the number of new factors is large, the study is by its very nature exploratory and its conclusions should only be regarded as hypotheses to be tested in a subsequent confirmatory study. Confirmatory studies can, however, address several factors. If regression modeling is used, the models should contain all of the new factors, as well as the factors representing the standard classification system. Multiple comparison adjustments should be used to account for the fact that several hypotheses are being tested.

SPLIT SAMPLE ANALYSES

It is possible to conduct an exploratory and confirmatory analysis within a single study. The data may be split into two groups: one group is used for exploratory analysis, and the remainer of the data are set aside. When the expoloratory analysis is entirely completed, then specific, focused hypotheses are formulated and the part of the data set aside are used for confirmatory analysis. There are two limitations to this approach: (1) it does not provide the confidence in reproducibility that confirmatory testing on an independent data set would provide, and (2) many data sets are not large enough for exploratory analysis, much less for splitting into two sets. For large data sets collected in a multi-institutional setting, however, this can be a useful approach. Otherwise, the investigators may not feel ready for a fully confirmatory analysis without some opportunity for refining their hypotheses.

SAMPLE SIZE

An important part of the process of planning a clinical trial is determining a sample size that will provide reliable results. Most prognostic factor studies are retrospective in the sense that they use data from patients who were accrued prior to the planning of the study. Consequently, in many cases the number of such patients for whom data and tissue is available is not under the control of the investigator. As a result, there really is no meaningful sample-size planning, and the number of cases is often very inadequate for obtaining reliable results.

The physician reading a prognostic factor study may be interested in knowing whether the number of cases studied is adequate for producing reliable results. When a simple hypothesis is being tested, the adequacy of the sample size can often best be assessed from the results by examining the confidence interval for the estimate of interest. Adequacy of sample size is more difficult to assess for prognostic factor studies, however. As indicated previously, we are often interested in estimating the prognostic effect of a factor within categories determined by the standard classification system. Consequently, an adequate sample size is needed within each such category. For assessing the effect of a binary prognostic factor on survival or disease-free survival, the number of "events" needed to have statistical power $1 - \beta$ for detecting a hazard ratio of δ is approximately

$$\frac{(z_{1-\alpha} + z_{1-\beta})^2}{(\log(\delta)^2 w(1 - w)}$$

where $z_{1-\alpha}$ equals 1.965 for 5% two-sided statistical significance, $z_{1-\beta}$ equals 1.28 for 90% statistical power, and $w : (1 - w)$ are the proportion of patients with and without the prognostic factor. For detecting a prognostic factor that occurs in half of the patients and has a hazard ratio of 2, the preceding formula indicates that about 87 events are needed in each category of the standard classification. If only 25% of the patients have the factor, then about 117 events per category are needed. If only 50% of the patients die (for survival) or recur (for disease-free survival) during the interval of follow-up, then the number of patients required is twice the number of events required. If only 25% of the patients fail, then the number of patients required is 4 times the number of events required. For detecting a hazard ratio of 3 instead of 2, the required number of events is reduced to 35 or 47, depending on w.

The preceding analysis, however, is for assessing a single prognostic factor. If several factors are being assessed in a confirmatory study, the significance level α in the previous formula should be reduced to reflect the number of tests being performed.

For exploratory studies, variable selection algorithms are often highly unstable with regard to the variables selected as "most important" unless the sample size is very large.[7,8] It is possible to use statistical resampling methods such as the "bootstrap" to assess whether the set of prognostic factors selected is stable.[9]

ESTIMATING PROGNOSTIC VALUE

In general we are more interested in whether a factor has a medically important effect on prognosis than on just whether the effect is zero, which is measured by statistical significance. For a focused confirmatory study, one can display survival curves for the levels of a prognostic factor within the categories of a standard classification. For exploratory studies, however, presentations of prognostic value are often heavily biased because the same data are used for selecting the prognostic variables, estimating the regression coefficients, and selecting the model, as for estimating the effect of the model. Typically after the variables are selected and regression coefficients determined, prognostic groups are determined based on cutpoints imposed on the prognostic index. The prognostic index is the "y variable" predicted by the regression model. Then survival curves are shown for these prognostic groups and the reader is impressed by the separation of the survival curves. Such curves are highly biased and misleading, however. Valid estimates of prognostic value require a split sample approach, a more sophisticated statistical resampling procedure, or a confirmatory study.

PUBLICATION BIAS

Publication bias is the tendency of journals to prefer manuscripts that claim to demonstrate positive findings. Publication bias has been discussed primarily in the context of clinical trials,[10] but it is probably more severe with regard to prognostic factor studies, particularly small prognostic factor studies. Large clinical trials are expensive and time-consuming endeavors, and the results are usually published regardless of the outcome. Of course, prominent journals may be more likely to accept the manuscript if the results are positive. Small methodologically weak clinical trials or prognostic factor studies are easier to dismiss by journals unless the results are strikingly positive. There are more small, inadequate clinical trials than large, adequate ones, and even more small, inadequate exploratory prognostic factor studies. The problem is compounded by an order of magnitude for prognostic factor studies, because of the near certainty of producing statistically significant prognostic factors by chance alone if enough factors, endpoints, cutpoints, and subsets are analyzed. Consequently, the literature is probably cluttered with false-positive studies that would not have been submitted or published if the results had come out differently. This link between sample size and publication bias should add to the skepticism with which we read reports of small prognostic factor studies, and reinforces the importance of requiring focused confirmatory studies before accepting the results into clinical practice.

CONCLUSION

We have mostly discussed prognostic factors in the context of regression models. Such models are very general. For example, neural network models are nonlinear regression models.[11] The most important principles for assessing prognostic factor models have little to do with the details of the models, such as whether they are based on neural networks, decision trees, proportional hazards, or whatever. The most important principles are the things that are most often forgotten in reporting prognostic factor studies. These principles are listed in Table 4.1.

As indicated earlier, before a prognostic factor or new classification system is adopted into clinical practice and used for therapeutic decision making, it is important that (1) at least one confirmatory study of the factor has been conducted; (2) any assays used have been determined to be reproducible between laboratories; (3) the factor has substantial predictive value beyond that of standard prognostic factors; and (4) the predictions have therapeutic implications. Based on past experience, we could also add that any new classification system that hopes to be widely used must be relatively simple and scientifically plausable. "Black box" predictive indices derived from complex models lack the scientific plausability needed for wide acceptance.

We expect that cancer treatment will move toward molecularly targeted therapies that will repair or compensate genomic disfunctions of cancer cells. The effects of such therapies may be more specific and less toxic to normal cells than are current drugs. Molecular classification systems will be needed in order to utilize these therapies effectively. Efficient translation of the fruits of the human genome project and developments in functional genomics and combinatorial chemistry to develop effective molecularly targeted therapies requires that we dramatically improve the way we do prognostic factor studies, giving greater emphasis to the conduct of large, definitive prospective confirmatory studies.

REFERENCES

1. Gasparini G, Pozza F, Harris AL: Evaluating the potential usefulness of new prognostic and predictive indicators in node-negative breast cancer patients. *J Natl Cancer Inst* 85:1206–19, 1993.

2. Hilsenbeck SG, Clark GM, McGuire WL: Why do so many prognostic factors fail to pan out? *Breast Cancer Res Treat* 22:197–204, 1992.

3. Altman DG, Lausen B, Sauerbrei W, Schumacher M: The dangers of using 'optimal' cutpoints in the evaluation of prognostic factors. *J Natl Cancer Inst* 86:829–35, 1994.

4. Simon R, Altman DG: Statistical aspects of prognostic factor studies in oncology. *Br J Cancer* 69:979–85, 1994.

5. Harrell FE, Lee KL, Mark DB: Multivariable prognostic models: issues in developing models, evaluating assumptions and adequacy, and measuring and reducing errors. *Stat Med* 15:361–87, 1996.

6. Harrell FE, Lee KL, Pollock BG: Regression models in clinical studies: determining relationships between predictors and response. *J Natl Cancer Inst* 80:1198–202, 1988.

7. Concato J, Peduzzi P, Holford TR: Importance of events per independent variable in proportional hazards regression analysis I. Background, goals, and general strategy. *J Clin Epidemiol* 48:1495–501, 1995.

8. Peduzzi P, Concato J, Feinstein AR: Importance of events per independent variable in proportional hazards regression analysis II. Accuracy and precision of regression estimates. *J Clin Epidemiol* 48:1503–10, 1995.

9. Altman DG, Anderson PK: Bootstrap investigation of the stability of a Cox regression model. *Stat Med* 8:771–83, 1989.

10. Begg CB, Berlin JA: Publication bias and dissemination of clinical research. *J Natl Cancer Inst* 81:107–15, 1989.

11. Faraggi D, Simon R: A neural network model for survival data. *Stat Med* 14:73–82, 1995.

CHAPTER 5

Artificial Neural Networks for Physicians: A Technology Introduction

DAVID M. RODVOLD, DAVID G. MCLEOD, JEFFREY M. BRANDT,
PETER B. SNOW, AND GERALD P. MURPHY

Artificial neural networks (ANNs) are the sole successfully deployed artificial intelligence (AI) applications that attempt to mimic the activities of the human brain and how it physically operates. The "artificial" in artificial neural nets is included to distinguish the computer-based systems from their biological counterparts. ANNs have become very common in a broad set of problem domains including medical, industrial, and financial applications. Within urology, the 1994 seminal paper by Snow et al.[1] established ANNs as a significant predictive technology in the prostate cancer arena. ANNs are well-established computational models, with research dating to the 1940s.[2,3]

Within AI, ANNs are generally contrasted with knowledge-based systems (also known as expert systems). Expert systems use a somewhat contrived structure composed of explicit knowledge rules, while ANNs provide a reasonably faithful representation of biological neural systems. ANNs are generally easier to construct than knowledge-based systems, but the simple rule structure of knowledge-based systems provides a more traceable chain of logic from the input to output.

There are a large number of different types of ANNs that computer science researchers apply to various problem types. However, one particular type of ANN architecture has emerged as the de facto standard in practice — the so-called "feedforward" network, which is described in detail below. Other types of networks that the reader may encounter will generally be some sort of a geometric construct, such as probabilistic neural networks or Kohonen networks. Probabilistic neural networks use a "nearest-neighbor" approach, where prospective cases are associated with the closest case that was available during network construction. Kohonen networks are a clustering technique, where similar

Prognostic Factors in Cancer, 2nd edition, Edited by Mary K. Gospodarowicz
ISBN 0-471-40633-3   Copyright © 2001 Wiley-Liss, Inc.

cases are identified as being members of the same group. This document does not address these more esoteric constructs, rather it focuses on the ubiquitous feedforward networks. An interested reader can find detailed information on various ANN paradigms in Lawrence[4] or Wasserman.[5]

WHAT IS AN ARTIFICIAL NEURAL NETWORK?

The primary primitive data structure in the human brain is the *neuron*, and there are roughly 10^{11} of them in the human brain. Extending from the neurons are tendril-like *axons*, which carry electrochemical signals from the body of the neuron. Thinner structures called *dendrites* protrude from the axons, and continue to propagate the signals from the neural cell bodies. Where the dendrites from two neurons meet, interneural signals are passed. These intersection points (numbering about 10^{15}) are called *synapses*. The strength of the synaptic connections between neurons dictates their level of interaction. When a biological neuron becomes activated (i.e., it "fires"), adjacent neurons that are strongly connected will also be activated. Figure 5.1 shows an extremely simplified representation of two connected biological neurons.

Artificial neural networks are computer programs that emulate some of the higher-level functions of the architecture just described. As in the human brain, there are neurons and synapses modeled, with various synaptic connection strengths (referred to as weights) for each connected pair of neurons. However, similar to many computer programs (and unlike the brain) there is a specific set of input and output neurons for each problem and each net. These input and output neurons correspond to the inputs to, and outputs from, a traditional computer program. The other (so-called "hidden") neurons, along with the synapses and

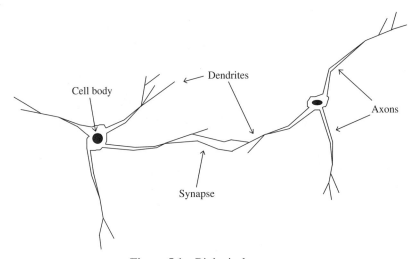

Figure 5.1 Biological neurons.

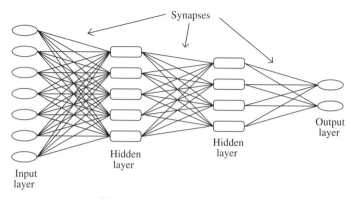

Figure 5.2   ANN architecture.

weights, correspond to the instructions in a traditional program. Figure 5.2 shows a representation of a multilayer perceptron artificial neural network, which is a popular type of feedforward network. The network shown has 7 input neurons, 2 output neurons, 2 hidden layers, 9 hidden neurons, and 63 synapses/weights. The synaptic weights contain the "intelligence" of the system.

Biological neurons are physically limited in the magnitude of the signal that can be passed on to adjacent neurons. An average biological neuron in the human brain is connected with about 10^4 of its neighbors, and its activation level is limited in such a way that, beyond some threshold, additional incoming signals have little or no effect on the outgoing signals. ANNs have a similar need to operate with signals restricted to a known finite range, usually with numeric values between zero and one, or between minus one and one. Artificial neural networks thus include some sort of activation function to limit the signal that is received from, and propagated to, adjacent neurons. There are a number of mathematical functions that are used for this, but they have the common characteristic that they take incoming signal strengths that may have a very large range and transform them to a much smaller and more easily managed range. These activation functions are often referred to as squashing functions (since they squash arbitrarily large ranges into preset limited ranges), and they include both linear and nonlinear functions. The input and output neurons associated with the ANN are subject to similar range restrictions and are scaled and shifted as necessary to ensure internal range consistency within the ANN. An additional neuron is also often included in a feedforward ANN, to ensure that some signal is available to all neurons regardless of the inputs from the other neurons. This additional neuron is usually referred to as the bias neuron, and always sends the maximum allowable value (usually the value of one) to all noninput neurons. Like other synaptic connections, the connections between the bias neuron and other neurons each have their own weights.

With this background established, the composition of a feedforward ANN is as follows:

- Number of input neurons
- Number of output neurons
- Scale and shift values for each input and output neuron
- Inclusion of a bias neuron
- Number of hidden layers
- Number of neurons in each hidden layer
- Connection weight for each pair of connected neurons
- Activation function(s) for each layer

Although the items on this list completely define a feedforward ANN, the list itself is hardly a satisfying description of how ANNs are created and used. The next section discusses these matters in detail.

HOW DO ARTIFICIAL NEURAL NETWORKS WORK?

Traditional computer programs consist of a set of explicit instructions wherein the program is told exactly what to do. ANNs operate under a fundamentally different assumption: the program is told what to *know* rather than what to *do*. This is accomplished during the training phase of ANN development. During training, the ANN learns the behavior of the desired system by being repeatedly exposed to historical data that characterizes the effect of interest.

The initial network configuration (number of hidden neuron layers, number of hidden neurons in each layer, activation function, etc.) is chosen by the system designer. There are no set rules to determine these network parameters, and currently trial and error based on experience seems to be the best method. Some commercial programs use automatic optimization techniques to find good network architectures.

The synaptic weights are initially randomized, so that the system initially consists of "white noise." Training data are then run through the network to see how many cases it gets correct (how a network is "fired" is described in detail below). A correct case is one where the network result is sufficiently close to the established output from the training database. Initially the number of correct cases will be very small. The network training module then examines the errors and adjusts the synaptic weights in an attempt to increase the number of correctly assessed training cases. Once the adjustments have been made, the training data are again presented to the network, and the entire process iterates. Eventually, the number of correct cases will reach a maximum, and the training iteration ends.

Once the training is complete, testing is performed. When creating the training database, some of the data are withheld from the system. Usually at least 10 to 20% of the available data are set aside to run through the trained network, to test the system's ability to correctly assess cases that it has not seen before. If the testing data are assessed with success similar to the training data, and if this performance is sufficient, the network is ready for actual use. If the testing data are not assessed with sufficient accuracy, the network parameters must be adjusted by the network designer, and the entire process is repeated until acceptable results are achieved. Figure 5.3 graphically shows how an ANN converges to a set of weights during training.

There are a number of algorithms used to train the synaptic weights of an ANN. The most popular method is called *backpropagation of errors*. The details of this algorithm are quite mathematically intensive and unimportant for the purposes of the discussion presented here. Other training algorithms that are commonly seen include the conjugate gradient descent method and the Levenberg-Marquardt algorithm.[6]

As noted, the type of ANN that we are concerned with is called a *feedforward network*. This terminology comes from the way in which the known input values are transformed into the desired output values. Figure 5.2 shows the architecture of a typical feedforward ANN, which in this case has seven inputs and produces two outputs. If the left-to-right direction is designated as forward, then the input signals propagate forward from the input neurons to the output neurons. During the firing of the network, there is no backward information flow through a feedforward ANN.

When the network fires, a series of mathematical operations occur that use the ANN definition information listed in the preceding section to transform inputs to outputs. To fire the network, the calculations for each layer must be completed before the next layer is begun. First, the input values are scaled and shifted into the appropriate range and the resulting values are stored in the input neurons. This completes the calculations for the input layer.

The next step is to calculate the values of the neurons in the first hidden layer. In the typical feedforward network shown in, neurons in adjacent layers are completely connected. In other words, there is a synapse between every neuron in the input layer and every neuron in the first hidden layer. In this example, since there are 7 input neurons and 5 neurons in the first hidden layer, there are 35 synapses between the first two layers of the ANN. Each synapse has a numeric weight that determines the strength of the connection between the two neurons. The value of a neuron in the first hidden layer is straightforward to calculate. It is the sum of the weighted neural values of the 7 neurons on the input layer.

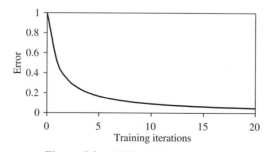

Figure 5.3   ANN training progress.

In other words, the value of each of the 5 neurons in the first hidden layer is the sum of 7 numbers. The 7 numbers are calculated by multiplying the value of each of the 7 input neurons by the corresponding synaptic weights. When these sums are complete, the values in each of the 5 neurons in the first hidden layer are squashed using the activation function, and are then ready for propagation to the next layer.

The ANN shown in Figure 5.2 has a second hidden layer. The procedure for calculating the values of these 4 neurons is the same as described in the previous paragraph, except here 20 synaptic weights are used to calculate the sums of 5 numbers needed by each of the 4 neurons in the second hidden layer. These summed values are then squashed and ready to be propagated to the output layer. The calculation for the output layer follows the same procedure, with eight synaptic weights available for calculating the output layer sums. After squashing the output layer, the output neurons will contain values in the range used by the neural network, either zero to one or minus one to one. To get the value of interest to the neural network user, these values must be transformed back into their original range. The scale and shift values for the output neurons are applied to the squashed values to produce the desired output of the neural network.

The calculations associated with firing an ANN seem tedious, and in fact are rarely performed manually. Rather, the ANNs are generally encoded into some computer application that can quickly and automatically calculate the outputs for any set of inputs. The branch of mathematics known as linear algebra[7] provides some numeric constructs that ease the computational burden somewhat. In particular, matrix multiplication is used to calculate the unsquashed values of the neurons, and linear transforms are used to aid in the shifting and scaling of the input and output neurons.

When ANN construction and training is complete, the trained systems must be put into some user-approachable format. Neural net "shell" programs provide facilities for both the construction and exercising of user-trained networks. These shell programs are generally stand-alone applications, and cannot be embedded within other applications. However, some shell programs provide the option of creating outputs of the trained network parameters that can be included in-line with other programs such as spreadsheets or custom-built applications.

WHY DO ARTIFICIAL NEURAL NETWORKS WORK?

The preceding sections have established some detail on what ANNs are and how they operate. The final step is to explain why ANNs are able to perform predictive tasks.

One predictive technique that is well-established within the medical community is statistical regression. Linear regression models are presented regularly in scholarly journals as approximations to data sets. The basic concept with linear regression is to fit an approximating straight line to a data set. The technique that is generally used for this is the method of least squares, wherein the sum of the squares of the residuals (distances from the data points to the approximating lines) is minimized.[8] The result of the least-squares approximation is estimators for two parameters, β_0 and β_1, which correspond to the y-axis intercept and slope of the regression line, respectively. The formula for the regression line is

$$y = \beta_0 + \beta_1 x$$

An example of a linear regression approximation is shown in Figure 5.4. In this figure, the data points are modeled by a regression line with parametric estimators of $\beta_0 = -1.17$ and $\beta_1 = 2.12$, so

$$y = -1.17 + 2.12x$$

The general linear regression model is a simple linear combination equation. A feedforward ANN can also be programmed to serve as a linear combination, by simply setting the number of input neurons to 1, the number of output neurons to 1, the activation function to be linear, and connecting a bias neuron. As an experiment, this was done, and a network was trained on the data in Figure 5.4 using backpropagation of errors for 100 training iterations. Table 5.1 shows the parameters of the trained ANN. A very simple equation can be constructed from these data to fire the ANN manually:

$$y = (((x^*\text{scale\_in} + \text{shift\_in})^*\text{weight} - \text{offset}) - \text{shift\_out})/\text{scale\_out}$$

When the appropriate values are substituted into the preceding equation, and the equation is reduced to minimal form, the equation derived by the ANN is

$$y = -1.19 + 2.10x$$

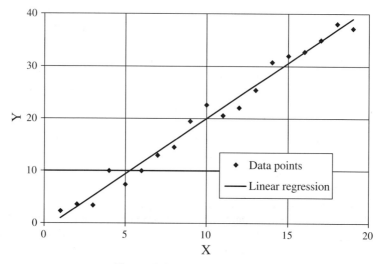

Figure 5.4 Linear regression.

TABLE 5.1   Trained ANN Parameters

Parameter	Value
Number of input neurons (n_in)	1
Number of output neurons (n_out)	1
Scale value for input neuron (scale_in)	0.0555555
Shift value for input neuron (shift_in)	−0.0555555
Scale value for output neuron (scale_out)	0.0279319
Shift value for output neuron (shift_out)	−0.0635376
Bias neuron inclusion (bias)	True
Number of hidden layers	0
Input-to-output synaptic weight (weight)	1.05405
Bias-to-output synaptic weight (bias)	0.0382502
Activation function (squash)	Linear

This line is almost identical to the line produced by linear regression. The minor differences in the parameters are attributable to the stochastic nature of ANN training algorithms. A plot comparing the two lines is not very illustrative, since the lines lie so close to each other as to be indistinguishable.

To understand why ANNs work, the significance of this demonstration cannot be overstated. The basic message is that, when restricted in specific ways, ANNs are actually linear regression models. In other words, ANNs are a superset of statistical linear regression. This effect has been demonstrated and documented in both the statistical[9] and ANN[10] arenas. The ways in which the parameters/weights are found in the two models differ somewhat, but in fact they share some fundamental similarities. Linear regression models generally use the method of least squares to find the values of β_0 and β_1, while ANNs use a training method such as backpropagation of errors. In assessing the error of the network during training, however, root-mean-square (rms) error is generally the metric of choice, which is very similar to the least-squares calculation used in regression.

The domain of statistics provides many models that exceed the performance of linear regression, and if ANNs were limited to this simple linear performance, there certainly would be no compelling reason to adopt them. Removing the restrictions placed on the network from the preceding example allows a much wider range of applications to be derived. In fact, linear regression is not the only statistical model that has a direct neural analog. Table 5.2 (adapted from Sarle[9]) lists the statistical equivalents of several ANN types.

Since there seems to be a demonstrable correspondence between ANNs and statistical techniques, it is logical to question why one technique should be chosen over the other. Indeed, neither technique is powerful enough to render the other obsolete. In general, statistical approaches are useful when attempting to scientifically quantify the performance of some system. In fact, no ANN analysis should be considered complete until a rigorous statistical analysis of the results has been performed. ANNs, conversely, are very useful when creating predictive models where the interrelationships and behavior of the

TABLE 5.2 Neural/Statistical Equivalents

ANN Model	Statistical Equivalent
Single linear perceptron	Linear regression
Simple linear perceptron	Multivariate multiple linear regression
Simple nonlinear perceptron	Logistic regression
Adaline network	Linear discriminant function
Functional link network	Polynomial regression
Multilayer perceptron	Simple nonlinear regression or multivariate multiple nonlinear regression

various problem parameters are unknown. Most statistical regression techniques require some a priori assumptions regarding the distribution(s) within the data set. ANN construction and training techniques allow users to create predictive models without explicitly specifying such information. Further, there are many neural models for which there is no particular statistical analog.

ARTIFICIAL NEURAL NETWORK ISSUES

Regardless of the power of neural networks to solve problems effectively, there are still issues associated with them of which potential users should be aware. One of the most often-heard criticisms aimed at ANNs and their practitioners is that scientific rigor is not often applied to analyses performed with ANNs. It is indeed true that the automated nature of many ANN tools can lull users into complacency when creating neural systems. There is often a tendency to merely plug in the data, turn the ANN training software on, and blindly accept the result. ANNs are powerful tools, and as such, must be used with great care. Rodvold[11] presents a software-development-process model for ANNS in critical applications that guides users from system specification, through data gathering, training, and deployment, finally to system validation and verification. By following this or a similar development process, developers can systematically avoid "bad science" when using ANNs.

Perhaps the most difficult task when creating an ANN is knowing exactly when it is "done." The previous discussions presented in this chapter showed fixed architectures with a set number of neurons, layers, and so on. While there are some broad rules of thumb regarding what an ANN should look like for a given project, there is still a great deal of uncertainty in determining the optimal architecture. If the network is too small for the problem, performance will suffer. If it is too large, performance may be artificially inflated by a network that is merely memorizing the data rather than generalizing trends (this effect is sometimes referred to as "overfitting"). Determining the balance between these effects is usually a highly iterative process. Some ANN shell programs have built-in facilities that aid the ANN developer in this process. When such tools are used, the resulting architecture should be critically inspected to ensure that the proposed solution is not inconsistent with known problem parameters.

Related to the issue of architecture optimization is the problem of "over-training" a network. While a network is being trained, the error of the predictions drops very rapidly at first, and then improvements begin to diminish. This is shown graphically in Figure 5.3. The large, early gains are made when the ANN is finding the "signal" contained in the data. The slower, later gains are accomplished only as the ANN memorizes the "noise" inherent in the data. The primary way to avoid this effect is to monitor ANN training, and when gains begin to diminish, the training can be manually interrupted. Alternatively, some ANN shells apply this method automatically and supply the user with the "earliest" network that encapsulates the desired effect.

It has been said that ANNs have tremendous "egos." When a trained ANN is asked a question, it will always give an answer. The mathematical construct for an ANN does not preclude any inputs from the user, even nonsensical or unique cases. The ANN will always return an answer for any set of inputs, even if it not "qualified" to assess the particular case. For prospective cases that are presented to an ANN that are reasonably similar to cases contained in the training database, ANNs are usually very good at generalizing or interpolating results. When deploying a trained ANN, however, safeguards must be included that prevent the ANN from being exercised for cases that are clearly outside its realm of expertise. This is usually accomplished by simply checking the inputs for prospective cases against the ranges for each input parameter that were present in the training database.

Finally, one particularly troubling aspect of ANN training is a sensitivity to initial conditions. It was mentioned earlier that ANN synaptic weights are generally randomized before training begins. Backpropagation of errors as a training paradigm is what is known as an "error surface traversal algorithm." In other words, as training occurs, the ANN moves from one trained state to another looking for ways to improve performance by adjusting weights. The weight adjustment algorithm is not exhaustive, though, and not all combinations of weights will be assessed for quality. Thus the final answer determined by the training algorithm will be determined partially by exactly what random values were contained in the initial untrained ANN. The end result is that the same network architectures, trained twice in a row, will result in two disparate sets of synaptic weights. While this is somewhat bothersome, it would not be truly troubling if the performance of the two networks was equivalent. In this case, it would be as if two doctors could reach the same diagnosis for a condition by following distinct chains of logic. However, the performance of two architecturally identical ANNs trained by backpropagation are often significantly different. The main problem is that backpropagation tends to get "stuck" in local error minima while searching for the global minimum. There are some modifications that have been attached to backpropagation to attempt to avoid this problem, but often the only way to deal with the issue is to train the same network architecture several times to assess the variance of the performance results, and then plan a training regimen based on estimated confidence intervals. The better solution at this time seems to be the use of newer training algorithms (such as the previously mentioned conjugate gradient descent method or Levenberg-Marquardt algorithm) that are less likely to yield locally optimized solutions. Another approach is to use nonrandom approaches in initializing ANN weights in an attempt to start the training in the neighborhood of the global minimum. The need for such alternate training algorithms should be considered when purchasing an off-the-shelf ANN shell.

ARTIFICIAL NEURAL NETWORK APPLICATIONS

In this section we discuss several applications in which ANNs have been used to estimate prognosis for individual patients. Some guidelines are suggested for reporting and comparing ANN analyses to other predictive technologies such as regression. The advantages and disadvantages of ANN technology compared with other predictive technologies are also discussed.

In recent years artificial neural networks have been used to estimate prognosis for individual patients. They have been used to predict recurrence of prostate cancer in the five years following treatment (surgery or radiation therapy). Inputs involve pretreatment clinical information and, where available, pathology information available as a result of treatment. Figure 5.5 shows the user interface for a neural network designed to predict a 10-year prognosis for brachytherapy treatment for prostate cancer with and without accompanying external beam radiation treatment. ANNs have been used to predict the pathological stage of a patient's prostate cancer given clinical data available from pretreatment information such as biopsy results.

ANNs have been developed that predict the likelihood of survival and nonrecurrence (disease-free survival) for five years following treatment for breast cancer. Input variables consist of demographics, family history, pathology results, and treatment provided. ANNs have been developed that predict five-year survival following treatment for colon cancer. A neural network has been developed that predicts short-term (less than a year) recurrence of cancer following initial surgery for women with advanced ovarian cancer.

Most prognostic medical applications of neural networks involve the prediction of a binary outcome such as survival (yes/no), recurrence (yes/no), and positive or negative biopsy. Tools that predict binary outcomes (neural networks, regression analyses, decision trees, etc.) should always report results as the area under the receiver operator characteristic (ROC) curve for validation or prospective cases not used to develop the model. The ROC curve is a plot of sensitivity (on the y-axis) vs. 1-specificity (on the x-axis). The ROC area is independent of outcome prevalence in the database used for model development. An area of 50% indicates the model is no better than random guessing at the outcome state. An area of 100% indicates the model is perfect in predicting the outcome state. Experience on the part of the authors indicates that predictive models that

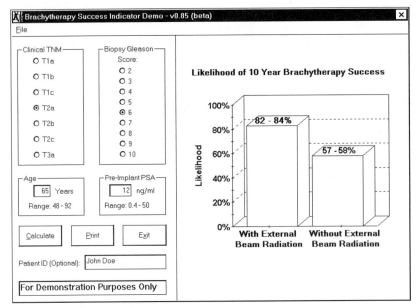

Figure 5.5 Brachytheraphy efficacy predictor output.

produce a ROC area in excess of approximately 80% for validation or prospective cases, will be clinically useful.

Additional useful results from ANNs or other predictive tools involve the reporting of the specificity, positive predictive value, and negative predictive value at high sensitivity. These are often clinically useful results. For example, at 95% sensitivity for identifying men with prostate cancer, the specificity of the model will determine the number of men on the average that must be biopsied to find a cancer.

ANNs have both advantages and disadvantages over other predictive technologies. When properly developed, they are generally the most accurate tool. Unlike rule-based or decision tree analyses that lump a patient into a bin with other more or less similar cases (with resulting loss of accuracy), the ANN and regression technologies treat patients on an individual basis with a continuously varying outcome prediction as input variables are changed.

ANN disadvantages center in two areas. First, because of the relatively large number of degrees of freedom associated with ANN architectures, they have a tendency to overfit training data, as has already been mentioned. This problem can be overcome in one of several ways, but care must be taken to document and report predictive accuracy on validation or prospective cases not used in the development of the network. The second disadvantage, the so-called "black box" problem, is not easily overcome. Whereas all the predictive technologies yield useful information about relative variable importance in predicting outcome, only rule-based systems and to some extent regression analyses yield insight into the underlying patterns in the data responsible for determining outcome. The reason for this is the distributed nature of information in the neural network. The hidden neurons and associated weights and biases (where information is stored) are not associated with any particular input variable, thus making insight into decision making a very difficult task. ANNs trade insight for accuracy.

SUMMARY

This report has presented some technical background in an attempt to help physicians understand the basic issues associated with ANNs. The primary messages that this chapter conveys are:

1. ANNs are complex numeric constructs, but no more so than many other accepted techniques used in the medical community.
2. ANNs bear a strong resemblance to many well-known statistical methods, but are usually easier to apply.
3. There are issues associated with ANNs that require users to apply rigorous engineering practices to their studies.

With this framework established, it should be easier for clinicians and researchers to interpret and assess many of the studies that are currently being published in oncologic and other medical domains.

REFERENCES

1. Snow PB, Smith DS, Catalona WJ: *Artificial neural networks in the diagnosis and prognosis of prostate cancer: a pilot study. J Urol* 152:1923–26, 1994.
2. Hebb D: *The organization of behavior.* New York, Wiley, 1949.
3. Pitts W, McCullogh W: How we know universals. *Bull Math Biophys* 9 (127): 1947.
4. Lawrence J: *Introduction to neural networks: computer simulations of biological intelligence.* Grass Valley (CA), California Scientific Software, 1991.
5. Wasserman PD: *Neural computing: theory and practice.* New York, Van Nostrand Reinhold, 1989.
6. Masters T: *Neural, novel & hybrid algorithms for time series prediction.* New York, Wiley, 1995.
7. Hoffman KM, Kunze RA: *Linear Algebra.* Englewood Cliffs (NJ), Prentice Hall, 1971.
8. Mendenhall W: *Introduction to probability and statistics.* Boston, Duxbury Press, 1987.
9. Sarle WS: Neural networks and statistical models. *Proc 19th Annu SAS Users Group Int Conf.* 1994.

10. Ripley BD: Statistical aspects of neural networks, in Barndorff-Nielsen OE, Jensen JL, Kendall WS (eds.): *Networks and chaos — statistical and probabilistic aspects*. London, Chapman & Hall, 1993, pp. 40–123.

11. Rodvold DM: A software development process model for artificial neural networks in critical applications. *Proc 1999 Int Joint Conf on Neural Networks (IJCNN'99)* Washington (DC), 1999.

CHAPTER 6

Tumor, Host, and Environment-related Prognostic Factors

BRIAN O'SULLIVAN, MARY K. GOSPODAROWICZ, and ROBERT
G. BRISTOW

In the current climate of knowledge in oncology, an understanding of factors that govern outcome in cancer patients is essential to achieve the maximum therapeutic benefit. Discipline in the approach to patient management allows the most advantageous application of current evidence and leads to best practice. To determine prognosis it is helpful to consider *tumor-related* prognostic factors that characterize the disease, *host-related* prognostic factors that typify the patient, and *environment-related* factors, which are external factors not directly related to either the disease or the patient (see Chapter 2).

In this chapter, we review the most common factors in each of these categories. The discussion will focus on prognostic factors that are relevant at the time of diagnosis and initial treatment. However we caution that, in the management of a cancer patient, determination of prognosis could be required repeatedly to take account of multiple episodes throughout the course of the disease. Frequently these situations reflect decision-making points (e.g., concerning adjuvant therapy, management of recurrent cancer, and palliative or terminal care). The diversity and impact of prognostic factors in each category will be demonstrated using examples from the recent literature. A comprehensive review of prognostic factors in distinct cancers follows in Part B of the book.

Most cancer literature equates prognosis with tumor characteristics. Cancer pathology and anatomic disease extent account for most variations in cancer outcome. Since screening and early detection allow for diagnosis of small localized cancers, however, environmental factors are likely to have a more pronounced impact on outcome. This is particularly so as treatment becomes more effective. In addition, these factors are easier to influence by applying currently existing knowledge compared to those factors at the host or tumor level

Prognostic Factors in Cancer, 2nd edition, Edited by Mary K. Gospodarowicz
ISBN 0-471-40633-3 Copyright © 2001 Wiley-Liss, Inc.

that are ingrained permanently in the phenotype of the case. The environmental factors are also the least studied despite evidence that they may have profound impact on outcome.[1] For example, we reviewed Medline® publications between December 1, 1998 and November 30, 1999 under the search terms "prognostic factors in cancer" and "human" and "English language." This revealed 21 of 983 papers on prognostic factors in cancer dealing with environment-related factors, as indicated by their titles. In contrast, the same search yielded 189 publications with titles focusing on genetic or molecular prognostic factors. It would seem from this initial and potentially superficial examination that a disproportionate neglect of prognostic factors other than those related to the tumor might exist. This warrants further evaluation, since it is possible that an alternative situation is that the nontumor factors are either too few in number, not relevant to patient outcome, or will soon be surpassed by an overwhelming influence of new factors that are being detected with modern techniques. We believe that the latter is unlikely in the foreseeable future and that all of these factors are highly relevant to the task of uncovering prognosis in cancer.

TUMOR-RELATED PROGNOSTIC FACTORS

Tumor-related prognostic factors are generally the main determinants of outcome in cancer patients (Table 6.1). The fundamental tumor-related prognostic factors relate to the histologic type and features, and the anatomic disease extent. With progress in our understanding of tumor biology, however, it is expected that molecular and genetic tumor characteristics will assume a much more important role in cancer diagnosis, treatment, and prognosis.

Pathology

Tumor pathology is crucial to the determination of prognosis in cancer. The histologic type defines the disease under consideration, but additional factors such as grade, pattern of growth, presence of lymphatic or vascular invasion, infiltration patterns, multifocality, and others, also affect the outcome.[2-4] Pathologic factors have been extensively studied in many tumors and are described in the disease-specific chapters of the second part of the book. Pathologic factors are also vulnerable to the modifications that take place when classification and terms are altered.

Anatomic Extent of Disease

The anatomic tumor extent is customarily recorded using the TNM classification according to criteria intended to categorize the size and/or depth of invasion of primary tumor, the presence of regional lymph-node metastasis, and the presence of distant metastasis. Pierre Denoix created the TNM classification over 50 years ago with the aims of describing disease extent, predicting prognosis, and helping to formulate treatment strategies.[5,6] The TNM classification has been revised

TABLE 6.1   Examples of Tumor-related Prognostic Factors

1. Pathology
   - Morphologic classification, for example, adenocarcinoma, squamous
   - Histologic grade
   - Growth pattern, for example, papillary vs. solid, cribriform vs.tubular vs. solid
   - Pattern of invasion, for example, perineural, small-vessel invasion
2. Anatomic tumor extent
   - TNM categories
   - Tumor bulk
   - Single vs. multifocal tumor
   - Number of sites of involvement
   - Tumor markers, for example, PSA, AFP, CEA
3. Tumor biology
   - Tumor markers, for example, her2neu, CD20
   - Proliferation indices, for example, S-phase fraction, MiB-1
   - Molecular markers: p53, rb, Bcl2
   - Genetic markers: t(2:5) translocation
4. Symptoms related to the presence of tumor
   - Weight loss
   - Pain
   - Edema
   - Fever
5. Performance status

periodically to make it more relevant to modern treatment approaches. Sometimes these revisions are substantial, bearing little resemblance to prior classifications in some diseases. For example, the most recent revisions to the TNM classification for testis and nasopharynx tumors involved substantial revisions and improved the clinical relevance of these classifications. The goals of staging are not only to describe the anatomic extent of disease, and indicate prognosis, but also to guide the choice of the most appropriate therapy. With multiple goals, no staging classification is likely to be perfect in satisfying any individual purpose and, in aiding the goals of cancer care, must strike a balance between what is not only feasible in the practical sense but also available for widespread use. Therefore, the determination of the predominant objective of the TNM classification is often based on consensus rather than on uniform criteria. Notwithstanding this, the TNM categories and stage groupings will continue to be extremely useful prognostic factors for the foreseeable future. However, several other descriptors of disease extent often improve the definition of outcomes further. Among those are tumor bulk (which may not be accounted for in TNM), the number of tumors, and the number of metastases.[7-9]

Symptoms

While they may be considered patient-related factors, the prime origin of symptoms in oncology is the invasive character of the tumor, the presence of disease burden in the host, or the elaboration of factors that may elicit as systemic response in the host. Consequently, symptoms are often forgotten tumor-related prognostic factors. In fact, the presence of symptoms is a very important prognostic factor in most patients with cancer.[10–13] Classic examples of the impact of symptoms are B-symptoms (night sweats, fever, and weight loss) in Hodgkin's disease. The presence of symptoms is usually associated with the presence of advanced disease, and in disease detected by screening or by intentional early detection efforts, symptoms are present.

Tumor Biology

Traditionally, the expression of cancer-related proteins were utilized solely as tumor markers (i.e., PSA, CEA) to reflect overall tumor burden, without the ability to characterize the behavior of the tumor. More recent results in cancer biology have highlighted the prognostic role of cancer-related proteins as gene products that have functional value in determining cancer causation and suppression (e.g., ras, src, c-myc, p53, pRB), tumor-cell apoptosis (e.g., the bcl-2/bax and caspase family of proteins), the normal and aberrant control of the cell cycle (i.e., p53, pRb, cyclins, p21/p27/p16; PCNA, Ki67), and finally, tumor mestastasis and angiogenesis (i.e., TIMP-1/2,CD44, VEGF, FGF, angiogenesis inhibitors).

In parallel, exciting developments are also occurring in molecular diagnostics, including the use of DNA microarray analyses, fluorescent flow cytometric and immunohistochemical analyses, and chromosomal analyses, including spectral karyotyping and comparative genomic hybridization (i.e., SKY, CGH). These new technologies have increased our ability to accurately determine genetic information pertaining to minimal tumor burden, aggressive tumor-cell growth, tumor-cell response following DNA-damaging or immunotherapies and a given tumor's propensity for metastatic spread. In order to deal with complicated bioinformatics, new strategies are required to combine multiple types of information from molecular technologies to try and summarize the genetic profile for each tumor.

Although the utility of these proteins is varied depending on the clinical situation, their prognostic use can perhaps be simplified into three main areas: (1) prediction of occult disease and the need for adjuvant therapy; (2) prediction of natural history and patient survival; and (3), molecular prediction of treatment response. It is becoming increasingly clear that no one specific gene sequence or expressed protein will predict the clinical behavior of tumors. This concept is represented in Figure 6.1, as specific proteins might overlap two or more of these categories for any given tumor site.

In the first prognostic category, decision making in the use of adjuvant therapies requires the accurate risk-determination of occult metastatic spread as a reflection of minimal disease burden. For example, adjuvant chemotherapy can be given on the basis of the adverse prognosis associated with the expression of a mutated p53 tumor suppressor protein, altered expression of the p27 cyclin-kinase inhibitor, or altered apoptosis-related bcl-2/bax protein ratios, in node-negative,

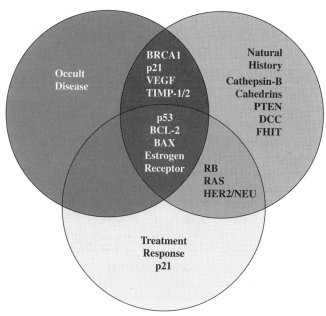

Figure 6.1 Shown are overlapping uses for selected protein biomarkers in the prognostic categories of occult disease, natural history, and treatment response. It logically follows that there would rarely be a prognostic biomarker that could predict for occult disease and treatment response but not the natural history of disease.

premenopausal, breast cancer.[14] Similar decisions about adjuvant therapy may be derived from molecular information based on the detection of small numbers of epithelial or hematopoietic tumor cells in the bone marrow determined using reverse-transcriptase polymerase chain reaction (RT-PCR) analyses. In these cases, specific mRNAs transcribed from aberrant epithelial or hematopoietic genes can be detected by RT-PCR, or a larger panel of mRNAs can be detected by "sequential analysis of gene expression" (SAGE), to compare normal and cancerous gene sequences.[15] Finally, micrometastases in the bone marrow can also be detected by antibodies directed against aberrant epithelial or hematopoietic gene products.[16-18] In this prognostic category, molecular factors dictate the potential for, and levels of, occult metastatic disease.

In the second category, altered expression of a combination of proteins may predict for the natural history of disease, and therefore disease-free or overall survival. It is known that tumors undergo multiple stages of tumor progression associated with specific changes in oncogenes (i.e., ras, src) and tumor suppressor genes (i.e., APC, DCC, p53). The acquisition of these genetic observations can have prognostic implication in bladder, prostate, and colon cancer, and can be associated with decreased overall survival.[19,20] Most investigators now agree that it is the accumulation of many changes, forming a "genetic aggregate," that determines the overall clinical behavior of a tumor, and these aggregates can be used by the clinician to improve estimates of patient survival.

Finally, predicting treatment response with molecular biomarkers is a conduit to novel cancer therapeutics and individualization of treatment. Both in radiotherapy and chemotherapy, mutations in the cell cycle and apoptotic proteins (i.e., p53, bax/bcl-2, pRB) have been associated with increased relapse rates or decreased local control following treatment.[21-23] Determination of a protein expression profile based on pretreatment biopsies may allow the triaging of patients into resistant or sensitive categories. It would be optimal to develop a prognostic "molecular therapeutic ratio" for each individual patient based on the expression profile within both normal and tumor tissues. Such information can then be utilized to triage patients appropriately to treatments that use specific pharmacologic agents to normalize intracellular signaling, or reinstitute normal protein function using gene therapy, and/or use immunotherapy directed against distinct tumor-specific proteins.[24]

The current limitation to the accurate use of genetic information relates to the multifactorial nature (i.e., cell, tumor, host) of cancer prognosis and tumor-cell heterogeneity. The interpretation of a given genetic analysis is complicated by the dynamic state of proteins whose expression can be altered in the tumor cell due to cell cycle position or oxygen/nutrient status. For example, intratumoral hypoxia, which is found in many tumors, can alter the expression of a number of prognostically important genes involved in angiogenesis, tumor response, and metastasis,[25] and can further be modulated by host factors (i.e., anemia, smoking history).

In the near future, a bioinformatics profile could include information from a DNA microarray and a sophisticated protein expression from a number of biopsies (to address intratumoral heterogeneity) to provide a molecular profile for each patient.[26,27] It is exciting that both the information and the technology are rapidly becoming available to develop molecular models of prognostication and lay the foundation for novel strategies of therapeutic intervention.

HOST-RELATED PROGNOSTIC FACTORS

Host- or patient-related prognostic factors are those factors present in the patient that are either indirectly or not related to malignancy, but through interference with the behavior of the tumor or their effect on treatment have a major impact on the outcome. These factors can generally be classified as demographic patient characteristics, comorbidity, and coexistent illness, especially those affecting the immune status, performance status related to comorbid illness, and factors that relate to the host mental state, attitude, and compliance with therapy (Table 6.2).

Demographics

Demographic factors shown to affect outcome in oncology include *age, gender,* and *ethnicity.* None of these factors can be influenced by treatment intervention, but many independently influence the outcome of other factors. Age has an

TABLE 6.2   Examples of Host-related Prognostic Factors

1. Demographics
   - Age
   - Race
   - Gender
   - Level of education
   - Socioeconomic status
   - Religion
2. Comorbidity
   - Constant
   - Inherited immune deficiency,
   - Von Recklinghausen disease
   - Changeable
   - Coexistent illness, for example, inflammatory bowel disease, collagen vascular disease
   - Weight
   - Cardiac status
   - Acquired immune deficiency
   - Infection
   - Mental health
3. Performance status
4. Compliance
   - Social reaction to illness
   - Influence of habits, drugs, alcohol, smoking
   - Belief in alternative therapies

impact on outcome. Older patients have poorer survival in Hodgkin's disease, lymphomas, glioblastoma, ovarian cancer, and many other tumors.[4,28–30] It is often unclear whether this difference in outcome is related to the biology of the disease, the ability to tolerate the optimal therapy, or difficulties in managing treatment complications and recurrence. Gender is less well defined as a prognostic factor, but the outcome in men has been reported to be inferior to that of women in Hodgkin's disease, malignant melanoma, and some other cancers.[28,31] In a large population-based study, the survival of women with cancer has been reported to be better than men in a large number of cancers.[32] Racial origin has been implicated in the outcome in prostate cancer, with African American patients having higher failure rates than the Caucasian patients following radical prostatectomy.[33] Race has also been shown to be an important factor in endometrial cancer, with worse survival in African American woman even when the outcomes were adjusted for stage and socioeconomic status.[34]

Comorbidity

Comorbid conditions may be inherited genetic diseases like neurofibromatosis, both a risk factor for neurogenic sarcoma and a prognostic factor for cancer outcome, von-Hippel Lindau disease, or the unfortunate occurrence of albinism in a "black" African. The latter, by rendering the individual entirely ill equipped for his or her environment, leads to the development of squamous carcinomas of the skin that present in advanced stage in this unfamiliar setting and beyond the ability to use curative surgery.[35] In addition, acquired states such as collagen vascular disease, infections, and diabetes are also important.[36] Comorbid conditions may reflect compromised cardiac, pulmonary, or renal function that by interference with therapy of cancer alters the outcomes.[13,37] The unique confounding interaction between histologic subtype and ethnic origin is prognostically important in carcinoma of the nasopharynx (see Chapter 13).

Immune Status

The host immune status is important since the outcomes of cancers in immuno-compromised patients are inferior to those observed in immunocompetent patients.[38] Examples of such situations include cancers in heart or kidney transplant patients, cancers in patients on long-term immunosuppressive therapy, and cancers in HIV infected patients.[39] The prognosis of patients with HIV-associated Kaposi sarcoma is dependent more on the status of the HIV infection than the extent of disease.

Mental State

A significant proportion of patients with cancer present late to the doctor because of widespread denial of illness or a diversity of beliefs and behavior.[40] Thus, the presence of depression or other mental illness may affect the outcome through delays in seeking medical attention and or lack of compliance with therapy. Depression was shown to be associated with a shorter survival in lung cancer patients.[41–43] Patients who present with late stages of cancer often have complicated medical and psychiatric problems labeled as "maladaptive delay or denial." In some, psychiatric problems may have either contributed to the delay in diagnosis or have interfered with treatment of the late-stage cancer. Multiple resources and multiple types of intervention are needed in order to help such patients negotiate the clinical environment.[44] This topic is discussed in greater detail elsewhere (see Chapter 8).

Prior Cancer and Treatment for Prior Cancer

A history of prior cancer and treatment of that cancer place survivors at risk for future events.[45–48] The prognostic impact of prior radiation exposure has been studied, but the management of second cancers has not been considered to the same extent.[49] This is discussed further in the chapter on soft tissue sarcomas, since these are the tumors most likely to occur following radiation exposure for a previous cancer (see Chapter 27). Cancer survivors face unique problems that are often related to treatment of their first cancer, and the prognostic factors related to the outcome following treatment for specific cancer need to be elucidated.[50–53]

The prognosis of metachronous cancers occurring in the same individual has been shown to be affected by the treatment of the first cancer.[54]

Performance Status

Performance status is a powerful prognostic factor in many cancers, especially those with advanced presentations that require treatment with chemotherapy, for example, lung cancer and bladder cancer.[55,56] Performance status may be due to the effect of the tumor on the patient: in that case, it should be considered a tumor-related prognostic factor. If due to advanced age, comorbidity from other illnesses or prior treatment, it should be considered a patient-related factor. The presence of renal disease, heart disease, or respiratory disease can compromise the outcome through interference with the physician's ability to perform surgery or to deliver full dose radiotherapy or chemotherapy.

Compliance

Compliance with a proposed screening or treatment plan can affect the survival of a patient or group of patients.[44,57,58] Unfortunately, patient compliance is not usually reported. In highly curable tumors such as germ-cell testicular cancers or Hodgkin's disease, a lack of compliance with recommended treatment might result in death of young people. Lack of compliance with screening recommendations in breast cancer may lead to delay in diagnosis, more advanced stage at diagnosis, and poorer survival. Limited available evidence documents the impact of patients' compliance on the outcomes in head and neck and endometrial cancer.[57,58]

ENVIRONMENT-RELATED PROGNOSTIC FACTORS

The impact of tumor-related prognostic factors such as histology and extent of disease has been widely acknowledged. The host-related factors have been less studied, but age, race, and performance status have been included in most discussions of the expected treatment outcomes. The environment-related factors, those that are external to the patient, have been less studied and frequently do not appear in the discussion of the expected outcomes. Numerous environmental factors affect the outcome for an individual or population of patients. To integrate the information from diverse sources we will consider factors that have a physician focus, a health care system focus, and a society focus. In each group, we consider factors that relate to treatment of cancer, to education, and to quality (Table 6.3).

Physician Focus

The choice of treatment modality, or more specifically, the treatment plan, has a profound impact on outcome. Inappropriate interventions can result in excessive

TABLE 6.3 Examples of Environment-related Prognostic Factors

	Related to		
	Treatment	Education	Quality
Physician	Choice of physician or specialty • Quality of diagnosis • Accuracy of staging Choice of treatment Expertise of physician: "narrow experts" Timeliness of treatment Ageism	Ignorance of medical profession Access to internet Knowledge, education of the patient Participation in clinical trials Participation in continuing education	Quality of treatment Skill of the physician Treatment verification
Health care system	Access to appropriate diagnostic methods Access to care • Distance • Waiting Lists • Monopoly control of access to care Availability of publicly funded screening programs	Continuing medical education Lack of audit of local results Access to internet Development of practice guidelines Dissemination of new knowledge	Quality of equipment Quality management in treatment facility Maintenance of health records Availability of universal health insurance Quality of diagnostic services Implementation of screening programs Promotion of error-free environment
Society focus	Preference for unconventional therapies Socioeconomic status Distance from cancer center Insurance status Access to transportation, car, etc. Ageism	Literacy Access to information	Access to affordable health insurance Nutritional status of the population

toxicity and compromised quality of life, at least, but failure to control cancer can also result in death. There are published data on the impact of physician's, or physicians', expertise and skill on outcomes in selected cancers. However, one can speculate that many other physician-dependent factors affect the manner in which cancer is diagnosed, staged, and treated. These factors may not involve the actual treatment, but relate to the education of physicians, access to current information, and quality of decision making and treatment delivery by physicians.

Expertise of Caregivers

The expertise of the treating physician is a prognostic factor, as it affects the outcome in cancer patients. There is increasing evidence that for many cancers, centers that do not treat a certain "critical mass" of patients may not achieve the optimal treatment outcome. This finding has occurred in several studies of advanced germ-cell testicular cancer in the United Kingdom and Europe; differences in outcome also have been observed when the outcomes in Surveillance, Epidemiology, and End Results (SEER) program data have been compared to the outcome achieved by the expert group at the Memorial Hospital.[59-62] There is much evidence that specialization in cancer care improves the outcomes.[63] Referral to a multidisciplinary team improved survival of patients with ovarian cancer in Scotland.[64] Gillis and Hole, in a study conducted in a geographically defined area, showed a 9% higher 5-year survival and 8% higher 10-year survival for patients with breast cancer cared for by a specialist surgeon rather than by nonspecialists.[65] There is conflicting evidence relating to the impact of the volume of physicians' work on the outcomes observed in their patients.[66,67]

Health Care System Focus

Ageism: Cancer in Old Age

Although more than a third of cancers are diagnosed in people over 75, this group is less extensively investigated and receives less treatment than younger patients.[68] The presence of ageism has also been a concern in screening programs for breast cancer.[69] Patients 75 years of age and older were less likely to have surgery or any other tumor-directed therapy in a population-based study of lung cancer.[70] These issues have been discussed in detail.[71] Other examples of discrimination against older patients includes the independent finding of less frequent use of breast conservation surgery in patients older than 70 years in a statewide population-based study. Also apparent were the absence of private insurance and care undertaken by older surgeons, both of which were independently significant.[72]

Racial Influences

Like older patients, African Americans seem not to gain the same access to treatment in comparison with other members of the U.S population.[73,74] Bach and colleagues noted that blacks are less likely to receive surgical treatment and have inferior survival compared to whites, in a population-based study of patients 65 years of age or older with resectable non-small-cell lung cancer (stage I or

II) between 1985 and 1993 in the SEER program (10,984 patients).[74] The rate of surgery was 12.7% lower for black compared to white patients, and the 5-year survival rate was lower for blacks (26.4% vs. 34.1% $p < 0.001$). Among the patients undergoing surgery, however, survival was similar for the two racial groups, as it was among those who did not undergo surgery.[74]

Access to Cancer Care

Remoteness from the Cancer Center
The issue of nonmedical factors affecting the choice of treatment has been recognized for many years. In their population-based study in two rural U.S. states, Greenberg and colleagues also noted that, in addition to the apparent discrimination against older patients, the treatment of patients varied according to their marital status, medical insurance coverage, and proximity to a cancer-treatment center. These discriminants were not based on apparent differences in tumor stage or functional status, although both these factors were also strongly predictive of the type of treatment.[70] A study of the rates of mastectomy versus breast conservation therapy and the use of radiotherapy and chemotherapy also showed that patients in districts far away from the cancer center were denied access to these treatments despite published guidelines showing them to be useful.[75] A study of the delivery of radiotherapy in Ontario, Canada, documented a lower use of radiotherapy in areas without easy access to a radiotherapy facility.[76]

Geographic Locations in Communities without Medical Resources
It is generally understood that medical care, as we understand it, involves attempts to uphold the highest standards for patients with cancer and other illnesses. Unfortunately, we cannot avoid the grim reality that much of the world's cancer burden exists in communities where medical resources are severely compromised. In these jurisdictions a complex situation exists whereby many prognostic factors conspire among each other to render a favorable prognosis unlikely. Thus combinations of factors such as poor understanding of the disease and its presenting symptoms, barely effective referral processes, inadequate communication, diagnostic and treatment resources, and associated comorbidities including other diseases and nutritional factors may all coexist.[77,78] These factors are mentioned in some of the chapters in Part B of the book. Examples include the late presentations of breast cancer,[79] Hodgkin's disease,[80] gastric cancer,[81] penile carcinoma,[82] head and neck cancers,[83,84] and skin cancers[35] in communities lacking resources to provide prompt care or jurisdictions that may serve populations that lack the opportunity or knowledge to achieve prompt diagnosis following the onset of initial symptoms.

Medical Records
The knowledge of prior medical interventions is crucial in providing high-quality care for cancer patients. The preservation of medical records of cancer patients is essential to the future of patients; for example, knowledge of the radiotherapy data

may have an impact on decision making years later. Missing data from medical records affects the quality of cancer registry data and potentially undermine interpretation of epidemiological studies and evaluation of care.[85,86] Currently, many records that may be essential in the future are being destroyed.[87,88]

Access to Internet

Improved public access to medical information already has an impact on cancer patients.[89] Many patients gather information about their recommended cancer treatments and expected outcomes, and question their physicians about them. This new self-advocacy is likely to improve the outcomes by empowering patients to become full partners in medical care.[90,91]

Participation in Clinical Trials

Patients who participate in clinical trials have been noted to have a better survival as compared to those treated outside a clinical trial.[92,93] Explanations suggested for these observations, at least in breast cancer, include observations that patients treated on clinical trials are more likely to receive standard-dose chemotherapy than other patients treated in the clinic, even when analysis has controlled for patient age and stage of disease.[94] Patients on trials are also more likely to receive better general support compared to other patients.[95]

Society Focus

Socioeconomic Status

Patients who are less wealthy are likely to be treated differently in health care systems that do not permit equal access to care.[96] In addition, although the reasons for this are likely multifactorial, cancer survival is linked to socioeconomic status, as demonstrated in studies of the socioeconomic determinants of health.[97-99] The report produced by the Office of National Statistics, the Cancer Research Campaign, and the London School of Hygiene and Tropical Medicine, suggested that over 12,700 deaths from cancer in the UK could be avoided every year if all patients shared the survival rates of the most affluent patients. A study of 3 million adults and 18,000 children with cancer showed that the most affluent patients were 5–16% more likely to be alive after 5 years than the most deprived patients. Interestingly, the effect of wealth was seen in survivors of adult cancers only; no effect was seen in childhood cancer patients.[100,101]

Mackillop and colleagues found that even in the Canadian health care system, which is designed to provide an equitable access to equivalent standards of care, community income was a significant factor for survival in all common cancers.[1] These authors detected differences in the association of socioeconomic status and cancer survival large enough to be medically and socially significant. For example, the difference in the 5-year survival between the top and bottom socioeconomic groups in cancer of the uterine cervix is almost as great as the difference between patients presenting with Stage I and Stage II disease. In breast cancer, the difference between the top and bottom survival curves for socioeconomic status is greater than the difference conferred by any available form of systemic adjuvant treatment in that disease. The prognosis of cutaneous melanoma has been found to be better for affluent people compared to less affluent individuals.[102] A study of possible socioeconomic and regional variation in the survival of children with acute lymphoblastic leukemia in England and Wales found little evidence of socioeconomic gradient in survival, but regional differences in survival were observed.[103] Review of cancer patient survival for six common cancer sites in The Netherlands showed that patients with a higher socioeconomic status had a better survival.[104] The reasons for these findings are uncertain and open to much unresolved speculation. In particular, physician influence may override the issues of patients' socioeconomic status in providing optimal treatment, as shown in a study of breast cancer therapy in three affiliated centers staffed by similarly trained surgeons, yet serving widely disparate populations.[105] Similarly, in a milieu of equal access to treatment, apparent decreased rates of breast conservation surgery were not explained by racial or socioeconomic factors, but were related instead to presentation with more advanced disease among African-American women.[106]

Nutrition

Evidence from patients with head and neck cancer, lymphoma, and leukemia suggests that the presence of poor nutrition is associated with adverse prognosis.[107–109] However, the assessment of the independent value of nutritional distortion can be difficult to evaluate. Thus, it is no surprise that the patient suffering from the cachexia of malignancy will be nutritionally compromised, but in this case, the tumor is more likely to have caused it rather than the patient's environment. In addition, distorted nutrition may not necessarily imply weight loss or starvation, let alone cachexia. A contrast is provided by the situation in breast cancer where obesity may be a risk factor for adverse prognosis. Relative weight was significantly associated with increasing risk of dying by 12% per kg/m^2. Other nutritional findings were also associated with increased risk of recurrence. These risks included such factors as baseline consumption of butter, margarine, lard, and beer.[110] The association of nutritional changes and outcome of breast cancer appears complex, however, and not consistent.[111] Other examples can be found in most cancer sites. For example, in prostate cancer, a bicity cohort study observed a consistent and significant inverse association between the premorbid intake of monounsaturated fat and risk of death. On the other hand, the authors acknowledge that inconsistent results for energy intake between both cities could potentially be attributed to nonrespondent bias.[112] In pediatric malignancy, conflicting views about the adverse prognosis of malnutrition are confounded by the adverse influence of socioeconomic circumstances. Studies conducted mainly in developing countries have shown malnutrition to be an important prognostic factor in such children. However, other socioeconomic conditions could affect the outcome of therapy in patients with malignancies such as acute lymphatic leukemia (ALL): these include access to communication, transportation, laboratory studies, and therapy.[113] Alternative evidence suggests that nutritional status at diagnosis, defined on the basis of the body-mass index, appears to have no effect on the prognosis in ALL. Therefore, at least in developed countries, it should not be considered an independent prognostic factor.[114] In lung cancer, both anthropometric (e.g., weight/height ratio) and biochemical nutritional parameters seem to be reliable indicators for the assessment of performance status and survival.[115] In addition, cytokine levels (IL-6 and IFN-gamma) have been suggested to be associated with compromised nutritional status and are prognostic for worse outcome in lung cancer.[116]

Education

Education, whether involving physicians, patients, or society at large, has a profound impact on the outcome in cancer patients. While it is obvious that physician education may affect treatment selection, it may be less apparent how it affects the outcome in cancer through its impact on patients, society, and health care system. Patient education may be of equal importance. Less educated patients are less likely to seek medical opinion, become informed, or participate, when invited, in prevention, screening, and early detection programs.[117] They are less likely to have access to the Internet, a powerful source of information about cancer treatment. Patients with poor education are less likely to question their physicians and the health care system.[118] Extremes exist, of course, although these may not be considered a concern in the developed world. Nevertheless, a recent study in Africa indicated that one of the greatest barriers to early referral in breast cancer was the fear of mastectomy. This unusual study of more than 2000 women revealed that delay in seeking medical attention was also associated with preferences for spiritual treatments (13.5%), denial (8.5%), preference for native doctors or herbalists (23.1%), and economic reasons (10.2%).[119] Many of these patients also presented with advanced-stage disease. Similar levels of ignorance were documented in relation to knowledge of carcinoma of the uterine cervix evident among women attending a general hospital clinic in Nigeria.[120] In fact, only 15% of these women had ever heard of cervical cancer.[120]

In health care systems in the developed world, continuing education results in optimization of treatment efforts. The development and dissemination of evidence-based practice guidelines leads to best practice patterns.[121–123] Support and value of continuing education by the health care system leads to improved quality and access to care.

Dissemination of New Knowledge

There is an unacceptable lag time between new evidence becoming available to practitioners and its implementation in daily medical practice. Development and effective dissemination of current evidence-based practice guidelines should decrease this delay and result in improved outcomes for patients with cancer.[90,124] Activities such as multidisciplinary tumor conferences, continuing medical education events, accreditation, and recertification also contribute to dissemination of information and its implementation into clinical practice.

Quality of Care

Quality of Treatment

Quality of treatment is under the direct control of treating physician, but factors such as the presence of local real time audit of treatment plans, tumor boards to validate staging and treatment decisions, and the completeness and accuracy of health records all contribute to outcomes.[125,126] The constraints on access to care in some health care systems may indirectly have a negative impact on the quality of care provided by individual physicians.

Quality Improvement Program and Reduction of Error in Medicine

Similar to industry, in medicine the presence of national and institutional quality-improvement initiatives is likely to lead to better results and increased patient satisfaction.[127–130]

Human errors in medicine are common and are responsible for a substantial morbidity and mortality associated with medical care.[131–134] In oncology, the errors may involve the diagnosis or the treatment of cancer.[133–135] The introduction of audit and the use of new technology-based applications to support human ability are aimed at lowering the error rates.[125,136] So far in medicine we lag substantially behind progress demonstrated in the aviation and other high-risk industries where fatality rates have become vanishingly small.[131] While the two are not equivalent, since the medical "industry" is dealing with an adverse subject population, they are also not comparable from the standpoint of preparedness. What is needed is proper design of equipment, support systems, safe job environment, controlled working hours, and organizational structure. One is left to conclude that the social structures in many counties seem less obsessed with safety in health care compared to industry standards. At the root of this is likely an issue of expectation on the part of society to severe illnesses, coupled with the imposition of standards of resource allocation by policymakers that must compromise between the availability of resources and the comprehensiveness of programs.

SUMMARY

Numerous prognostic factors affect the outcomes in cancer. The preceding scheme for classification of prognostic factors into tumor-, host-, and environment-related factors is helpful in illustrating the scope of prognostic factors and bringing attention to the factors rarely considered in cancer patients. With continuous improvements in cancer diagnosis and treatment, environment-related factors would become more important. Even now, the attempts to compare treatment results in diverse patient groups are hampered by the lack of data on the environment-related factors.[137–139] A broader understanding of cancer biology may revolutionize the approach to cancer prevention, diagnosis, and treatment. Until this progress is translated into clinical benefit, however, attention to the quality of cancer diagnosis and treatment is needed to optimize what is currently achievable.

REFERENCES

1. Mackillop WJ, Zhang-Salomons J, Groome PA, et al.: Socioeconomic status and cancer survival in Ontario. *J Clin Oncol* 15:1680–9, 1997.

2. Fielding LP, Pettigrew N: College of American Pathologists conference XXVI on clinical relevance of prognostic markers in solid tumors. Report of the Colorectal Cancer Working Group. *Arch Pathol Lab Med* 119:1115–21, 1995.

3. Gelb AB: Renal cell carcinoma: current prognostic factors. Union Internationale Contre le Cancer (UICC) and the American Joint Committee on Cancer (AJCC). *Cancer* 80:981–6, 1997.

4. Friedlander ML: Prognostic factors in ovarian cancer. *Semin Oncol* 25:305–14, 1998.

5. Sobin LH, Fleming ID: *TNM classification of malignant tumors*, 5th ed. (1997). Union Internationale Contre le Cancer and the American Joint Committee on Cancer. *Cancer* 80:1803–4, 1997.

6. Gospodarowicz M, Benedet L, Hutter R, et al.: History and international developments in cancer staging. *Cancer Prev. Control* 2:262–8, 1998.

7. Dubben HH, Thames HD, Beck-Bornholdt HP: Tumor volume: a basic and specific response predictor in radiotherapy. *Radiother Oncol* 47:167–74, 1998.

8. Millan-Rodriguez F, Chechile-Toniolo G, Salvador-Bayarri J, et al.: Multivariate analysis of the prognostic factors of primary superficial bladder cancer. *J Urol* 163:73–8, 2000.

9. Sabbatini P, Larson SM, Kremer A, et al.: Prognostic significance of extent of disease in bone in patients with androgen-independent prostate cancer. *J Clin Oncol* 17:948–57, 1999.

10. Feinstein AR, Wells CK: A clinical severity staging system for patients with lung cancer. *Medicine* 69:1–33, 1990.

11. Feldman JG, Saunders M, Carter AC, et al.: The effects of patient delay and symptoms other than a lump on survival in breast cancer. *Cancer* 51:1226–9, 1983.

12. Piccirillo JF, Feinstein AR: Clinical symptoms and comorbidity: significance for the prognostic classification of cancer. *Cancer* 77:834–42, 1996.

13. Pugliano FA, Piccirillo JF, Zequeira MR, et al.: Clinical-severity staging system for oral cavity cancer: five-year survival rates. *Otolaryngol Head Neck Surg* 120:38–45, 1999.

14. Wu J, Shen ZZ, Lu JS, et al.: Prognostic role of p27Kip1 and apoptosis in human breast cancer. *Br J Cancer* 79:1572–8, 1999.

15. Lal A, Lash AE, Altschul SF, et al.: A public database for gene expression in human cancers. *Cancer Res* 59:5403–7, 1999.

16. Braun S, Pantel K: Micrometastatic bone marrow involvement: detection and prognostic significance. *Med Oncol* 16:154–65, 1999.

17. Lambrechts AC, van't Veer LJ, Rodenhuis S: The detection of minimal numbers of contaminating epithelial tumor cells in blood or bone marrow: use, limitations and future of RNA-based methods. *Ann Oncol* 9:1269–76, 1998.

18. Pantel K, Cote RJ, Fodstad O: Detection and clinical importance of micrometastatic disease. *J Natl Cancer Inst* 91:1113–24, 1999.

19. Harding MA, Theodorescu D: Prognostic markers in localized prostate cancer: from microscopes to molecules. *Cancer Metastasis Rev* 17:429–37, 1998.

20. Kinzler KW, Vogelstein B: Lessons from hereditary colorectal cancer. *Cell* 87:159–70, 1996.

21. Bristow RG, Benchimol S, Hill RP: The p53 gene as a modifier of intrinsic radiosensitivity: implications for radiotherapy. *Radiother Oncol* 40:197–223, 1996.

22. Harris EE, Kao GD, Muschel RJ, et al.: Potential applications of cell cycle manipulation to clinical response. *Cancer Treat Res* 93:169–90, 1998.

23. Kastan MB: Molecular determinants of sensitivity to antitumor agents. *Biochim Biophys Acta* 1424:R37–42, 1999.

24. Bussemakers MJ: Changes in gene expression and targets for therapy. *Eur Urol* 35:408–12, 1999.

25. Dachs GU, Chaplin DJ: Microenvironmental control of gene expression: implications for tumor angiogenesis, progression, and metastasis. *Semin Radiat Oncol* 8:208–16, 1998.

26. Friend SH: How DNA microarrays and expression profiling will affect clinical practice. *BMJ* 319:1306, 1999.

27. Merlino G, Helman LJ: Rhabdomyosarcoma — working out the pathways. *Oncogene* 18:5340–8, 1999.

28. Hasenclever D, Diehl V: A prognostic score for advanced Hodgkin's disease. International Prognostic Factors Project on Advanced Hodgkin's Disease. *N Engl J Med* 339:1506–14, 1998.

29. A predictive model for aggressive non-Hodgkin's lymphoma. The International Non-Hodgkin's Lymphoma Prognostic Factors Project. *N Engl J Med* 329:987–94, 1993.

30. Burger PC, Green SB: Patient age, histologic features, and length of survival in patients with glioblastoma multiforme. *Cancer* 59:1617–25, 1987.

31. Chang AE, Karnell LH, Menck HR: The National Cancer Data Base report on cutaneous and noncutaneous melanoma: a summary of 84,836 cases from the past decade. The American College of Surgeons Commission on Cancer and the American Cancer Society. *Cancer* 83:1664–78, 1998.

32. Micheli A, Mariotto A, Rossi AG, et al.: The prognostic role of gender in survival of adult cancer patients. EUROCARE Working Group. *Eur J Cancer* 34:2271–8, 1998.

33. Moul JW, Douglas TH, McCarthy WF, et al.: Black race is an adverse prognostic factor for prostate cancer recurrence following radical prostatectomy in an equal access health care setting. *J Urol* 155:1667–73, 1996.

34. Connell PP, Rotmensch J, Waggoner SE, et al.: Race and clinical outcome in endometrial carcinoma. *Obstet Gynecol* 94:713–20, 1999.

35. Yakubu A, Mabogunje O: Skin cancer of the head and neck in Zaria, Nigeria. *Acta Oncol* 34:469–71, 1995.

36. Neumann HP, Bender BU, Berger DP, et al.: Prevalence, morphology and biology of renal cell carcinoma in von Hippel-Lindau disease compared to sporadic renal cell carcinoma. *J Urol* 160:1248–54, 1998.

37. Peipert JF, Wells CK, Schwartz PE, et al.: Prognostic value of clinical variables in invasive cervical cancer. *Obstet Gynecol* 84:746–51, 1994.

38. DeMario MD, Liebowitz DN: Lymphomas in the immunocompromised patient. *Semin Oncol* 25:492–502, 1998.

39. Pham SM, Kormos RL, Landreneau RJ, et al.: Solid tumors after heart transplantation: lethality of lung cancer. *Ann Thorac Surg* 60:1623–6, 1995.

40. Phelan M, Dobbs J, David AS: 'I thought it would go away': patient denial in breast cancer. *J R Soc Med* 85:206–7, 1992.

41. Spiegel D: Cancer and depression. *Br J Psychiatry Suppl* 109–16, 1996.

42. Buccheri G: Depressive reactions to lung cancer are common and often followed by a poor outcome. *Eur Respir J* 11:173–8, 1998.

43. Faller H, Bulzebruck H, Drings P, et al.: Coping, distress, and survival among patients with lung cancer. *Arch Gen Psychiatry* 56:756–62, 1999.

44. Kunkel EJ, Woods CM, Rodgers C, et al.: Consultations for 'maladaptive denial of illness' in patients with cancer: psychiatric disorders that result in noncompliance. *Psychooncology* 6:139–49, 1997.

45. Van Leeuwen FE, Stiggelbout AM, van den Belt-Dusebout AW, et al.: Second cancer risk following testicular cancer: a follow-up study of 1,909 patients. *J Clin Oncol* 11:415–24, 1993.

46. Travis LB, Curtis RE, Glimelius B, et al.: Second cancers among long-term survivors of non-Hodgkin's lymphoma. *J Natl Cancer Inst* 85:1932–7, 1993.

47. Hoppe RT: Hodgkin's disease: complications of therapy and excess mortality. *Ann Oncol* 8(Suppl 1):115–8, 1997.

48. Eng C, Li FP, Abramson DH, et al.: Mortality from second tumors among long-term survivors of retinoblastoma. *J Natl Cancer Inst* 85:1121–8, 1993.

49. Wolden SL, Hancock SL, Carlson RW, et al.: Management of breast cancer after hodgkin's disease. *J Clin Oncol* 18:765, 2000.

50. Bower JE, Ganz PA, Desmond KA, et al.: Fatigue in breast cancer survivors: occurrence, correlates, and impact on quality of life. *J Clin Oncol* 18:743, 2000.

51. Crom DB, Chathaway DK, Tolley EA, et al.: Health status and health-related quality of life in long-term adult survivors of pediatric solid tumors. *Int J Cancer Suppl* 83:25–31, 1999.

52. Hancock SL, Hoppe RT, Horning SJ, et al.: Intercurrent death after Hodgkin disease therapy in radiotherapy and adjuvant MOPP trials [published erratum appears in *Ann Intern Med* 114(9):810, 1991]. *Ann Intern Med* 109:183–9, 1988.

53. Loge JH, Abrahamsen AF, Ekeberg, et al.: Fatigue and psychiatric morbidity among hodgkin's disease survivors. *J Pain Symptom Manage* 19:91–99, 2000.

54. Dolan R, Vaughan C, Fuleihan N: Metachronous cancer: prognostic factors including prior irradiation. *Otolaryngol Head Neck Surg* 119:619–23, 1998.

55. Kappen HJ, Neijt JP: Advanced ovarian cancer. neural network analysis to predict treatment outcome. *Ann Oncol* 4(Suppl 4):31–4, 1993.

56. Turesson I, Abildgaard N, Ahlgren T, et al.: Prognostic evaluation in multiple myeloma: an analysis of the impact of new prognostic factors. *Br J Haematol* 106:1005–12, 1999.

57. Cathcart CS, Dunican A, Halpern JN: Patterns of delivery of radiation therapy in an inner-city population of head and neck cancer patients: an analysis of compliance and end results. *J Med* 28:275–84, 1997.

58. Obermair A, Hanzal E, Schreiner-Frech I, et al.: Influence of delayed diagnosis on established prognostic factors in endometrial cancer. *Anticancer Res* 16:947–9, 1996.

59. Collette L, Sylvester RJ, Stenning SP, et al.: Impact of the treating institution on survival of patients with "poor-prognosis" metastatic nonseminoma. European Organization for Research and Treatment of Cancer Genito-Urinary Tract Cancer Collaborative Group and the Medical Research Council Testicular Cancer Working Party. *J Natl Cancer Inst* 91:839–46, 1999.

60. Feuer EJ, Sheinfeld J, Bosl GJ: Does size matter? Association between number of patients treated and patient outcome in metastatic testicular cancer. *J Natl Cancer Inst* 91:816–8, 1999.

61. Harding MJ, Paul J, Gillis CR, et al.: Management of malignant teratoma: does referral to a specialist unit matter?. *Lancet* 341:999–1002, 1993.

62. Aass N, Klepp O, Cavallin-Stahl E, et al.: Prognostic factors in unselected patients with nonseminomatous metastatic testicular cancer: a multicenter experience. *J Clin Oncol* 9:818–26, 1991.

63. Selby P, Gillis C, Haward R: Benefits from specialised cancer care. *Lancet* 348:313–8, 1996.

64. Junor EJ, Hole DJ, Gillis CR: Management of ovarian cancer: referral to a multi-disciplinary team matters. *Br J Cancer* 70:363–70, 1994.

65. Gillis CR, Hole DJ: Survival outcome of care by specialist surgeons in breast cancer: a study of 3786 patients in the west of Scotland. *BMJ* 312:145–8, 1996.

66. Parry JM, Collins S, Mathers J, et al.: Influence of volume of work on the outcome of treatment for patients with colorectal cancer. *Br J Surg* 86:475–81, 1999.

67. Sainsbury R, Haward B, Rider L, et al.: Influence of clinician workload and patterns of treatment on survival from breast cancer. *Lancet* 345:1265–70, 1995.

68. Siu LL, Shepherd FA, Murray N, et al.: Influence of age on the treatment of limited-stage small-cell lung cancer. *J Clin Oncol* 14:821–8, 1996.

69. Sutton GC: Will you still need me, will you still screen me, when I'm past 64? *BMJ* 315:1032–3, 1997.

70. Greenberg ER, Chute CG, Stukel T, et al.: Social and economic factors in the choice of lung cancer treatment. A population-based study in two rural states. *N Engl J Med* 318:612–7, 1988.

71. Mayer RJ, Patterson WB: How is cancer treatment chosen? *N Engl J Med* 318:636–8, 1988.

72. Kotwall CA, Covington DL, Rutledge R, et al.: Patient, hospital, and surgeon factors associated with breast conservation surgery. A statewide analysis in North Carolina. *Ann Surg* 224:419–26; discussion 426–9, 1996.

73. King TE, Jr., Brunetta P: Racial disparity in rates of surgery for lung cancer. *N Engl J Med* 341:1231–3, 1999.

74. Bach PB, Cramer LD, Warren JL, et al.: Racial differences in the treatment of early-stage lung cancer. *N Engl J Med* 341:1198–205, 1999.

75. Sainsbury R, Rider L, Smith A, et al.: Does it matter where you live? Treatment variation for breast cancer in Yorkshire. The Yorkshire Breast Cancer Group. *Br J Cancer* 71:1275–8, 1995.

76. Mackillop WJ, Groome PA, Zhang-Solomons J, et al.: Does a centralized radiotherapy system provide adequate access to care? *J Clin Oncol* 15:1261–71, 1997.

77. Ameh EA, Sabo SY, Muhammad I: Late presentation of cancers in Zaria: an intractable problem. *Trop Doct* 28:166–8, 1998.

78. Martin WM: Radiotherapy and oncology in Papua New Guinea—how it differs from Western practice. *Australas Radiol* 34:238–40, 1990.

79. Anim JT: Breast cancer in sub-Saharan African women. *Afr J Med Sci* 22:5–10, 1993.

80. AbuElHassan MS, Ahmed ME, A/Gadir AF, et al.: Differences in presentation of Hodgkin's disease in Sudan and Western countries. *Trop Geogr Med* 45:28–9, 1993.

81. Koong HN, Chan HS, Nambiar R, et al.: Gastric cancers in Singapore: poor prognosis arising from late presentation. *Aust N Z J Surg* 66:813–5, 1996.

82. Nath S, Desai G, Munkonge L: Carcinoma of penis in Zambia: associated problems in management. *Cent Afr J Med* 38:108–11, 1992.

83. Oji C: Late presentation of orofacial tumours. *J Craniomaxillofac Surg* 27:94–9, 1999.

84. Sani A, Said H, Lokman S: Carcinoma of the larynx in Malaysia. *Med J Malaysia* 47:297–302, 1992.

85. Vickers N, Pollock A: Incompleteness and retrieval of case notes in a case note audit of colorectal cancer. *Qual Health Care* 2:170–4, 1993.

86. Smith SJ, Muir KR, Wolstenholme JL, et al.: Continued inadequacies in data sources for the evaluation of cancer services. *Br J Cancer* 75:131–3, 1997.

87. Hawkins MM, Craft AW: Retaining personal medical records of children who have had chemotherapy and radiotherapy. *BMJ* 308:1654–5, 1994.

88. Melton LJ, III: The threat to medical-records research. *N Engl J Med* 337:1466–70, 1997.

89. Pergament D, Pergament E, Wonderlick A, et al.: At the crossroads: the intersection of the Internet and clinical oncology. Oncology (Huntingt on) 13:577–83; discussion 583–6, 1999.

90. Haynes RB: Using informatics principles and tools to harness research evidence for patient care: evidence-based informatics. MEDINFO 9(Pt 1):33–6, 1998.

91. Jadad AR: Promoting partnerships: challenges for the internet age. *BMJ* 319:761–4, 1999.

92. Stiller CA: Centralised treatment, entry to trials and survival. *Br J Cancer* 70:352–62, 1994.

93. Karjalainen S, Palva I: Do treatment protocols improve end results? A study of survival of patients with multiple myeloma in Finland. *BMJ* 299:1069–72, 1989.

94. Weijer C, Freedman B, Fuks A, et al.: What difference does it make to be treated in a clinical trial? A pilot study. *Clin Invest Med* 19:179–83, 1996.

95. Skrutkowska M, Weijer C: Do patients with breast cancer participating in clinical trials receive better nursing care? *Oncol Nurs Forum* 24:1411–6, 1997.

96. Dolan JT, Granchi TS, Miller CC, III, et al.: Low use of breast conservation surgery in medically indigent populations. *Am J Surg* 178:470–4, 1999.

97. Kogevinas M, Porta M: Socioeconomic differences in cancer survival: a review of the evidence. *IARC Sci Publ*: 177–206, 1997.

98. Lamont DW, Symonds RP, Brodie MM, et al.: Age, socio-economic status and survival from cancer of cervix in the West of Scotland 1980–87. *Br J Cancer* 67:351–7, 1993.

99. Dickman PW, Auvinen A, Voutilainen ET, et al.: Measuring social class differences in cancer patient survival: is it necessary to control for social class differences in general population mortality? A Finnish population-based study. *J Epidemiol Community Health* 52:727–34, 1998.

100. Cancer Survival Trends in England and Wales, 1971–1995: Deprivation and NHS Region. London, The Stationery Office Publications Centre, 1999.

101. Anderson P: Study demonstrates link between cancer survival and wealth. *BMJ* 318:1163, 1999.

102. MacKie RM, Hole DJ: Incidence and thickness of primary tumours and survival of patients with cutaneous malignant melanoma in relation to socioeconomic status. *BMJ* 312:1125–8, 1996.

103. Schillinger JA, Grosclaude PC, Honjo S, et al.: Survival after acute lymphocytic leukaemia: effects of socioeconomic status and geographic region. *Arch Dis Child* 80:311–7, 1999.

104. Schrijvers CT, Mackenbach JP: Cancer patient survival by socioeconomic status in seven countries: a review for six common cancer sites [corrected] [published erratum appears in *J Epidemiol Community Health* 48(6):554, 1994]. *J Epidemiol Community Health* 48:441–6, 1994.

105. Heimbach JK, Biffl WL, Mitchell EL, et al.: Breast conservation therapy in affiliated county, university, and private hospitals. *Am J Surg* 178:466–9, 1999.

106. Velanovich V, Yood MU, Bawle U, et al.: Racial differences in the presentation and surgical management of breast cancer. *Surgery* 125:375–9, 1999.

107. Aviles A, Yanez J, Lopez T, et al.: Malnutrition as an adverse prognostic factor in patients with diffuse large cell lymphoma. *Arch Med Res* 26:31–4, 1995.

108. Van Bokhorst-de van der S, van Leeuwen PA, Kuik DJ, et al.: The impact of nutritional status on the prognoses of patients with advanced head and neck cancer. *Cancer* 86:519–27, 1999.

109. Brookes GB: Nutritional status — a prognostic indicator in head and neck cancer. *Otolaryngol Head Neck Surg* 93:69–74, 1985.

110. Hebert JR, Hurley TG, Ma Y: The effect of dietary exposures on recurrence and mortality in early stage breast cancer. *Breast Cancer Res Treat* 51:17–28, 1998.

111. Jain M, Miller AB: Tumor characteristics and survival of breast cancer patients in relation to premorbid diet and body size. *Breast Cancer Res Treat* 42:43–55, 1997.

112. Kim DJ, Gallagher RP, Hislop TG, et al.: Premorbid diet in relation to survival from prostate cancer (Canada). *Cancer Causes Control* 11:65–77, 2000.

113. Gomez-Almaguer D, Ruiz-Arguelles GJ, Ponce-de-Leon S: Nutritional status and socio-economic conditions as prognostic factors in the outcome of therapy in childhood acute lymphoblastic leukemia. *Int J Cancer Suppl* 11:52–5, 1998.

114. Weir J, Reilly JJ, McColl JH, et al.: No evidence for an effect of nutritional status at diagnosis on prognosis in children with acute lymphoblastic leukemia. *J Pediatr Hematol Oncol* 20:534–8, 1998.

115. Lai SL, Perng RP: Impact of nutritional status on the survival of lung cancer patients. *Chung Hua I Hsueh Tsa Chih (Taipei)* 61:134–40, 1998.

116. Martin F, Santolaria F, Batista N, et al.: Cytokine levels (IL-6 and IFN-gamma), acute phase response and nutritional status as prognostic factors in lung cancer. *Cytokine* 11:80–6, 1999.

117. Mazur DJ, Hickam DH: Five-year survival curves: how much data are enough for patient-physician decision making in general surgery? *Eur J Surg* 162:101–4, 1996.

118. Rubenstein L: Targeting health advocacy efforts toward the older population. *Cancer* 68:2519–24, 1991.

119. Ajekigbe AT: Fear of mastectomy: the most common factor responsible for late presentation of carcinoma of the breast in Nigeria. *Clin Oncol (R Coll Radiol)* 3:78–80, 1991.

120. Ajayi IO, Adewole IF: Knowledge and attitude of general outpatient attendants in Nigeria to cervical cancer. *Cent Afr J Med* 44:41–3, 1998.

121. Grol R, Zwaard A, Mokkink H, et al.: Dissemination of guidelines: which sources do physicians use in order to be informed? *Int J Qual Health Care* 10:135–40, 1998.

122. Browman GP: Evidence-based paradigms and opinions in clinical management and cancer research. *Semin Oncol* 26:9–13, 1999.

123. Woolf SH, Grol R, Hutchinson A, et al.: Clinical guidelines: potential benefits, limitations, and harms of clinical guidelines. *BMJ* 318:527–30, 1999.

124. Sackett DL, Rosenberg WM: The need for evidence-based medicine. *J R Soc Med* 88:620–4, 1995.

125. Brundage MD, Dixon PF, Mackillop WJ, et al.: A real-time audit of radiation therapy in a regional cancer center. *Int J Radiat Oncol Biol Phys* 43:115–24, 1999.

126. Vanderpump MP, Alexander L, Scarpello JH, et al.: An audit of the management of thyroid cancer in a district general hospital. *Clin Endocrinol (Oxford)* 48:419–24, 1998.

127. Johnston PG, Daly PA, Liu E: The NCI All Ireland Cancer Conference. *Oncologist* 4:275–277, 1999.

128. Hermens RP, Hak E, Hulscher ME, et al.: Improving population-based cervical cancer screening in general practice: effects of a national strategy. *Int J Qual Health Care* 11:193–200, 1999.

129. McGivney WT, Barker ML, Bost JE, et al.: Panel discussion. Data needs in cancer. *Oncology (Huntingt)* 12:147–56, 1998.

130. Frolich A, Bernstein K, Vingtoft S, et al.: Quality development based on informatics in health care: steps in the Danish national strategy illustrated by four cases. MEDINFO 8(Pt 2):1632, 1995.

131. Berwick DM, Leape LL: Reducing errors in medicine. *BMJ* 319:136–7, 1999.

132. Fiorino C, Reni M, Bolognesi A, et al.: Set-up error in supine-positioned patients immobilized with two different modalities during conformal radiotherapy of prostate cancer. *Radiother Oncol* 49:133–41, 1998.

133. Ash D, Bates T: Report on the clinical effects of inadvertent radiation underdosage in 1045 patients. *Clin Oncol (R Coll Radiol)* 6:214–26, 1994.

134. Quekel LG, Kessels AG, Goei R, et al.: Miss rate of lung cancer on the chest radiograph in clinical practice. *Chest* 115:720–4, 1999.

135. Lee AH, Mead GM, Theaker JM: The value of central histopathological review of testicular tumours before treatment. *BJU Int* 84:75–8, 1999.

136. Bates DW, Teich JM, Lee J, et al.: The impact of computerized physician order entry on medication error prevention. *J Am Med Inform Assoc* 6:313–21, 1999.

137. Berrino F, Gatta G, Chessa E, et al.: Introduction: the EUROCARE II Study. *Eur J Cancer* 34:2139–53, 1998.

138. Berrino F, Micheli A, Sant M, et al.: Interpreting survival differences and trends. *Tumori* 83:9–16, 1997.

139. Survival of Cancer Patients in Europe: The EUROCARE-2 study. *IARC Sci Publ*: 1–572, 1999.

CHAPTER 7

Prognostic Factors in Cancer Patient Care

MARY K. GOSPODAROWICZ and BRIAN O'SULLIVAN

The activities of clinical practice of medicine include the processes of diagnosis, treatment, and follow-up care.[1] Interspersed throughout is the fundamental activity of prognostication. Whatever the situation, physicians are asked daily about the foreseeable outcome of the disease, expected results of treatment, and possible complications. The care of patients with cancer involves a series of steps, starting with the initial assessment, leading to the diagnosis, treatment, and assessment of outcomes. In each of these steps, and in all forms of physician–patient interaction, the ability to communicate the prognosis or to predict the probable outcome is critical.

The modern approach to patient management endorses clinical practice based on scientific evidence from experiments or observations. To facilitate consistent management, and to facilitate audit; evidence- or consensus-based clinical practice guidelines are developed for patient groupings based according to defined and reproducible characteristics and reliable predictions of different outcomes.[2,3] The necessity of grouping patients with similar characteristics to guide treatment and to anticipate the outcome has been recognized as far back as the seventeenth century.[4] The development of a prognostic classification for infections was followed by classifications for other diseases. In cancer, a formal staging classification (the TNM system) has been in use for over 50 years.[5] Cancer presents a formidable challenge for classification because it comprises a very heterogeneous group of diseases. The fundamental elements required to characterize each cancer are the organ of origin, the histologic type, and in addition numerous prognostic factors that characterize the tumor, the patient, and the environment surrounding the patient (see Chapters 2 and 6). Knowledge of prognostic factors is essential to all aspects of cancer care. Beginning with the diagnosis, and extending through the process of treatment planning, outcome

Prognostic Factors in Cancer, 2nd edition, Edited by Mary K. Gospodarowicz.
ISBN 0-471-40633-3 Copyright © 2001 Wiley-Liss, Inc.

assessment, and planning of support measures, it is essential to be familiar with issues that concern prognosis. Moreover, the knowledge, familiarity, and comprehension of this information are necessary to communicate with patients and their caregivers. Well-informed patients are better equipped to face the future and become partners in our efforts to improve outcomes through the generation of new knowledge through participation in clinical research in an informed manner.

In the process of diagnosis, the knowledge of factors that discriminate for more advanced disease presentations helps to reduce the need for unnecessary tests, while knowledge of the likely failure pattern leads to site-specific tests to rule out metastasis. For example, a low prostatic-specific antigen (PSA) level predicts for the presence of localized prostate cancer and obviates the need for extensive staging investigations.[6] In the process of understanding prognosis, a compilation of prognostic factors is analyzed to predict the future outcome. The international consensus on prognostic factor classifications in non-Hodgkin's lymphoma and germ-cell testis tumors are examples of wide use of multiple prognostic factors in the decision making and outcome assessment of these tumors.[7,8]

PROCESS OF CLINICAL DECISION MAKING

Knowledge of prognostic factors is essential for a number of steps in the decision-making process and in the comprehensive management of patients with cancer. In approaching the patient with cancer, physicians must make an assessment that would permit the generation of a therapeutic plan. To conduct an appropriate assessment, the physician must consider all relevant prognostic factors, and understand the milieu around the patient.

Determining the Goals of Treatment

The first step in the decision-making process involves judgment regarding the predominant goal of management. For example, current evidence suggests that all patients diagnosed with Hodgkin's disease should be considered candidates for curative therapy.[9] In contrast, in elderly patients with glioblastoma, with poor performance status and comorbidity, the goal of treatment should generally be palliation and supportive care.[10] Therefore, the goals of treatment may range from cure of cancer and long-term disease control to symptom control or palliation. A determination of detailed cancer pathology, extent of disease, and relevant host-related prognostic factors is an essential step in the decision making. Assessment of all these factors will allow the physician to determine the goals of treatment with greater precision and tailor the interventions in a manner relevant to the individual patient's cause.

Selection of Appropriate Treatment Modality

The second step in the decision-making process involves the selection of an appropriate treatment modality to achieve a desired goal. For example, chemotherapy is the appropriate treatment modality in a patient with advanced-stage diffuse large-cell lymphoma, while surgery is the only curative treatment option for a patient with localized renal cell cancer.[11,12] Careful evaluation of relevant prognostic factors in the context of the planned treatment facilitates prediction of the probable outcome. In some cases, knowledge of prognostic factors allows the physician to tailor the treatment to the disease severity. For example, stage I and II Hodgkin's disease patients without adverse prognostic factors can be treated successfully with radiation therapy alone, while those with adverse prognostic features (bulky mediastinal mass, mixed cellularity histology, age over 50 years) are better managed with chemotherapy and radiation.[13,14] Patients with stage II seminoma and small retroperitoneal lymph nodes have an excellent outcome when treated with radiation therapy alone, while those with bulky retroperitoneal disease require chemotherapy to achieve a similar outcome.[15] Knowledge of prognostic factors may also allow clinicians to select treatments that allows preservation of organs or function without compromising cure and survival. In the majority of cases of soft tissue sarcoma, a high rate of limb preservation can be achieved without major compromise in local control or survival.[16] In some this can be accomplished with surgery alone, but in others with adverse factors, radiotherapy is needed. Similarly, in selected cases of muscle-invasive bladder cancer, normal bladder function can be preserved with chemotherapy and radiation, while such treatment in unselected cases results in unacceptably high local failure and subsequent cystectomy rates.[17]

Decision Making for Long-term Survivors

Only minimal attention is paid to the cancer survivors, and there is paucity of information in the literature, insufficient research, and lack of attention to this group in cancer control programs. Except for the survivors of childhood cancers, few studies address the long-term health problems. Increased risk of delayed complications, and new cancers in adult cancer survivors are well documented.[18–22] Cancer survivors are at risk for second cancers, which at present constitute almost 14% of all new cancer cases in the U.S. Surveillance, Epidemiology, and End Results (SEER) program (L. Travis, personal communication, 2000). Care of these patients is more complex in part because of the long-term effects of treatments for the first cancer. The preservation of medical records of cancer patients is therefore essential. A current trend is to destroy medical records early.[23] The knowledge about potential risks of further disease in cancer survivors may allow for better health records retention policies.

PROCESS OF COMMUNICATING PROGNOSIS

Information Needs of Cancer Patients

Most patients with cancer desire information regarding the diagnosis, planning of treatment, and expected outcomes. In a study of information needs of women with breast cancer, the most highly ranked information categories were those related to the probability of cure and spread of disease.[24] In a study of Scottish patients with cancer, 79% of patients wanted as much information as possible and 96% had a need or an absolute need to know if they had cancer. Most patients also wanted to know the chance of cure (91%) and about side effects of treatment (94%). Patients from more affluent areas wanted more information than those from deprived areas.[25] In a study of cancer patients in South Africa, more than 75% indicated that they would like to receive detailed information about possible side effects; they also wished to understand how to minimize the side effects of different diagnostic and therapeutic interventions. Eighty percent wanted to be informed about the potential for success in their specific cancer. In addition, 78.5% wished to be informed about their individual prognosis and survival.[26]

Further studies suggest that physicians should attempt to consider the degree to which a patient with cancer desires information, and how active a role he or she wishes to take in making treatment decisions.[24,27,28] In addition, health professionals should be aware that the informational needs of patients and family members change throughout the course of care and therefore should be revisited periodically. Health care organisations should ensure that ongoing assessment of informational needs and education are a routine part of comprehensive cancer patient care. In this effort, the knowledge of factors that help to predict cancer outcomes will maximize patient comprehension and retention of information, encourage patient participation in health decision making, and foster dialogue with patients and families. Recognition of prognostic needs of patients will encourage health care organizations to ensure that ongoing informational needs assessment and education are a routine part of comprehensive cancer patient care.[28] Having determined patients' needs for information, the availability of high-quality health information may be important to the outcome, as misinformation can lead the patient to select inappropriate intervention, and not miss an opportunity to derive the benefit. Patients require access to evidence-based information of good quality so they can take an active part in decisions about their health care.[29,30]

Communication of Expected Outcomes

After selecting the appropriate treatment modality and treatment course, an appreciation of prognostic factors allows the clinician to more accurately predict the outcome in terms of the initial response to treatment, ultimate local tumor control, control of cancer, survival, and likelihood of treatment-induced complications. When applicable, all of these outcomes should be discussed with a patient and his or her family and are an essential step in the process of informed consent to treatment.[31,32] Such an open process of discussion about issues in general and specific knowledge about treatment efficacy may be most effective in alleviating anxiety and in reassuring family and caregivers. In turn, this permits family members to provide a more constructive support and plan for the immediate and the long-term future. The recognition of adverse prognostic factors that predict for high complication rates, or treatment failure, allows the health care team and caregivers to anticipate the need for physical or emotional support and provides an opportunity for planning for future resources. Patients are initially mostly interested in the overall success of cancer treatment, but in the course of their disease, the outcomes of interest also include the probability of pain or suffering, loss of function or independence, and institutionalization or hospitalization.[33]

Patients are known to overestimate their survival probability and select toxic therapies in an expectation of prolongation of life.[34] A more accurate prediction could empower the patient to make decisions that would not compromise survival, but would improve the quality of life and decrease suffering in cases where aggressive treatment has not been shown to be of benefit.

Promoting Autonomous Decision Making

Assisting patients with cancer to obtain information enables them to assume a more active role in treatment decision making and can go a long way to decreasing their levels of anxiety and depression.[35] Men given information assumed a significantly more active role in treatment decision making, and had a lower state of anxiety levels than those that were poorly informed.[35] Generally, patients want to be informed and participate in medical decisions. Knowledge of available treatments and their outcomes may encourage them to seek organ-preserving treatments even if they are associated with somewhat inferior outcomes.[36] In oncology care this remains their right, and it is the clinician's duty to respect it and to inform them of the limitations, risks, or advantages of any given treatment approach.

Process of Informed Consent for Medical Research

Patients who volunteer for medical research can face additional risks, which are not encountered outside the research project. The degree of such risks can often be known only after the research has been completed. When a research project involves new treatment, however, it can also offer potential benefits that would not be available outside a study protocol. To protect patients from unethical use of medical experimentation, the Declaration of Helsinki (1964) developed recommendations to guide physicians in biomedical research involving human subjects, and was adopted by the World Medical Assembly in 1964.[37] The Helsinki declaration states:

> In any research on human beings, each potential subject must be adequately informed of the aims, methods, anticipated benefits and potential hazards of the study and the discomfort it may entail. He or she should be informed that he or she is at liberty to abstain from participation in the study and that he or she is free to withdraw his or her consent to participation at any time. The physician should then obtain the subject's freely given informed consent, preferably in writing.

PLANNING SUPPORT MEASURES

Knowledge of disease characteristics permits planning for special needs. For example, extensive nasopharyngeal cancer may be optimally treated with conformal radiation therapy that allows safe delivery of high-dose radiation therapy around the sensitive structures in the base of the skull, including brain stem, spinal cord, and optic chiasm.[38] In some cases of head and neck cancer, an understanding of local disease extent, comorbidity, performance status, and treatment plan allows for selection of patients who will require feeding gastrostomy as a support measure.[39] Also, patients with socioeconomic difficulties may require supportive care to facilitate treatment attendance. Hospice support may need to be planned for patients with symptomatic metastatic disease, where the expected treatment outcome is at best short-term palliation. For patients who have difficulty accepting medical opinion and worry excessively about treatment effects and outcomes, contact with a patient support group may be of benefit.[40]

PROMOTING GOOD MEDICAL PRACTICE

Clinical Practice Guidelines

Clinical guidelines are defined as "systematically developed statements, which assist clinicians and patients in making decisions about appropriate treatment for specific conditions".[3,41] All clinical guidelines aim to promote "best practices" that improve the outcomes of treatment. The principal benefit of guidelines is to improve the quality of care received by patients. Clinical guidelines offer explicit recommendations for clinicians who are uncertain about how to proceed, overturn the beliefs of doctors accustomed to outdated practices, improve the consistency of care, and provide authoritative recommendations that reassure practitioners about the appropriateness of their treatment policies.[2,41–43] Clinical guidelines inform patients and the public about what their clinicians should be doing. Increasingly, lay guidelines summarize the benefits and harms of available options, along with estimates of the probability or magnitude of potential outcomes, and enable patients to make more informed health care choices and to consider their personal needs and preferences in selecting the best option. Most importantly, clinical guidelines can also help patients by influencing public policy. Guidelines call attention to underrecognized health problems, clinical services, and preventive interventions and to neglected patient populations and high-risk groups. Services that were not previously offered to patients may be made available as a response to newly released guidelines.

CREATING NEW KNOWLEDGE FOR PATIENT BENEFIT

The benefit derived from knowledge of prognostic factors extends beyond current patients. The assessment of outcome permits identification of groups of patients who do not respond to currently available therapy. Such patients should become eligible for clinical trials of new therapies, and prognostic factors are therefore essential to the conduct of randomized clinical trials.[44,45] First, prognostic factors are used to define eligibility criteria for entry into the trial, to define criteria for patient stratification to ensure balance is maintained in randomized trials, and to permit explanations to be formulated about observed differences in outcomes in trials. Knowledge of prognostic factors is also indispensable for the interpretation of the results of retrospective trials, and in attempting to contrast historical experience with current results. Although prospective randomized trials are the gold standard in clinical research, they are not always practical. In uncommon conditions, or for uncommon events, only descriptive evidence is available. In such circumstances, attempts to characterize patients according to prognostic variables are important.

TABLE 7.1   Role of Prognostic Factors in Patient Care

I. Process of decision making
  A. Select goal(s) of treatment
    • Cure, prolongation of life, control of cancer, preservation of organ and function, palliation of symptoms
  B. Tailor treatment plan to disease severity and with the goal to achieve the planned outcome
  C. Select appropriate treatment modality and intensity
    • Single modality, multimodality therapy
  D. Select adjuvant treatment
  E. Care of cancer survivors, follow-up care
II. Communication of prognosis
  A. Assist the patient in the process of informed consent
  B. Predict the outcome in terms of response, survival, organ preservation, complications, quality of life
  C. Promote autonomous decision making: patient empowerment
III. Planning support measures
  A. Identify sources needed to support the patient
  B. Need for special techniques, for example, conformal radiotherapy
  C. Need for supportive interventions, for example, gastrostomy tube, G-CSF in chemotherapy
  D. Supportive care: nursing, psychosocial
  E. Hospice support
  F. Patient support group
IV. Promoting good medical practice
  A. Promote good medical practice
  B. Develop clinical practice guidelines
  C. Assist in audit of medical practice
V. Creating new knowledge for patient benefit
  A. Encourage clinical trial participation
  B. Retrospective reviews of treatment results: historical controls

---

SUMMARY

Prognostic factors play an essential role in cancer patient care (Table 7.1). The determination of prognosis depends on the accurate assessment of prognostic factors and the appropriate choice of therapeutic and supportive intervention. This knowledge can then be applied to communicate the prognosis to the patient, caregivers, and support team. Knowledge and understanding of the variables that predict for a given outcome are essential to the understanding of the observed variations in treatment outcomes. This knowledge and understanding is required not only in the individual medical practice, but also at the institutional, local, regional, and national level, since the outcomes obtained from one group of patients cannot be inferred to apply to another group if one can have no confidence that the groups are comparable. This principle governs much of the knowledge generated from clinical research and that determines the treatment choices we normally offer patients.

REFERENCES

1. Rizzi DA: Medical prognosis — some fundamentals. *Theor Med* 14:365–75, 1993.
2. Shekelle PG, Woolf SH, Eccles M, et al.: Clinical guidelines: developing guidelines. *BMJ* 318:593–6, 1999.
3. Browman GP: Evidence-based paradigms and opinions in clinical management and cancer research. *Semin Oncol* 26:9–13, 1999.
4. Gospodarowicz M, Benedet L, Hutter R, et al.: History and international developments in cancer staging. *Cancer Prev Control* 2:262–8, 1998.
5. Sobin LH, Fleming ID: *TNM classification of malignant tumors*, 5th ed. (1997). Union Internationale Contre le Cancer and the American Joint Committee on Cancer. *Cancer* 80:1803–4, 1997.
6. Sassine AM, Schulman C: Clinical use of prostate-specific antigen in the staging of patients with prostatic carcinoma. *Eur Urol* 23:348–51, 1993.
7. A predictive model for aggressive non-Hodgkin's lymphoma. The International Non-Hodgkin's Lymphoma Prognostic Factors Project. *N Engl J Med* 329:987–94, 1993.
8. International germ cell consensus classification: a prognostic factor-based staging system for metastatic germ cell cancers. International Germ Cell Cancer Collaborative Group. *J Clin Oncol* 15:594–603, 1997.
9. Sieber M, Ruffer U, Jostin A, et al.: Treatment of Hodgkin's disease: current strategies of the German Hodgkin's Lymphoma Study Group. *Ann Oncol* 10 (Suppl 6):23–9, 1999.
10. Ushio Y: Treatment of gliomas in adults. *Curr Opin Oncol* 3:467–75, 1991.
11. Fisher RI: Diffuse large-cell lymphoma. *Ann Oncol* 11 (Suppl 1):29–33, 2000.
12. Motzer RJ, Russo P, Nanus DM, et al.: Renal cell carcinoma. *Curr Probl Cancer* 21:185–232, 1997.
13. Gospodarowicz MK, Sutcliffe SB, Clark RM, et al.: Analysis of supradiaphragmatic clinical stage I and II Hodgkin's disease treated with radiation alone. *Int J Radiat Oncol Biol Phys* 22:859–65, 1992.

14. Gospodarowicz MK, Sutcliffe SB, Bergsagel DE, et al.: Radiation therapy in clinical stage I and II Hodgkin's disease. The Princess Margaret Hospital Lymphoma Group. *Eur J Cancer* 28A:1841–6, 1992.

15. Warde P, Gospodarowicz M, Panzarella T, et al.: Management of stage II seminoma. *J Clin Oncol* 16:290–4, 1998.

16. O'Sullivan B, Wylie J, Catton C, et al.: The local management of soft tissue sarcoma. *Semin Radiat Oncol* 9:328–48, 1999.

17. Shipley WU, Kaufman DS, Heney NM, et al.: An update of combined modality therapy for patients with muscle invading bladder cancer using selective bladder preservation or cystectomy. *J Urol* 162:445–50; discussion 450–1, 1999.

18. Herold AH, Roetzheim RG: Cancer survivors. *Prim Care* 19:779–91, 1992.

19. Gotay CC, Muraoka MY: Quality of life in long-term survivors of adult-onset cancers. *J Natl Cancer Inst* 90:656–67, 1998.

20. Byrne J: Long-term genetic and reproductive effects of ionizing radiation and chemotherapeutic agents on cancer patients and their offspring. *Teratology* 59:210–5, 1999.

21. Ferrell BR, Dow KH, Leigh S, et al.: Quality of life in long-term cancer survivors. *Oncol Nurs Forum* 22:915–22, 1995.

22. Li FP, Stovall EL: Long-term survivors of cancer [editorial; comment]. *Cancer Epidemiol Biomarkers Prev* 7:269–70, 1998.

23. Hawkins MM, Craft AW: Retaining personal medical records of children who have had chemotherapy and radiotherapy. *BMJ* 308:1654–5, 1994.

24. Degner LF, Kristjanson LJ, Bowman D, et al.: Information needs and decisional preferences in women with breast cancer. *JAMA* 277:1485–92, 1997.

25. Meredith C, Symonds P, Webster L, et al.: Information needs of cancer patients in west Scotland: cross sectional survey of patients' views. *BMJ* 313:724–6, 1996.

26. McLoughlin HA, Oosthuizen BL: The information needs of cancer patients in the Pretoria and Witwatersrand area. *Curationis* 19:31–5, 1996.

27. Sutherland HJ, Llewellyn-Thomas HA, Lockwood GA, et al.: Cancer patients: their desire for information and participation in treatment decisions. *J R Soc Med* 82:260–3, 1989.

28. Harris KA: The informational needs of patients with cancer and their families. *Cancer Pract* 6:39–46, 1998.

29. Charnock D, Shepperd S, Needham G, et al.: DISCERN: an instrument for judging the quality of written consumer health information on treatment choices. *J Epidemiol Community Health* 53:105–11, 1999.

30. Shepperd S, Charnock D, Gann B: Helping patients access high quality health information. *BMJ* 319:764–6, 1999.

31. Gramlich EP, Waitzfelder BE: Interactive video assists in clinical decision making. *Methods Inf Med* 37:201–5, 1998.

32. Gamble K: Communication and information: the experience of radiotherapy patients. *Eur J Cancer Care (Engl)* 7:153–61, 1998.

33. Christakis NA, Sachs GA: The role of prognosis in clinical decision making. *J Gen Intern Med* 11:422–5, 1996.

34. Weeks JC, Cook EF, O'Day SJ, et al.: Relationship between cancer patients' predictions of prognosis and their treatment preferences. *JAMA* 279:1709–14, 1998.

35. Davison BJ, Degner LF: Empowerment of men newly diagnosed with prostate cancer. *Cancer Nurs* 20:187–96, 1997.

36. McNeil BJ, Weichselbaum R, Pauker SG: Speech and survival: tradeoffs between quality and quantity of life in laryngeal cancer. *N Engl J Med* 305:982–7, 1981.

37. Declaration of Helsinki (1964). *BMJ* 313:1448–49, 1996.

38. Verhey LJ: Comparison of three-dimensional conformal radiation therapy and intensity-modulated radiation therapy systems. *Semin Radiat Oncol* 9:78–98, 1999.

39. Van Bokhorst-de van der S, van Leeuwen PA, Kuik DJ, et al.: The impact of nutritional status on the prognoses of patients with advanced head and neck cancer. *Cancer* 86:519–27, 1999.

40. Christakis NA: Predicting patient survival before and after hospice enrollment. *Hosp J* 13:71–87, 1998.

41. Woolf SH, Grol R, Hutchinson A, et al.: Clinical guidelines: potential benefits, limitations, and harms of clinical guidelines. *BMJ* 318:527–30, 1999.

42. Feder G, Eccles M, Grol R, et al.: Clinical guidelines: using clinical guidelines. *BMJ* 318:728–30, 1999.

43. Haycox A, Bagust A, Walley T: Clinical guidelines—the hidden costs. *BMJ* 318:391–3, 1999.

44. Sather HN: The use of prognostic factors in clinical trials. *Cancer* 58:461–7, 1986.

45. Simon R: Importance of prognostic factors in cancer clinical trials. *Cancer Treat Rep* 68:185–192, 1984.

CHAPTER 8

Psychosocial Factors in Prognosis

CLAIRE V.I. EDMONDS and ALASTAIR J. CUNNINGHAM

Physicians often encounter patients' belief that psychological factors can predict survival from cancer. However, the research literature is filled with methodological shortcomings and results are often contradictory and problematic.[1-3] The present brief review discusses psychosocial factors that have shown a relatively consistent relationship to survival in cancer patients.[4-6]

QUALITY OF LIFE

A variety of measures have been used to assess a complex property labeled *quality of life* (QoL). Some of these measures, such as Karnofsky Performance Status[7] and Functional Living Index for Cancer (FLIC)[8] effectively have a single global scale, while newer instruments such as the European Organization for Research and Treatment of Cancer-QLQ-C30 (EORTC-QLQ-C30)[9] allow for the assessment, both separately and globally, of components such as physical, psychological, social, and functional factors. The development of these scales reflects the increasing use of QoL as an outcome measure in clinical trials of chemotherapeutic agents.

When assessing the role that psychosocial factors may play in the prediction of survival, it is important first to test for and then take into account known biological predictors of survival such as age and extent of disease; this has been done in all of the studies in this section.

Among the early studies using global measures, Kukull et al. found a symptom distress measure predictive of survival in patients with advanced lung cancer,[10] and Ganz et al. and Ruckduschel et al. showed that a more global QoL instrument (FLIC) predicted survival in the same population of patients.[11,12] Coates and his colleagues found that QoL (assessed by six linear analog scales) was significantly related to survival in metastatic breast cancer patients enrolled in a chemotherapy

Prognostic Factors in Cancer, 2nd edition, Edited by Mary K. Gospodarowicz
ISBN 0-471-40633-3   Copyright © 2001 Wiley-Liss, Inc.

trial, independently of the medical intervention itself.[13] More recent research with multifactor measures demonstrated that several subscales of the EORTC-QLQ-C30 (overall physical condition, global QoL, and social functioning) were each independent predictors of survival in a relatively large, heterogeneous population of cancer patients.[14] Wisloff et al. also found that survival in newly diagnosed multiple myeloma patients was predicted by the EORTC-QLQ-C30 and that, 12 months after diagnosis, the physical functioning subscale and the World Health Organization (WHO) status were at least as important for survival as having obtained a response to chemotherapy.[15] Cognitive failure, fatigue, and global health status, as assessed by the Therapy Impact Scale, independently predicted survival in a sample of terminal cancer patients with mixed diagnoses.[16] Kaasa et al. also found that QoL and, specifically, general symptoms of fatigue, loss of appetite, insomnia and pain, as well as psychological well-being and stage of disease, predicted survival in lung cancer patients enrolled in a clinical trial.[17] In fact, patients with high levels of psychosocial functioning lived twice as long as those with low levels. The authors suggest, however, that this might have been confounded with the extent of disease. In contrast, Dancey et al. reported that while the EORTC-QLQ-C30 was predictive of survival overall for the whole sample, in the subset of patients with low QoL, those with poor social functioning lived longer than those with better social functioning.[18]

In sum, while there appears to be some survival advantage to higher QoL, it is not entirely clear whether this reflects some specific psychosocial influences or is an indirect effect of physical health status.

PSYCHOSOCIAL FACTORS AND BONE MARROW TRANSPLANTATION

Possibly because of the extreme emotional stress of the bone marrow transplant (BMT) procedure, there have been a number of studies on psychological factors in this population of patients. In an early study, Neuser found that patients scoring high on the striving for recognition and help subscale of the Personality Research Form had a higher chance of survival one year later; however, medical variables were not controlled for.[19] Colon et al., in a retrospective analysis, used pre-BMT psychiatric evaluations and found that stage of disease, depressed mood, and poor social support all independently predicted for length of survival.[20] In a study specifically designed to use psychological factors as predictors, Andrykowski et al. determined that a combination of medical and psychological factors predicted poorer duration of survival, specifically, poorer quality of bone marrow match, anxious preoccupation as a coping style, and lower QoL during recovery from the procedure were related to shorter duration of survival.[21] Low symptom distress, high hopefulness and low acceptance were predictive of better survival in combination with several medical variables in a more recent study by Molassiotis et al.[22] Not all studies have shown a relationship; neither mental adjustment to cancer nor depression prior to BMT predicted survival in a study by Murphy et al.[23]

As with the QoL area, it appears that psychological factors, specifically coping style, may be associated with duration of survival after a BMT procedure, but more research is required to clarify this relationship.

SOCIAL SUPPORT

A long-standing and popular area of research has been the impact of social support on chronic illness in general and cancer specifically.[24] Cancer patients who report having good social support, better relationships and confidants, and involvement in social activities have been found to survive better than those who do not.[25-29] One study suggests that social support may be more protective for patients with earlier disease than for those with more advanced illness.[30] Married subjects may have better survival rates from cancer,[31] and similarly, death of a spouse has been related to cancer onset and poorer survival rates.[32,33] Conversely, among patients with poor prognoses, Cassileth et al. found that single patients were more likely to survive longer.[34] Negative results also include a study by Barraclough et al., who found that lack of a confidant did not increase the risk of relapse in breast cancer patients.[35]

Overall, the research points in the direction that social support is related to survival, although some contrary results have been reported.

STRESS AND COPING

In spite of widespread popular belief, the evidence is inconsistent for an effect of stressful life events on the progression of cancer. There are many design problems in the early studies that appeared to show an effect of stress causing more rapid disease progression[36,37] (reviewed by Fox[3,38]). In studies by Ramirez et al. and Forsen et al., severe stress was related to earlier death.[39,40] However, a number of studies have found no relationship between stress and subsequent disease progression. While self-reported stress was related to initial tumor size in one study, stress did not predict subsequent relapse.[41] In primary breast cancer patients, severe life events, social difficulties, depression, and lack of confidants were not related to disease progression.[35] In a large epidemiological study, women who had experienced the severe stress of the death of a child were

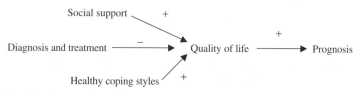

Figure 8.1 The impact of social support and coping styles on survival may be mediated through quality of life.

not more likely to develop cancer, nor to succumb to it if they did have cancer, than matched controls.[42] A very recent study on breast cancer patients also found that stressful life events did not confer greater risk of relapse.[43]

Depression was also thought to be a risk factor for developing cancer on the basis of longitudinal research by Shekelle and colleagues.[44] More recent, larger prospective studies have failed to support this relationship.[45-48] In terms of disease progression, depression has not been found to increase relapse rate in patients with either breast cancer[35,49] or hematological and colorectal cancers.[50]

In contrast to stress and depression, coping styles, and repression in particular, have been associated with differences in rate of disease progression in cancer patients. In an early study, Blumberg et al. identified defensiveness and an inability to discharge negative emotions as a risk factor for progression.[51] Derogatis et al. found that dysphoria, anxiety, and dissatisfaction predicted better survival one year after a diagnosis of metastatic breast cancer.[52] Dean and Surtees also showed that increased psychiatric symptoms after diagnosis of breast cancer predicted longer survival.[53] Jensen found that repressive coping styles predicted progression in breast cancer patients.[54] Temoshok et al. also observed that suppression of negative emotions was related to more serious disease in melanoma patients,[55] and in two experimental studies cancer patients were more likely than control subjects to use repressive coping when faced with an experimental stressor.[56,57] Negative studies have also been reported, finding no relationship between distress and coping styles in cancer patients and subsequent survival.[50,58,59]

In an influential, although small study by Greer and colleagues, patients' emotional adjustment to primary breast cancer was assessed three months after their initial surgery. These emotional responses were divided into several categories: fighting spirit, denial, stoic acceptance, and helplessness–hopelessness. It was found that reactions of fighting spirit were related to better survival at 5-, 10-, and 15-year follow-up; however, disease staging was not taken into account.[60-62] Further controlled research with both breast and lymphoma patients demonstrated that responses of denial and fighting spirit were predictive of better disease-free interval and survival rates than responses of stoic acceptance and helplessness–hopelessness.[63] In a very recent study of 578 patients with breast cancer, the same research group was unable to find a protective effect for fighting spirit, but replicated their earlier findings that helplessness–hopelessness as well as depression scores predicted poorer survival.[64] Other researchers have also examined the effect of these coping styles on survival. Stein et al. reported that nursing home cancer patients who reacted to placement with helplessness–hopelessness were observed to die more quickly.[65] DiClemente and Temoshok also found that stoic acceptance in women and helplessness–hopelessness in men predicted relapse in patients with malignant melanoma.[66] Negative results include the study by Cassileth and colleagues in which helplessness–hopelessness was not a significant predictor in patients with advanced cancer.[34]

While the evidence for stress promoting cancer progression is equivocal, it does appear that certain coping styles, notably an attitude of helplessness and repression of emotion, may be poor prognostic indicators. More research is needed to better understand how different reactions such as helplessness–hopelessness and depression relate to each other, and to define the role of coping in survival.

INTERVENTION STUDIES

With the publication of several intervention studies, another avenue has opened up to understanding the effect of psychosocial factors on cancer progression. Survival advantages were reported by both Spiegel et al. and Fawzy et al. in randomized trials of psychosocial interventions for cancer patients.[67,68] Contrary results have also been published by Morganstern et al., Ilnyckyj et al., and Cunningham et al.[69–71] These studies were not designed to test specific prognostic factors, but positive results in the former two studies suggest that social support and coping, which are amenable to change through psychotherapy, may be relevant to survival. More studies of this kind are underway.

While the impact of psychotherapy on survival has not been unambiguously demonstrated, there is a growing consensus that psychosocial interventions reliably enhance QoL in cancer patients.[72–74] The various findings in this brief review might be brought together in the following tentative model: Starting from the observation that QoL affects prognosis and that support and certain coping styles may improve QoL, we suggest that QoL may mediate the effects of these psychosocial variables on survival (see Fig. 8.1).

CONCLUSIONS

Quality of life has an impact on survival in a number of studies, and more specific psychosocial factors may play a role in the duration of survival from BMT. While social support has usually been found to be protective, the effects of depression and stress are not consistent. Coping styles may also be related to prognosis, and in particular, a repressive style may be a poor prognostic factor. It is important to note that associations between psychosocial factors and survival are usually small compared to biological prognostic factors. On the other hand, psychosocial factors are amenable to improvement while presenting biomedical factors (such as age and location of metastatic spread) are often fixed. It is also important to note that many of these psychosocial variables are difficult to measure, that there are few standardized instruments, and that the field, on the whole, is filled with design problems that obscure the relationships. Psychosocial variables and physical health are likely to be interrelated in dynamic and complex ways. However, it is possible that social support and coping skills may influence survival through QoL. To summarize, a good QoL, accessible social support, and less repressive coping style can be considered as positive psychosocial prognostic indicators.

REFERENCES

1. Stam HJ, Steggles S: Predicting the onset or the progression of cancer from psychological characteristics: psychometric and theoretical issues. *J Psychosoc Oncol* 5(2):35–46, 1987.

2. Levenson JL, Bemis C: The role of psychological factors in cancer onset and progression. *Psychosomatics* 32(2):124–32, 1991.

3. Fox BH: The psychological epidemiology of cancer incidence and prognosis. *Chronic Dis Can* 16(1):S19–27, 1995.

4. Gross J: Emotional expression in cancer onset and progression. *Soc Sci Med* 28(12):1239–48, 1989.

5. Mulder CL, Van Der Pompe G, Spiegel D, et al.: Do psychological factors influence the course of breast cancer? *Psycho-Oncology* 1(1):155–67, 1992.

6. Garssen B, Goodkin K: On the role of immunological factors as mediators between psychosocial factors and cancer progression. *Psychiatry Res* 85:51–61, 1999.

7. Karnofsky DA, Burchenal JH: The clinical evaluation of chemotherapeutic agents in cancer, in Macleod CM (ed.): *Evaluation of chemotherapeutic agents*. New York, Columbia University Press, 1949.

8. Schipper H, Clinch J, McMurray A, et al.: Measuring the quality of life of cancer patients: The Functional Living Index-Cancer: development and validation. *J Clin Oncol* 2:472–83, 1984.

9. Aaronson NK, Ahmedzai S, Bergman B, et al.: The European Organization for Research and Treatment of Cancer QLQ-C30: a quality-of-life instrument for use in international clinical trials in oncology. *J Natl Cancer Inst* 85(5):365–76, 1993.

10. Kukull WA, McCorkle R, Driever M: Symptom distress, psychosocial variables and survival from lung cancer. *J Psychosoc Oncol* 4(1/2):91–104, 1986.

11. Ganz RA, Haskell CM, Figlin RA, et al.: Estimating the quality of life of patients with metastatic lung cancer using the Karnofsky performance status and the Functional Living Index-Cancer. *Cancer* 61:849–56, 1988.

12. Ruckdeschel JC, Piantadosi A: Quality of life in lung cancer surgical adjuvant trials. *Chest* 106(6):324S–28S, 1994.

13. Coates A, Gebski V, Signorini D, et al.: Prognostic value of quality of life scores during chemotherapy for advanced breast cancer. *J Clin Oncol* 10(12):1833–8, 1992.

14. Coates A, Porzsolt F, Osoba D: Quality of life in oncology practice: prognostic value of EORTC QLQ-30 scores in patients with advanced malignancy. *Eur J Cancer* 33(7):1025–30, 1997.

15. Wisloff F, Hjorth M: Health-related quality of life assessed before and during chemotherapy predicts for survival in multiple myeloma. *Br J Haematol* 97:29–37, 1997.

16. Tamburini M, Brunelli C, Rosso S, et al.: Prognostic value of quality of life scores in terminal cancer patients. *J Pain Symptom Manage* 11(1):32–41, 1996.

17. Kaasa S, Mastekaasa A, Lund E: Prognostic factors for patients with inoperable non-small-cell lung cancer, limited disease. *Radiother Oncol* 15:235–42, 1989.

18. Dancey J, Zee B, Osoba D, et al.: Quality of life scores: an independent prognostic variable in a general population of cancer patients receiving chemotherapy. *Qual Life Res* 6:151–8, 1997.

19. Neuser J: Personality and survival time after bone marrow transplantation. *J Psychosom Res* 32:451–5, 1988.

20. Colon EA, Callies AL, Popkin MK, et al.: Depressed mood and other variables related to bone marrow transplantation survival in acute leukemia. *Psychosomatics* 32:420–5, 1991.

21. Andrykowski MA, Brady MJ, Henslee-Downey PJ: Psychosocial factors predictive of survival after allogeneic bone marrow transplantation for leukemia. *Psychosom Med* 56:432–9, 1994.

22. Molassiotis A, Van Den Akker OBA, Milligan DW, et al.: Symptom distress, coping style and biological variables as predictors of survival after bone marrow transplantation. *J Psychosom Res* 42(3):275–85, 1997.

23. Murphy KC, Jenkins PL, Whittaker JA: Psychosocial morbidity and survival in adult bone marrow transplant recipients — a follow-up study. *Bone Marrow Transplant* 18:199–201, 1996.

24. House JS, Landis KR, Umberson D: Social relationships and death. *Science* 241:540–5, 1988.

25. Weisman AD, Worden JW: Psychosocial analysis of cancer deaths. *Omega* 6:61, 1976.

26. Funch DP, Marshall J: The role of stress, social support and survival from breast cancer. *J Psychosom Res* 27:77–83, 1983.

27. Hislop TG, Waxler NE, Coldman AJ, et al.: The prognostic significance of psychosocial factors in women with breast cancer. *J Chron Dis* 40:729–35, 1987.

28. Waxler-Morrison N, Hislop TG, Meares B, et al.: Effects of social relationships on survival for women with breast cancer: a prospective trial. *Soc Sci Med* 33(2):177–83, 1991.

29. Maunsell E, Brisson J, Duschenes L: Social support and survival among women with breast cancer. *Cancer* 76(4):631–7, 1995.

30. Ell K, Nishimoto R, Morvay T, et al.: A longitudinal analysis of psychological adaptation among survivors of cancer. *Cancer* 63:406–13, 1989.

31. Goodwin JS, Hunt WC, Rey CR, et al.: The effects of marital status on stage, treatment and survival of cancer patients. *Advances* 5(4):12–17, 1987.

32. Neale AV, Tilley BC, Vernon SW: Marital status, delay in seeking treatment and survival from breast cancer. *Soc Sci Med* 23(3):305–12, 1986.

33. Courtney JG, Longnecker MP, Theorell T, et al.: Stressful life events and the risk of colorectal cancer. *Epidemiology* 4(5):4007–14, 1993.

34. Cassileth BR, Walsh WP, Lusk EJ: Psychosocial correlates of cancer survival: a subsequent report 3 to 8 years after cancer diagnosis. *J Clin Oncol* 6:1753–59, 1988.

35. Barraclough J, Pinder P, Cruddas M, et al.: Life events and cancer prognosis. *BMJ* 304:1078–81, 1992.

36. Evans E: *A psychological study of cancer.* New York, Dodd Mead, 1926.

37. LeShan L, Worthington RE: Some recurrent life history patterns observed in patients with malignant disease. *J Nerv Men Dis* 124:460–5, 1956.

38. Fox BH: Premorbid psychological factors as related to cancer incidence. *J Behav Med* 1(1):45, 1978.

39. Ramirez AJ, Craig TKJ, Walson JP, et al.: Stress and relapse of breast cancer. *BMJ* 298:291–3, 1989.

40. Forsen A: Psychosocial stress as a risk for breast cancer. *Psychother Psychosom* 55:176–85, 1991.

41. Giraldi T, Rodani MG, Cartei G, et al.: Psychosocial factors and breast cancer: a 6-year Italian follow-up study. *Psychother Psychosom* 66:229–36, 1997.

42. Kvikstad A, Vatten LJ: Risk and prognosis of cancer in middle-aged women who have experienced the death of a child. *Int J Cancer* 67:165–9, 1996.

43. Maunsell E, Brisson J, Mondor M, et al.: Stressful life events and survival after breast cancer. (Abst. 281 4th Int Congr of Psycho-Oncology). *Psycho-Oncology* 7(4) Suppl: 1998.

44. Shekelle RB, Raynor WJ, Ostfeld AM, et al.: Psychological depression and 17 year risk of death from cancer. *Psychosom Med* 43(2):117–25, 1981.

45. Kaplan GA, Reynolds P: Depression and cancer mortality and morbidity: prospective evidence from the Alameda County study. *J Behav Med* 11(1):1–13, 1988.

46. Hahn RC, Petitti DB: Minnesota Multiphasic Personality Inventory-rated depression and the incidence of breast cancer. *Cancer* 61:845–8, 1988.

47. Zonderman AB, Costa PT, McCrae RR: Depression as a risk for cancer morbidity and mortality in a nationally representative sample. *JAMA* 262:1191–5, 1989.

48. Linkins RW, Comstock GW: Depressed mood and development of cancer. *Am J Epidemiol* 132(5):962–72, 1990.

49. Jamison RN, Burish TG, Wallston KA: Psychogenic factors in predicting survival of breast cancer patients. *J Clin Oncol* 5:768–72, 1987.

50. Richardson JL, Shelton DR, Krailo M, et al.: The effects of compliance with treatment on survival among patients with hematologic malignancies. *J Clin Oncol* 8(2):356–64, 1990.

51. Blumberg EM, West PM, Ellis FW: A possible relationship between psychological factors and human cancer. *Psychosom Med* 16(4):227–86, 1954.

52. Derogatis LR, Abeloff MD, Melisaratos N: Psychological coping mechanisms and survival time in metastatic breast cancer. *JAMA* 242:1504–8, 1979.

53. Dean C, Surtees PG: Do psychological factors predict survival in breast cancer? *J Psychosom Res* 33(5):561–9, 1989.

54. Jensen MR: Psychobiological factors predicting the course of breast cancer. *J Pers* 55:317–42, 1987.

55. Temoshok L, Heller BW, Sagebiel RW, et al.: The relationship of psychosocial factors to prognostic indicators in cutaneous malignant melanoma. *J Psychosom Res* 29:139–54, 1985.

56. Kneier AW, Temoshok L: Repressive coping reactions in patients with malignant melanoma as compared to cardiovascular disease patients. *J Psychosom Res* 28(2):145–55, 1984.

57. Pettingale KW, Watson M, Greer S: The validity of emotional control as a trait in breast cancer patients. *J Psychosoc Oncol* 2(314):21–30, 1984.

58. Buddeburg C, Wolf C, Sieber M, et al.: Coping strategies and course of disease of breast cancer patients. *Psychother Psychosom* 55:151–7, 1991.

59. Tross S, Herndon J, Korzun A, et al.: Psychological symptoms and disease-free and overall survival in women with stage II breast cancer. *JNCI* 88(10):661, 1996.

60. Greer S, Morris T, Pettingale KW: Psychological response to breast cancer: effect on outcome. *Lancet* ii:785–7, 1979.

61. Pettingale KW, Morris T, Greer S, et al.: Mental attitudes to cancer: an additional prognostic factor. *Lancet* i:750, 1985.

62. Greer S, Morris T, Pettingale KW, et al.: Psychological response to breast cancer and 15 year outcome. *Lancet* i:49–50, 1990.

63. Morris T, Pettingale K, Haybittle J: Psychological response to cancer diagnosis and disease outcome in patients with breast cancer and lymphoma. *Psycho-Oncology* 1:105–14, 1992.

64. Watson M, Haviland JS, Greer S, et al.: Influence of psychological response on survival in breast cancer: a population-based cohort study. *Lancet*, 354:1331–6, 1999.

65. Stein S, Linn MW, Stein EM: Psychological correlates of survival in nursing home cancer patients. *The Gerontologist* 29(2):224–8, 1989.

66. DiClemente RJ, Temoshok L: Psychological adjustment to having cutaneous malignant melanoma as a predictor of follow-up clinical status. *Psychosom Med* 47:81, 1985.

67. Spiegel D, Bloom JR, Kraemer HC, et al.: Effect of psychosocial treatment on survival of patients with metastatic breast cancer. *Lancet* 2:888–91, 1989.

68. Fawzy FI, Fawzy NW, Hyun CS, et al.: Malignant melanoma. Effects of an early structured psychiatric intervention, coping and affective state on recurrence and survival 6 years later. *Arch Gen Psychiatry* 50:681–9, 1993.

69. Morganstern H, Gellert GA, Walter SD, et al.: The impact of a psychosocial support program on survival with breast cancer: the importance of selection bias in program evaluation. *J Chronic Dis* 37(4):273–82, 1984.

70. Ilnyckyj A, Farber J, Cheang MC, et al.: A randomized controlled trial of psychotherapeutic intervention in cancer patients. *Ann R Coll Physicians Surg Can* 27:93–6, 1994.

71. Cunningham AJ, Edmonds CVI, Jenkins GP, et al.: A randomized controlled trial of the effects of group psychological therapy on survival in women with metastatic breast cancer. *Psycho-Oncology* 7:508–17, 1998.

72. Anderson BL: Psychological interventions for cancer patients to enhance the quality of life. *J Consult Clin Psychol* 60:552–68, 1992.

73. Meyer TJ, Mark MM: Effects of psychosocial intervention with adult cancer patients: a meta-analysis of randomized experiments. *Health Psychol* 14(2):101–8, 1995.

74. Cunningham AJ, Edmonds CVI: Group psychological therapy for cancer patients: a point of view, and discussion of the hierarchy of options. *Int J Psychiatry Med* 26(1):51–82, 1996.

CHAPTER 9

The Role of Prognostic Factors in Cancer Research

PATTI A. GROOME and WILLIAM J. MACKILLOP

Knowledge about how the characteristics of the individual patients and their diseases will shape their future is useful when they are making decisions about their lives and when they and their doctors are making treatment decisions. When a patient's prognosis changes, new evaluation occurs that can affect further decisions about management. In all instances, knowledge about prognosis improves the quality of decisions by reducing uncertainty. In this chapter, we discuss the role of known prognostic factors in clinical research where the research products facilitate either direct or indirect improvement in the quality of clinical decision making.

Figure 9.1 depicts the uses of the output of various types of clinical research and the role that prognostic factors play in that research. In research that focuses on outcome prediction, formal consideration of the combined role of known prognostic factors through the development of predictive tools can improve the clinician's ability to prognosticate. In research on treatment effectiveness, consideration of known prognostic factors allows the researcher to isolate the effect more efficiently through case selection or through the control of prognostic differences between the treatment and control groups. When subgroups defined by important prognostic factors are analyzed separately, the researcher is able to determine whether treatment is equally effective across the groups, enhancing the clinician's ability to apply research findings to different patients. In research about cancer progression and treatment resistance, identification of clinical prognostic factors can provide a starting point for better understanding of these mechanisms and possibly even disease causation, which may lead to the development of new interventions. Last, in health services research, consideration of the variations in the distributions of prognostic factors among populations of patients permits the study of health system effects.

Prognostic Factors in Cancer, 2nd edition, Edited by Mary K. Gospodarowicz
ISBN 0-471-40633-3   Copyright © 2001 Wiley-Liss, Inc.

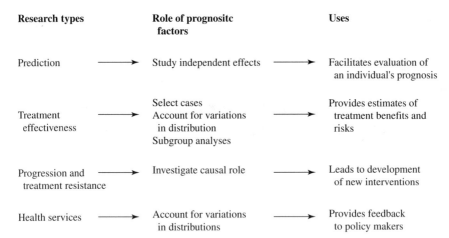

Research types	Role of prognositc factors	Uses
Prediction ⟶	Study independent effects ⟶	Facilitates evaluation of an individual's prognosis
Treatment effectiveness ⟶	Select cases Account for variations in distribution Subgroup analyses ⟶	Provides estimates of treatment benefits and risks
Progression and treatment resistance ⟶	Investigate causal role ⟶	Leads to development of new interventions
Health services ⟶	Account for variations in distributions ⟶	Provides feedback to policy makers

Figure 9.1 The role of prognostic factors in the various kinds of clinical research and the contribution of each to patient care.

STUDIES OF OUTCOME PREDICTION

The ability to predict outcome accurately provides the patient with a more realistic expectation of the future. Better understanding of a patient's prognosis can guide choices related to how aggressively the disease should be treated.

Prediction occurs in two other health-related domains that should not be confused with prognostic prediction. At the level of the population, the incidence of a disease varies by the risk factors (as distinct from prognostic factors) that describe that population. At the level of the individual, the diagnosis of disease is often partly determined by considering risk factors that predispose a patient to having the disease in question. Distinct from risk assessment, prognostic factors predict outcome after the diagnosis.

To properly assess prognosis, studies should simultaneously consider all of the relevant prognostic factors that have been identified. When new prognostic factors are being assessed for their contribution to prognosis they must be considered in the context of other known factors in order to assess the independent contribution of the new factor. Much of the knowledge about the role of prognostic factors in prediction is not based on such multivariable consideration of all relevant factors, but instead relies on information from univariate analyses.

A number of data sources can be used, including secondary use of clinical trial data, cohort data, or data from case series, but the data must be of high quality. Inaccuracy affects the usefulness of prognostic information. Errors or inconsistencies can occur due to interobserver variability, variability in the degree of information gathering, and inappropriate variable definitions. Using stage assignment as an example, random or systematic error can be produced when different observers with different skill sets assign stage. If we are comparing two populations of patients who were staged by different types of raters, with different skill sets, the group that is less skilled may introduce more random error and/or make systematic errors in assignment. Even in the presence of accurate stage assignment, if one study group is subject to more diagnostic imaging than another, upstaging of the former is likely, invoking a systematic bias known as *stage migration.*[1,2]

Predictive modeling combines information about prognostic factors to refine the assessment of prognosis by considering the combined, independent effects of those factors. The goal is to shift the predicted outcome probability away from ambivalence (a probability of 0.5) toward certainty (a probability of 1 or 0). Formal development and use of predictive models is rare in clinical practice. Although such analyses are preferred, it must be recognized that even when the most refined predictive model is used, all a physician can do is make a prediction of average outcome for a specific subgroup of patients into which the patient falls. There will always be variability of outcome within any subgroup. That is, we will never be able to predict with certainty whether a given patient will or will not experience a particular outcome (a probability of 1 or 0).

The relevant prognostic factors will vary depending on the purpose at hand. First, prognostic factors can play a role in the prediction of some outcomes and not others. For example, age may play a minimal role in predicting local control when other prognostic factors are taken into account, and weight loss may play a role in predicting palliative outcomes, whereas it may have no predictive value when the outcome is local control. Second, the prognostic factors of interest can actually relate to a competing risk rather than outcomes of the index disease. For instance, we might study comorbid diseases as prognostic factors for early, other-cause death in patients with curable prostate cancer. Third, a prognostic factor may be able to distinguish those who will benefit from treatment from those who will not. This is true in the decision to use tamoxifen in breast cancer, where knowledge of estrogen receptor status affects the decision. Fourth, when making prediction of future outcome, the factor need only make an independent contribution, the goal being maximal precision in the prediction. For this purpose, therefore, the factor need not be causally related to outcome; being a marker of risk status is sufficient. Fifth, when making predictions for patients whose disease type and severity overwhelms their future, the role of other prognostic factors may become unimportant. This can happen both in the case of advanced, severe disease and in the case of diseases that are highly curable in that the predicted probabilities of outcome, using information about disease severity only, are close to 0 and 1, respectively. Last, despite the needs of the study, the choice of prognostic factors that can be considered for development of a useful prediction tool is often constrained by the data that are available. Unfortunately, the inability to account for known prognostic factors increases the variance observed within prognostic subgroups, thereby decreasing the accuracy of prediction away from certainty (probability of 1 or 0) for a specific case.

The most important consideration for the development of a predictive tool is its usefulness to the clinician. The concept of medical meaningfulness was defined by

Wood as "the extent to which knowledge of a patient's case type alone — without other information about the individual patient — conveys clinical expectations and enables clinicians to exchange information about those expectations."[3] The opinions of clinicians about the usefulness of a prognostic model are important, as they are almost always the intended users. Nonsensical associations that do not fit with understood biologic and social effects, even if they are predictive, will rightly be considered invalid by clinicians. Such models are likely unstable, meaning that they would not be repeatable in other, similar settings. Also, patients who are grouped using a predictive tool based on their prognostic similarity may not actually have similar medical profiles. The clinical usefulness and interpretability of such predictive tools are then compromised. Intuitive understanding of the reasons for grouping certain patients is therefore necessary for clinical acceptance of a given prognostic scoring or grouping system.

Predictive studies can be conducted using data from most study designs. Secondary analyses using data from a clinical trial can assess the ability of collected prognostic variables to predict outcome, although the patients enrolled in trials are usually not representative of all patients with the disease. Only the control or standard treatment patients can be studied, and treatment assignment can be considered as a control variable. Data from case series and cohort studies can also be used. Ideally, a cohort of patients representing all persons with the disease should be assembled to achieve valid prediction. At least, the study population should consist of an inception cohort (patients identified at a similar time in the course of their disease) that was followed for a sufficient time to determine the outcome of interest.[4,5] Although a case control study can assess the relative importance of prognostic factors on outcome, data from these studies cannot be used to assess absolute risk unless the study population is nested within a defined cohort.

In all study designs, the contribution made by individual prognostic factors is often determined using statistical significance. The magnitude of the association between a prognostic factor and the outcome, however, does not address that factor's ability to predict that outcome. The percent variance explained is a more appropriate approach for this purpose.[6-10] Percent variance explained can be calculated for all the common multivariable models, which, in general, involves a comparison of predicted to observed values. This measure can be used to assess both the contribution of individual variables and also the predictive ability of the entire model.[7,11-13] After a predictive model is defined, model validation should occur by using one of various approaches to splitting the data into training and test sets and/or by independent validation on another data set entirely. Different statistical techniques are used to derive predictive models, including multivariable modeling, recursive partitioning, conjunctive consolidation, and neural networks.

Multivariable modeling uses whichever approach is relevant for the outcome of interest (for example, Cox regression is a common choice when survival outcomes are being assessed[14]). Problems with small numbers are mediated through the underlying mathematical model, which makes assumptions about the relationship among the effects. These approaches allow the investigator to compute the independent effects of various prognostic factors as long as the model assumptions are not violated (for example, Cox regression requires that the survival curves distinguished by the study variables be proportional to each other). The prognostic factor effects can then be combined to calculate the probability of outcome for specific patient types. Assigning prognosis in the clinical setting using the output from a multivariable model requires some mathematical manipulation and arbitrary allocation of missing variable values. Also, without reference to the input values, it is not apparent what kind of case is being described for a given prognostic score. That is, patients with differing clinical characteristics can achieve the same score.[15] Sometimes, models are used to define prognostic groups, often by the number of factors present, but this approach may be subject to problems with variation in prognosis among the members of the group and may not reflect an adequate clinical description of patient type. Multivariable approaches are described in more detail in Chapter 3.

Recursive partitioning involves multiple splits to isolate prognostically similar groups. These are tree-based approaches, which are transparent to the clinician. They may, however, ignore important variables when the effects of those variables do not provide any further useful partitions from what has already been defined. As discussed in Chapter 3, these approaches can also lead to unstable results and so careful validation is important. Assumptions about linear relationships among variables are avoided and the approach is useful for identifying complex interactions that may be missed with regression techniques. The resulting trees are easy to use in clinical practice.

Conjunctive consolidation, which has been proposed by Feinstein,[15] uses stratified analysis to combine categories both within levels of a given variable (which he labels sequential sequestration) and the combinations of these major variables (which he labels conjunctive consolidation). The criteria for combining in both instances include both biologic coherence and statistical homogeneity, or *isometry*. Compromises in meeting both criteria are necessary in order to produce a reasonable number of clinically useful prognostic categories. The approach is very labor intensive and will be affected more than the mathematical modeling approach by subjective decisions of the developer.

Like recursive partitioning, neural networks use information about prognostic factors with fewer restrictive mathematical assumptions than multiple regression techniques. Neural networks can handle the complex interactions that occur when we are trying to predict a biologic process. Obstacles to their use include: difficulties identifying factors that are not playing a role in prediction, which can lead to the collection of unnecessary data elements; difficulties interpreting the output of a neural network, which is only directly interpretable as a probability under certain circumstances,[16] and the inability to assign confidence levels to the output. Details of the method are presented in Chapter 3.

The use of neural networks for clinical prediction is still in the developmental stages. Physicians may have more problems accepting predictions from a neural network than from trees or regression models because the origin of the predictions (how the prognostic factors are used to make the prediction) are not apparent.

Recent work attempts to mitigate this problem.[17] Problems interpreting the role of specific prognostic factors will likely persist, however, due to the complex transformations that are usually made to the input values.[16]

STUDIES OF TREATMENT EFFECTIVENESS

The most common goal of clinical research on patients with cancer is to identify management strategies that alter important outcomes for the better. Both experimental and observational analytic study approaches can be used for this purpose.[18,19] Although experimental approaches are preferred, they are not feasible in every situation. Even so, the use of observational analytic designs (cohort and case control) to assess intended treatment effects is uncommon.

Much of what is known about outcomes of treatment is based on descriptive studies of case series, despite the fact that formal tests of treatment effectiveness cannot be conducted in these studies because the design precludes an explicit control group. Such studies are subject to problems of external validity because they are single institution series, usually from tertiary-care teaching institutions, whose patient populations are not representative because of referral bias.

Prognostic factors have a role in all three study designs. In both analytic approaches (randomized trials and observational studies), prognostic factors are considered in subject selection, determination of the consistency of treatment effectiveness among subgroups, and extrapolation of results.[18] In descriptive studies (case series), prognostic description of the study population and consideration of important prognostic subgroups also plays a role because this information allows a clinician to consider whether a given patient is like those in the series. If so, similar outcomes may occur with use of the recommended treatment.

The choice of prognostic factors to include in research depends on the purpose of the study. For instance, the stage of disease progression under study can affect the choice of relevant prognostic factors. In palliative care studies, weight loss and symptomatic status would play an important role in the evaluation of outcome, whereas these factors would be less important in curative treatment studies where the study population comprises cases with early disease.

When considering research findings in relation to an individual patient for the purpose of treatment selection, one often discovers that important prognostic variables have not been considered in the presentation of study results. When trying to assess the benefit-to-risk, or therapeutic, ratio of a given treatment alternative for a given patient, the physician may know that certain aspects of the patient's disease or health status will play a role that cannot be assessed from the evidence available. That is, the therapeutic ratio for this patient may be different from what was presented as the study result. One solution would be for researchers to consider all important prognostic subgroups in the design of clinical trials or observational studies, conduct formal assessment of the consistency of treatment and adverse outcome effects, and present the results of subgroup analyses when needed. Conversely, researchers should acknowledge the limitations to generalizability of their study results, reminding clinicians that the results may not apply to certain types of patients.

Often, there are trade-offs when conducting treatment effectiveness research between the inclusion of a wide range of patients with enough subjects in each subgroup to perform meaningful analyses and study resource limitations. More importantly, there are also trade-offs between the level of prognostic detail a study can consider and the number of patients available in such subgroups. Even if researchers are willing to limit subject selection to a very homogeneous study population, or even if they have the resources to assess subgroup effects, the number of subjects available may be limited. The increasing use of meta-analysis, which combines results across many studies (usually clinical trials), is one vehicle that could be used to deal with this dilemma. This is especially true if the original data were obtained. Then the consistency of the therapeutic ratio across subgroups could be addressed.

Inappropriate groupings may occur among the levels of a given prognostic factor when a researcher seeks to increase the size of a study population, or when groups have been defined without regard to variability among the members. If inappropriate stage groupings are used to select study subjects, the prognosis for some may lie outside the intended target group for the study. If a grouping scheme creates groups whose members have very different prognoses, the ability to control for stage differences in the analyses is compromised.

If prognostic factors are ignored when comparing outcomes of treatment, study results can be biased in a number of ways. There can be confounding by indication, which occurs when the treatment a patient receives is dependent on the disease severity or underlying health status (treatment selection bias). Patients can self-select by being more or less likely to be compliant or to seek help initially (self-selection bias). The patients seen in a particular institution can vary from the general population of patients with that disease (referral bias). The effect of each of these biases is partly or wholly due to systematic differences in prognosis between those who receive treatment and those who do not. To control for these biases in analytic studies, the researcher must ensure that the control group is prognostically similar to the treated group either through randomization, matching, or statistical analysis. Accounting for prognostic factors in analytic studies permits isolation of the effect of treatment.

In a clinical trial, randomization is conducted to attempt to control not only for known, but also for unknown prognostic factors. This is the single most important reason that this study design is preferred. In such studies, prognostic factors only need to be considered when subgroup analyses are planned or in the unlikely (unlucky) event that the treatment and control groups differ by known prognostic factors. In observational studies, consideration of prognostic factors is crucial and many argue that control of these factors may not be possible.[4] The threat of unknown factors looms large, as does the possibility that a given factor could completely confound the study of a treatment effect (all patients of a certain type only get one treatment). To minimize the bias due to differences in prognosis, some advocate an approach to observational study design that mimics the randomized trial as closely as possible, particularly regarding the use of admission criteria. [18] In any event, it is difficult to critically appraise such studies due to the necessarily complex designs and analyses. This is, possibly, one reason that these designs are not often used to assess intended treatment effects.[19]

An alternative observational analytic design that may be more likely to avoid the unknown prognosis problem is the instrumental variables approach, which has been adopted from econometrics.[19–22] This approach takes advantage of the variations in clinical opinion about best treatment that can occur when evidence is lacking. When difference in clinical opinion adheres (roughly) to some way of grouping patients that is not associated with outcome, the natural experiments that result can be exploited to learn about the marginal effect of the differences in the treatment distributions on outcome. Geography often defines such study groups (as the instrumental variable) when the use of treatment varies systematically among regions either due to local clinical culture[23] or due to differences in access.[24] The assumption of no direct effect of the instrumental variable on outcome needs to be carefully considered.[25,26] Bias can result if there are differences between the patient populations on factors other than treatment that can affect outcome. Such differences might be due to case mix, overall life expectancy, or the health system itself. Since this approach is population-based, data collection is problematic. The approach lends itself to the use of existing large administrative and clinical data sets, but these usually contain less information about prognosis than desired, so that the ability to examine the assumption of similar case mix may be compromised. This study design has not yet been widely used, but the increasing proliferation of electronic data collection will enhance its feasibility.

Thus when a hypothesis about the effectiveness of a given treatment is tested, the reasoning regarding the role of prognostic factors is the same no matter which analytic approach is used. Outcomes are observed following the use of some therapy in a group of patients with the same diagnosis. The presence of an appropriate control group allows the researcher to establish whether, and to what extent, the association between therapy and outcome is causal and not explained by some factor other than treatment. Avoiding bias using the experimental design means that the control group is drawn from the same population as the experimental group. Avoiding bias in observational designs means that an attempt is made to identify cases that were treated differently but arose from a similar patient population. The control group in an observational study could be concurrent or historical. Note, however, that the use of historical controls is more problematic, as new knowledge not related to the treatment being assessed may confound the association. Statistical adjustment for differences in prognostic factor distributions is almost always necessary in observational studies. In descriptive studies, such as case series, controls are imaginary cases based on the investigator's, or the reader's, synthesis of previous experience and reports in the literature. The product in this instance is the probability of the outcome rather than relative effectiveness.

When the critical outcome of the illness always occurs in the absence of therapy, it may not be necessary to carry out an analytic study. That is, as with the study of outcome prediction, the role of prognostic factors becomes much less important when the disease itself dictates the outcome, even to the point that there is no need for an explicit control group. In these instances, deviations from the previous pattern of behavior of the disease among treated cases can fairly be attributed to the treatment itself. Actually, this is the reasoning used in nonrandomized clinical Phase II studies in cancer, where we are comfortable that the disease would have progressed inexorably without therapy, and therefore shrinkage of tumor occurring in a treated group can fairly be attributed to the treatment. Similar reasoning was also applied to the evaluation of cytotoxic chemotherapy in previously uniformly lethal entities such as nonseminomatous testicular cancer, acute leukemia, and the lymphomas.

As the prediction of outcome becomes more uncertain, the importance of prognostic factors increases. With this comes a need for more data collection on each case, more careful identification of cases, the inclusion of a control group, and more sophisticated analyses. Larger study samples are needed to establish that an observed difference is actually due to treatment, or that the sample size problem can be alleviated through subject selection because the more similar the study subjects are on prognosis, the more easily a treatment effect can be isolated. At the same time, subject selection can reduce the generalizability of the study findings if prognosis is associated with treatment effectiveness. This problem is not exclusive to observational studies because the identification of a study population with uniform prognostic profiles is not achieved through randomization, but through the use of entry criteria and/or stratification. The efficiency of the clinical research process for assessing treatment effectiveness therefore depends on maximizing the use of prognostic factors to minimize the variance in treatment effectiveness due to these prognostic factors.

STUDIES OF DISEASE PROGRESSION AND TREATMENT RESISTANCE

Prognostic factors that predict disease progression or resistance to treatment may have a causal relationship to outcome. Any factors that play such a role become legitimate targets for interventions designed to modify the natural history of the disease or reduce treatment resistance. One example of such a factor would be the prognostic association between hypoxia and the outcome of radiotherapy. Such observations lead to hypotheses that can be tested using various research techniques, both experimental (on cells, animals, or humans) and observational. The hypoxia observation contributed to an increased understanding of the role that oxygen plays in radiation sensitivity and the subsequent use of hyperbaric oxygen, high linear energy transfer (LET) radiotherapy, and hypoxic cell sensitizers.

Prognostic factors that modify outcome may also be associated with a cause of the disease. One line of inquiry in etiologic cancer research, for instance, is to understand at the cellular and molecular levels the events that determine the natural history of the disease. The possibility that such prognostic factors are markers for disease progression may also point to underlying mechanisms leading to the occurrence of disease. In a similar manner, risk factors for disease may also predict poor prognosis.

HEALTH SERVICES RESEARCH

Health services research is "the scientific inquiry that produces knowledge about the resources, provision, organizing, financing, and policies of health services at the population level."[27] Study of health system processes is the first step to improvement of those processes that then lead to better patient care.

The clinically relevant goals of health services research involve the provision of information about the effectiveness, efficiency, and appropriateness of medical care. Prognostic factors must be an integral part of such studies. Models that describe health services research acknowledge this point,[27,28] but the work that is most clinically relevant, outcomes research and the study of practice variations, often does not adequately address variations in prognosis or the role of prognostic factors.

Outcomes studies assess quality of care by making comparisons across hospitals, individual or groups of physicians, health plans, and health systems. Similarity of case mix between the compared populations is addressed through a process known as *risk adjustment*, which is accomplished using knowledge about the prognostic characteristics of diagnostic codes in administrative data.[28] Because of sample size problems and the desire to study the quality of the entire system, risk adjustment is more often accomplished using statistical approaches than through restricting the selection of study subjects.

When practice patterns are compared across populations (geographic or secular), assumptions of case mix similarity must be defended and procedure rates are often adjusted for the most accessible prognostic information: age and sex. These studies are compromised by unobserved variations in rate of disease among communities. Interestingly, the existence of cancer registries provides the opportunity to control for rate differences because the study population can be restricted to those with the disease. Practice patterns can be studied within the cancer patient population using administrative data that have been linked to these registries.[29-31]

Control for prognostic factors in health services research is necessary so that the causes of practice and outcome variations can be isolated. Study factors that can have an impact on outcome include: compromised availability of resources, variability in clinical judgement, patient expectation or demand, and prevailing custom.[32] Some study factors are, in other contexts, prognostic factors. For instance, compromised access to care may be occurring only in disadvantaged groups. Those socioeconomic factors that identify such groups may be recognized prognostic factors for many adverse outcomes. Compromised access may be the more proximal reason for the higher rates of adverse outcomes. For example, if we find that lower socioeconomic status predisposes breast cancer patients to worse survival, further investigation may identify the cause as higher stage of disease at presentation, which points to problems in access to screening and/or awareness of the importance of breast self examination. Conversely, we may find that those patients whose breast cancer was not identified by a screening mammography were more likely to come from socioeconomically disadvantaged groups. In either case, the modifiable cause is access to screening mammography and education about breast self-examination.

SUMMARY

Known prognostic factors play a role in clinical research through their ability to predict outcome, identify like cases, confound the effects of study variables, and cause disease progression or even the disease itself. When designing a clinical research study, inclusion of prognostic factors as study variables must be considered and all potentially relevant prognostic factors should be included in the list of study variables. The collection of these data along with the formal use of control groups allows the researcher to address prognostic bias. Proper consideration of prognostic factors in clinical research improves the evidence that then results in better patient care across all aspects: better prognostication, better treatment decisions, and an improved health care system.

REFERENCES

1. Bradford Hill A: Principles of medical statistics. *Lancet* 1937.
2. Feinstein AR: The Will Rodgers phenomenon: stage migration and new diagnostic techniques as a source of misleading statistics for survival in cancer. *N Engl J Med* 312:1604–8, 1985.
3. Wood WR, Ament RP, Kobrinski KJ: A foundation for hospital case mix measurement. *Inquiry* 18:247–54, 1981.
4. Sackett DL, Haynes B, Guyatt G, et al.: *Clinical epidemiology: a basic science for clinical medicine.* 2d ed. Boston, Little, Brown, 1991.
5. Laupacis A, Wells G, Richardson WS, Tugwell P: Users' guides to the medical literature: V. How to use an article about prognosis. *JAMA* 272:234–7, 1994.
6. Korn EL, Simon R: Measures of explained variation for survival data. *Stat Med* 9:487–503, 1990.
7. Korn EL, Simon R: Explained residual variation, explained risk, and goodness of fit. *Am Stat* 45:201–6, 1991.
8. Schemper M: The relative importance of prognostic factors in studies of survival. *Stat Med* 12:2377–82, 1993.
9. Henderson R: Problems and prediction in survival-data analysis. *Stat Med* 14:161–84, 1995.
10. Krongrad A, Lai H, Lai S: Variation in prostate cancer survival explained by significant prognostic factors. *J Urol* 158:1487–90, 1997.

11. Kleinbaum DG, Kupper LL: *Applied regression analysis and other multivariable methods*. Boston, Duxbury Press, 1978.

12. Schemper M, Stare J: Explained variation in survival analysis. *Stat Med* 15:1999–2012, 1996.

13. Mittlbock M, Schemper M: Explained variation for logistic regression. *Stat Med* 15:1987–97, 1996.

14. Cox DR: Regression models and life-tables. *J R Stat Soc B* 34:187–202, 1972.

15. Feinstein AR, Wells CK: A clinical-severity staging system for patients with lung cancer. *Medicine* 69:1–33, 1990.

16. Tu JV: Advantages and disadvantages of using artificial neural networks versus logistic regression for predicting medical outcomes. *J Clin Epidemiol* 49:1225–31, 1996.

17. Clark GM, Hilsenbeck SG, Ravdin PM, et al.: Prognostic factors: rationale and methods of analysis and integration. *Breast Cancer Res Treat* 32:105–12, 1994.

18. Feinstein AR: *Clinical epidemiology: the architecture of clinical research*. Philadelphia, Saunders, 1985.

19. Selby JV: Case-control evaluations of treatment and program efficacy. *Epidemiol Rev* 16:90–101, 1994.

20. Imbens A, Angrist J: Identification and estimation of local average treatment effects. *Econometrica* 62:467–76, 1994.

21. Newhouse JP, McClellan M: Econometrics in outcomes research: the use of instrumental variables. *Annu Rev Public Health* 19:17–34, 1998.

22. McClellan M, McNeil B, Newhouse JP: Does more intensive treatment of acute myocardial infarction in the elderly reduce mortality? *JAMA* 272:859–66, 1994.

23. Groome PA, Mackillop WJ, Rothwell D, et al.: The management and outcome of glottic cancer: a population-based comparison between Ontario, Canada and the SEER areas of the United States. *J Otolaryngol* 29:67–77, 2000.

24. McClellan M, McNeil B, Newhouse JP: Does more intensive treatment of acute myocardial infarction in the elderly reduce mortality? *JAMA* 272:859–66, 1994.

25. Naylor CD: Ecological analysis of intended treatment effects: caveat emptor (editorial). *J Clin Epidemiol* 52:1–5, 1999.

26. Groome PA, Mackillop WJ: Re: Uses of ecologic studies in the assessment of intended treatment effects (letter). *J Clin Epidemiol* 52:903, 1999.

27. Shi L: *Health services research methods*. Albany (NY), Delmar, 1997.

28. Lezzoni LI: *Risk adjustment for measuring healthcare outcomes*, 2d ed. Chicago, Health Administration Press, 1997.

29. Potosky AL, Riley GF, Lubitz JD, et al.: Potential for cancer related health services research using a linked medicare-tumor registry database. *Med Care* 31:732–48, 1993.

30. Mackillop WJ, Groome PA, Zhang-Salomons J, et al.: Does a centralized radiotherapy system provide adequate access to care? *J Clin Oncol* 15:1261–71, 1997.

31. Mackillop WJ, Dixon P, Zhou Y, et al.: Variations in the management and outcome of non-small cell lung cancer in Ontario. *Radiother Oncol* 32:106–15, 1994.

32. Anderson TV, Mooney G, (eds.): *The challenges of medical practice variations*. London, Macmillan, 1990.

CHAPTER 10

Measuring the Accuracy of Prognostic Judgments

WILLIAM J. MACKILLOP, EMMA BARTFAY, PATTI A. and GROOME

> The practical test of a true science is the power it confers of prevision, or of knowing now what will follow hereafter. When we can prognosticate with certainty, medicine will have become a science.
>
> — H. Hartshorne, *A system of medicine*

Prognosis can be defined as, "a forecasting of the probable course and termination of an illness."[1] In the clinical practice of oncology the prognosis is important because it may determine the optimal choice of treatment, and because patients often want to know what is going to happen to them in order to prepare themselves for the future (see Chapter 1). Given that prognostic judgments are used as a basis for important decisions, we need to know how accurate they are. We may not yet be able to achieve the "certainty" in prognosis that Hartshorne envisaged as a characteristic of the scientific medicine,[2] but we should at least be able to measure the predictive value of our prognostic judgments, and take this into account in our decision making. It is generally accepted today that we should not place reliance on the results of diagnostic tests without knowing their accuracy, and the same principle should apply to prognostic judgments. However, while modern textbooks of clinical epidemiology deal thoroughly with methods for measuring the accuracy of diagnostic tests,[3,4] much less has been written about how to measure the accuracy of prognosis.

Although there is a very extensive literature about prognostic factors in cancer, there have been very few reports relating to the accuracy of prognostic judgments in practice in individual cases. In this chapter, we are concerned mainly with the quality of prognostic judgments at the level of the individual patient. This is much more of a challenge than predicting the outcome of groups of cases. Once

Prognostic Factors in Cancer, 2nd edition, Edited by Mary K. Gospodarowicz
ISBN 0-471-40633-3 Copyright © 2001 Wiley-Liss, Inc.

the average outcome of a specific medical problem has been established in a large group of cases, the average outcome in another large group of similar cases may be predicted with great precision. However, a precise knowledge of the average outcome of an illness may have little or no predictive value in the individual case. For example, if a large group of patients with a specific stage of a specific cancer has been observed to have a 5-year survival of 50% then we can be confident that if a large group of similar cases is managed in the same way in future, it will also have a 5-year survival of about 50%. When we try to use this information to predict the outcome in the next case of this illness that we encounter, however, it translates into a probability of 5-year survival of 0.5; In other words, it leaves us in a state of complete uncertainty.

The main objectives of this chapter are to describe methods that can be used to measure the accuracy of prognosis at the level of the individual case, and to review what little is known about the accuracy of prognostic judgments in oncology. We end by considering factors that may limit the degree of "certainty" that we can ever expect to achieve in prognosis in oncology.

DEFINITIONS

The quality of prognostic judgments in medicine can be described using the terminology that is generally used to describe the quality of judgments and measurements in other fields. The terms *accuracy* or *accurate* are commonly employed to describe the closeness of a measurement or judgment to the true value of the quantity of interest,[5] and the same terms can also be used to describe how close a prognostic judgment comes to the outcome that is subsequently observed.[6,7] The term accurate can also be used to describe an instrument for making measurements.[5] The degree of accuracy of the instrument is measured by how closely, on average, its measurements approximate the corresponding true values in a series of observations.[5] Similarly, the term accuracy can be applied to the performance of a clinician in predicting the outcome of an illness.[6,7] The accuracy of the prognosticator is measured by how closely the predictions approximate the observed outcomes in a series of cases.[6,7] The accuracy of a measuring instrument is determined by the extent to which it is affected by *random* and *systematic error*. The term *precision* is used to describe the extent to which a measuring instrument is free of random error,[5,8] and the term *calibration* is used to describe the extent to which it is free of systematic error.[6,9] These concepts can also be useful in describing prognostic judgments. The term *discrimination* is used to describe the extent to which a test or judgment distinguishes between two states. It is a concept borrowed from the signal-detection theory that has been widely used to evaluate diagnostic tests.[10,11] In the field of prognosis it has been used to measure the ability of prognostic judgment to distinguish between those patients who will be alive, and those patients who will be dead at a specified time in the future.[12,13]

TYPES OF PROGNOSTIC JUDGMENT

A prediction about the life expectancy of an incurable patient can be stated in months or years, and the outcome can be measured in the same units. Here, both the prediction and the outcome take the form of a continuous variable, and the accuracy of a prediction in an individual case is measured by how close it comes to the observed outcome. The accuracy of a series of such judgments is described by the average closeness of the predictions to the observed outcomes.[5] In contrast, predictions about the outcome of treatment in potentially curable patients are usually stated in terms of the chance of surviving, or of remaining disease-free, at some future time.[6,7] Here, the prediction takes the form of a probability expressed on a scale from 0 to 1, or from 0% to 100%. The outcome, however, is dichotomous; the patient either dies or does not die. The accuracy of such predictions is also measured by how close the prediction comes to the observed outcome, but a somewhat different approach is required to describe the accuracy of a series of such predictions.

In the following section, we deal first with ways of describing the accuracy of predictions concerning outcomes that take the form of a continuous variable, and then address the more complex issues involved in measuring the accuracy of predictions concerning dichotomous outcomes.

DESCRIBING THE ACCURACY OF PROGNOSIS

Outcomes Described by a Continuous Variable

Graphical Methods

The Scatter Plot   The relationship between predictions of duration of survival and the actual duration of survival in a series of cases can be described using a scatter plot of the type shown in Figure 10.1. This example comes from a prospective study of 468 terminally ill patients in which doctors provided a survival estimate at the time of referral to a hospice program.[14] The dots corresponding to cases in which the predictions were correct, lie along the diagonal. Dots above the diagonal correspond to cases in which survival was underestimated, and dots below the diagonal correspond to cases in which survival was overestimated. The average closeness of the dots to the line is a measure of the average accuracy of the judgments. In the series of cases illustrated in Figure 10.1, the dots are widely dispersed, indicating that the predictions are imprecise. There are obviously more dots above the diagonal than below it, indicating that these predictions were also poorly calibrated and that they systematically overestimated survival in this group of patients.

An alternative, and perhaps preferable approach, would be to plot the difference between the predicted survival and the observed survival as a function of the observed survival. This method has been used to describe the degree of agreement between two sets of observations, and may provide a clearer

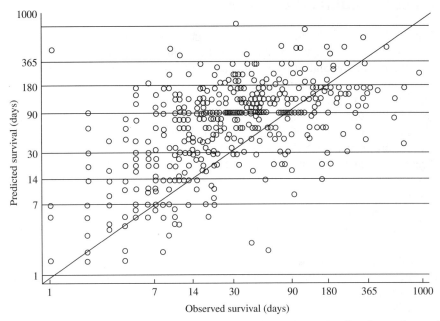

Figure 10.1 Predictions of survival in terminally ill patients. Predicted vs. observed survival in 468 terminally ill hospice patients. The diagonal line represents perfect prediction. Patients above the diagonal line are those in whom survival was overestimated; patients below the line are those in whom survival was underestimated. (From Christakis and Lamont.[14])

impression of the degree of random and systematic variation between predictions and outcomes.[15,16]

Quantitative Methods

The accuracy of this type of prediction can be quantified in terms applied to describe forecasts in other settings: the mean absolute error (MAE); the mean absolute percentage error (MAPE); the root-mean-square error (RMSE); and the root-mean-square percentage error (RMSPE).[17-19] Where p_i is the predicted value of the variable, and a_i is its actual value, these quantities are defined as follows:

The mean absolute error

$$\text{MAE} = \frac{\sum_{i=1}^{n} |p_i - a_i|}{n}$$

The mean absolute percentage error

$$\text{MAPE} = \frac{\sum\limits_{i=1}^{n} |100(p_i - a_i)/a_i|}{n}$$

The root-mean-square error

$$\text{RMSE} = \sqrt{\frac{\sum\limits_{i=1}^{n} (p_i - a_i)^2}{n}}$$

The root-mean-square percentage error

$$\text{RMSPE} = \sqrt{\frac{\sum\limits_{i=1}^{n} (100(p_i - a_i)/a_i)^2}{n}}$$

The unit-free measures, MAPE and RMSPE, are used more frequently in forecasting.[19]

Dichotomous Outcomes

Graphical Methods

The relationship between probabilistic predictions and dichotomous outcomes can also be displayed graphically.

The Reliability Diagram Figure 10.2 illustrates the results of a study in which doctors were asked to predict the probability of cure in a hundred recently diagnosed cases of cancer.[7] Five years later, these predictions were compared with the observed disease-free survival. The results are shown in what is referred to as a *calibration curve* or reliability diagram.[6] Each dot here corresponds to a subgroup of cases rather than an individual case. Patients were first classified into subgroups according to the probability of survival assigned to them (see Caption to Fig. 10.2). The actual outcome for each subgroup was then determined, and plotted against the average probability predicted for the subgroup. Dots corresponding to groups of cases in which average outcome exactly matched the average prediction lie on the diagonal line of perfect calibration. Points above the diagonal line represent subgroups in which the probability of cure was underestimated, and points below the diagonal line represent subgroups in which the probability of survival was overestimated. In the series of cases illustrated in Figure 10.2, the clinicians' predictions of the probability of cure were well calibrated. This type of analysis is simple to do, easy to understand, and useful

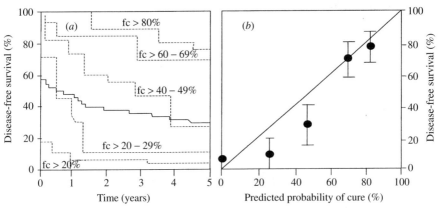

Figure 10.2   Calibration of doctors' estimates of probability of cure. (*a*) Disease-free survival of all 98 patients (——) and of subgroups of patients defined by their doctors' estimates of their probability of cure (- -). Two patients who died of other causes with no evidence of cancer were censored in this analysis. The number of patients in each prognostic subgroup were as follows: $f_c = 0\%$, $n = 42$; $f_c \geq 0$–19%, $n = 6$; $f_c = 20$–39%, $n = 11$; $f_c = 40$–59%, $n = 12$; $f_c = 60$–79%, $n = 13$; and $f_c \geq 80\%$, $n = 14$. (*b*) The mean estimated probability of cure of each subgroup is plotted against the observed disease-free survival rate at 5 years ($\pm$S.E.). The solid diagonal line represents perfect calibration. (From Mackillop and Quirt.[7])

in revealing systematic errors in prognostic judgments.[6] However, it does not describe individual outcomes as a function of individual predictions, and random errors are obscured by the averaging of outcomes within subgroups.

The Covariance Graph   Figure 10.3 illustrates the same data in the form of a covariance graph. This graph shows the relationship between prediction and outcome for each case individually.[20] The upper panel of Figure 10.3 shows a frequency distribution of the estimates of probability of cure that were initially assigned to patients who subsequently remained alive and free of recurrence for 5 years. The lower panel of Figure 10.3 shows a frequency distribution of the estimates of probability of cure initially assigned to those who subsequently developed a recurrence or died within 5 years.[7] Although the modes of the distributions in the upper and lower panels are widely separated, the distributions overlap, and there is no cutoff point in the predictions that perfectly separates curable from incurable patients. These results are similar to those of a diagnostic test that produces higher values in subjects who have a given disease than for those who do not, but which does not perfectly distinguish between them. The specificity of such a test can be increased by increasing the arbitrary decision criterion used to distinguish "positive" from "negative" results, but this is achieved only at the expense of a concurrent decrease in sensitivity. These concepts, which have been widely used in diagnosis,[3,4] are also applicable to prognosis.[12,13] By way of illustration, consider the vertical dotted line in

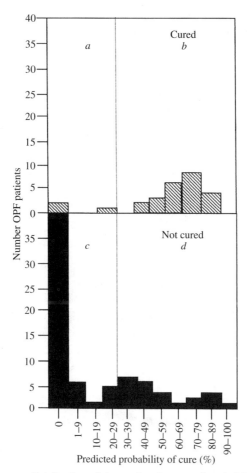

Figure 10.3   Frequency distribution of doctors' estimates of probability of cure. Patients were subgrouped according to their outcome, then further subgrouped based on their assigned probability of cure. The upper panel (*a, b*) shows doctors' estimates of probability of cure for patients alive and cancer-free at five years, and the lower panel (*c, d*) shows doctors' estimates of the probability of cure for patients "not cured" (dead, or alive with cancer at 5 years). An arbitrary cutoff point, or decision criterion, to the right of which patients might be labeled curable, and to the left of which patients might be labeled incurable, is shown as a vertical dotted line. (From Mackillop and Quirt.[7])

Figure 10.3 as the cutoff point, or decision criterion, to the right of which patients are labeled curable, and to the left of which they are labeled incurable. Area (*b*) of Figure 10.3 contains the subgroup of 5-year disease-free survivors that would be classified as curable on the basis of this decision criterion. These true predictions of cure are equivalent to the true positives in a diagnostic test. Similarly, the predictions in area (*c*) are true predictions of failure or true negatives, those in area (*a*) are false predictions of failure or false negatives, and those in area

(d) are false predictions of cure or false positives. The sensitivity of these prognostic judgments is given by $b/(b+a)$, and the specificity by $c/(c+d)$. As the decision criterion is moved to the right, specificity increases while the sensitivity decreases.

The ROC Curve   The relationship between sensitivity and specificity, as the decision criterion is changed, is shown in the receiver operating characteristic (ROC) curve displayed in Figure 10.4. The area under the ROC curve (A_{ROC}) is a measure of the discrimination of the prognostic judgments.[21,22] For these data $A_{ROC} = 0.91 \pm 0.09$, which indicates that there is a probability of 0.91 that the doctor, in assessing any randomly selected pair of cancer patients, one of whom is curable and the other not, will assign a higher probability of cure to the curable patient. An area of 1.0 indicates perfect discrimination, whereas an area of 0.5 indicates no discrimination.[21,22]

Scoring Rules

The Brier Score   Weather forecasters have developed rules for scoring the accuracy of individual forecasts, depending on how closely they match the observed outcome.[23,24] One example is the Brier score. Where p_i is the predicted probability of cure and y_i the actual outcome for patient i, and where $y_i = 1$ if the patient is cured and $y_i = 0$ if the patient is not cured, the Brier score for

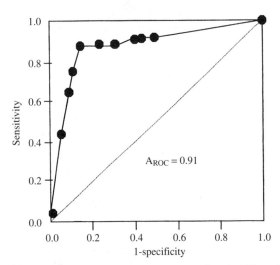

Figure 10.4   The discrimination of doctors' estimates of probability of cure. The ROC curve was constructed from the crude data shown in Figure 10.3, using each probability of cure estimate as a decision criterion. Sensitivity = $b/(a+b)$, and specificity = $c/(c+d)$, where a, b, c, and d are as defined in Figure 10.3. The dashed diagonal line shows the relationship that would be observed if there were no discrimination ($A_{ROC} = 0.5$). (From Mackillop and Quirt.[7])

patient i may be expressed as

$$B_i = (p_i - y_i)^2$$

and the average Brier score for a group of n patients is given by

$$\overline{B} = \frac{\sum_{i=1}^{n} (p_i - y_i)^2}{n}$$

The Brier score can range from 0 for a perfect prediction to 1 for the worst possible prediction. This scoring system has been applied to clinical forecasts in a variety of different settings.[25,26] This approach is useful in studies of prognosis because statistical methods have been developed to compare the accuracy of two sets of predictions, based on their Brier scores,[27,28] and because a set of Brier scores can be decomposed into separate components that reflect the skill of the prognosticator and the difficulty of the task.[29-31]

Comparing the Accuracy of Forecasts Using the Brier Score   Spiegelhalter has provided a method to test the accuracy of a set of judgments based on the Brier score.[27] The null hypothesis is that the predictions accurately reflect the outcomes, and the test statistic is

$$z = \frac{\overline{B} - E_0(\overline{B})}{\sqrt{V_0(\overline{B})}}$$

where

$$E_0(\overline{B}) = \frac{\sum_{i=1}^{n} p_i(1 - p_i)}{n}$$

is the expected value for the Brier score under H_0, and

$$V_0(\overline{B}) = \frac{\sum_{i=1}^{n} p_i(1 - p_i)(1 - 2p_i)^2}{n^2}$$

is the variance for the Brier score. Hence, z is an approximately standard normal test statistic under H_0.

Redelerier extended the approach to compare accuracy of two sets of predictions.[28] Where p_{1i} and p_{2i} represent the estimated probabilities of cure in the first and second sets of predictions, respectively, and D_1 and D_2 are the differences between the observed and expected Brier scores for the first and second sets of judgments, respectively, we can test the null hypothesis that the two sets of judgments are equally close to their respective expected values, H_0: $D_1 = D_2$. The test statistic is given by

$$z = \frac{D_1 - D_2}{\sqrt{V_{D_1 - D_2}}}$$

where

$$D_1 - D_2 = \frac{2 \sum_{i=1}^{n} (p_{1i} - p_{2i}) \pi_i - (p_{1i} - p_{2i}) y_i}{n}$$

and

$$V_{D_1 - D_2} = \frac{4 \sum_{i=1}^{n} (p_{1i} - p_{2i})^2 \pi_i (1 - \pi_i)}{n^2}$$

is the variance associated with the difference between D_1 and D_2.* If the calculated value of z is larger than the corresponding value in the standard normal table, we reject the null hypothesis and conclude that there is evidence to suggest a difference in accuracy between the two sets of judgments.

Decompositions of the Brier Score   The purpose of decomposing the Brier score is to partition it into components that reflect separately the difficulty of the task and the skill of the forecaster. Methods for decomposing the Brier score were first developed by Murphy, 30 years ago for the purpose of analyzing performance in weather forecasting.[29-31] We will describe here Yates' decomposition,[20,26] a method that we have used previously to analyze prognostic judgments in oncology.[7] It can be viewed in terms of three components: bias, slope, and scatter,[26]

$$B = \overline{d}(1 - \overline{d}) + (\text{bias})^2 + \overline{y}(1 - \overline{y})(\text{slope})(\text{slope} - 2) + \text{scatter}$$

where bias $= \overline{d} - \overline{p}$, is the difference between the actual rate $(\overline{d})$ and the average judgment $(\overline{p})$. It is a measure of overall calibration, and can be thought of as a measure of the doctors' knowledge about the behavior of the disease. This term is also referred to as *reliability-in-the-large*.

The equation slope $= \overline{p}_1 - \overline{p}_0$ is the difference between the average probability of event predicted for those who did have the event $(\overline{p}_1)$ and the average probability of event predicted for those who did not have the event $(\overline{p}_0)$. The larger the value of slope, the better the predictions are at distinguishing between

---

* In the equations π_i is the true (but unknown) probability that $y_i = 1$. In order to use this method to compare the Brier scores, we must first estimate π_i. One option is to assign a value from an external source; another option is to set it equal to the observed frequency in a population. A third option is to use the average of the two estimated probabilities.

patients who will be cured and those who will not be cured. It is a measure of discrimination,

$$\text{scatter} = \frac{N_1 \text{var}(p_1) + N_0 \text{var}(p_0)}{N_1 + N_0}$$

The pooled variance of the two groups is an index of noise, or random error, and, $\bar{d}(1 - \bar{d})$ is the outcome variance. This last variance is beyond the control of the prognosticator, but contributes to the difficulty of the task.

Logistic Regression

Logistic regression is often used as a method for making predictions about binary outcomes in medicine.[32] It can also be used to investigate the relationship between the predicted probability of an outcome and the observed outcome.[10] If we denote the probability of event $(Y = 1)$ with a set of k covariates to be $\Pr(Y = 1 | x_1, x_2, \ldots, x_k)$, the logistic model can be written as

$$\Pr(Y = 1 | x_1, x_2, \ldots, x_k) = \frac{\exp\left(\alpha + \sum_{j=1}^{k} \beta_j x_j\right)}{1 + \exp\left(\alpha + \sum_{j=1}^{k} \beta_j x_j\right)}$$

or

$$\log\left\{\frac{\Pr(Y = 1 | x_1, \ldots, x_k)}{\Pr(Y = 0 | x_1, \ldots, x_k)}\right\} = \alpha + \sum_{j=1}^{k} \beta_j x_j$$

where α is a constant and β_j are the regression coefficients for the k covariates.

When assessing the accuracy of prognosis, the left-hand side of the equation is the logit transformation of the actual probability of the event. One of the covariates on the right-hand side of the equation is the estimated probability of the outcome of interest, and there may or may not be other covariates. A number of methods are available to determine how much of the variance in the outcome is explained by the predicted probabilities. For a useful review of these, see Mittlbock and Schemper.[33]

MEASURING THE ACCURACY OF PROGNOSTIC JUDGMENTS IN ONCOLOGY

Prospective Cohort Studies

Prospective studies of the accuracy of prognosis in oncology can take a long time to complete because the outcomes of interest may not be apparent for several years. This is probably the reason why so few studies of prognostic judgment have been done in the field of cancer medicine, in contrast to the much larger number in critical-care medicine where outcomes are often evaluable within a few days. Most of the few prospective studies of the accuracy of prognosis in oncology have been done in the terminally ill population, where the necessary follow-up time is relatively short.

Pseudoprospective Studies

One approach that can be used to circumvent the requirement for prolonged follow-up is to identify study cases retrospectively after the outcome of interest has declared itself. The cases are then documented carefully, and doctors who are blinded to the outcome are asked to give their prognosis based on the findings at the time of diagnosis.[34,35] One other advantage of the use of case scenarios like this is that it enables the investigator to explore variations in the prognoses assigned by different doctors in the same case. In real life, it is much more difficult to obtain multiple, independent predictions in the same case.[7] Case scenarios, however, necessarily present the clinical findings from the perspective of the investigator, whereas in actual practice different clinicians will choose for themselves what information they will take into consideration, and what they will ignore in reaching their judgments.[7] This study design may therefore underestimate interobserver variation.

Retrospective Studies

Another way of avoiding the need for prolonged follow-up is to study predictions of outcome that have been collected in the past for other purposes. When this approach is taken, it is important to ensure that the forecasts are not biased. It is not, for example, valid to use predictions of duration of survival that were assigned as part of the process for admission to a hospice program, if the expected duration of survival is a criterion for admission to the program.

HOW ACCURATE ARE PROGNOSTIC JUDGMENTS IN ONCOLOGY?

Studies of Predictions of the Duration of Survival

There have been several studies of the accuracy of clinical predictions about the duration of survival in cancer patients in the terminal and preterminal phases of the illness. All these have shown that there is a lot of random error in that judgment. Several have shown poor calibration with a systematic tendency to overestimation of the duration of survival,[14,36,37] while others have not found evidence of bias.[7] Most of these studies have been too small to provide sufficient power to identify characteristics of the doctor or the patient that are associated with the accuracy of the judgments. One larger scale study, the results of which were shown in Figure 10.1, demonstrated that doctors with more clinical experience were more accurate in their judgments, and also that prognostic judgments were more accurate when the doctor had known the patient for a longer of time. One other interesting observation from one of our own studies is that, toward the end of the patient's life, the accuracy of prognostic judgments increases. This phenomenon may be regarded as an example of what meteorologists call the "horizon effect," meaning that short-term forecasts are usually more accurate than long-term forecasts.[7]

Studies of Predictions of the Probability of Cure

Case Scenarios

We have used case scenarios to study variability in prognostic judgments in the field of lung cancer.[38] We asked practicing oncologists that treated lung cancer to predict survival in non-small-cell lung cancer based on written descriptions of the history, clinical findings, and results of the investigations in three typical cases. Figure 10.5 illustrates oncologists' judgments about the probability of 5-year survival in the case of a patient who had undergone a lobectomy for a

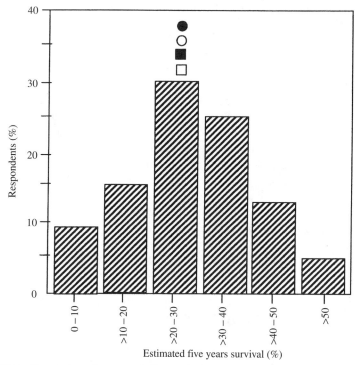

Figure 10.5 Doctors' estimates of the probability of 5-year survival for stage II non-small-cell lung cancer. The histogram shows the probability of 5-year survival assigned to the case by 234 practicing oncologists. The 5-year survival reported in the literature for similar patients is provided for comparison: (■) Slack;[39] (○) Shields;[40] (●) Shields;[41] (□) Lung Cancer Study Group.[42] (From Raby et al.[38])

Stage II squamous cancer of the lung, and in whom clear resection margins had been achieved. The mode of the doctors' estimates of 5-year survival corresponds to the results reported in the literature for similar cases that had been managed in the same way,[39-42] but the distribution of the estimates was very broad (mean 31% ± SD 13.4%; coefficient of variation, 42%). This implies that there was significant disagreement about the natural history of Stage II non-small-cell lung cancer even among doctors who are specialized in the care of this disease. We found similar levels of disagreement respecting the prognosis of patients with Stage III and Stage IV non-small-cell lung cancer.[38]

Clinical Studies

There have been many studies of probabilistic judgments of prognosis in acute-care medicine,[12,13,43-45] but there has been little comparable work in the chronic diseases, and almost none in oncology. In the study that provided the results illustrated in Figures 10.2, 10.3 and 10.4, we compared physicians' estimates of the probability of cure at the time of initiation of treatment with subsequent outcome, measured in terms of 5-year, disease-free survival.[7] This first study was done in a miscellaneous group of cases. We have since repeated the exercise in two other prospective cohort studies, one in lung cancer,[46] and the other in head and neck cancer.[47] The predictions in each of these studies were generally well calibrated, although in the head and neck cancer study we found a systematic overestimation of the probability of 5-year survival among patients with advanced cancers.

Table 10.1 shows that the discrimination of doctors' predictions concerning the probability of cure of patients with cancer in our study was as good as short-term forecasts in acute-care medicine,[12,43-45] and better than cardiologists' 3-year infarct-free survival forecasts.[34,35] Furthermore, while prognosis is generally thought to be more of an art and less of a science than diagnosis, the level of discrimination of long-term forecasts in oncology compares very favorably with that of some diagnostic judgments.[25] Table 10.1 also shows that the accuracy of prognostic judgments in cancer medicine compare very favorably with the accuracy of forecasts in other spheres. The discrimination of predictions of 5-year disease-free survival reported here were, for example, better than the discrimination of short-term weather predictions.[48]

Unfortunately, we can identify no other studies of this kind in the world literature. It is therefore impossible to reach any general conclusions about the accuracy of predictions of the probability of cure in the routine practice of cancer medicine.

THE LIMITS OF PROGNOSTIC JUDGMENT

In interpreting the results of studies of the accuracy of prognostic judgments in oncology, it is important that we consider how accurately we can ever expect to predict the outcome of cancer. The outcome of an illness can only be predicted to the extent that it is predetermined. The maximum achievable accuracy of prognosis will fall short of 100% to the extent that the outcome of interest is determined by random events.

TABLE 10.1 The Discrimination of Human Judgments in Various Fields

Forecasters	Context	Prediction	Sources of Information	Area Under ROC Curve A_{ROC}	Reference
Senior cardiologists	Patients with ≥ obstruction of ≥ 1 major coronary artery	Probability of 3-year survival	Written case descriptions	0.74	35
Cardiology fellows	Patients with ≥ 75% obstruction of ≥ 1 major coronary artery	Probability of 3-year survival	Written case descriptions	0.80	34
Board-certified critical-care fellows	Medical intensive-care-unit patients 24 hours after admission	Probability of surviving until discharge	The patient The patient's chart Results of tests	0.899 ± 0.36 (SE)	44
Critical-care fellows	Patients in a medical/surgical intensive care unit within 24 hours of admission	Probability of surviving until discharge	The patient The patient's chart Results of tests	0.856 ± 0.028 (SE)	43
Experienced intensive care unit physicians	Patients in a medical intensive care unit within 24 hours of admission	Probability of surviving until discharge	The patient The patient's chart Results of tests	0.85	15
Attending intensive care unit physicians	Patients in a medical intensive care unit within 24 hours of admission	Probability of surviving until discharge	The patient The patient's chart Results of tests	0.89	14
Doctors who order blood cultures	Hospitalized patients who had a blood culture	Probability of a positive culture	The patient The patient's chart	0.687 ± 0.073 (SE)	25
Meteorologists	Weather	Probability of rain within next 12 hours	Current meteorological data	0.871	48
Meteorologists	Weather	Probability of rain in 5 to 6 days	Current meteorological data	0.728	48

From what we know about the biology of cancer, it appears unlikely that the course of the illness is ever completely determined at the time of diagnosis. Genetic plasticity is a characteristic of neoplasia, and tumors evolve stepwise by random mutation and natural selection.[49] There is no theoretical reason to believe that it is possible to predict when a metastatic, or drug-resistant, clone will develop, and these are the events that often determine the outcome of the illness. Furthermore, there are sound theoretical reasons to believe that it is impossible to predict whether a given dose of chemotherapy or radiotherapy will cure a particular case. Cell killing by cytotoxic agents involves random processes, and most exhibit first-order kinetics of cell killing.[50] It is therefore partly a matter of chance whether or not the last clonogenic cell is eliminated by a given dose of radiation or chemotherapy.[50] In studies using identical tumors transplanted into genetically identical laboratory animals, it has repeatedly been shown that it is possible to define a dose of radiation or chemotherapy that eradicates the cancer in 50% of the animals, and yet fails to cure it in the other 50%. This dose is referred to as the 50% tumor control dose (TCD_{50}), and it has often been used to measure the sensitivity of tumors to cytotoxic agents. It is taken for granted in this context that the outcome in the individual animal is determined by random processes after the treatment is administered, and not by preexisting differences among the animals.

How, then, do we interpret a 50% cure rate following radiotherapy in a specific group of patients with squamous cancer of the oropharynx? The outcomes may have been entirely predetermined. Half the patients may have started treatment with a 100% probability of cure, while the other half started with a 0% probability of cure. If the molecular basis of these differences in radiocurability could have been identified, then the outcome could have been accurately predicted in every case. However, the outcome may not have been predetermined at all. All the patients may have started out with a 50% chance of cure, and the different outcomes that they experienced might have been decided by chance during treatment. In this case, the outcomes were entirely unpredictable. In fact, any combination of predetermination and chance could have produced the same results, and the predictability of the outcomes could therefore have ranged from 0% to 100%.

The difference between cancer outcomes that are predetermined, but as yet unknown, and those that that have yet to be decided, is analogous to the difference between the "scratch and win" feature on a lottery ticket that determines if it's a winner or a loser at the time you buy it, and the random draw that determines winners and losers after the fact. The extent to which cancer outcomes are established by the random draw sets the outer limits of the predictability of the prognosis in oncology.

CONCLUSIONS

Prognosis is important in cancer medicine and it is therefore important to measure the accuracy of prognostic judgments in routine practice. There are methods available for measuring the accuracy of prognosis that are entirely appropriate to the study of cancer, but so far, there have been very few studies of the accuracy of prognosis in oncology. The few investigations that have been done show that the accuracy of prognostic judgments in oncology seems to be comparable with that of other types of human judgment, but more research is needed before any general conclusions can be drawn. There are good reasons to believe that it will never be possible to prognosticate with certainty. The goal of prognostic factors research can only be to minimize uncertainty. There is little possibility of eliminating it.

REFERENCES

1. *Webster's encyclopedic unabridged dictionary of the english language.* New York, Portland House, 1989.
2. Hartshorne JH: in Reynolds JR (ed.): *A system of medicine.* Vol. 1. Philadelphia, Henry C. Lea's Son 1880, pp. 21–32.
3. Sackett DL, Haynes RB, Guyatt GH, Tugwell P: *Clinical epidemiology: a basic Science for clinical medicine.* Toronto, Ont., Canada, Little, Brown, 1991.
4. Feinstein AR: Symptomatic patterns, biological behaviour, and prognosis in cancer of the lung. *Ann Intern Med* 61:27–39, 1964.
5. Sokal RR, Rohlf FJ: *Biometry.* San Francisco, Freeman, 1969.
6. Poses RM, Cebul RD, Centor RM: Evaluating of physicians' probabilistic judgments. *Med Decis Making* 8:223–240, 1988.
7. Mackillop WJ, Quirt CF: Measuring the accuracy of prognostic judgments in oncology. *J Clin Epidemiol* 50(1):21–9, 1997.
8. Rothman KJ: *Modern epidemiology.* Boston, Little, Brown, 1986.
9. Liechtenstein S, Fischoff B, Phillips LD: Calibration of probabilities: the state of the art in 1980, in Kahneuman D, Slovick P, Tversky A (eds.): *Judgment under uncertainty: heuristics and biases.* Cambridge, Cambridge University Press, 1982; pp. 306–34.
10. Swets JA: ROC analysis applied to the evaluation of medical imaging techniques. *Invest Radiol* 14:109–21, 1979.
11. Griner PF, Mayewski RJ, Mushlin AI: Selection and interpretation of diagnostic tests and procedures: principles and applications. *Ann Intern Med* 94:553, 1981.
12. McClish DK, Powell SH: How well can physicians estimate mortality in a medical intensive care unit? *Med Decis Making* 9:125–32, 1989.
13. Knaus WA, Wagner DP, Lynn J: Short-term mortality predictions for critically ill hospitalized adults: science and ethics. *Science* 254:389–94, 1991.
14. Christakis NA, Lamont EB: Extent and determinants of error in doctors' prognoses in terminally ill patients: prospective cohort study. *BMJ*, 320:469–79, 2000.
15. Altman DG, Bland JM: Measurement in medicine: the analysis of method comparison studies. *Statistician* 32:307–17, 1983.
16. Bland JM, Altman DG: Statistical methods for assessing agreement between two methods of clinical measurement. *Lancet* 1:307–10, 1986.

17. Ahlburg D: How accurate are the U.S. Bureau of the Census projections of total live births? *J Forecast* 1:365–74, 1982.

18. Mahmoud E: Accuracy in forecasting: a survey. *J Forecast* 3:139–59, 1984.

19. Martin CA, Witt SF: Forecasting tourism demand: a comparison of the accuracy of several quantitative methods. *Int J Forecast* 5:7–19, 1989.

20. Yates JF: External correspondence: decompositions of the mean probability score. *Org Behav Human Perform* 30:132–56, 1982.

21. Bamber D: The area above the ordinal dominance graph and the area below the receiver operating characteristic graph. *J Math Psychol* 12:387–415, 1975.

22. Hanley JA, McNeil BJ: The meaning and use of the area under a receiver operating characteristic (ROC) curve. *Radiology* 143:29–36, 1982.

23. Winkler RL, Murphy AH: "Good" probability assessors. *J Appl Meteorol* 7:751–60, 1968.

24. Brier GW: Verification of forecasts expressed in terms of probability. *Mon Weather Rev* 78:1–3, 1950.

25. Poses RM, Anthony M: Availability, wishful thinking, and physicians' diagnostic judgments for patients with suspected bacteremia. *Med Decis Making* 11(3):159–68, 1991.

26. Arkes HR, Dawson NV, Speroff T, et al.: The covariance decomposition of the probability score and its use in evaluating prognostic estimates. *Med Decis Making* 15(2):120–31, 1995.

27. Spiegelhalter DJ: Probabilistic prediction in patient management and clinical trials. *Stat Med* 5:421–33, 1986.

28. Redelerier DA, Bloch DA, Hickam DH: Assessing predictive accuracy: how to compare Brier scores. *J Clin Epidemiol* 44(11):1141–6, 1991.

29. Murphy AH: Scalar and vector partitions of the probability score: Part I. Two-state situation. *J Appl Meteorol* 11:273–82, 1972.

30. Murphy AH: Scalar and vector partitions of the probability score: Part II. N-state situation. *J Appl Meteorol* 11:1183–92, 1972.

31. Murphy AH: A new vector partitions of the probability score. *J Appl Meteorol* 12:595–600, 1973.

32. Muller ME, Langefeld CD, Tierney WM, et al.: Validation of probabilistic predictions. *Med Decis Making* 13:49–58, 1993.

33. Mittlbock M, Schemper M: Explained variation for logistic regression. *Stat Med* 15:1987–97, 1996.

34. Lee KL, Pryor DB, Harrell FE, et al.: Predicting outcome in coronary disease: statistical models versus expert clinicians. *Am J Med* 80:553–60, 1986.

35. Kong DF, Lee KL, Harrell FE, et al.: Clinical experience and predicting survival in coronary disease. *Arch Intern Med* 149:1177–81, 1989.

36. Forster LF, Lynn J: Predicting life span for applicants to inpatient hospice. *Arch Intern Med* 148:2540–3, 1988.

37. Parkes CM: Accuracy of predictions of survival in later stages of cancer. *BMJ* 2:29–31, 1972.

38. Raby B, Pater J, Mackillop WJ: Does knowledge guide practice? Another look at the management of non-small cell lung cancer. *J Clin Oncol* 13:1904–11, 1995.

39. Slack NH: Bronchogenic carcinoma: nitrogen mustard as a surgical adjuvant, and factors influencing survival. *Cancer* 25:987–1002, 1970.

40. Shields TW, Humphrey EW, Eastridge CE, et al.: Adjuvant cancer chemotherapy after resection of carcinoma of the lung. *Cancer* 40:2057–62, 1977.

41. Shields TW, Higgins GA, Humphrey EW, et al.: Prolonged intermittent adjuvant chemotherapy with CCNU and hydroxyurea after resection of carcinoma of the lung. *Cancer* 50:1713–21, 1982.

42. Lung Cancer Study Group: Effects of postoperative mediastinal radiation on completely resected Stage II and Stage III epidermoid cancer of the lung. *N Engl J Med* 315:1377–81, 1986.

43. Poses RM, Bekes C, Copare FJ, Scott WE: The answer to "What are my chances, doctor?" depends on whom is asked: prognostic disagreement and inaccuracy for critically ill patients. *Crit Care Med* 17:827–833, 1989.

44. Brannen AL, Godfrey LJ, Goetter WE: Prediction of outcome from critical illness: a comparison of clinical judgment with a prediction rule. *Arch Intern Med* 149:1083–6, 1989.

45. Dolan JG, Bordley DR, Mushlin AI: An evaluation of clinicians' subjective prior probability estimates. *Med Decis Making* 6:216–3, 1986.

46. Quirt CF, Mackillop WJ: The accuracy of predictions of life expectancy in lung cancer. *Clin Invest Med* 19(4): 1996.

47. Quirt CF, Hall S, Dixon P, et al.: Measuring the accuracy of prognostic judgments in head and neck cancer. *Clin Invest Med* 20(4): 1997.

48. Stanski HR, Wilson LJ, Burrows WR: Survey of common verification methods in meteorology. *Environment Canada Atmospheric Environment Service Research Report*, No. (MSRB): 89–5, 1989.

49. Nowell P: Mechanisms of tumour progression. *Cancer Res* 46:2203–7, 1986.

50. Skipper HE, Schabel FM, Wilcox WS: Experimental evaluation of potential anti-cancer agents XIII: on the criteria and kinetics associated with "curability" of experimental leukemia. *Cancer Chemother Rep* 35:1–15, 1964.

PROGNOSTIC FACTORS IN SPECIFIC CANCERS

HEAD AND NECK TUMORS

CHAPTER 11

Oral Cavity, Pharynx, and Larynx Cancer

JEAN-LOUIS LEFEBVRE, ERIC LARTIGAU, AHMED KARA, and JÉRÔME SARINI

Cancers of the oral cavity, pharynx, and larynx occur with a yearly incidence of around 500,000 new cases. They are frequent in developed countries, about equally in North America and the European Community where they have a particularly high incidence in France. Most of these cancers are squamous-cell carcinomas (SCCs) occurring in rather debilitated patients after a long history of tobacco consumption and alcohol abuse. The vast majority of patients are males aged around 50 years, but there is a tendency to an increasing incidence in females and young adults. In addition, the sociocultural profile of patients suffering from head and neck SCC is often poor. In general, SCCs of the head and neck often proliferate rapidly, are locally aggressive, and carry a high tendency to metastasize to cervical lymph nodes. In presentations with very large lymph nodes, or when lymph nodes are very numerous, the possibility of distant metastasis increases significantly. This natural history explains why that these SCCs are most often diagnosed at an advanced stage, requiring combined therapies. The outcome for this patient population is poor for several reasons: the risk of failure for the index tumor; the risk of developing subsequent SCCs along the upper aerodigestive tract, esophagus, and lung; and the frequency of intercurrent diseases. The risks from comorbity and second cancers arise almost exclusively from the common etiologic association with alcohol and tobacco abuse. SCCs of the oral cavity, pharynx, and larynx are a major public health problem. Apart from large campaigns against tobacco use and alcohol abuse and information that may encourage earlier diagnosis, efforts should be made to assess prognostic factors capable of predicting both outcome and the response to various treatments. In turn, this should help select appropriate therapeutic protocols.

Prognostic Factors in Cancer, 2nd edition, Edited by Mary K. Gospodarowicz
ISBN 0-471-40633-3   Copyright © 2001 Wiley-Liss, Inc.

TUMOR-RELATED PROGNOSTIC FACTORS

Macroscopic Tumor Characteristics

The various primary sites within this group of head and neck tumors carry different prognoses. Review of a series of 5161 successive new cases (treated with either curative or palliative intent at Centre Oscar Lambret) showed a 3-year and 5-year overall survival, respectively, of 41% and 30% for oral cavity, 24% and 14% for oropharynx, 19% and 12% for hypopharynx, 50% and 40% for larynx cancer. These significant differences in survival derived from differences in clinical stage, performance status, and the therapeutic options at presentation. In addition, those diseases with the highest association with combined alcohol and tobacco abuse (e.g., hypopharyngeal and sugraglottic lesions) generally had a worse prognosis because of comorbidities (e.g., liver disease and second cancers) compared to disease where smoking is the sole etiologic factor (e.g., early glottic cancer).

Endophytic tumors are often considered to carry a poorer prognosis than exophytic ones. This is probably influenced by the fact that endophytic tumors are diagnosed at a much more advanced stage. The anatomic complexity of the head and neck and the presence of difficult to assess anatomic spaces that provide natural routes for deep tumor spread may explain the significant rates of local failure. Modern imaging has considerably improved the evaluation of tumor extension allowing an improved customization of the treatment.

Another factor is the clinical appearance of tumors. The cancer may appear as a sole well-defined mucosal change or as multicentric changes with a mix of cancerous and precancerous lesions. In such situations, the exact definition of the tumor extension may be difficult, in particular in the case of submucosal extension of the disease with different loci separated by a normal mucosa. Recurrences around the treated area are more frequent in the latter case.

Histologic Characteristics

As already mentioned, most of the oral cavity, oropharynx, and larynx cancers are SCCs. Grading of differentiation has been, for a long time, considered to be of prognostic relevance. To date, no convincing data are available as to the prognostic significance of well-differentiated or moderately differentiated tumors. Discrepancies in reporting tumor grade are explained by the heterogeneity of the tumors and the frequent associated infection. Tumor grade may also vary in different parts of the same tumor, or a biopsy fragment may not be representative of the entire tumor. The individual observer's interpretation of the findings may also vary. In contrast, a consensus does exist for the poorly differentiated SCC subtype, which has a higher metastasizing potential but a better sensitivity to radiotherapy and chemotherapy. In tumors with a basaloid component, the prognosis seems to be particularly poor due to the high incidence of distant metastases. In the case of lesions manifesting a sarcomatoid component, the prognosis is also poorer, while the verrucous SCCs carry a better prognosis due in large part to the rarity of metastasis. Other histologic types comprise the glandular carcinomas and adenoid cystic carcinoma, the latter carrying a metastatic potential, sometimes many years after the initial treatment.

Extent of the Disease

Local Extension   Local extent classification varies according to the primary site. For oral and oropharyngeal SCC, the definition of local extension, according to the International Union Against Cancer–American Joint Committee on Cancer (UICC–AJCC TNM) 5th classification (see Appendix 11A), is mainly based on the tumor size: T1 for lesions of less than 2 cm in diameter, T2 for lesions between 2 and 4 cm, and T3 for lesions over 4 cm. For larynx and hypopharynx SCC, the T classification is based on an anatomic definition: T1 for tumor confined to one subsite, T2 for tumors extending to several subsites, while T3 relates to a fixity of the true vocal cord, although the 5th edition TNM, for the first time, also includes size as a component of the hypopharynx classification.[1] Whatever the primary site, T4 are generally those tumors infiltrating "deep" tissues outside the organ. Small degrees of mucosal extension are no longer regarded as T4 in the TNM. This may generate some confusion, in particular when T4 are defined on imaging that is able to detect subclinical extensions. As a result a T4 (on imaging) may be smaller than a T3 (on clinical assessment), and subsequently have a better prognosis. Other than this consideration there is no doubt that, in the vast majority of the cases, the bigger the primary tumor, the poorer its prognosis. In the Centre Oscar Lambret series, the 3-year and 5-year overall survivals were 62% and 48% for T1, 43% and 31% for T2, 27% and 19% for T3, 21% and 13% for T4. The survival differences were nonsignificant between T1 and T2 categories, or between T3 and T4, but were significant between T1–2 as compared to T3–4. Nevertheless, a rare but intriguing situation is observed in early-stage oral cancers in patients without tobacco or alcohol history, which behave inexplicably aggressively with a very poor prognosis. Finally, the TNM classification does not refer to tumor thickness, which has been reported as predictive of local recurrence if not ultimate survival. A critical depth of 2 mm has been recommended for consideration.[2]

Lymph-Node Involvement   It is widely accepted that lymph-node involvement is certainly the most important clinical prognostic factor. The TNM classification refers to the absence (N0) or the presence of lymph-node metastasis, to the size (below 3 cm, 3 to 6 cm, and over 6 cm), to the number of involved lymph nodes and to their location in the neck (homolateral or contralateral or bilateral). Again, the use of imaging and other diagnostic tools such as fine-needle aspiration biopsy (in particular when guided by ultrasounds) provide variation to the definition of N0 necks from one institution to another, and subsequently to the prediction of the risk for clinically false-negative necks. In our experience, in the already mentioned study, the presence of at least one palpable lymph node reduced the 5-year survival to at least half of the expected rate.

More importantly, the histological evaluation of the lymph-node involvement, on neck dissection specimen, is a very important source of prognostic data. In a series of 1331 consecutive patients from Centre Oscar Lambret[3] who underwent a neck dissection (followed by postoperative irradiation in case of nodal involvement), the mortality rate was significantly lower in patients without lymph-node involvement (59%) when compared to patients with lymph-node metastases (77%, $p = 0.000001$), and in patients with lymph-node involvement without extracapsular extension (R − ve 74%) compared to those with extracapsular spread (R + ve 82%, $p = 0.009$). Another study of 914 patients from Institut Gustave Roussy[4] found a significant differences in 5-year survivals (N − ve R − ve — 71%; N + ve R − ve — 47%; N + ve R + ve — 27%; $p < 0.001$). The number of positive lymph nodes (LN+) as well as their location in the neck, irrespective of the presence or not of a extracapsular extension, appeared in both studies to have a significant impact on prognosis. In our study, the mortality rate was 65% when there were less than three positive lymph nodes vs. 84% when there were three or more involved lymph nodes ($p < 0.02$) and 66% in the absence of positive lymph nodes in the lower third of the neck (infraomohyoid level or Level IV) versus 80% when this level was involved ($p = 0.0009$). A multifactorial evaluation revealed that, irrespective of T classification, the presence of an extracapsular extension, or of three or more positive lymph nodes, or of lymph-node involvement in Level IV, had a similar impact on prognosis with a risk of nodal recurrences two times higher and a risk of distant metastases three times higher when compared with patients without one of these three types of nodal involvement.

Clinical aspect and imaging of lymph nodes are also of interest. As a general rule, necrotic lymph nodes are less chemo- and radioresponsive,[5] probably due to tumor hypoxia.[6]

Stage Grouping

If stage I (T1N0M0) and stage II (T2N0M0) are a homogenous groups, stages III and IV mix together completely different clinical situations that carry very different prognosis. Reviewing 3714 previously untreated SCC, we found a median survival of 89 months in stage I patients, 46 months in stage II, 19 months in stage III, and 11 months in stage IV. Within the stage III group, a median survival was 42 months for T1-2N1 patients, 21 months for T3N0 patients, and 13 months for T3N1 patients. Within the stage IV group, median survival was 16 months for T4N0-1M0 patients, 11 months for T1-3N2-3M0 patients, and 4 months for M1 patients. In addition, within each group and subgroup, median survival varied according to the primary site. As far as survival is concerned, the prognostic value of stage grouping must be handled with caution. In contrast, it is unquestionable that the lower the stage, the higher the risk of metachronous cancer. In our review, risk of dying from a second primary was four times higher for stage I when compared to stage IV; half the stage I oral SCC patients developed a second primary.

Tumor Biology A great deal of scientific excitement has been generated over the past 15 years in biological research for head and neck cancers. The apparent stagnation in outcomes despite important advances has led to the conclusion that treatment and follow-up policies should no longer be defined only by clinical data. Research has mainly focused on two goals: to predict the response to treatment (to avoid ineffective therapies), or to predict the outcome (to fine-tune the follow-up). Another subject is the effort to identify biomarkers to predict the efficacy of an intervention for which the endpoints require a very long-term evaluation (chemoprevention of second primary tumors). Frequently, the predictive value of these factors was identified on univariate analysis only, and most of the potential molecular markers remain investigational. To date, there are no really consistent data about the prognostic reliability of a single biological assay, and a panel of different tests will be necessary to identify the exact biological profile of a tumor.

p53 An impressive series of papers has been published in recent years regarding the identification of p53 protein in cancer and its potential use as a prognostic factor for tumor outcome. Most of the published data are controversial. Some authors have found a predictive positive value of p53 protein overexpression as regards to survival,[7,8] while other authors concluded that there was no significant correlation.[9–14] These results may be explained by the heterogeneity of tumors and the mixture, in published papers, of different tumor sites. However, when some studies focused on a specific tumor site, there were no converging conclusions for overall survival,[15–17] as for the impact of Tp53 gene mutations.[18,19]

If p53 overexpression and Tp53 gene mutation did not appear to be indisputable prognostic parameters as regards survival, there are nonetheless consistent data about prediction of treatment response. Overexpression of p53 on surgical margins[20] that appeared to be free of disease on pathological evaluation, had the same deleterious outcome on local control as positive margins. On the other hand, p53 is required for radiation-induced apoptosis. As a result, it was hypothesized that tumors lacking a functional p53 gene would be radioresistant. Actually, it was found that p53 mutation was able to reduce hypoxic cell death, conferring hypoxia-mediated radioresistance.[21] This should lead to the conclusion that p53 mutation is associated with biologically aggressive tumor, possibly resistant both to irradiation and to chemotherapeutic agents. To contradict this, overexpression of p53 was found to be predictive of chemosensitivity in some studies.[22] Finally, antibodies to p53 could correlate with local control and survival.[23,24] All these inconsistencies can be explained by the heterogeneity in laboratory assays.

Epidermal Growth Factor Receptor

Hyperexpression of epidermal growth-factor receptor (EGFR) correlates with tumor size and stage, and appears to be predictive of an unfavorable outcome: poorer survival, shorter disease-free interval, and higher recurrence rates after irradiation.[25–27] Patients with high EGFR and transforming growth factor (TGF) alpha levels did poorly compared with patients having low or moderate levels.[28] The combination of antibodies to the EGFR with radiation could improve tumor curability by increasing radiosensitivity and promoting apoptosis.[29]

Angiogenesis-related Markers and Tumor Oxygenation In vitro studies have shown that inhibition of vascular endothelial growth factor (VEGF) engenders tumor regression. While in one study,[30] VEGF staining correlated with nodal metastasis, in another study it failed to show correlation between VEGF staining and either lymph-node metastasis or overall survival.[31] In one study, a correlation was observed between image cytometric quantification of factor VIII (immunostaining) and lymph-node metastases.[32] In conclusion, it has not yet been established whether VEGF is predictive for local recurrence. Tissue oxygenation is known to play a role in the tumor response to radiotherapy. Tumor hypoxia can be evaluated by direct measurement using the polarographic technique. In advanced head and neck tumors, a correlation was found in multivariate analysis between tumor oxygenation and local tumor control.[33] Local tumor control at 2 years was 36% for poorly oxygenated tumors (% pO_2 values < 2.5 mmHg) versus 70% for well-oxygenated tumors ($p = 0.01$).These observations have been confirmed by other groups.[34]

Cell Kinetics It has been postulated that fast tumor regrowth (repopulation) during treatment (mostly radiotherapy) was able to compensate for the induced cell loss. In vivo labeling with bromodeoxyuridine (BrdUrd) or iododeoxyuridine (IdUrd) can evaluate tumor growth through flow cytometry or immunohistochemistry. The labeling index (LI), the S-phase duration, and the potential doubling time of the tumor population (Tpot) are calculated. Despite initial interest, most published data did not demonstrate a relation between Tpot and treatment outcome after radiotherapy, either conventional or with modified fractionation (accelerated, hyperfractionated). For example, large data sets with long follow-up (>36 months) found no correlation between cell kinetics and tumor outcome.[35,36] This was confirmed by the results from the Gray Laboratory with the CHART protocol, where no significant association between cell kinetics parameters and local-regional control or survival was observed.[37] The best way to define tumor proliferation could be to use the labeling index alone or antigens associated with proliferation (p105, Ki-67, and PCNA).[38]

On a related theme, tumors that do not have excessive proliferation characteristics prior to treatment, can be induced to accelerated repopulation during radiotherapy.[39,40] It appears that proliferation may begin after a lag phase of three to four weeks, which has implications for optimal design of radiotherapy fractionation schedules, including especially the duration of treatment and the undesirability of interrupting the course once it is under way.[40] It is conceivable that the same problem my also occur with other cancer treatments as well.

Cyclin D1 During the cell cycle, complexes of cyclin D1 and cyclin-dependent kinases (cdk4 and cdk6) mediate progression through G1. Overexpression of cyclin D1 shortens the G1 interval and subsequently accelerates cell proliferation and increases the overall tumor aggressiveness by desensitizing cellular proliferation to inhibitory signals. Cyclin D1 overexpression or amplification predicted poor overall or cause-specific survival in most of the series.[41,42] However, at least two large series reported no clear correlation between 11q13 amplification and tumor control.[43,44]

Loss of Heterozygosity and DNA Ploidy   Many loci have been studied, but unfortunately there is little information linking loss of heterozygosity (LOH) to local control and to radiosensitivity, even if LOH at 8p or 3p loci appeared predictive of a poor outcome in some studies. A reduced number of disease-free and overall survivals have been correlated to LOH at chromosome 3p in patients with oral cancer,[45] and at chromosome 8p23 for supraglottic tumors treated with surgery.[46] It has been suggested that the presence of two tumor suppressor genes, (3p and 8p), whose loss correlates could explain tumor recurrence, is of prognostic significance.

DNA aneuploidy is considered to be associated with poor prognosis. It is correlated either to an increase in local recurrence or a decrease in survival.[47] The correlation between aneuploidy and radioresistance has been described for head and neck tumors, but remains controversial as it is for most of the molecular markers tested as prognostic factors for local recurrence and radioresistance.[48]

HOST-RELATED PROGNOSTIC FACTORS

There are so many interactions between age, gender, socioeconomic level, and stage of disease at presentation, access to health system, and choice of therapeutic protocols that the individual influences of demographic characteristics on outcome are difficult to separate. In addition, the comorbid conditions of most of these patients require clinicians to use suboptimal therapies at times, since these would be the only ones that could be safely used in some of these patients. In general, females carry a slightly better prognosis, but this advantage seems to exist mainly for early-stage diseases. Since these diseases are cured in the majority of cases, one can suggest that this apparent better prognosis only reflects the difference in life expectancy between both sexes. In a retrospective review of 4610 successive patients from Centre Oscar Lambret, 194 were below 40 years and 273 over 75 years in age at presentation. We did not find significant differences in tumor-related causes of death regardless of age. There were fewer treatment-related deaths in young adults and a higher proportion of deaths from intercurrent diseases in old patients.

Performance status is a frequent parameter in decision making for head and neck cancer. Tobacco consumption and alcohol abuse have generated comorbidities, such as liver cirrhosis, cardiovascular diseases, and chronic pulmonary dysfunction, that do not allow complex therapies and may contraindicate some chemotherapeutic regimens or certain surgical procedures potentially generating aspiration during the immediate postoperative courses. As a result, these comorbid situations may influence the prognosis either directly due to the occurrence of deaths from intercurrent disease or indirectly due to the modification of treatment planning. Another issue is the tolerance to treatment, which is compromised by a poor performance status. An European Organization for Research and Treatment of Cancer (EORTC) study of altered fractionation irradiation in oropharyngeal SCC showed that the improvement in survival was achieved only in patients with a Karnofsky index over 90.[49] It is very common to note in patients that tobacco smoking continuation and alcohol abuse during treatment increase the occurrence of high-grade complications that may lengthen the overall treatment time, compromise the therapeutic sequence, and subsequently alter its efficiency.[50]

Heredity is rarely assessed in head and neck oncology. Having the same lifestyle as parents seems more determining in risk of developing a head and neck cancer than a particular genetic profile. However, there are published data showing that a chromosomic instability may predispose to the risk of multiple primary tumors.[51]

ENVIRONMENT-RELATED PROGNOSTIC FACTORS

Socioeconomic factors are probably the most difficult parameter to assess in head and neck patients. Clearly at least three out of four patients live in the poorest strata of the society (in terms of income and educational level), in particular patients with pharyngeal SCC. In our experience, one-third of patients lived alone at time of diagnosis, 15% were unemployed, and 15% were incapacitated. This poor sociocultural profile may explain that these patients delayed consulting a physician. In addition, tobacco and alcohol consumption produces a chronic inflammation of the upper aerodigestive tract that masks symptoms for a long time. Whatever the explanation of the delay to diagnosis, this delay leads to a diagnosis at an advanced stage, and is the real cause of the poor outcome. In contrast, the socioeconomic status may have a direct impact on the outcome during the follow-up. There are important sequels of treatments that compromise the social and domestic rehabilitation of the patient. Return to occupation is rarely achieved due to the consequences of treatment on the one hand, and, on the other hand, an economic environment that does not favor considering these patients as potential workers. In essence, employers may well choose to reserve these job positions for other healthy individuals who are not burdened with the problems of head and neck oncology treatments. In turn, the social isolation that results does not encourage patients to change their lifestyle, and indirectly predisposes them to recurrences or metachronous cancers.

Quality of care is also an important issue. Optimal decision making is based on a thorough evaluation of the disease, including panendoscopy, modern imaging, and biological tests. Care supply and access to care are obvious criteria for an appropriate treatment selection. To this extent, it is clear that the quality of care is directly linked to the wealth of the country the patients live in. Thereafter, the process of decision making is of importance. There are two major options for treatment: surgery and radiotherapy. More recently, chemotherapy has been integrated in therapeutic protocols, even in protocols with curative intent. Treatment selection of a single modality therapy or of a combined protocol must be made after completion of a fair anticipation of functional and cancer related results. A multidisciplinary discussion is warranted to guarantee the best choice of treatment. Having access to a comprehensive medical structure (a private or a public structure, a comprehensive center, or a well-organized network) and offering such an opportunity increases chances of cure. Finally, early-stage diseases most often require single-modality therapy (function-preservation surgery or definitive irradiation). To ensure both local control and optimal functional outcome requires expertise. In contrast, combined modality therapies are frequently needed for advanced diseases. The patient's preparation for treatment, the treatment itself, and posttreatment course management require the combined expertise of the treatment team. A minimum mass of annually treated patients is necessary to get this expertise. In addition, clinical research is carried out in large medical structures, offering chances to be enrolled in innovative therapy approaches.

SUMMARY

The anatomic extent of disease and tumor grade are the most important tumor-related prognostic factors in oral cavity, oropharynx, and larynx cancers. Because of the high prevalence of tobacco and alcohol consumption in these patients, however, associated comorbid conditions and performance status have a profound impact on the outcome. Appendix 11B provides a summary of the prognostic factors in these SCC of the head and neck.

███████ **APPENDIX 11A**

TNM Classification Oral Cavity, Oropharynx, and Larynx

T Category — Primary Tumor

TX Primary tumor cannot be assessed

T0 No evidence of primary tumor

Tis Carcinoma in situ

Lip, Oral Cavity, Oropharynx

T1 Tumor 2 cm or less in greatest dimension

T2 Tumor more than 2 cm but not more than 4 cm in greatest dimension

T3 Tumor more than 4 cm in greatest dimension

T4 Lip: Tumor invades adjacent structures (e.g., through cortical bone, inferior alveolar nerve, floor of mouth, skin of face)

    Oral cavity: Tumor invades adjacent structures (e.g., through cortical bone, into deep (extrinsic) muscle of tongue, maxillary sinus, skin. Superficial erosion alone of bone/tooth socket by gingival primary is not sufficient to classify as T4)

    Oropharynx: Tumor invades adjacent structures (e.g., pterygoid muscle(s), mandible, hard palate, deep muscle of tongue, larynx)

Hypopharynx

T1 Tumor limited to one subsite of hypopharynx and 2 cm or less in greatest dimension

T2 Tumor involves more than one subsite of hypopharynx or an adjacent site, or measures more than 2 cm but not more than 4 cm in greatest diameter without fixation of the hemilarynx

T3 Tumor measures more than 4 cm in greatest dimension or with fixation of hemilarynx

T4 Tumor invades adjacent structures (e.g., thyroid/cricoid cartilage, carotid artery, soft tissues of neck, prevertebral fascia/muscles, thyroid, and/or esophagus)

Supraglottic Larynx

T1 Tumor limited to one subsite of the supraglottis with normal vocal cord mobility

T2 Tumor invades mucosa of more than one adjacent subsite of supraglottis or base of tongue, vallecula, medial wall of pyriform sinus) without fixation of the larynx

T3 Tumor limited to larynx with vocal cord fixation and/or invades any of the following: postcricoid area, preepiglottic tissues

T4 Tumor extends through the thyroid cartilage, and/or extends into soft tissues of the neck, thyroid, and/or esophagus

Glottic Larynx

T1 Tumor limited to the vocal cord(s) (may involve anterior or posterior commissures) with normal mobility

    T1a Tumor limited to one vocal cord

    T1b Tumor involves both vocal cords

T2 Tumor extends to the supraglottis and/or subglottis, and/or with impaired vocal cord mobility

T3 Tumor limited to the larynx with vocal cord fixation

T4 Tumor invades through the thyroid cartilage and/or to other tissues beyond the larynx (e.g., trachea, soft tissues of the neck, including thyroid, pharynx)

Subglottic Larynx

T1 Tumor limited to the subglottis

T2 Tumor extends to the vocal cord(s) with normal or impaired mobility

T3 Tumor limited to the larynx with vocal cord fixation

T4 Tumor invades through the cricoid or thyroid cartilage and/or extends to other tissues beyond the larynx (e.g., trachea, soft tissues of neck, including thyroid, esophagus)

N Category — Regional Lymph Nodes

NX Regional lymph nodes cannot be assessed

N0 No regional lymph-node metastasis

N1 Metastasis in a single ipsilateral lymph node, 3 cm or less in greatest dimension

N2 Metastasis in a single ipsilateral lymph node, more than 3 cm but not more than 6 cm in greatest dimension; or in multiple ipsilateral lymph nodes, none more than 6 cm in greatest dimension; or in bilateral or contralateral lymph nodes, none more than 6 cm in greatest dimension

    N2a Metastasis in a single ipsilateral lymph node more than 3 cm but not more than 6 cm in greatest dimension

    N2b Metastasis in multiple ipsilateral lymph nodes, none more than 6 cm in greatest dimension

    N2c Metastasis in bilateral or contralateral lymph nodes, none more than 6 cm in greatest dimension

N3 Metastasis in a lymph node more than 6 cm in greatest dimension

M Category — Distant Metastasis

MX Distant metastasis cannot be assessed

M0 No distant metastasis

M1 Distant metastasis

Stage — Grouping

0	Tis	N0	M0
I	T1	N0	M0
II	T2	N0	M0
III	T1	N1	M0
	T2	N1	M0
	T3	N0,N1	M0
IVA	T4	N0,N1	M0
	Any T	N2	M0
IVB	Any T	N3	M0
IVC	Any T	Any N	M1

Source: Sobin LH, Wittekind Ch (eds.): *TNM classification of malignant tumors*, 5th ed. Union Internationale Contre le Cancer Wiley-Liss, New York, 1997.

■■■■■■■ **APPENDIX 11B**

Prognostic Factors in Cancers of the Oral Cavity, Oropharynx, and Larynx

Prognostic Factors	Tumor Related	Host Related	Environment Related

Essential	Tumor size
	Nodal
	extension
		Performance status
		Comorbidities
		Compliance
		Tobacco and alcohol
		  consumption
			Multidisciplinary decision
			  making
			Care supply
			Imaging

Additional	Histologic grading	Social environment	Access to comprehensive care

New and
promising
	P53 mutations
	EGFR
	Angiogenesis-
	  oxygenation
	Cell kinetics
		Mutagen sensitivity	Research and development
			  (technology, drugs, surgical
			  procedures, etc.)

REFERENCES

1. Sobin LH, Fleming ID: *TNM classification of malignant tumors*, 5th ed. Union Internationale Contre le Cancer and the American Joint Committee on Cancer. *Cancer* 80:1803–4, 1997.

2. Spiro RH, Huvos AG, Wong GY, et al.: Predictive value of tumor thickness in squamous carcinoma confined to the tongue and floor of the mouth. *Am J Surg* 152:345–50, 1986.

3. Lefebvre JL, Buisset E, Ton Van J, et al.: Les facteurs pronostiques chirurgicaux. Impact des donnees histopathologiques, in Demard, F (ed): *Facteurs pronostiques des carcinomes des voies aero-digestives superieures*. Paris, Masson, 1997, pp 141–5.

4. Mamelle G, Pampurik J, Luboinski B, et al.: Lymph node prognostic factors in head and neck squamous cell carcinomas. *Am J Surg* 168:494–8, 1994.

5. Munck JN, Cvitkovic E, Piekarski JD, et al.: Computed tomographic density of metastatic lymph nodes as a treatment-related prognostic factor in advanced head and neck cancer. *J Natl Cancer Inst* 83:569–75, 1991.

6. Lartigau E, Randrianarivelo H, Martin L, et al.: Oxygen tension measurements in human tumours: the Institut Gustave-Roussy experience. *Radiat Oncol Invest* 1:285–91, 1994.

7. Sauter ER, Ridge JA, Litwin S, et al.: Pretreatment p53 protein expression correlates with decreased survival in patients with end-stage head and neck cancer. *Clin Cancer Res* 1:1407–12, 1995.

8. Shin DM, Lee JS, Lippman SM, et al.: p53 expressions: predicting recurrence and second primary tumors in head and neck squamous cell carcinoma. *J Natl Cancer Inst* 88:519–29, 1996.

9. Sittel C, Ruiz S, Volling P, et al.: Prognostic significance of Ki-67 (MIB1), PCNA and p53 in cancer of the oropharynx and oral cavity. *Oral Oncol* 35:583–9, 1999.

10. Ahomadeghe JC, Barrois M, Fogel S: High incidence of p53 alterations (mutation, deletion, overexpression) in head and neck primary tumors and metastases; absence of correlation with clinical outcome. Frequent protein overexpression in normal epithelium and in early non-invasive lesions. *Oncogene* 10:1217–27, 1995.

11. Dolcetti R, Doglioni C, Maestro R, et al.: p53 over-expression is an early event in the development of human squamous-cell carcinoma of the larynx: genetic and prognostic implications. *Int J Cancer* 52:178–82, 1992.

12. Koch WM, Brennan JA, Zahurak M, et al.: p53 mutation and locoregional treatment failure in head and neck squamous cell carcinoma. *J Natl Cancer Inst* 88:1580–6, 1996.

13. Nylander K, Schildt EB, Eriksson M, et al.: PCNA, Ki-67, p53, bcl-2 and prognosis in intraoral squamous cell carcinoma of the head and neck. *Anal Cell Pathol* 14:101–10, 1997.

14. Riethdorf S, Friedrich RE, Ostwald C, et al.: p53 gene mutations and HPV infection in primary head and neck squamous cell carcinomas do not correlate with overall survival: a long-term follow-up study. *J Oral Pathol Med* 26:315–21, 1997.

15. Gluckmann JL, Stambook PJ, Pavelic ZP: Prognostic significance of p53 protein accumulation in early stage T1 oral cavity cancer. *Oral Oncol* 30B:281, 1994.

16. Franck LJ, Bur ME, Garb J, et al.: p53 tumor suppressor oncogene expression in squamous cell carcinoma of the hypopharynx. *Cancer* 73:181–6, 1994.

17. Caminero MJ, Nunez F, Suarez C, et al.: Detection of p53 protein in oropharyngeal carcinoma. Prognostic implications. *Arch Otolaryngol Head Neck Surg* 122:769–72, 1996.

18. Nogueira CP, Dolan RW, Gooey J, et al.: Inactivation of p53 and amplification of cyclin D1 correlate with clinical outcome in head and neck cancer. *Laryngoscope* 108:345–50, 1998.

19. Erber R, Conradt C, Homann N, et al.: TP53 DNA contact mutations are selectively associated with allelic loss and have a strong clinical impact in head and neck cancer. *Oncogene* 16:1671–9, 1998.

20. Brennan JA, Mao L, Hruban RH, et al.: Molecular assessment of histopathological staging in squamous-cell carcinoma of the head and neck. *N Engl J Med* 332:429–35, 1995.

21. Graeber TG, Osmanian C, Jacks T, et al.: Hypoxia-mediated selection of cells with diminished apoptotic potential in solid tumours. *Nature* 379:88–91, 1996.

22. Bradford CR, Zhu S, Wolf GT, et al.: Overexpression of p53 predicts organ preservation using induction chemotherapy and radiation in patients with advanced laryngeal cancer. Department of Veterans Affairs Laryngeal Cancer Study Group. *Otolaryngol Head Neck Surg* 113:408–12, 1995.

23. Bourhis J, Lubin R, Roche B, et al.: Analysis of p53 serum antibodies in patients with head and neck squamous cell carcinoma. *J Natl Cancer Inst* 88:1228–33, 1996.

24. Lavielle JP, Rignini C, Reyt E, et al.: Implication of p53 alteration and anti p53 antibody response in head and neck squamous cell carcinoma. *Oral Oncol* 34:84–92, 1998.

25. Santini J, Formento JL, Francoual M, et al.: Characterization, quantification, and potential clinical value of the epidermal growth factor receptor in head and neck squamous cell carcinomas. *Head Neck* 13:132–9, 1991.

26. Dassonville O, Formento JL, Francoual M, et al.: Expression of epidermal growth factor receptor and survival in upper aerodigestive tract cancer. *J Clin Oncol* 11:1873–8, 1993.

27. Miyaguchi M, Olofsson J, Hellquist HB: Expression of epidermal growth factor receptor in glottic carcinoma and its relation to recurrence after radiotherapy. *Clin Otolaryngol* 16:466–9, 1991.

28. Grandis JR, Melhem MF, Gooding WE, et al.: Levels of TGF-alpha and EGFR protein in head and neck squamous cell carcinoma and patient survival. *J Natl Cancer Inst* 90:824–32, 1998.

29. Huang SM, Bock JM, Harari PM: Epidermal growth factor receptor blockade with C225 modulates proliferation, apoptosis, and radiosensitivity in squamous cell carcinomas of the head and neck. *Cancer Res* 59:1935–40, 1999.

30. Moriyama M, Kumagai S, Kawashiri S, et al.: Immunohistochemical study of tumour angiogenesis in oral squamous cell carcinoma. *Oral Oncol* 33:369–74, 1997.

31. Salven P, Heikkila P, Anttonen A, et al.: Vascular endothelial growth factor in squamous cell head and neck carcinoma: expression and prognostic significance. *Mod Pathol* 10:1128–33, 1997.

32. Williams JK, Carlson GW, Cohen C, et al.: Tumor angiogenesis as a prognostic factor in oral cavity tumors. *Am J Surg* 168:373–80, 1994.

33. Nordsmark M, Overgaard M, Overgaard J: Pretreatment oxygenation predicts radiation response in advanced squamous cell carcinoma of the head and neck. *Radiother Oncol* 41:31–9, 1996.

34. Brizel DM, Sibley GS, Prosnitz LR, et al.: Tumor hypoxia adversely affects the prognosis of carcinoma of the head and neck. *Int J Radiat Oncol Biol Phys* 38:285–9, 1997.

35. Bourhis J, Dendale R, Hill C, et al.: Potential doubling time and clinical outcome in head and neck squamous cell carcinoma treated with 70 GY in 7 weeks. *Int J Radiat Oncol Biol Phys* 35:471–6, 1996.

36. Hoyer M, Jorgensen K, Bundgaard T, et al.: Lack of predictive value of potential doubling time and iododeoxyuridine labelling index in radiotherapy of squamous cell carcinoma of the head and neck. *Radiother Oncol* 46:147–55, 1998.

37. Wilson GD, Dische S, Saunders MI: Studies with bromodeoxyuridine in head and neck cancer and accelerated radiotherapy. *Radiother Oncol* 36:189–97, 1995.

38. Toffoli G, Franchin G, Barzan L, et al.: Brief report: prognostic importance of cellular DNA content in T1–2 N0 laryngeal squamous cell carcinomas treated with radiotherapy. *Laryngoscope* 105:649–52, 1995.

39. Withers HR, Peters LJ, Taylor JM, et al.: Local control of carcinoma of the tonsil by radiation therapy: an analysis of patterns of fractionation in nine institutions [see comments]. *Int J Radiat Oncol Biol Phys* 33:549–62, 1995.

40. Roberts SA, Hendry JH: Time factors in larynx tumor radiotherapy: lag times and intertumor heterogeneity in clinical datasets from four centers. *Int J Radiat Oncol Biol Phys* 45:1247–57, 1999. ·

41. Bellacosa A, Almadori G, Cavallo S, et al.: Cyclin D1 gene amplification in human laryngeal squamous cell carcinomas: prognostic significance and clinical implications. *Clin Cancer Res* 2:175–80, 1996.

42. Akervall JA, Michalides RJ, Mineta H, et al.: Amplification of cyclin D1 in squamous cell carcinoma of the head and neck and the prognostic value of chromosomal abnormalities and cyclin D1 overexpression. *Cancer* 79:380–9, 1997.

43. Fortin A, Guerry M, Guerry R, et al.: Chromosome 11q13 gene amplifications in oral and oropharyngeal carcinomas: no correlation with subclinical lymph node invasion and disease recurrence. *Clin Cancer Res* 3:1609–14, 1997.

44. Muller D, Millon R, Velten M, et al.: Amplification of 11q13 DNA markers in head and neck squamous cell carcinomas: correlation with clinical outcome. *Eur J Cancer* 33:2203–10, 1997.

45. Partridge M, Emilion G, Langdon JD: LOH at 3p correlates with a poor survival in oral squamous cell carcinoma. *Br J Cancer* 73:366–71, 1996.

46. Scholnick SB, Haughey BH, Sunwoo JB, et al.: Chromosome 8 allelic loss and the outcome of patients with squamous cell carcinoma of the supraglottic larynx. *J Natl Cancer Inst* 88:1676–82, 1996.

47. Joensu H: DNA flow cytometry in the prediction of survival and response to radiotherapy in head and neck cancer. A review. *Acta Oncol* 29:513–16, 1990.

48. Smith BD, Haffty BG: Molecular markers as prognostic factors for local recurrence and radioresistance in head and neck squamous cell carcinoma. *Radiat Oncol Investig* 7:125–44, 1999.

49. Horiot JC, Le Fur R, N'Guyen T, et al.: Hyperfractionation versus conventional fractionation in oropharyngeal carcinoma: final analysis of a randomized trial of the EORTC cooperative group of radiotherapy. *Radiother Oncol* 25:231–41, 1992.

50. Browman GP, Wong G, Hodson I, et al.: Influence of cigarette smoking on the efficacy of radiation therapy in head and neck cancer. *N Engl J Med* 328:159–63, 1993.

51. Cloos J, Steen I, Joenje H, et al.: Association between bleomycin genotoxicity and non-constitutional risk factors for head and neck cancer. *Cancer Lett* 74:161–5, 1993.

CHAPTER 12

Paranasal Sinus Cancer

JOHN N. WALDRON and IAN J. WITTERICK

Malignant disease arising in the maxillary, ethmoid, frontal, or sphenoid sinuses, collectively known as the paranasal sinuses, is rare.[1] Paranasal sinus cancer represents less than 5% of all head and neck malignancy, which in turn comprises less than 10% of malignancy overall. The majority of paranasal sinus cancers arise within the maxillary sinus (70–80%) followed by the ethmoid sinus (10–20%). Because of this, much of the literature (including the present chapter) focuses on data derived from description of tumors arising at these two sites. Cancers arising in the sphenoid or frontal sinuses are extremely rare. The outcome of patients presenting with paranasal sinus cancer is generally poor, with most centers reporting 5-year survival rates in the range of 30–40%.[2–6]

As with any rare disease, the task of reliably identifying and validating independent prognostic factors for paranasal sinus cancer is complicated by the lack of prospectively collected data and the variability of data reported in the retrospective literature that spans many decades, with most series containing relatively small numbers of patients. Reports frequently describe patients with a wide range of tumor extent and histology treated with variable treatment approaches. Outcomes are often analyzed and reported with respect to different endpoints. Prognostication and empiric management recommendations are regularly based on conclusions drawn from the comparison of inhomogeneous treatment groups. In this chapter we attempt to identify prognostic factors that are supported by currently available data and, of equal importance, those that do not enjoy this support.

TUMOR-RELATED PROGNOSTIC FACTORS

Extent of the Primary Tumor

The extent of the primary tumor is the most important prognostic factor for cancer of the paranasal sinuses. Very few papers describe actual tumor size or volume

Prognostic Factors in Cancer, 2nd edition, Edited by Mary K. Gospodarowicz.
ISBN 0-471-40633-3   Copyright © 2001 Wiley-Liss, Inc.

as it relates to outcome. Instead, paranasal sinus tumors are more often described in terms of their extent relative to the sinus of origin and the surrounding normal anatomic structures. An assortment of systems for describing the extent of tumor have been proposed.[7-15] In 1933 Ohngren described maxillary tumor location relative to a plane defined by a line drawn between the angle of the mandible and the medial canthus.[7] This was in part prompted by the limits of surgical resectability of tumors extending posterosuperior to this line into orbit, ethmoids, and pterygopalatine fossa. Ohngren's line subsequently formed the basis for the initial versions of both the American Joint Committee on Cancer (AJCC) and the International Union Against Cancer (UICC) staging classifications of maxillary tumors.[16] Advances in both imaging and surgical technique over recent decades have led to refinement and unification of these staging systems.[14,15] Le et al. (1999) compared the 1997 version of the UICC/AJCC staging system to the earlier 1977 version for 97 patients with carcinomas of the maxillary antrum and concluded the 1997 version was superior in predicting both survival and local control.[6] Appendix 12A outlines the 1997 UICC/AJCC classification for describing primary tumor extension for tumors arising in the maxillary and ethmoid sinuses. Due to their exceptional rarity, there is no formal staging system for cancers arising in the sphenoid or frontal sinuses.

Clinical outcome in terms of survival and local control of paranasal sinus cancer is strongly correlated with primary tumor extent, irrespective of the system used to describe it.[6,17-20] We have reviewed 180 cases of paranasal sinus cancer managed at the Princess Margaret Hospital between 1976 and 1993.[5] All tumors were of malignant epithelial histology and managed with curative intent. Tumor extent was described using both the 1997 UICC staging criteria (Appendix 12A.) and a scoring system based on the cumulative number of sites of involvement beyond the sinus of origin, for the latter, each site of involvement is given a score of one. The sites are as follows:

Nasal cavity	Intracranial
Face subcutaneous	Brain
Skin	Ethmoid sinus
Oral cavity	Sphenoid sinus
Orbit erosion	Nasopharynx
Orbit erosion and displacement of contents	Frontal sinus
Posterior to antrum (pterygoids/infratemporal fossa)	Maxillary sinus

Figure 12.1 illustrates outcome in terms of actuarial cause-specific survival and its relationship to disease extent as described by these two methods. It is clear from these data that prognosis is strongly linked to disease extent and that for advanced tumors further refinement may be possible by a cumulative description of sites of involvement beyond the original sinus. The reader is cautioned, however, that this method of prognostication awaits validation by application to other clinical series.

Adverse outcome has been associated with extension of the primary sinus tumor to specific anatomic areas, including orbit, the infratemporal or

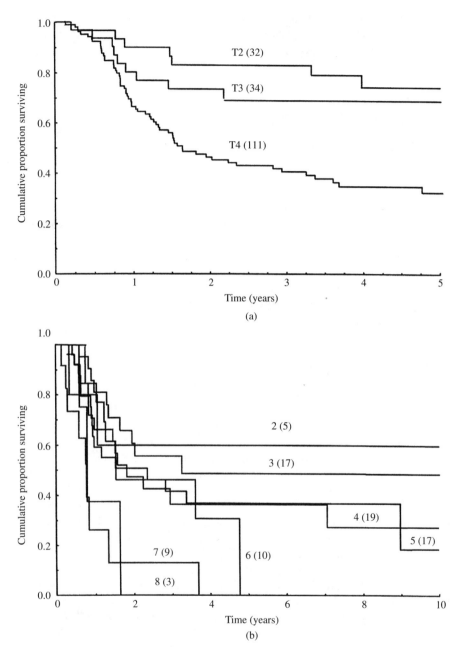

Figure 12.1 Actuarial cause-specific survival for epithelial paranasal sinus cancer. (*a*) Disease extent according to 1997 UICC T categories T2–T4. (*b*) Disease extent for T4 category patients according to cumulative numbers of sites of involvement beyond the sinus of origin as defined in the list on page 000. Patient numbers in each group listed in parenthesis.

pterygopalatine fossa, and the cranium.[21] It remains unproven if extension of tumor to these sites represents independent adverse prognostic features or are simple surrogates for bulky disease. Furthermore, it should be noted that the impact of contemporary surgical and high-precision radiation techniques has yet to be fully described in relation to disease extending to these anatomic regions previously considered inoperable or difficult to irradiate to high doses.

Several important caveats should be considered in terms of the methods of staging paranasal sinus cancer. The potential for stage migration exists with the widespread availability of advanced imaging methods such as thin-cut-spiral computed tomography (CT) and magnetic resonance imaging (MRI), which may allow radiologic detection of tumor extension that would have been missed previously.[22,23] Similarly, positron emission tomography (PET) may provide a major impact on both the staging and assessment of treatment response in this disease.[24] The emergence and refinement of endoscopic sinus surgery now permits visualization and biopsy of anatomic structures that previously could only be accessed with much more invasive procedures. A common pitfall is the comparison of patients staged based on the pathologic analysis of surgical specimens with those staged clinically, as this has been shown to lead to stage migration.[25] Hence future reporting of results should include clear descriptions of the methods used to determine disease extent, and great care should be taken in drawing conclusions in cohorts of patients evaluated with less sophisticated techniques.

Tumor Site of Origin

Most patients with paranasal sinus cancer present with locally advanced disease. Some authors have observed difficulty in defining the specific site of origin of advanced primary tumors that may involve a number of anatomic structures. Tumors arising in the maxillary antrum or ethmoid sinuses will often extend into the nasal cavity. Prior to the advent of widespread CT or MRI, such tumors were often classified as "sinonasal." The distinction as to the specific site of origin of these sinonasal tumors does have an impact on prognosis since a nasal site of origin predicts a more favorable outcome compared to sinus cancer[17–19,26] and results from papers that do not distinguish the two should be interpreted with caution. Similarly, it is important to distinguish tumors arising within the palate with secondary extension to the maxillary sinus from those arising within the antrum and extending inferiorly, since outcome for palate tumors is superior.[27] Those reports that have compared the sinus of origin (maxillary verses ethmoid) have concluded that outcomes are equally poor for these two sites and more dependent on the extent of disease than the particular site of origin.[17,26]

Presenting Symptoms and Signs

The most common symptoms of paranasal sinus cancer at presentation include pain, facial swelling, nasal obstruction, nasal discharge or epistaxis, and oral cavity symptoms due to extension through hard palate. Symptoms of advanced disease with pterygoid, infratemporal fossa, skull base, or orbital involvement can include trismus, cranial neuropathies, and diplopia.[17] Ominous signs include facial erythema and induration, suggesting involvement of the overlying skin, and proptosis, suggesting gross orbital involvement.[28] Time between symptom onset and diagnosis can vary between a few weeks and several years with a median in the range of 6 months. The delay in diagnosis can be attributed to a low index of suspicion and the fact that the early symptoms of paranasal sinus cancer often mimic benign nasal and sinus disease. Interpretation of the relationship between the length of symptoms prior to diagnosis and eventual outcome is confounded by a number of issues. By their nature, early-stage sinus tumors are confined to the sinus of origin and are often asymptomatic, and by the time symptoms begin the disease is often extensive. Thus while a short interval between symptom onset and diagnosis may be considered favorable in terms of a timely onset of treatment, it does not always translate into an increased likelihood for cure. In fact, a rapid onset of symptoms may be indicative of a rapidly growing aggressive histology. Conversely, a lengthy interval between symptom onset and diagnosis need not indicate an advanced neglected disease, but rather a tumor with slow growth and a long natural history such as an adenoid cystic carcinoma.[29]

Regional Lymph Node Involvement

Regional lymph-node involvement in the neck is documented in 10 to 15% of patients at presentation.[5,30] Many series report that the presence of lymph-node involvement in the neck at diagnosis is uniformly associated with very poor survival, with 5-year rates of <10%.[3,21,30,31] Although the majority of these patients die as a consequence of failure at the primary site, they seem to have similar rates of local control to those presenting without any lymph-node involvement. The particularly poor survival in these patients is related to an excess subsequent risk of developing regional failure in the neck or, more importantly, distant metastasis.[6,31]

Histologic Type

A wide assortment of histologic types of tumor can arise within the paranasal sinuses.[32] By far the most common is squamous-cell carcinoma, which accounts for 60–75% in most series, with the remainder composed of undifferentiated tumors, adenoid cystic tumors, and adenocarcinomas. Other tumor types, including lymphomas, plasmacytomas, esthesioneuroblastomas, melanomas, and sarcomas, are so rare as to preclude discussion here. However, the clinician should be aware that the management strategy, and ultimate prognosis, of these extremely rare tumors often differs considerably from the more common carcinomas on which the following discussion focuses.

There are important clinicopathologic differences between the four main types of carcinomas arising in the paranasal sinuses. Adenocarcinomas may develop at any site, but are relatively more common in the ethmoid sinus where a definitive link has been established between this disease and occupational exposure to wood dust.[33,34] Many case series have demonstrated an improved outcome for patients with adenocarcinomas as compared to those with squamous or undifferentiated tumors.[31,35,36] It remains unclear if this effect is independent of stage.[20] Alvarez et al. (1995) examined 41 cases of squamous carcinoma and 34 cases of adenocarcinoma arising in the paranasal sinuses. Their multivariate analysis showed no difference in outcome between these two groups.[4] Adenoid cystic cancer arises more often in the maxillary antrum. It is characterized by a long natural history that often manifests as superior short-term survival rates compared to the other epithelial cancers.[19] This seemingly favorable behavior is qualified by the fact that over time this tumor displays a relentless pattern of recurrence both locoregionally or distantly such that the majority of patients will relapse if followed long enough.[37-41] Up to 20% of paranasal sinus tumors are classified histologically as undifferentiated.[32] Although these tumors may simply represent one end of the spectrum of differentiation of classic squamous or adenocarcinomas, a number of authors have described them as forming a distinct clinicopathologic entity termed sinonasal undifferentiated carcinoma.[42,43] Clinically these tumors are characterized by aggressive local spread, rapid growth, and an increased likelihood to metastasize distantly, which ultimately translates into very poor survival.[19,20,31] For carcinomas, in general, worse outcome has been associated with dedifferentiation.[3,17,19,44]

Biologic Factors

A literature is beginning to accumulate describing the relationship between molecular biologic parameters and outcome in cancers of the paranasal sinus. Some examples of such research include the use of flow cytometry to measure cellular DNA content in squamous carcinomas of the maxillary antrum, which has demonstrated improved outcome for aneuploid tumors.[45] Point mutations within the ras oncogene of adenocarcinomas of the ethmoid are associated with a poorer outcome[46] independent of the tumor stage. Increased cell proliferation in sinonasal tumors may be associated with the inhibition of expression of p27, a cyclin-dependent kinase inhibitor.[47] There seems little doubt that in the decades to come molecular biologic parameters will form an important basis for prognostication and guidance of therapy for cancers of the paranasal sinuses. The data available thus far must be considered preliminary.

PATIENT-RELATED PROGNOSTIC FACTORS

Cancers of the paranasal sinuses arise most commonly in the fifth and sixth decades of life. The male-to-female ratio is about 2 to 1. Of five series in which the influence of patient-related variables on outcome has been examined using multiple regression analysis,[2-6] two have demonstrated significantly better survival in younger patients[3,6] and one has concluded that female patients fare better.[6] Unlike other head and neck cancers, baseline hemoglobin has not correlated with outcome.[5,48] The incidence of paranasal sinus cancers is higher in Japan, South America, India, and the Philippines than in Europe or North

America.[49] The exact reason for this is unknown, though it is probably related to a combination of genetic and environmental influences. Japanese specialists have published an extensive literature describing the treatment of patients with maxillary sinus cancer, and for the most part patient outcomes are similar to those in European and North American series.[50,51] Less literature is available from other countries. The impact of socioeconomic status on outcome in this disease can only be speculated upon. Given the strong relationship between disease extent and outcome, it may be presumed that superior treatment results would be obtained for patients with access to a medical infrastructure that would facilitate early detection and state of the art treatment.

ENVIRONMENT-RELATED PROGNOSTIC FACTORS

Treatment-related Prognostic Factors

Management strategies for cancer arising in the paranasal sinuses have evolved empirically. There are no randomized clinical trials comparing the treatment options for this disease. Consequently, a variety of treatment approaches are practiced and advocated throughout the world. These usually consist of some combination or sequence of surgery, radiation, and possibly chemotherapy. Treatment offered seems more often dictated by locally available expertise and patterns of practice than an evidence-based approach. Most authors advocate a combined modality approach that consists of radical surgical resection, followed by postoperative radiation. Many retrospective series in the literature report improved outcome for patients offered a planned combined approach as compared to those treated with radiation alone.[4,19] However, in most of these series there are significant imbalances in the treatment groups due to patient selection. When the characteristics of treatment groups are reported, it is often noted that patients treated with radiation alone have a higher burden of advanced disease, making conclusions concerning best therapeutic approach difficult to interpret. Of the five series that have controlled for case selection by performing multivariate analysis of outcome with respect to treatment modality[36-52] one has concluded that surgery followed by postoperative radiation is superior to radiation alone.[6] It is important to realize that given the rarity of this disease recent treatment advances with high-precision radiation and advanced surgical techniques have outpaced the ability to report results with significant numbers of patients. Thus, the potential benefits of these interventions are underreported in the literature.

Radiation Therapy for Paranasal Sinus Cancer

The use of radiation alone has been shown in many contemporary series to cure approximately 30% of patients with cancers of the paranasal sinus.[17,20,31,48] Analysis of the relationship between radiation dose and outcome for patients with paranasal sinus cancer is difficult due to the small numbers of patients in most series, the variable addition of other therapies such as surgery and chemotherapy, and finally the fact that for any one series a wide enough ranges of doses may not have been given to establish a dose–response relationship. When such data are available the results must be interpreted with caution, since patients given lower doses may have been treated with palliative intent for very advanced tumors or even had their treatment stopped at a lower dose due to ill health or tumor progression. Nevertheless, a few papers have demonstrated that patients receiving higher doses of radiation, usually >65 Gy, have improved survival.[2,3,6,53] Tumor repopulation during prolonged courses of radiation may adversely effect outcome. Two series have demonstrated that prolongation of overall treatment times greater than 50 days is associated with poor outcome.[6,53] The failure of radiation to control disease may result from inadequate coverage of tumor during a course of radiation due to a failure to appreciate the full extent of the tumor and/or failure to devise and deliver a plan sufficient to cover the tumor. The use of CT and MRI has improved the ability to determine tumor extent,[23] and the use of CT scans for treatment planning has been shown to improve outcome due to improved tumor coverage.[54]

The delivery of high doses of radiation to tumors of the paranasal sinuses is complicated by the proximity of these tumors to an assortment of critical normal structures including the eyes, optic nerves and chiasm, brain, brainstem, and spinal cord. The radiation dose these structure can safely tolerate is considered lower than that required to eradicate carcinomas.[55] Ocular toxicity because of radiation treatment for paranasal sinus cancers has been frequently reported, since with conventional planning and treatment techniques it is often impossible to avoid irradiating the ipsilateral eye.[56] Shielding of the eye in cases with orbital invasion has resulted in treatment failure.[57] Within the last decade there has been a rapid advance in the development of techniques to deliver high-precision radiation therapy whereby CT and MRI images are linked directly to advanced treatment planning and delivery computer programs. This made possible the delivery of radiation to complex target volumes with very little dose to the surrounding normal tissues. Such techniques include stereotactic radiation therapy (SRT), intensity-modulated radiation therapy (IMRT),[58] and tomotherapy.[59] These technologies should allow radiation dose escalation and the addition of concurrent cytotoxic or biologic therapies with reduced acute and/or late radiation toxicity.

When radiation is combined with surgery it can be delivered either preoperatively or following surgical resection. There are compelling arguments for and against each approach.[20,60] The majority of patients treated with a combined modality approach are managed with surgery followed by postoperative radiation, although there is no conclusive evidence that one approach is superior to the other in terms of survival.[1,61]

Surgery for Paranasal Sinus Cancer

Surgical resection of paranasal sinus cancers can be offered as part of the primary treatment approach or reserved for the salvage of patients failing radiation.

Resection of paranasal sinus cancers is indicated when the tumor can be safely excised with clear margins and acceptable morbidity in the absence of distant metastases. A wide variety of surgical approaches can be offered, depending on the exact location and extent of the tumor. The development and refinement of new surgical techniques such as combined craniofacial approaches, new reconstructive techniques including microvascular free flaps,[62,63] and prosthetic devices[64] has allowed patients previously deemed unresectable to undergo successful resection.[65] The full impact of such techniques on survival is difficult to demonstrate specifically, since many series will group patients treated over a time span of decades during which these advanced approaches were in development. Since the majority of patients dying of paranasal sinus cancer do so because of local failure, it seems logical to conclude that surgical strategies designed to improve local control should translate into improved survival.

Numerous surgical series have demonstrated that negative surgical margins are associated with improved survival.[66–70] The ability to achieve negative margins has been facilitated by advances in skull-base surgery that have suggested improved survival in paranasal sinus cancers previously considered hopeless.[65,71,72] Significant improvements in survival for ethmoidal carcinomas have occurred primarily due to the advent of anterior skull-base surgery, allowing complete resection with negative margins.[10,13,73–75] Extension to the pterygopalatine fossa and/or infratemporal fossa have been considered risk factors for local recurrence due to the difficulty in surgical resection of these areas with clear margins.[21,28,76] With the advent of craniofacial surgery, including subtemporal approaches, en bloc resection of the pterygopalatine fossa and infratemporal fossa with clear margins is now possible.

Indications for orbital exenteration as part of definitive resection of paranasal sinus cancer vary among surgeons and have included bone erosion adjacent to the orbit, periorbital invasion, invasion of the infraorbital nerve, and invasion of the posterior orbit or orbital apex. Surgical consensus has changed from almost routine exenteration decades ago to the current approach of selective preservation. Some authors believe that the only reason for orbital exenteration is frank invasion of the orbital fat or musculature.[77] There currently seems to be general agreement that bone erosion itself does not constitute an absolute indication for orbital exenteration.[21,76,77] Four series have compared orbital sparing operations versus procedures combined with orbital exenteration and found no differences in 5-year survival rates.[76–78] In 1996, McCary et al. reported good results in a series of patients with sinonasal malignancies with orbital involvement treated by preoperative radiation therapy and orbital sparing procedures.[79]

Management of the Neck

The need for treatment of the neck with surgery and/or radiation in patients presenting with lymph-node involvement is self-evident; however, such treatment in node-negative patients remains controversial. Some authors cite rates of nodal recurrence as high as 38% as justification for elective neck treatment.[80,81] Most series note rates of neck recurrence in the 10–15% range.[5,17,61] Patients who fail in the neck very often have concomitant failure at the primary and/or distant sites. When appropriate, neck salvage with surgery and/or radiation remains a curative option. Therefore at this time there is little evidence that treating the neck prophylactically has a survival benefit, providing patients have undergone appropriate staging investigations. Nevertheless, it must be kept in mind that nodal failure in the untreated neck may emerge as a survival-limiting event if strategies to improve control at the primary site are successful.

Chemotherapy

The use of systemic chemotherapy has not been demonstrated to improve survival for patients with paranasal sinus cancer. Initial enthusiasm for the use of both intra-arterial and topical application of 5-flurouracil in the Japanese literature has not resulted in a significant survival advantage.[82] Meta-analysis of the role of concurrent chemotherapy and radiation in head and neck cancers in general has suggested a benefit in terms of local control and overall survival,[83] suggesting that this may be a promising avenue of research for advanced paranasal sinus cancers.

SUMMARY

The relevance of the prognostic factors with respect to the proposed grouping system defined earlier in this volume is illustrated in Appendix (12B). The only clearly established essential prognostic factor for epithelial cancers of the paranasal sinuses is the extent of disease at diagnosis. The presence of advanced local or nodal disease strongly predicts for a poor outcome with conventional treatments. Additional predictors of outcome include histopathological subtype and differentiation, patient age, gender, and treatment-related factors, such as the establishment of clear surgical margins and the delivery of higher doses of radiation over shorter overall treatment times. Finally, with recent technical and biological developments new and promising prognostics factors will include the identification of molecular biologic markers for the prediction of response and the guidance of therapy, which should include experimental approaches combining high-precision radiation therapy with dose escalation ideally integrated with state-of-the-art surgical resection, and concurrent therapy with cytotoxic and/or biologic agents. Since the prospect of randomized clinical trials in this disease is remote, it remains critical that patient groups within Phase I and II clinical trials be uniformly staged and described to facilitate comparison to others. Whatever the specifics of the treatment approach, the management of these rare tumors remains complex, and when appropriate patients should be referred to centers with the necessary expertise to offer aggressive state-of-the-art treatment.

■■■■■ **APPENDIX 12A**

TNM Classification of Cancers of the Paranasal Sinus

Maxillary Sinus

T1 Tumor limited to the antral mucosa with no erosion or destruction of bone.

T2 Tumor causing bone erosion or destruction, except for the posterior antral wall, including extension into the hard palate and/or the middle nasal meatus.

T3 Tumor invades any of the following: bone of the posterior wall of maxillary sinus, subcutaneous tissues, skin of cheek, floor or medial wall of orbit, infratemporal fossa, pterygoid plates, ethmoid sinuses.

T4 Tumor invades orbital contents beyond the floor or medial wall, including any of the following: the orbital apex, cribriform plate, base of skull, nasopharynx, sphenoid, frontal sinuses.

Ethmoid Sinus

T1 Tumor confined to the ethmoid with or without bone erosion.

T2 Tumor extends into the nasal cavity.

T3 Tumor extends to the anterior orbit, and/or maxillary sinus.

T4 Tumor with intracranial extension, orbital extension including apex, involving sphenoid, and/or frontal sinus and/or skin of external nose.

Regional Lymph Nodes (N)

NX Regional lymph nodes cannot be assessed.

N0 No regional lymph node metastasis.

N1 Metastasis in a single ipsilateral lymph node, 3 cm or less in greatest dimension.

N2 Metastasis in a single ipsilateral lymph node, more than 3 cm but not more than 6 cm in greatest dimension; or in multiple ipsilateral lymph nodes, none more than 6 cm in greatest dimension; or in bilateral or contralateral lymph nodes, none more than 6 cm in greatest dimension.

    N2a Metastasis in a single ipsilateral lymph node more than 3 cm but not more than 6 cm in greatest dimension.

    N2b Metastasis in multiple ipsilateral lymph nodes, none more than 6 cm in greatest dimension.

    N2c Metastasis in bilateral or contralateral lymph nodes, none more than 6 cm in greatest dimension.

N3 Metastasis in a lymph node more than 6 cm in greatest dimension.

Distant Metastasis (M)

MX Distant metastases cannot be assessed.

M0 No distant metastasis.

M1 Distant metastasis.

Source: Sobin LH, Wittekind Ch (eds.): *TNM classification of malignant tumors*, 5th ed. Union Internationale Contre le Cancer Wiley-Liss, New York, 1997.

▬▬▬ **APPENDIX 12B**

Prognostic Factors for Survival in Paranasal Sinus Cancer

Prognostic Factors	Tumor Related	Host Related	Environment Related
Essential	Primary tumor extent Lymph-node involvement		
Additional	Histopathological type Histologic grade	Age Gender	Radiation dose Total time of treatment Surgical margins
New and Promising	Molecular biologic markers		High-precision dose escalated RT Concurrent cytotoxic or biologic therapies Ideal integration with advanced surgical techniques

REFERENCES

1. Osguthorpe JD: Sinus neoplasia. *Arch Otolaryngol Head Neck Surg* 120:19–25, 1994.
2. Kondo M, Ogawa K, Inuyama Y, et al.: Prognostic factors influencing relapse of squamous cell carcinoma of the maxillary sinus. *Cancer* 55:190–6, 1985.
3. Giri SP, Reddy EK, Gemer LS, et al.: Management of advanced squamous cell carcinomas of the maxillary sinus. *Cancer* 69:657–61, 1992.
4. Alvarez I, Suarez C, Rodrigo JP, et al.: Prognostic factors in paranasal sinus cancer. *Am J Otolaryngol* 16:109–14, 1995.
5. Waldron J, O'Sullivan B, Cummings B, et al.:: Paranasal sinus cancer: A retrospective analysis of 180 cases managed at a single institution. *Clin Invest Med* 19:83, 1996.
6. Le QT, Fu KK, Kaplan M, et al.: Treatment of maxillary sinus carcinoma: A comparison of the 1997 and 1977 American Joint Committee on cancer staging systems. *Cancer* 86:1700–11, 1999.
7. Ohngren LG: Malignant tumors of the maxillo-ethmoidal region. *Acta Otolaryngol Suppl* 19:101–106, 1933.
8. Lederman M: Tumors of the upper jaw: Natural history and treatment. *J Laryngol Otol* 84:369–401, 1970.
9. Sakai S, Hamasaki Y: Proposal for the classification of carcinoma of the paranasal sinuses. *Acta Oto-Laryngol* 63:42–8, 1967.

10. Parsons JT, Mendenhall WM, Mancuso AA, et al.: Malignant tumors of the nasal cavity and ethmoid and sphenoid sinuses. *Int J Radiat Oncol, Biol, Phys* 14:11–22, 1988.

11. Zamora RL, Harvey JE, Sessions DG, et al.: Clinical classification and staging for primary malignancies of the maxillary antrum. *Laryngoscope* 100:1106–11, 1990.

12. Carinci F, Farina A, Padula E, et al.: Primary malignancies of the nasal fossa and paranasal sinuses: Comparison between UICC classification and a new staging system. *J Craniofacial Surg* 8:405–12, 1997.

13. Cantu G, Solero CL, Mariani L, et al.: A new classification for malignant tumors involving the anterior skull base. *Arch Otolaryngol Head Neck Surg* 125:1252–7, 1999.

14. Flemming ID, Cooper JS, Henson DE, et al. (eds): *AJCC cancer staging manual*, 5th ed. Philadelphia, Lippincott, 1997.

15. Sobin LH, Wittekind C, (eds): *UICC TNM classification of malignant tumors*, 5th ed. New York, Wiley-Liss, 1997.

16. Chandler JR, Guillamondegui OM, Sisson GA, et al.: Clinical staging of cancer of the head and neck: A new "new" system. *Am J Surg* 132:525–528, 1976.

17. Logue JP, Slevin NJ: Carcinoma of the nasal cavity and paranasal sinuses: An analysis of radical radiotherapy. *Clin Onco* 3:84–9, 1991.

18. Parsons JT, Kimsey FC, Mendenhall WM, et al.: Radiation therapy for sinus malignancies. [Review]. *Otolaryngol Clin of N Am* 28:1259–68, 1995.

19. Harbo G, Grau C, Bundgaard T, et al.: Cancer of the nasal cavity and paranasal sinuses. A clinico-pathological study of 277 patients. *Acta Oncol* 36:45–50, 1997.

20. Waldron JN, O'Sullivan B, Warde P, et al.: Ethmoid sinus cancer: Twenty-nine cases managed with primary radiation therapy. *Int J Radiat Oncol Biol Phys* 41:361–9, 1998.

21. Gullane PJ, Conley J: Carcinoma of the maxillary sinus. A correlation of the clinical course with orbital involvement, pterygoid erosion or pterygopalatine invasion and cervical metastases. *J Otolaryngol* 12:141–5, 1983.

22. Kondo M, Ando Y, Inuyama Y, et al.: Maxillary squamous cell carcinomas staged by computed tomography. *Int J Radiat Oncol Biol Phys* 12:111–6, 1986.

23. Maroldi R, Farina D, Battaglia G, et al.: MR of malignant nasosinusal neoplasms. Frequently asked questions. *Eur J Radiol* 24:181–90, 1997.

24. Slevin NJ, Collins CD, Hastings DL, et al.: The diagnostic value of positron emission tomography (PET) with radiolabelled fluorodeoxyglucose (18F-FDG) in head and neck cancer. *J Laryngol Otol* 113:548–54, 1999.

25. Robin PE, Powell DJ. Diagnostic errors in cancers of the nasal cavity and paranasal sinuses. The essential role of surgery. *Arch Otolaryngol* 107:138–40, 1981.

26. McNicoll W, Hopkin N, Dalley VM, et al.: Cancer of the paranasal sinuses and nasal cavities. Part II. Results of treatment. *J Laryngol & Otol* 98:707–18, 1984.

27. Truitt TO, Gleich LL, Huntress GP, et al.: Surgical management of hard palate malignancies. *Otolaryngol Head Neck Surg* 121:548–52, 1999.

28. Weymuller E, Jr., Reardon EJ, Nash D. A comparison of treatment modalities in carcinoma of the maxillary antrum. *Arch Otolaryngol* 106:625–9, 1980.

29. Miller RH, Calcaterra TC. Adenoid cystic carcinoma of the nose, paranasal sinuses, and palate. *Arch of Otolaryngol* 106:424–6, 1980.

30. Robin PE, Powell DJ: Regional node involvement and distant metastases in carcinoma of the nasal cavity and paranasal sinuses. *J Laryngol Otol* 94:301–9, 1980.

31. Neal AJ, Habib F, Hope-Stone HF: Carcinoma of the maxillary antrum treated by preoperative radiotherapy or radical radiotherapy alone. *J Laryngol Otol* 106:1063–6, 1992.

32. Weber AL, Stanton AC: Malignant tumors of the paranasal sinuses: radiologic, clinical, and histopathologic evaluation of 200 cases. *Head Neck Surg* 6:761–76, 1984.

33. Hadfield EH, Macbeth RG: Adenocarcinoma of ethmoids in furniture workers. *Ann Otol Rhinol Laryngol* 80:699–703, 1971.

34. Klintenberg C, Olofsson J, Hellquist H, et al.: Adenocarcinoma of the ethmoid sinuses. A review of 28 cases with special reference to wood dust exposure. *Cancer* 54:482–8, 1984.

35. Saunders SH, Ruff T: Adenocarcinoma of the para-nasal sinuses. *J Laryngol Otol* 90:157–66, 1976.

36. Knegt PP, de Jong PC, van Andel JG, et al.: Carcinoma of the paranasal sinuses. Results of a prospective pilot study. *Cancer* 56:57–62, 1985.

37. Tran L, Sidrys J, Horton D, et al.: Malignant salivary gland tumors of the paranasal sinuses and nasal cavity. The UCLA experience. *Am J Clin Oncol* 12:387–92, 1989.

38. Jones AS, Hamilton JW, Rowley H, et al.: Adenoid cystic carcinoma of the head and neck. *Clin Otolaryngol* 22:434–43, 1997.

39. Konno A, Ishikawa K, Numata T, et al.: Analysis of factors affecting long-term treatment results of adenoid cystic carcinoma of the nose and paranasal sinuses. *Acta Otolaryngol Suppl* 537:67–74, 1998.

40. Kim GE, Park HC, Keum KC, et al.: Adenoid cystic carcinoma of the maxillary antrum. *Am J Otolaryngol* 20:77–84, 1999.

41. Naficy S, Disher MJ, Esclamado RM: Adenoid cystic carcinoma of the paranasal sinuses. *Am J Rhinol* 13:311–4, 1999.

42. Levine PA, Frierson H, Jr., Stewart FM, et al.: Sinonasal undifferentiated carcinoma: A distinctive and highly aggressive neoplasm. *Laryngoscope* 97:905–8, 1987.

43. Houston D, Gillies E: Sinonasal undifferentiated carcinoma: A distinctive clinico-pathologic entity. *Adv Anat Pathol* 6:317–23, 1999.

44. Miyaguchi M, Sakai S, Takashima H, et al.: Lymph node and distant metastases in patients with sinonasal carcinoma. *J Laryngol Otol* 109:304–7, 1995.

45. Halvorson DJ, Day S, Christian DR, Jr., et al.: Flow cytometry and squamous cell carcinoma of the maxillary sinus: A possible prognostic indicator for multimodality intervention. *Oncology* 56:248–52, 1999.

46. Perez P, Dominguez O, Gonzalez S, et al.: ras gene mutations in ethmoid sinus adenocarcinoma: Prognostic implications. *Cancer* 86:255–64, 1999.

47. Saegusa M, Nitta H, Hashimura M, et al.: Down-regulation of p27Kip1 expression is correlated with increased cell proliferation but not expression of p21waf1 and p53, and human papillomavirus infection in benign and malignant tumors of sinonasal regions. *Histopathology* 35:55–64, 1999.

48. Haylock BJ, John DG, Paterson IC: The treatment of squamous cell carcinoma of the paranasal sinuses. *Clin Oncol* 3:17–21, 1991.

49. Ayiomamitis A, Parker L, Havas T: The epidemiology of malignant neoplasms of the nasal cavities, the paranasal sinuses and the middle ear in Canada. *Arch Oto-Rhino-Laryngol* 244:367–71, 1988.

50. Sakai S, Fuchihata H, Hamasaki Y: Treatment policy for maxillary sinus carcinoma. *Acta Oto-Laryngologica* 82:172–81, 1976.

51. Shibuya H, Horiuchi J, Suzuki S, et al.: Maxillary sinus carcinoma: Result of radiation therapy. *Int J Radiat Oncol Biolo Phys* 10:1021–6, 1984.

52. Jakobsen MH, Larsen SK, Kirkegaard J, et al.: Cancer of the nasal cavity and paranasal sinuses. Prognosis and outcome of treatment. *Acta Oncol* 36:27–31, 1997.

53. Pearlman AW, Abadir R: Carcinoma of maxillary antrum: The role of pre-operative irradiation. *Laryngoscope* 84:400–9, 1974.

54. Tsujii H, Kamada T, Matsuoka Y, et al.: The value of treatment planning using CT and an immobilizing shell in radiotherapy for paranasal sinus carcinomas. *Int J Radiat Oncol Biol Phys* 16:243–9, 1989.

55. Emami B, Lyman J, Brown A, et al.: Tolerance of normal tissue to therapeutic irradiation. *Int J Radiat Oncol Biol Phys* 21:109–122, 1991.

56. Nakissa N, Rubin P, Strohl R, et al.: Ocular and orbital complications following radiation therapy of paranasal sinus malignancies and review of literature. *Cancer* 51:980–6, 1983.

57. Bush SE, Bagshaw MA: Carcinoma of the paranasal sinuses. *Cancer* 50:154–8, 1982.

58. Purdy JA: 3D treatment planning and intensity-modulated radiation therapy. *Oncology (Huntington)* 13:155–68, 1999.

59. Mackie TR, Balog J, Ruchala K, et al.: Tomotherapy. *Semin Radiat Oncol* 9:108–17, 1999.

60. Waldron JN, O'Sullivan B: The principles of radiation oncology, in Pollock RE (ed.): *Manual of clinical oncology*, 7th ed. New York, Wiley-Liss, 251–74, 1999.

61. Sisson G, Sr., Toriumi DM, Atiyah RA: Paranasal sinus malignancy: A comprehensive update. *Laryngoscope* 99:143–50, 1989.

62. Yoza S, Gunji H, Ono I: Primary maxillary reconstruction after radical maxillectomy using a combined free flap and secondary dynamic suspension. *J Craniofacial Surg* 8:65–73, 1997.

63. Kyutoku S, Tsuji H, Inoue T, et al.: Experience with the rectus abdominis myocutaneous flap with vascularized hard tissue for immediate orbitofacial reconstruction. *Plast Reconstr Surg* 103:395–402, 1999.

64. Hochman M: Reconstruction of midfacial and anterior skull-base defects. *Otolaryngol Clin N Am* 28:1269–77, 1995.

65. Janecka IP, Sen C, Sekhar L, et al.: Treatment of paranasal sinus cancer with cranial base surgery: Results. *Laryngoscope* 104:553–5, 1994.

66. Kraus DH, Sterman BM, Levine HL, et al.: Factors influencing survival in ethmoid sinus cancer. *Arch Otolaryngol Head Neck Surg* 118:367–72, 1992.

67. Wax MK, Yun KJ, Wetmore SJ, et al.: Adenocarcinoma of the ethmoid sinus. *Head Neck* 17:303–11, 1995.

68. Bilsky MH, Kraus DH, Strong EW, et al.: Extended anterior craniofacial resection for intracranial extension of malignant tumors. *Am J Surg* 174:565–8, 1997.

69. Rutter MJ, Furneaux CE, Morton RP: Craniofacial resection of anterior skull base tumors: factors contributing to success. *Aust NZ J Surg* 68:350–3, 1998.

70. Mouriaux F, Martinot V, Pellerin P, et al.: Survival after malignant tumors of the orbit and periorbit treated by exenteration. *Acta Ophthalmol Scand* 77:326–30, 1999.

71. Catalano PJ, Hecht CS, Biller HF, et al.: Craniofacial resection. An analysis of 73 cases. *Arch Otolaryngol Head Neck Surg* 120:1203–8, 1994.

72. McCutcheon IE, Blacklock JB, Weber RS, et al.: Anterior transcranial (craniofacial) resection of tumors of the paranasal sinuses: Surgical technique and results. *Neurosurgery* 38:471–9, 1996.

73. Bridger GP: Radical surgery for ethmoid cancer. *Arch Otolaryngol* 106:630–4, 1980.

74. Ketcham AS, Van Buren JM. Tumors of the paranasal sinuses: A therapeutic challenge. *Am J Surg* 150:406–13, 1985.

75. Shah JP, Kraus DH, Arbit E: Craniofacial resection for tumors involving the anterior skull base. *Otolaryngol Head Neck Surg* 106:386–393, 1992.

76. Som ML: Surgical managment of carcinoma of the maxilla. *Arch Otolaryngol* 99:270–273, 1974.

77. Perry C, Levine PA, Williamson BR, et al.: Preservation of the eye in paranasal sinus cancer surgery. *Arch Otolaryngol Head Neck Surg* 114:632–4, 1988.

78. Xuexi W, Pingzhang T, Yongfa Q: Managment of the orbital contents in radical surgery for squamous cell carcinoma of the maxillary sinus. *Chin Med J (Engl)* 108:123–5, 1995.

79. McCary WS, Levine PA, Cantrell RW: Preservation of the eye in the treatment of sinonasal malignant neoplasms with orbital involvement. A confirmation of the original treatise. *Arch Otolaryngol Head Neck Surg* 122:657–9, 1996.

80. Jiang GL, Ang KK, Peters LJ, et al.: Maxillary sinus carcinomas: Natural history and results of postoperative radiotherapy. *Radiother & Oncol* 21:193–200, 1991.

81. Paulino AC, Fisher SG, Marks JE: Is prophylactic neck irradiation indicated in patients with squamous cell carcinoma of the maxillary sinus? *Int J Radiat Oncol Biol Phys* 39:283–9, 1997.

82. Tsujii H, Kamada T, Arimoto T, et al.: The role of radiotherapy in the management of maxillary sinus carcinoma. *Cancer* 57:2261–6, 1986.

83. Bourhis J, Pignon JP: Meta-analyses in head and neck squamous cell carcinoma. What is the role of chemotherapy? *Hematol Oncol Clin N Am* 13:769–75, vii, 1999.

CHAPTER 13

Nasopharyngeal Carcinoma

BRIAN O'SULLIVAN and VINCENT CHONG

Nasopharyngeal carcinoma (NPC) is unusual in several ways. Its epidemiology, associated with ethnicity, genetic predisposition, viral, and environmental dietary exposure, is unique in itself. In addition, the predilection for certain geographic areas, with relative sparing of adjacent regions is noteworthy. Unjustly perhaps, NPC poses a formidable public health hazard to countries that are relatively compromised in their ability to provide the technical diagnostic and therapeutic approaches considered to be necessary for optimal management today. However, what sets it apart from most diseases is the anatomic challenge it presents to the oncology team because of the proximity of the nasopharynx to critical anatomic structures and the high predilection for distant metastasis once the primary and regional lymph-node areas are extensively involved, which is all too frequent.

In this chapter we discuss prognostic factors of importance in the management of NPC using the classification proposed earlier in this book (see Chapter 2). Factors will be considered by whether they relate to the *disease* itself, the patient (or *host*), or the *environment* which influences the opportunity for optimal treatment and diagnosis. The classification may not always apply since, in the case of NPC, there may be overlap among factors and arbitrary placement of factors may be necessary. We will also attempt to categorize the available evidence into factors which are essential to our ability to treat the disease (*essential* factors), those which add valuable information about the disease but do not affect treatment decisions (*additional* factors), and finally those that are being described and may provide important understanding of disease behavior and therapeutic approaches in future years. In the interest of relevance to the treatment of the disease, and for brevity, the discussion of the final group of factors (those termed *new and promising*), will be restricted to experience of patient outcome. Therefore, preclinical studies will not receive attention.

Prognostic Factors in Cancer, 2nd edition, Edited by Mary K. Gospodarowicz
ISBN 0-471-40633-3   Copyright © 2001 Wiley-Liss, Inc.

Special attention to the classification of stage of disease will be given. This is because for NPC anatomic features are so important that a relevant and reproducible system of classification merits attention above other prognostic factors. In fact, few diseases received the same level of attention in the preparation of the 5th edition (TNM) stage classification of the International Union Against Cancer (UICC)[1] and the American Joint Committee on Cancer (AJCC[2]). A major revision of the NPC stage was accomplished by a substantial collaborative consultation among radiation oncologists in Southeast Asia, with support from diagnostic radiologists, pathologists, and surgeons there and elsewhere.

TUMOR-RELATED FACTORS

Anatomic Extent

Anatomy and Routes of Spread

The Local Issues (normal and tumor anatomy)   Understanding the normal anatomy and routes of spread of NPC is pivotal to appreciation of the management and prognosis of NPC. The salient issues will be summarized, but greater detail is available.[3,4] The anatomy is best approached from the vantage of the radiologist, because contemporary treatment is guided almost exclusively by accurate imaging using computerized tomography (CT), or preferably magnetic resonance imaging (MRI) where available.[5] The most important issue to appreciate is that the location of the nasopharynx in the lee of the skull base provides great opportunity for tumor to extend into regions of relative inaccessibility. Because of this, radiotherapy, with or without chemotherapy, forms the mainstay of management.

The nasopharynx is a fibromuscular sling hanging from the skull base and its shape is maintained by a stiff aponeurosis (the pharyngobasilar fascia) formed from the most cephalad extension of the pharyngeal musculature. The nasopharyngeal space communicates directly with the nasal cavity anteriorly and the oropharynx inferiorly. It is beneath the sphenoid sinus of the skull base. Mucosa lines the space and several structures are related to it. Both eustachian tubes enter through lateral openings in the pharyngobasilar fascia termed the sinus of morgani. The pharyngeal end of each tube creates an elevation called the torus tubarius on each side of the nasopharynx. Behind and above each torus is a recess in the lateral mucosa called the fossa of Rosenmuller where most NPC originates. The parapharyngeal space (PPS) separates the wall of the nasopharynx from the masticator space (or infratemporal fossa). It is a thin region comprising loose areolar tissue and if breached by laterally extending tumor, invasion of the masticator muscles or of the mandibular nerve may result. Invasion of the PPS is found in approximately 70% of cases,[6] which presents an immediate treatment challenge because the PPS lies directly in the region of shielding needed to protect the spinal cord in most traditional radiotherapy planning. Therefore, specific radiotherapy techniques are needed.

The carotid space (CS) is located behind the PPS, and therefore even further in the undertreated shielded region designed to protect the spinal cord from a traditionally fashioned radiation beam. The CS forms the most lateral compartment of the nasopharynx and tumor can readily extend back to the neurovascular structures adjacent to the lateral vertebral bodies and clivus, since its path is not impeded. Superolateral to the fossa of Rosenmuller, and within the pharyngobasilar fascia, lies the foramen lacerum through part of which runs the carotid artery as it traverses the skull base. Tumor entering this region has ready access to the cavernous sinus, a grave prognostic sign. Lateral to the foramen lacerum and outside the pharyngobasilar fascia lies the foramen ovale just above the PPS. Tumor breaching the PPS can readily extend through the foramen ovale intracranially without bone destruction, as manifested on MRI, yet invisible to CT.[3] This is the most common route of intracranial spread. Skull-base erosion is considered to be present in up to one-third of the cases.[3] A component of the fifth cranial nerve is commonly compressed at this point, resulting in facial pain, but further infiltration of these nerves may result in denervation. These manifestations are also grave, as are the findings of palsies of the remaining cranial nerves in the cavernous sinus, the region of the jugular foramen and the orbital fissures and related anatomy.

A local primary NPC tumor may escape destruction by radiotherapy for several reasons. In addition to the intrinsic sensitivity to radiotherapy, tumor size is also relevant (because of the number of clonogens which may survive the radiotherapy course), as is its shape (which may result in extension into regions in front or behind structures which must be protected from the high-dose volume, e.g., the spinal cord, brain stem, and optic nerves and optic chiasma). Finally, any invasive character is important, with involvement of bone, muscle, nerves, and vessels in an aggressive and infiltrating character which are likely surrogates for biologically aggressive disease.

Metastases Cervical adenopathy is very common in NPC (seen in 75%).[6] Typically both the anterior deep cervical lymph nodes (Levels I, II, III and IV), and Level V are at risk. The retropharyngeal lymph nodes are the primary echelon, but are bypassed in about 35% of cases. Distant metastasis is also frequent in NPC (evident in approximately 5% to 41% of case) compared to other head and neck sites where the rate of 5% to 24% is seen, depending on the series.[3] They are seen in bone (most frequently), lung, and liver.

The Stage of Disease The main tumor prognostic factors are encompassed by the stage of disease as captured in TNM (see Appendix 13A). The most recent edition of TNM incorporated a major revision to the NPC classification.[1,2] One of the components which was included for the first time was the presence of PPS involvement because of its prognostic relevance and the technical problems in treating this region with radiotherapy.

- *Parapharyngeal Involvement* Subdivision, based on prognosis, of the degree of parapharyngeal extension has been promoted by authors in different ways.[7–9] One system involved classification based on the lateral extension across the PPS,[7] another separated the pre- versus poststyloid components of the PPS,[8] while another subdivided the PPS into paranasopharynx versus paraoropharynx.[10] Another assertion was that poststyloid involvement was caused by infiltration from the upper cervical lymph nodes rather than direct extension of the primary tumor.[11]

Clearly, putative differences in prognostic estimates relate in part to differences in definition, but also to differences in the radiation techniques employed to address this potentially unfavorable presentation of disease. Evidence exists that specific attention to the technical delivery of radiation treatment may significantly improve the poor prognostic outcome of parapharyngeal extension, although this interpretation may also be influenced by the use of chemotherapy in certain studies, and again the definition used to describe it.[12]

Although different degrees of parapharyngeal involvement may still represent different orders of prognosis, it is included as a subcategory within T2 (as T2b) in the 5th edition TNM. The rationale for this decision is discussed elsewhere.[13]

- *Advanced T-Category Disease* The T4 category now includes extension to extreme soft tissue areas such as the infratemporal fossa (masticator space) or hypopharynx, in addition to gross intracranial extension and/or cranial nerve involvement, which are associated with a significantly more sinister prognosis.[14] Bone involvement alone is classified as T3 disease.

- *Summary of Modifications to T-Categories in 5th Edition TNM* The 4th Edition TNM suffered from "lumping" of a heterogeneous population of patients in the T4 category and an irrelevant "splitting" of the most favorable prognostic T-category into T1 and T2. Finally, posterolateral extension into the PPS had not previously been recognized in the UICC/AJCC TNM, nor had the real magnitude of tumor extending into the masticator space (or infratemporal fossa), orbit, or hypopharynx. Extreme extensions of this type may be surrogates for bulk of disease,[15] and may also be associated with more aggressive disease. The omission of PPS involvement previously was a serious weakness because of its distinct impact on outcome depending on radiotherapy techniques for the reasons discussed earlier and will be revisited under Environment-Related Factors.

- *Classification of Regional Lymph Nodes (N categories)* Size (greatest diameter $\leq$ 6 cm vs. >6 cm), level (upper-mid vs. supraclavicular), and laterality (unilateral vs. bilateral) are significant factors for distant failure and cancer-specific death and have been included as the criteria for N-categorization in the new TNM.[13] When adjusted for other parameters, there are no significant differences between unilateral and contralateral involvement, upper and mid-level of neck, and nodal size <3 cm and >3 to <6 cm.[13] Multiplicity and fixation are not included in the new TNM due to a combination of factors, including varied statistical significance, absence of definition, and interrelationship with other parameters of lymph-node description.[13,16,17]

- *Stage Groups* The 10-year disease-specific survival (DSS) for the 5th Edition TNM provide a relatively distinct outcome by different stages, with the corresponding rates being 77% (Stage I), 65% (Stage II), 54% (Stage III),

TABLE 13.1   Stage-Grouping and 10-Year Actuarial Disease-Specific Survival (DSS) in T and N Subsets Using the 1997 5th Edition TNM for a Series of 4514 Cases of Nasopharyngeal Carcinoma

Proportion by Stage (%)	TN Subset	Stage	DSS(%)
Stage I: 10%	T1N0M0	I	77
Stage II: 21%	T2N0M0	II	78
	T1N1M0	II	64
	T2N1M0	II	57
Stage III: 30%	T3N0M0	III	68
	T3N1M0	III	54
	T1N2M0	III	48
	T2N2M0	III	51
	T3N2M0	III	39
Stage IV: 39%	T4N0M0	IVA	39
	T4N1M0	IVA	26
	T4N2M0	IVA	20
	T1N3M0	IVB	36
	T2N3M0	IVB	29
	T3N3M0	IVB	31
	T4N3M0	IVB	15

Source: Reproduced with modification and permission from Reference 13.

and 29% (Stage IV) from the robust data set of almost 5000 patients which was used to develop the classification.[13] These data are also shown in greater detail by T- and N-category combinations and stage group (Table 13.1).

Anatomic Features Beyond the 5th Edition TNM

- *Tumor Volume*   Since the publication of the 5th edition, a classification based on tumor volume instead of strict anatomic extent alone has become available.[18] A large primary tumor volume (>60 cc) was associated with significantly poorer local control (5-year local control rate: 56%) and disease-specific survival (5-year survival rate: 53%). Large lymph-node tumor volumes (>30 cc) were also associated with significantly higher distant failure rate (5- year distant relapse-free survival rate: 54%) and lower disease-specific survival (5-year survival rate: 40%). The authors concluded that the primary tumor volume carried greater prognostic value than Ho's staging classification.[18]

- *The Influence of "Tumor Invasion"*   A recent small series of cases imaged by MRI appears to complicate the conclusion by Chua and colleagues concerning the influence of primary tumor volume.[19] No apparent relationship between tumor volume determined by MRI and local control when the tumor volume was more than 20 cc. All patients without invasion of the pharyngobasilar fascia had local control. Deep tumor infiltration appeared more prognostic than tumor volume.[19]

In a recent study of 218 patients, 87 had nasal involvement, one of the components of TNM.[20] Of these, 60 showed a pattern of mucosal infiltration (MI), while 27 had an exophytic protruding (EP) component. Multivariate analysis demonstrated that infiltration of nasal fossa mucosa was an independent prognostic factor for primary control and freedom from progression. The authors concluded that differentiation into infiltrating versus exophytic type is of value in predicting the outcome of treatment and suggest that only the infiltrating group should be considered "nasal involvement" in the staging of NPC.[20]

Subdivision of the Parapharynx   Recently, and subsequent to the publication of the 5th Edition TNM, the Singapore group have again advocated a subdivision in the PPS at the C1/C2 vertebral interspace paraoropharyngeal involvement versus paranasopharyx in a population-based CT staged series report.[6] In the overall analysis, parapharyngeal involvement appeared to be prognostically unimportant, probably because of boosting with a "parapharyngeal boost technique" if this component of disease was bulky.[6] However, a prognostic distinction was noted on subset analysis in the Cox model when the PPS was subdivided into paraoropharyngeal versus paranasopharyx involvement (Table 13.2). It is possible this may have resulted from the fact that tumor with paraoropharyngeal involvement is bulkier and similar to the observations concerning tumor volume.[18] Nevertheless, it may be of interest when evaluating prognostic factors in the future.

Tumor Factors Other than Anatomic Extent

Pathology
Histologic Subtype   The World Health Organization (WHO) subdivides NPC histology into Type 1 keratinizing squamous-cell carcinomas (WHO-1), nonkeratinizing (WHO-2), and undifferentiated carcinomas (WHO-3).[21] The presence or absence of keratin in biopsy specimens has been correlated with tumor behavior, locoregional control, patterns of failure, and survival of patients irradiated

TABLE 13.2   Multivariate Analysis of Prognostic Factors for Patients with Nasopharyngeal Carcinoma: Factors in the Final Cox Model

Factor	Hazard Ratio	95% CI	p-Value
Age	1.026/year	1.015–1.028	<0.0001
Lymph node level	1.71/level	1.49 –1.97	<0.0001
Cranial nerve involvement	2.14	1.49 –1.97	0.0001
Orbit involvement	2.50	1.42 –4.40	0.004
Paranasopharyngeal involvement	1.38	1.05 –1.80	0.02
Nasal involvement	1.47	1.07 –2.02	0.02

Source: Table modified and reproduced with permission from Reference 6.

Abbreviation: CI: confidence interval.

for NPC ($P = 0.001$).[22] Patients with keratinizing squamous-cell cancers, even though they had a lower incidence of lymphatic and distant metastases, had a poorer survival rate because of a higher incidence of deaths from uncontrolled primary tumors and nodal metastases ($P = 0.001$).[22] In addition, 5069 NPC cases from the U.S. National Cancer Data Base (NCDB) were grouped by their histologic types and patient ethnic ancestry.[23] The study showed that WHO-1 carcinomas comprised 75% of the U.S. NPC cases and were found most often in U.S.-born, non-Hispanic whites. WHO-2 and WHO-3 NPC carcinomas comprised the remaining 25% and were more common in people of Asian ancestry. Histologic composition correlated with survival. Thus Asians had the highest proportion of radioresponsive WHO-2 and WHO-3 carcinomas and better survival (5-year relative survival: 65%) than African-Americans and Hispanic and non-Hispanic whites (5-year relative survival: 37%), who had the greatest number of less radioresponsive WHO-I tumors.[23] Also, the distinction between *host* versus *tumor* prognostic factors in this instance becomes blurred, since they are so clearly associated.

Other Pathologic Features Numerous small studies have shown varying differences in prognosis.

Moderate or marked density of dendritic cells (S100+) are associated with longer survival than those without such infiltration. The same study indicated that a significant relationship between monocytic and macrophagic cells (lysozyme+) within the tumor and survival was also present.[24]

Local infiltration of T-lymphocyte subsets revealed a trend toward better prognosis in cases with no or slight stromal T8 lymphocyte cell infiltration.[25]

Markers of Prognostic Value in NPC As with many cancers the search for biologic markers to predict prognosis in NPC has been ongoing. Unfortunately, hypothesis testing prospective studies from which to prove independent significance are essentially unavailable. Generally, the reports are also weakened by methodologic problems, including small patient cohorts, retrospective design, and evaluation of only components of the potential stage profile. Finally, although it is accepted that techniques for biologic evaluation may vary among different laboratories, to date the studies also lack consistency. As noted earlier, preclinical studies using cell lines or animal models will not be addressed. The positive early reports of the past decade are mentioned even if these have not translated into universal clinical usage but where evidence to refute the findings or their relevance is not apparent.

Biologic Markers in Tumor Tissue

- *The P53 Tumor Suppressor Gene* Studies of altered expression of the p53 suppression gene have not been as enlightening in NPC compared to other tumors. Uncertainty exists about the degree of detection or expression of p53 in NPC in the first instance, and even if p53 is detectable there appears to be little clinical evidence at the present time that it can be implicated in prognosis.[26–30] In contrast it is suggested that the low frequency of p53 mutations detected previously in NPC could relate to the molecular techniques used to screen for mutations, and that these mutations may lie outside the typical exon "hot spot" regions of the gene.[27,31] Correlative studies also suggest that p53 has a role in regulating tumor apoptosis[32] and that patients with tumors positive for p53 tend to be resistant to radiotherapy and have a poorer prognosis ($p = 0.05$).[33]

- *Tumor Angiogenesis* Recently, Roychowdhury and colleagues correlated clinical data with immunohistochemical evaluation of archival tissue from 30 NPC patients treated at the University of California at San Francisco between 1956 and 1990. "Intense tumor angiogenesis," defined by microvessel counts per field correlated with the development of distant metastasis ($p = 0.03$), shorter overall survival ($p = 0.02$), and disease-free survival ($P = 0.05$). The conclusions were that tumor angiogenesis and the presence of strong c-erbB2 expression may be predictive in addition to other clinical characteristics, including stage of disease.[29] Others have also reported that alterations of microvessel parameters were significantly linked to metastasis.[34] The relationship of vascular endothelial growth factor (VEGF) with angiogenesis and lymph-node metastasis has also been explored. A significant correlation between both increased microvessel count and VEGF expression and the progression of regional lymph-node metastasis suggests a VEGF mediated effect on angiogenesis.[35] In contrast, serum levels of VEGF are not predictive for outcome (see later).[36]

- *Other Evaluations of Tumor Tissue* Contradictory information is available about the expression of the apoptosis-related protein bcl-2. This has not been found to be prognostic by some,[32,33] but as noted earlier, was by Roychowdhury et al.[29]

Another study examining the expression of c-myc and ras oncogenes found no influence of ras p21 expression, but overexpression of the c-myc oncogene correlated with a poor prognosis ($p < 0.05$).[37]

The level of Ki-67, a marker of proliferation, has generally not been prognostic.[29,32,33] Proliferative activity assessed by mitotic index and proliferating cell nuclear antigen (PCNA) showed prognostic discrimination when T4 cases (UICC 4th Edition) were excluded from a subset of "advanced" cases.[38] Similarly, Chan and colleagues found that a higher PCNA labeling index (LI) was associated with a poorer disease-free survival.[39]

The prognosis of NPC patients with HLA-DR expression was better than those without ($P < 0.01$).[40] The positive rate of HLA-DR gradually decreased with tumor progression, showing difference among tumors in different clinical stages ($p < 0.05$).

Downregulation of the cadherin-catenin cell adhesion complex may play a role in cancer invasion and metastasis. Zheng and colleagues noted that reduced expression of E-cadherin and beta-catenin expression was associated with a shorter survival ($p < 0.001$). In advanced NPC patients (Ho Stages IV and V), a significant difference in survival was observed in tumors with higher versus lower levels of E-cadherin expression ($p = 0.0224$, log-rank test).[41]

The expression of latent membrane protein-1 (LMP1) correlated with clinical and follow-up data. LMP1-positive tumors grew faster and more expansively than LMP1-negative tumors. Paradoxically, LMP1-negative tumors recurred at a higher frequency, and showed an increased tendency to metastasize.[42] Serum anti-LMP-1 antibodies are mentioned below.

Additional results suggest that the absence of nm23-H1 protein expression was significantly associated with lymph-node metastasis, recurrence, and distant metastasis in NPC. This study involved a Cox regression on 231 patients studied for expression of nm23-H1 on paraffin-embedded specimens as well as mRNA expression in fresh tissues from 78 cases investigated by in situ hybridization and reverse-transcriptase polymerase chain reaction (RT-PCR).[43]

The prognostic significance of soluble interleukin-2 receptor was assessed in 295 patients with NPC and 97 age-matched controls. Soluble interleukin-2 receptor levels in NPC cases were elevated and correlated with clinical staging. The significance of these observations 10 years later remains uncertain.[44]

Serum Markers in Patients with NPC A variety of studies exist about the prognostic association of levels of "markers". Apart from the difficulty of determining independent significance, another problem with such reports is that one must differentiate those markers that can emulate the biologic behavior of the tumor from those representing a greater burden of disease elaborating larger amounts of the marker. Alternatively the marker may be a host response to the presence of disease (e.g., raised liver enzymes in the presence of liver metastases). In some situations several of these mechanisms may exist, although it may not yet be possible to infer which applies.

A variety of different serum markers have been studied, but space does not permit a detailed discussion of each. They include CYFRA 21-1 (a fragment of cytokeratin expressed by simple epithelia and their malignant counterparts),[45,46] serum ferritin,[47] serum copper,[48] IgA VCA titer.[49] Other recent serum-level assessments of prognostic relevance include the evaluation of serum lactic dehydrogenate (LDH),[50] transforming growth factor beta 1 (TGF-beta 1),[51] serum levels of anti-EBV/VCA gig and Ina,[52] serum anti-LMP-1 antibodies,[53] and serum levels of tissue polypeptide antigen (TPA).[54]

Many of these factors are reported to be associated with advanced stage of disease, or may predict those who will develop metastasis, or are restricted to those with distant metastasis. Some predict for poorer survival, but do not control for other known factors. In the case of LDH, the level correlated with responsiveness to systemic chemotherapy. In the case of some it remains uncertain what their role should be, since they were described a decade ago without further commentary, yet have not become standard assessment tools in the management of NPC.[48,54]

The Impact of Local Recurrence on Distant Failure Although strictly a time-dependent variable representing an outcome of initial treatment, it is tempting to consider whether failure at the primary site in NPC enhances the risk of distant metastasis. Kong and colleagues reported that patients with locoregional relapse had significantly higher distant metastases rate than patients with locoregional control using time-adjusted statistical models.[55] An alternative hypothesis is that patients who fail at the primary have a biologically unfavorable disease would have failed at distant sites anyway. Separating these issues is problematic and methodologically challenging. The use of time-dependent adjustment in a Cox model may not be able to completely control for this bias (see Chapter 2).

HOST-RELATED FACTORS

NPC often strikes the young and "healthy" compared to other head and neck cancers where alcohol- and tobacco-associated diseases are common. Therefore it affects people with little predisposition other than ethnicity and geography, and these would not normally be expected to influence prognosis. Consequently, most patients with NPC do not have typical associated comorbidity led to the development of the disease. However, certain comments are still valid concerning the environment in which the patient is diagnosed and treated.

Ethnicity

This issue was mentioned earlier under Tumor-related Factors and will not be repeated in detail. The patient with a WHO-1 tumor with keratinisation is more likely to be a Caucasian than of Asian ancestry[13,23] and can expect a different response to treatment (see earlier).[22,23] The WHO-1 patient is also more likely to be treated in a different *environment*, typically outside of Southeast Asia. Whether or not this provides less opportunity for disease control because of inexperience among the clinicians who are likely to provide care is unknown. Alternatively, on average such a patient may experience a greater opportunity for cure because of easier potential access to expensive diagnostic and treatment resources. Such issues are mentioned in the Environment-related section below.

Age

Age is a prognostic factor in NPC. The disease is exceptionally rare in the young, and large series of children with NPC are not available.[56] Survival declines with age at diagnosis, and this is evident in numerous reports.[57] A recent report indicated a hazard ratio of 1.026/year for the independent effect of age (Table 13.2). On the other hand, the rate of distant metastasis in children was noted to be as high as 81% in Egypt.[58]

Gender

Gender is an inconsistent prognostic factor in NPC. No evidence of difference in age-standardized survival was apparent between men and women in the recent EUROCARE study.[57] Similarly gender was not prognostic in the Singapore study as evidenced by its absence in their final multivariate model (Table 13.2),[6] nor was it in the huge series reported recently from Hong Kong (4514 cases).[13]

Symptoms and Performance Status

As with histology and ethnicity, patient symptoms and performance status are not necessarily *host* factors and could also relate to the influence of the *tumor*. Nevertheless, they will be considered here. Information concerning performance status and outcome is not readily available, although cases with good status had the most favorable outcome in a nationwide study.[59] Performance status is also of significant importance in the management of recurrent NPC where long-term control is still possible.[60] Also, cases being enrolled in randomized trials of aggressive therapies are often restricted to those with better status, implying that other patients may have less opportunity to benefit from experimental therapies may report improved outcome.[61] The previously described series from San Francisco also showed that a duration of symptoms of fewer than 6 months correlated with a shorter disease-free survival ($p = 0.05$).[29]

Comorbidity

The ability of patients to tolerate treatment and to survive beyond the time a cancer may be cured can be profoundly influenced by associated illnesses. In the case of the former, the systemic treatments in current use or investigation have resulted in death directly from chemotherapy despite the restriction of those studies to better performance status patients.[61,62] In a series of NPC patients treated with aggressive combination chemotherapy at the Princess Margaret Hospital, 3 of 7 drug-related deaths were from fulminant hepatitis attributed to reactivation of hepatitis B.[63] Therefore, the high incidence of hepatitis in some geographic regions where NPC is also common may pose problems if chemotherapy is to be considered. The recent EUROCARE study noted poor survival for NPC in Scotland and Estonia compared to other European countries. Although the reasons for this may be multifactorial, the suggestion was made that this is probably due to the influence of alcohol-related comorbidity.[57]

ENVIRONMENT-RELATED FACTORS

The contemporary era has brought significant change to the management of NPC. Many of these changes may be difficult to provide in those countries where the need is greatest from the point of view of the incidence of the disease. Specifically, diagnostic and staging equipment have become very expensive, and optimal treatment for NPC often requires highly technical radiotherapy. In addition, chemotherapy may be both effective and toxic and the support system to provide it safely may not be readily available in many countries.

Diagnosis, Staging, and Disease Monitoring

The critical anatomic issues have already been discussed, including the fact that these issues generally demand high-quality imaging to determine disease extent for accurate target delineation. At this time it appears that MRI is the superior modality in NPC.[3,5] Evidence of improved outcome is as yet unavailable, since MRI is a relatively new modality. Previous evidence is available of "changing stage" of disease when CT became more widely available,[64] and was elegantly shown to improve survival overall.[65] Recent evidence suggests that the early diagnosis of recurrence, including distinguishing it from radiation fibrosis, may be enhanced by both the wider use of MRI and potentially by newer diagnostic modalities such as 99mTc-sestamibi (MIBI) SPECT imaging.[66,67] Of course, any potential advantages such imaging modalities may provide in facilitating earlier salvage therapy cannot be realized where they are unavailable. This applies to many, though not all, regions where NPC has its highest incidence.

Radiotherapy treatment

External Beam

- *Radiotherapy Dose-Fractionation*   Both the primary and the regional lymphatics need to be treated adequately. A full discussion of radiotherapy treatment is not possible in this text and the issues of radiotherapy dose fractionation are discussed elsewhere.[68,69] It is axiomatic that the treatment should be provided according to appropriate radiobiological principles to obtain optimal results. The discussion will concentrate more on potential detriments associated with not being able to provide timely treatment, treatment disruption for any reason, where it is not provided, or where treatment expertise is limited.

- *Interruption of Treatment*   The effect of treatment interruption and prolonged overall radiotherapy treatment time was investigated in almost 700 NPC patients. The hazard rate for locoregional failure increased by 3.3% for each day of interruption.[55] Thus interruptions and prolonged treatment adversely affect outcome in radiotherapy for NPC and is presumably due to repopulation of tumor clonogens during treatment. Every effort should be made to keep treatment on schedule, and interruptions for whatever reasons should be minimized.[55]

- *Adequacy of Tumor Coverage*   As implied before, in NPC there is the requirement for adequacy of coverage of disease while still protecting normal tissues where long-term damage may have devastating consequences. Although evidence that dose can be conformed to the required target has been present for some time,[70] little has been published concerning the outcome of newer radiotherapy techniques. This is an evolving field, and recently techniques involving sophisticated computer software and hardware have become available to permit very precise dose deposition in NPC by varying the intensity of the beam through intensity-modulated radiotherapy IMRT.[71,72] Detailed descriptions of some of the radiotherapy requirements have also been published as it relates to NPC.[73–75] The evidence for benefit is as yet indirect, but compelling data indicate that locoregional control rates of 71% are achieved where the radiotherapy margin was <1 cm compared to 91%

where the margin was ≥ 1 cm,[76] reinforcing that it is important to ensure that adequate tumor coverage by the radiotherapy fields exists.

- *Delay in Initiation of Radiotherapy*   Almost no attention has been paid to the potential detriment that delay in initiation of radiotherapy may have on the outcome of NPC. The only study to confront the issue addressed T1-category NPC patients. Delay in initiation of treatment to the primary target did not affect the control rate at irradiated sites, but there was a trend toward increase in failures at untreated sites that were deemed clinically too serious to be ignored.[77] This study, addressing only T1-category patients, was potentially underpowered to detect an effect, if one was present. Evidence from a study of tonsillar carcinoma suggests that the effect is only readily evident in the larger tumors and would be difficult to see in "early" disease.[78] Limitation in access to timely cancer treatment, especially radiotherapy, may therefore compromise outcome.

Brachytherapy   While not universally employed in the management of NPC, evidence exists that augmentation of the doses to superficial disease appears to have the potential for improved outcome.[79–82] As indicated below, it is also useful for recurrent disease because of the ability to focus dose to a restricted target area.[83]

Chemoradiotherapy

The role of chemotherapy in NPC has been considered for many years, generally with induction chemotherapy, which has not shown a survival advantage. Recently an Intergroup randomized trial evaluated concurrent cisplatin during radiotherapy, followed by adjuvant cisplatin combined with fluorouracil in locally advanced disease. The experimental arm experienced a significant improvement in 3-year survival rate ($p = 0.005$).[61] Difficulties include the small size of the trial and the exceptionally poor 3-year survival in the radiotherapy-alone control arm (46%). This raises the question about its applicability to Asian patients who almost exclusively compose WHO-2 and WHO-3 histologies. In contrast, the Intergroup trial was undertaken in North America, where the histology mix is different. Also, in an environment where experience in the technical delivery of radiotherapy for NPC is not as great as it would be in Asia, an alternative explanation is that concurrent chemotherapy may overcome potential limitations of underdosage in the target volume. What are awaited are long-term late toxicity studies, since the critical issue is safety of concurrent chemoradiotherapy to vulnerable anatomy in the skull-base region, and little is known about the true degree of late toxicities of this approach.[84]

Influence of Country of Treatment

Most of what has been stated up to this point applies to the delivery of care in environments where high standards of research, investigation, and treatment are available for NPC. Unfortunately this is not universally the case. All cases of nasopharyngeal carcinoma had cervical lymphadenopathy at presentation at a center in Kenya. Of these, 70.6% had N3 disease. The average period of delay between the first medical attention at a primary health care facility and the first appointment at the national hospital was 8.7 months. Inherent inefficiency in the referral system was deemed a major contributing factor to the advanced stage at presentation.[85] It can be assumed that may countries suffer from similar socioeconomic and infrastructure problems.

Further evidence of compromise in outcome due to the environment where a patient is treated comes from the EUROCARE study. This study was mentioned earlier under Host-Related factors.[57] Here variations in survival are described for adults with NPC diagnosed and treated in Europe from 1978 to 1989. The causes of these differences are difficult to determine since stage data were unavailable. However, possibilities include access to timely care, compromised diagnosis and staging (including accurate tumor definition for treatment), and less experience or skill in planning and delivery of radiotherapy. The possibility that comorbidity may have confounded the outcome has already been mentioned.[57]

Management of Recurrence

Patients recurring at the local site may be salvaged with further treatment. The major barrier to retreatment is toxicity and the challenge is to accomplish it safely. Generally radiotherapy is used, but surgery is indicated in selected cases[86-89] and in some cases may be preferable to radiotherapy.[90] Histology, and interval to recurrence were independent prognostic factors for overall survival, but only histology and presence of complications were significant for local-regional progression-free rate.[91] The protective effect of long latency in apparently reducing the risk of distant metastasis has also been studied in a multivariate analysis of 847 cases of recurrent NPC.[92] In another study of reirradiation, the 3-year and 5-year overall survival rates were 46% and 36%, respectively.[60] A multivariate analysis revealed older age, recurrent T3-4 disease, and palliative treatment to be unfavorable factors in predicting overall survival. For performance-adjusted survival the unfavorable factors were similar except that baseline Karnofsky performance status <70 substituted for older age. A high complication rate was also observed after reirradiation, with 34% of patients developing neurological sequel.[60] Lee et al. demonstrated that the major determinant of posttreatment complications related to the severity of damage in the initial treatment course and the time interval between the initial course and the radiotherapy for recurrence.[93] Yet another recent study of reirradiation showed that intracranial invasion and/or cranial nerve palsy and re-treatment dose ($\geq$50 Gy) yielded significantly better survival, in addition to latency beyond 2 years since initial diagnosis.[94]

In addition to conventional external beam alone and surgery, recurrent NPC is a logical candidate for selected treatments to attempt to deliver a high dose while protecting normal tissues from injury. The main approaches that have been taken are the use of brachytherapy for a component of the course,[83,95] or stereotactic radiotherapy approaches.[94,96,97] Suggestions of benefit have also been made for conformal external beam radiotherapy, which resulted in fewer severe complications with no brain necrosis cases in contrast to conventional radiotherapy.[94]

This topic is placed under *environment-related* prognostic factors because the skill and experience of the treatment team is important to permit early diagnosis and management in a systematic way. It is probable that in centers with little experience of primary management of NPC, the likelihood of having a coherent protocol for recurrent disease would be even more remote.

SUMMARY

This review of prognostic factors in NPC provides a brief summary of the current state of knowledge. It is apparent that, while NPC offers a significant model in oncology for environmental, genetic, and infectious factors in its causation, it remains an enigma in terms of prognosis. The dominant themes continue to be the complex nature of the anatomic site where the disease originates and the presence of critical adjacent anatomy which may be injured by high dose radiotherapy. For this reason, the development of a relevant staging system to be used worldwide was an important step forward. However, the complexity and expense of the treatment, including support for radiotherapy and chemotherapy toxicity, and the cost of radiotherapy and staging equipment, makes it difficult to provide the same opportunity for cure in all countries where this disease is diagnosed. This is especially true in countries where resources are limited. Apart from anatomic details of the disease, these *environmental* factors probably govern the outcome of these patients even more than the subtleties of the other factors we have discussed. For this reason, an attempt to stratify the different factors in levels of relevance is provided as well, with essential factors for treatment implementation being tabulated ahead of other factors (see Appendix 13B). Meanwhile it is hoped that the future will bring the promise of a better understanding of treatment and prognosis through discoveries of molecular alterations in this rare disease. So far these findings are preliminary and remain largely in the experimental domain at the present time.

■■■■■■■ **APPENDIX 13A**

Nasopharynx TNM Classification

T — Primary Tumor

T1 Tumor confined to nasopharynx

T2 Tumor extends to soft tissue of oropharynx and/or nasal fossa
   T2a without parapharyngeal extension
   T2b with parapharyngeal extension

T3 Tumor invades bony structures and/or paranasal sinuses

T4 Tumor with intracranial extension and/or involvement of cranial nerves, infratemporal fossa, hypopharynx, or orbit

N — Regional Lymph Nodes

NX Regional lymph nodes cannot be assessed

N0 No regional lymph-node metastasis

N1 Unilateral metastasis in lymph node(s), 6 cm or less in greatest dimension, above supraclavicular fossa

N2 Bilateral metastasis in lymph node(s), 6 cm or less in greatest dimension, above supraclavicular fossa

N3 Metastasis in lymph node(s)
   N3a greater than 6 cm in dimension
   N3b in the supraclavicular fossa

Nasopharynx Stage Grouping

Stage 0	Tis	N0	M0
Stage I	T1	N0	M0
Stage IIA	T2a	N0	M0
Stage IIB	T1	N1	M0
	T2a	N1	M0
	T2b	N0, N1	M0
Stage III	T1	N2	M0
	T2a, T2b	N2	M0
	T3	N0, N1, N2	M0
Stage IVA	T4	N0, N1, N2	M0
Stage IVB	Any T	N3	M0
Stage IVC	Any T	Any N	M1

Source: Sobin LH, Wittekind Ch (eds.): *TNM classification of malignant tumors*, 5th ed. Union Internationale Contre le Cancer Wiley-Liss, New York, 1997.

Summary Table of Prognostic Factors in Nasopharyngeal Carcinoma

Prognostic Factors	Tumor Related	Host	Environment Related
Essential	TNM stage (including presence of metastases) WHO histologic subtype	Performance status Comorbidity	Available imaging (MRI & CT) Adverse geographic location for many reasons Adequacy of coverage by RT (need for conformal techniques in some presentations) Experienced team, including for salvage diagnosis and retreatment Compromised support for chemotherapy toxicity when indicated
Additional	Tumor volume Tumor infiltration Local failure on risk of distant metastasis Parapharyngeal space subdivision	Ethnicity Age Symptoms	Treatment interruption Available technical radiotherapy Treatment delay
New and promising	Dentritic cell density Lysozyme + tumor Angiogenesis p53 (debatable) c-myc oncogene HLA-DR expression E-cadherin/betacatenin LMP1 + tumor nm23-H1 expression interleukin 2 receptor CYFRA 21-1 level Serum LDH Serum copper Serum ferritin Serum TPA		New imaging to identify recurrence (PET, etc.)

REFERENCES

1. Sobin LH, Wittekind C (eds.): *UICC TNM classification of malignant tumors*, 5 ed. New York, Wiley, 1997.

2. Fleming I, Cooper J, Henson D, et al. (eds.): *AJCC cancer staging manual*, 5th ed. Philadelphia, Lippincott-Raven, 1997.

3. Chong VFH, Mukherji SK: Carcinoma of the nasopharynx. *Semin Ultrasound CT MRI* 19(6):449–62, 1998.

4. Chong VF, Mukherji SK, Ng SH, et al.: Nasopharyngeal carcinoma: Review of how imaging affects staging. *J Comput Assist Tomogr* 23(6):984–93, 1999.

5. Ng SH, Chang TC, Ko SF, et al.: Nasopharyngeal carcinoma: MRI and CT assessment. *Neuroradiology* 39(10):741–6, 1997.

6. Heng DM, Wee J, Fong KW, et al.: Prognostic factors in 677 patients in Singapore with nondisseminated nasopharyngeal carcinoma. *Cancer* 86(10):1912–20, 1999.

7. Sham JS, Choy D.: Prognostic value of paranasopharyngeal extension of nasopharyngeal carcinoma on local control and short-term survival. *Head Neck* 13(4):298–310, 1991.

8. Min H, Hong M, Ma J, et al.: A new staging system for nasopharyngeal carcinoma in China. *Int J Radiat Oncol Biol Phys* 30(5):1037–42, 1994.

9. Tsao S.: Staging, in Chong V, Tsao S, (eds.): *Nasopharyngeal carcinoma. Singapore*, Armour, 1997, 77–89.

10. Tsao S: A new working staging system for nasopharyngeal carcinoma (NPC), in Tursz T, Pagano J, Ablashi D, et al.: (eds.): *The Epstein-Barr virus and associated diseases*, Vol 225. Libby Eurotext, 1993, 727–34.

11. Guan XX. Invasion of poststyloid space and metastasis of deep upper cervical lymph node in nasopharyngeal carcinoma. *Chung Hua Chung Liu Tsa Chih* 12(2):117–9, 1990.

12. Teo P, Tsao S, Shiu W, et al.: A clinical study of 407 cases of nasopharyngeal carcinoma in Hong Kong. *Int J Radiat Oncol Biol Phys* 17:515–30, 1989.

13. Lee AW, Foo W, Law SC, et al.: Staging of nasopharyngeal carcinoma: From Ho's to the new UICC system. *Int J Cancer* 84(2):179–87, 1999.

14. Sham J, Cheung Y, Choy D, et al.: Cranial nerve involvement and base of the skull erosion in nasopharyngeal carcinoma. *Cancer* 68:422–6, 1991.

15. King AD, Lam WW, Leung SF, et al.: MRI of local disease in nasopharyngeal carcinoma: Tumour extent vs tumour stage. *Br J Radiol* 72(860):734–41, 1999.

16. Johns M, Neal D, Cantrell R: Staging of cervical lymph node metastasis: Comparison of two systems. *Ann Otol Rhinol Laryngol* 93:330–2, 1984.

17. Lee AW, Foo W, Poon YF, et al.: Staging of nasopharyngeal carcinoma: Evaluation of N-staging by Ho and UICC/AJCC systems. Union Internationale Contre le Cancer. American Joint Committee for Cancer. *Clin Oncol (R Coll Radiol)* 8(3):146–54, 1996.

18. Chua DT, Sham JS, Kwong DL, et al.: Volumetric analysis of tumor extent in nasopharyngeal carcinoma and correlation with treatment outcome. *Int J Radiat Oncol Biol Phys* 39(3):711–9, 1997.

19. Sakata K, Hareyama M, Tamakawa M, et al.: Prognostic factors of nasopharynx tumors investigated by MR imaging and the value of MR imaging in the newly published TNM staging. *Int J Radiat Oncol Biol Phys* 43(2):273–8, 1999.

20. Lin ZX, Li DR, Chen ZJ, et al.: What is the significance of nasal involvement in nasopharyngeal carcinoma? *Int J Radiat Oncol Biol Phys* 45(4):907–14, 1999.

21. Shanmugaratnam K, Sobin LH: Histological typing of upper respiratory tract tumours. International Histological Classification of Tumours No 19. Geneva, WHO, 1978.

22. Reddy SP, Raslan WF, Gooneratne S, et al.: Prognostic significance of keratinization in nasopharyngeal carcinoma. *Am J Otolaryngol* 16(2):103–8, 1995.

23. Marks JE, Phillips JL, Menck HR: The National Cancer Data Base report on the relationship of race and national origin to the histology of nasopharyngeal carcinoma. *Cancer* 83(3):582–8, 1998.

24. Gallo O, Bianchi S, Giannini A, et al.: Correlations between histopathological and biological findings in nasopharyngeal carcinoma and its prognostic significance. *Laryngoscope* 101(5):487–93, 1991.

25. Hsu MM. Local infiltration of T-lymphocyte subsets as a prognostic indicator in patients with nasopharyngeal carcinoma. *Ear Nose Throat J* 69(8):543–7, 1990.

26. Spruck CHd, Tsai YC, Huang DP, et al.: Absence of p53 gene mutations in primary nasopharyngeal carcinomas. *Cancer Res* 52(17):4787–90, 1992.

27. Porter MJ, Field JK, Lee JC, et al.: Detection of the tumour suppressor gene p53 in nasopharyngeal carcinoma in Hong Kong Chinese. *Anticancer Res* 14(3B):1357–60, 1994.

28. Sheu LF, Chen A, Tseng HH, et al.: Assessment of p53 expression in nasopharyngeal carcinoma. *Hum Pathol* 26(4):380–6, 1995.

29. Roychowdhury DF, Tseng A, Jr., Fu KK, et al.: New prognostic factors in nasopharyngeal carcinoma. Tumor angiogenesis and C-erbB2 expression. *Cancer* 77(8): 1419–26, 1996.

30. Gulley ML, Burton MP, Allred DC, et al.: Epstein-Barr virus infection is associated with p53 accumulation in nasopharyngeal carcinoma. *Hum Pathol* 29(3):252–9, 1998.

31. Lung ML, Hu Y, Cheng Y, et al.: p53 inactivating mutations in Chinese nasopharyngeal carcinomas. *Cancer Lett* 133(1):89–94, 1998.

32. Harn HJ, Hsieh HF, Ho LI, et al.: Apoptosis in nasopharyngeal carcinoma as related to histopathological characteristics and clinical stage. *Histopathology* 33(2):117–22, 1998.

33. Masuda M, Shinokuma A, Hirakawa N, et al.: Expression of bcl-2-, p53, and Ki-67 and outcome of patients with primary nasopharyngeal carcinomas following DNA-damaging treatment. *Head Neck* 20(7):640–4, 1998.

34. Qian CN, Min HQ, Liang XM, et al.: Primary study of neovasculature correlating with metastatic nasopharyngeal carcinoma using computer image analysis. *J Cancer Res Clin Oncol* 123(11/12):645–51, 1997.

35. Wakisaka N, Wen QH, Yoshizaki T, et al.: Association of vascular endothelial growth factor expression with angiogenesis and lymph node metastasis in nasopharyngeal carcinoma. *Laryngoscope* 109(5):810–4, 1999.

36. Qian CN, Zhang CQ, Guo X, et al.: Elevation of serum vascular endothelial growth factor in male patients with metastatic nasopharyngeal carcinoma. *Cancer* 88(2):255–61, 2000.

37. Porter MJ, Field JK, Leung SF, et al.: The detection of the c-myc and ras onco-genes in nasopharyngeal carcinoma by immunohistochemistry. *Acta Otolaryngol* 114(1):105–9, 1994.

38. Faccioli S, Cavicchi O, Caliceti U, et al.: Cell proliferation as an independent predictor of survival for patients with advanced nasopharyngeal carcinoma. *Mod Pathol* 10(9):884–94, 1997.

39. Chan AT, Ho S, Teo PM, et al.: Assessment of proliferating cell nuclear antigen in nasopharyngeal carcinoma tissue and its relation to clinical findings. *Oral Oncol* 33(1):13–8, 1997.

40. Liu B, Su Z, Chen S: A study of HIA-DR antigen expression in nasopharyngeal carcinoma and its relation with clinical pathology and prognosis. *Chung Hua Ping Li Hsueh Tsa Chih* 25(3):162–4, 1996.

41. Zheng Z, Pan J, Chu B, et al.: Downregulation and abnormal expression of E-cadherin and beta-catenin in nasopharyngeal carcinoma: close association with advanced disease stage and lymph node metastasis. *Hum Pathol* 30(4):458–66, 1999.

42. Hu LF, Chen F, Zhen QF, et al.: Differences in the growth pattern and clinical course of EBV-LMP1 expressing and non-expressing nasopharyngeal carcinomas. *Eur J Cancer* 31A(5):658–60, 1995.

43. Guo X, Min HQ, Zeng MS, et al.: nm23-H1 expression in nasopharyngeal carcinoma: Correlation with clinical outcome. *Int J Cancer* 79(6):596–600, 1998.

44. Hsu MM, Ko JY, Chang YL: Elevated levels of soluble interleukin 2 receptor and tumor necrosis factor in nasopharyngeal carcinoma. *Arch Otolaryngol Head Neck Surg* 117(11):1257–9, 1991.

45. Ho S, Leung WT, Yuen J, Johnson PJ: Serum levels of CYFRA 21–1 in nasopha-ryngeal carcinoma and its possible role in monitoring of therapy. *Eur J Cancer B Oral Oncol* 32B(6):377–80, 1996.

46. Lin WY, Yen TC, Cheng KY, Wang SJ: The value of CYFRA 21–1, a new tumor marker, in nasopharyngeal carcinoma. *Neoplasma* 45(1):21–4, 1998.

47. Ho S, Leung SF, Leung WT, et al.: Strong association between hyperferritinaemia and metastatic disease in nasopharyngeal carcinoma. *Eur J Cancer B Oral Oncol* 32B(4):242–5, 1996.

48. Lian SL, Hsu HY, Lin SM: Serum copper and zinc levels in patients with nasopha-ryngeal carcinoma. *Taiwan I Hsueh Hui Tsa Chih* 88(3):236–9, 1989.

49. Ho S, Teo P, Kwan WH, et al.: Staging and IgA VCA titre in patients with nasopharyngeal carcinoma: Changes over a 12-year period. *Oral Oncol* 34(6):491–5, 1998.

50. Liaw CC, Wang CH, Huang JS, et al.: Serum lactate dehydrogenase level in patients with nasopharyngeal carcinoma. *Acta Oncol* 36(2):159–64, 1997.

51. Xu J, Menezes J, Prasad U, Ahmad A: Elevated serum levels of transforming growth factor beta1 in Epstein-Barr virus-associated nasopharyngeal carcinoma patients. *Int J Cancer* 84(4):396–9, 1999.

52. Liu MT, Yeh CY: Prognostic value of anti-Epstein-Barr virus antibodies in nasopha-ryngeal carcinoma (NPC). *Radiat Med* 16(2):113–7, 1998.

53. Xu J, Ahmad A, DA, M, et al.: Analysis and significance of anti-latent membrane protein-1 antibodies in the sera of patients with EBV-associated diseases. *J Immunol* 164(5):2815–22, 2000.

54. Sundram FX, Aw SE, Toh HJ, Chua ET: Significance of tissue polypeptide antigen (TPA) levels in nasopharyngeal cancer. *Ann Acad Med Singapore* 19(2):156–60, 1990.

55. Kwong DL, Sham JS, Chua DT, et al.: The effect of interruptions and prolonged treatment time in radiotherapy for nasopharyngeal carcinoma. *Int J Radiat Oncol Biol Phys* 39(3):703–10, 1997.

56. Wolden SL, Steinherz PG, Kraus DH, et al.: Improved long term survival with combined modality therapy for pediatric nasopharynx cancer. *Int J Radiat Oncol Biol Phys* 46:859–64, 2000.

57. Jiong L, Berrino F, Coebergh JWW, Group at EW: Variation in survival for adults with nasopharyngeal cancer in Europe. *Eur J Cancer* 34(14):2162–6, 1998.

58. Zaghloul MS, Dahaba NM, Wahab AA, et al.: Nasopharyngeal carcinoma in children and adolescents: Successful role of retrieval therapy. *Tumori* 79:123–7, 1993.

59. Kajanti M, Flander M, Grenman R, et al.: Treatment results of nasopharyngeal cancer—A nationwide survey from Finland. *Acta Oncol* 35(6):697–702, 1996.

60. Chua DT, Sham JS, Kwong DL, et al.: Locally recurrent nasopharyngeal carcinoma: Treatment results for patients with computed tomography assessment. *Int J Radiat Oncol Biol Phys* 41(2):379–86, 1998.

61. Al-Sarraf M, LeBlanc M, Giri PG, et al.: Chemoradiotherapy versus radiotherapy in patients with advanced nasopharyngeal cancer: Phase III randomized Intergroup study 0099. *J Clin Oncol* 16(4):1310–7, 1998.

62. International Nasopharynx Cancer Study Group: Preliminary results of a randomized trial comparing neoadjuvant chemotherapy (cisplatin, epirubicin, bleomycin) plus radiotherapy vs. radiotherapy alone in Stage IV (>or = N2, M0) undifferentiated nasopharyngeal carcinoma: A positive effect on progression-free survival. VUMCA I trial. *Int J Radiat Oncol Biol Phys* 35(3):463–9, 1996.

63. Siu LL, Czaykowski PM, Tannock IF: Phase I/II study of the CAPABLE regimen for patients with poorly differentiated carcinoma of the nasopharynx. *J Clin Oncol* 16(7):2514–21, 1998.

64. Kraiphibul P, Atichartakarn V, Clongsusuek P, et al.: Changes in T-staging of nasopharyngeal carcinoma by CT-scan. *J Med Assoc Thai* 72(12):661–5, 1989.

65. Yamashita S, Kondo M, Inuyama Y, Hashimoto S: Improved survival of patients with nasopharyngeal squamous cell carcinoma. *Int J Radiat Oncol Biol Phys* 12(307–12), 1986.

66. Kostakoglu L, Uysal U, Ozyar E, et al.: Monitoring response to therapy with thallium-201 and technetium-99m-sestamibi SPECT in nasopharyngeal carcinoma. *J Nucl Med* 38(7):1009–14, 1997.

67. Pui MH, Du JQ, Yueh TC, Zeng SQ: Imaging of nasopharyngeal carcinoma with Tc-99m MIBI. *Clin Nucl Med* 23(1):29–32, 1998.

68. Lee AW, Chan DK, Fowler JF, et al.: Effect of time, dose and fractionation on local control of nasopharyngeal carcinoma. *Radiother Oncol* 36(1):24–31, 1995.

69. Geara FB, Sanguineti G, Tucker SL, et al.: Carcinoma of the nasopharynx treated by radiotherapy alone: Determinants of distant metastasis and survival. *Radiother Oncol* 43(1):53–61, 1997.

70. Leibel SA, Kutcher GJ, Harrison LB, et al.: Improved dose distributions for 3D conformal boost treatments in carcinoma of the nasopharynx. *Int J Radiat Oncol Biol Phys* 20(4):823–33, 1991.

71. De Neve W, De Gersem W, Derycke S, et al.: Clinical delivery of intensity modulated conformal radiotherapy for relapsed or second-primary head and neck cancer using a multileaf collimator with dynamic control [published erratum appears in *Radiother Oncol* 52(1):89, 1999]. *Radiother Oncol* 50(3):301–14, 1999.

72. Verhey LJ: Comparison of three-dimensional conformal radiation therapy and intensity-modulated radiation therapy systems. *Semin Radiat Oncol* 9(1):78–98, 1999.

73. LoSasso T, Chui CS, Kutcher GJ, et al.: The use of a multi-leaf collimator for conformal radiotherapy of carcinomas of the prostate and nasopharynx [see Comments]. *Int J Radiat Oncol Biol Phys* 25(2):161–70, 1993.

74. Pommier P, Lapeyre M, Ginestet C, et al.: Conformal radiotherapy in cancer of the upper aerodigestive tract. *Cancer Radiother* 3(5):414–24, 1999.

75. Cheung KY, Choi PHK, Chau RMC, et al.: The roles of multileaf collimators and micro-multileaf collimators in conformal and conventional nasopharyngeal carcinoma radiotherapy treatments. *Med Phys* 25(10):2077–85, 1999.

76. Jian JJ, Cheng SH, Prosnitz LR, et al.: T classification and clivus margin as risk factors for determining locoregional control by radiotherapy of nasopharyngeal carcinoma. *Cancer* 82(2):261–7, 1998.

77. Lee AW, Chan DK, Fowler JF, et al.: T1 nasopharyngeal carcinoma: The effect of waiting time on tumor control. *Int J Radiat Oncol Biol Phys* 30(5):1111–7, 1994.

78. Mackillop WJ, Bates J, O'Sullivan B, Withers HR: The effect of delay in treatment on local control by radiotherapy. *Int J Radiat Oncol Biol Phys* 34(1):243–50, 1996.

79. Chang JT, See LC, Tang SG, et al.: The role of brachytherapy in early-stage nasopharyngeal carcinoma. *Int J Radiat Oncol Biol Phys* 36(5):1019–24, 1996.

80. Levendag PC, Schmitz PI, Jansen PP, et al.: Fractionated high-dose-rate brachytherapy in primary carcinoma of the nasopharynx. *J Clin Oncol* 16(6):2213–20, 1998.

81. Slevin NJ, Wilkinson JM, Filby HM, Gupta NK: Intracavitary radiotherapy boosting for nasopharynx cancer. *Br J Radiol* 70:412–4, 1997.

82. Teo PM, Leung SF, Lee WY, Zee B: Intracavitary brachytherapy significantly enhances local control of early T-stage nasopharyngeal carcinoma: The existence of a dose-tumor-control relationship above conventional tumoricidal dose. *Int J Radiat Oncol Biol Phys* 46(2):445–58, 2000.

83. McLean M, Chow E, O'Sullivan B, et al.: Re-irradiation for locally recurrent nasopharyngeal carcinoma. *Radiother Oncol* 48(2):209–11, 1998.

84. Baron-Hay S, Clifford A, Jackson M, Clarke S: Life threatening laryngeal toxicity following treatment with combined chemoradiotherapy for nasopharyngeal cancer: A case report with review of the literature. *Ann Oncol* 10(9):1109–12, 1999.

85. Oburra HO: Late presentation of laryngeal and nasopharyngeal cancer in Kenyatta National Hospital. *East Afr Med J* 75(4):223–6, 1998.

86. Fee WE, Jr., Gilmer PA, Goffinet DR: Surgical management of recurrent nasopharyngeal carcinoma after radiation failure at the primary site. *Laryngoscope* 98(11):1220–6, 1988.

87. Wei WI, Ho CM, Yuen PW, et al.: Maxillary swing approach for resection of tumors in and around the nasopharynx. *Arch Otolaryngol Head Neck Surg* 121(6):638–42, 1995.

88. Morton RP, Liavaag PG, McLean M, Freeman JL: Transcervico-mandibulo-palatal approach for surgical salvage of recurrent nasopharyngeal cancer. *Head Neck* 18(4):352–8, 1996.

89. Hsu MM, Ko JY, Sheen TS, Chang YL: Salvage surgery for recurrent nasopharyngeal carcinoma. *Arch Otolaryngol Head Neck Surg* 123(3):305–9, 1997.

90. Teo PM, Kwan WH, Chan AT, et al.: How successful is high-dose (> or = 60 Gy) reirradiation using mainly external beams in salvaging local failures of nasopharyngeal carcinoma? [see Comments]. *Int J Radiat Oncol Biol Phys* 40(4):897–913, 1998.

91. Hwang JM, Fu KK, Phillips TL: Results and prognostic factors in the retreatment of locally recurrent nasopharyngeal carcinoma. *Int J Radiat Oncol Biol Phys* 41(5):1099–111, 1998.

92. Lee AW, Foo W, Law SC, et al.: Recurrent nasopharyngeal carcinoma: The puzzles of long latency. *Int J Radiat Oncol Biol Phys* 44(1):149–56, 1999.

93. Lee AW, Foo W, Law SC, et al.: Total biological effect on late reactive tissues following reirradiation for recurrent nasopharyngeal carcinoma. *Int J Radiat Oncol Biol Phys* 46(4):865–72, 2000.

94. Chang JT, See L, Liao C, et al.: Locally recurrent nasopharyngeal carcinoma. *Radiother Oncol* 54(2):135–42, 2000.

95. Orecchia R, Leonardi MC, Krengli M, et al.: External radiotherapy plus intracavitary brachytherapy for recurrent chordoma of the nasopharynx. *Acta Oncol* 37(3):301–4, 1998.

96. Cmelak AJ, Cox RS, Adler JR, et al.: Radiosurgery for skull base malignancies and nasopharyngeal carcinoma [see Comments]. *Int J Radiat Oncol Biol Phys* 37(5):997–1003, 1997.

97. Kocher M, Voges J, Staar S, et al.: Linear accelerator radiosurgery for recurrent malignant tumors of the skull base. *Am J Clin Oncol* 21(1):18–22, 1998.

■■■■■■ CHAPTER 14

Salivary Gland Cancers

JOSEPH CALIFANO and RONALD H. SPIRO

Malignant salivary gland tumors are remarkable for their relative infrequency as compared to other solid tumors, and their wide diversity in histologic appearance, clinical presentation, and biologic behavior. By virtue of the slow growth rates of some of these tumors, posttreatment surveillance must continue for a decade or more in order to accrue reliable data regarding locoregional control and survival. Fortunately, useful prognostic information can be derived from assessment of clinical stage, and tumor histology.

TUMOR-RELATED FACTORS

Anatomic Site of Origin

Most salivary gland tumors arise from the paired major salivary glands, with the parotid gland accounting for 70% of the total. In our experience, 25% of those tumors arising in the parotid gland are malignant.[1] As the size of the salivary gland of origin decreases, however, the risk of malignancy increases, so that approximately 50% of submandibular gland tumors and almost all sublingual gland tumors and minor salivary gland tumors treated in our hospital prove to be malignant. Because most published reports are based on the experience at academic and tertiary referral centers, they usually include a higher proportion of malignant tumors than is likely to be encountered in the general population. Nonetheless, the risk of malignancy certainly varies according to site of origin of the tumor.

Histologic Subtype

It is important to remember that identification of these tumors can be a significant challenge to pathologists, and classification systems may vary between reporting centers. The prevalent histologic types of salivary gland malignancy

Prognostic Factors in Cancer, 2nd edition, Edited by Mary K. Gospodarowicz
ISBN 0-471-40633-3   Copyright © 2001 Wiley-Liss, Inc.

1	Mucoepidermoid grade 1	(72 PTS. 58 Censored)
2	Mucoepidermoid other	(132 PTS. 57 Censored)
3	Acinic-cell carcinoma	(56 PTS. 46 Censored)
4	Adenoidcystic	(53 PTS. 20 Censored)
5	Malignant mixed tumours	(67 PTS. 25 Censored)
6	Adeno carcinoma	(47 PTS. 21 Censored)
7	Squamous or anaplastic carcinoma	(34 PTS. 8 Censored)

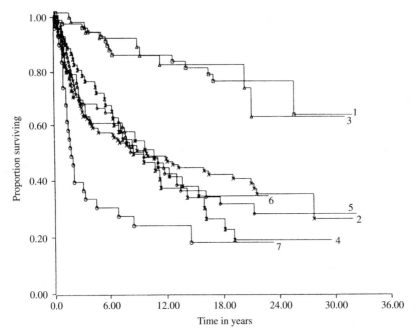

Figure 14.1 Cumulative survival for salivary gland malignancies by histology.[1] Note that survival curves overlap for several tumor types.

and their associated Kaplan-Meier survival curves are depicted in Figure 14.1.[2,3] Most studies indicate that low-grade mucoepidermoid carcinoma and acinic-cell carcinoma have a more favorable prognosis, and squamous-cell carcinoma, salivary duct carcinoma, and anaplastic carcinoma have a relatively poor survival. The remaining histopathologic types fall in an intermediate group in terms of survival. As already mentioned, follow-up requirements differ according to histology. Recurrence may occur more than 10 years following treatment for some salivary gland tumors (Fig. 14.1). In patients with adenoid cystic carcinoma in particular, disease-related deaths could occur after more than 20 years of follow-up. This explains why disease-free survival may differ significantly from cumulative survival. The indolent clinical course seen in many patients with adenoid cystic carcinoma is often characterized by a long, disease-free interval, and/or slow growth of pulmonary metastases.

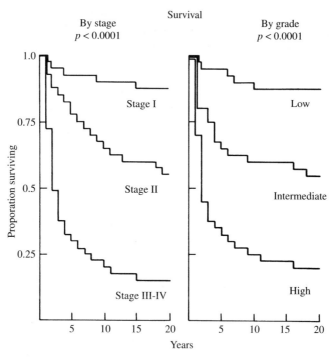

Figure 14.2 Cumulative survival curves for salivary gland malignancy according to stage and grade.[1] Significant differences are apparent.

Extent of Disease

Clinical stage is by far the best predictor of survival and is determined by tumor size and the presence or absence of cervical nodal and distant metastasis.[1,4,5] T Category increases, regardless of size, when there is extension of tumor into skin, adjacent soft tissues or bone, or when the facial nerve is involved. Significant differences in survival, according to tumor stage, are shown in Figure 14.2, the TNM indicated are those prior to the 5th Edition. Facial nerve paralysis in patients with parotid gland carcinoma is an indicator of extremely poor prognosis, with 5-year survival rates varying between 0% and 15% in those patients who present with paralysis.[6-8] The importance of facial nerve invasion was recognized in the recently modified TNM classification (5th Edition) shown in Appendix 14A. If the facial nerve is involved, such cases are automatically classified as T4 disease, and this is a change from previous editions of TNM.

Tumor Grade

Tumor grade also appears to have an influence on survival (Fig. 14.2).[1,9] We and others have classified mucoepidermoid carcinoma into high-, intermediate-, and low-grade tumors. In our experience, adenocarcinomas and acinic-cell carcinoma can also be graded, but this is not true for other histologic subtypes.[10] This is a complex and occasionally confusing issue. For example, adenoid cystic carcinoma can be classified as low, intermediate, or high grade depending on whether the tumor has "bland" tubular/cribriform features, a more prognostically ominous solid morphology, or a combination of both patterns. Despite other reports to the contrary, however, we are unable to substantiate significant survival differences when adenoid cystic carcinoma is graded in this fashion.[4] Although tumor control is less often achieved in patients with other high-grade lesions,[1,4] the evidence suggests that the decision to treat with adjuvant external-beam radiation therapy should not be based on tumor grade alone.

Minor Salivary Glands

Historically, it has been thought that tumors originating in minor salivary glands have a worse prognosis than those originating in the major glands. Because they may arise in obscure sites, minor salivary tumors tend to be more advanced at the time of diagnosis. They also have a greater propensity to invade adjacent bone when compared to major salivary tumors, particularly in the palate where they most commonly arise. This also holds true for minor salivary tumors arising in the paranasal sinuses, which are inherently more difficult to resect with adequate, generous margins due to their proximity to cranial and orbital structures. Bony involvement is an indicator of poor prognosis in univariate analysis.[6] Using the staging system employed for squamous-cell carcinoma in identical sites, multivariate analysis confirms that tumor extent (i.e., stage) is clearly the most significant predictor of local control in patients with minor salivary gland carcinoma. Stage for stage, however, there are no significant survival differences when comparing patients treated for malignant major or minor salivary gland tumors.[7,11]

Residual Disease

Adequacy of surgical resection is another important prognostic factor. The presence of microscopic tumor at the border of resection portends poorer local control in multiple studies.[12-14] Adjunctive external beam radiation therapy is indicated when microscopic residual disease is suspected, especially when dealing with a high-grade neoplasm.

Perineural Spread

Perineural spread, when present in squamous-cell carcinoma, carries a poor prognosis as well, but it is unclear whether this is a reflection of the inherently aggressive nature of these tumors, or of persistent disease present in neural tissue beyond the border of resection.[8,12,15] The incidence of perineural tumor spread in adenoid cystic carcinoma is notoriously high. As some authors have correctly emphasized, however, local control is most significantly reduced when tumor extends in and around major "named" nerves.[13] Pain may be an indicator of perineural tumor extension, and experience suggests that this symptom has ominous implications for survival when associated with any malignant tumor.[6,14]

Molecular Factors

As yet there are no single laboratory or molecular biologic parameters that clearly identify tumors and or patients with poor prognosis, although this remains an active area of research.

HOST-RELATED FACTORS

Age and Gender

Parotid neoplasms in younger patients tend more frequently to be benign; when younger patients present with malignant neoplasms, these tumors tend to be lower-grade and less aggressive neoplasms.[16] In childhood, for example, low-grade mucoepidermoid carcinoma is the most common malignant salivary gland tumor.[17] Male gender also seems to indicate an adverse prognosis in those patients with parotid cancer as well.

Influence of Geography on the Host

Some studies have indicated a high incidence of anaplastic salivary gland cancer and nasopharyngeal cancer in Inuit populations from Greenland, perhaps in part due to Epstein-Barr virus (EBV).[18] EBV has also been described as a possible etiologic agent in the development of lymphoepithelial carcinoma of the salivary gland in Chinese populations.[19,20] At this time, there are no other significant host-related factors that predict risk of salivary gland malignancy, presumably due to the low incidence of these neoplasms in the general population. Specific commentary on whether tumors arising in different geographic regions have different prognosis because of host and/or environmental factors is not possible. Also, it must be acknowledged that, in the context of geographic and patient factors, the distinction of what might relate to a host phenotype versus the influence of the environment where that patient lives (e.g., access to timely and expert treatment and assessment, adequate nutrition and performance status, adequate support, compliance with treatment, etc.) becomes blurred.

ENVIRONMENT-RELATED FACTORS

Prior Surgical Intervention

As indicated earlier, the presence of positive or close margins after surgical resection is a poor prognostic indicator and an indication for adjuvant external-beam radiation therapy. As a corollary, prior open biopsy has a negative impact on local control. Definitive surgery in this setting often necessitates a more extensive resection, and postoperative radiation therapy may be indicated as well.

Previous Radiation Exposure

While not prognostic factors for outcome for a given salivary cancer in the strict sense, certain environmental exposures do increase the risk of developing this lesion and in that way are prognostic. In the process it is recognized that a patient affected in this way may now have acquired a host-related prognostic factor rather than an environment-related factor if there is prognostic distinction due to the presence of the factor. For example, ionizing radiation exposure has been linked to the development of both benign and malignant salivary gland neoplasms. The data that support these conclusions come from studies of survivors of the Hiroshima and Nagasaki atomic bombings and patients exposed to therapeutic and diagnostic radiation of the head and neck.[21] Atomic bomb survivors have a dose-related increased risk of developing malignant salivary gland tumors in general (mucoepidermoid carcinoma in particular) as well as benign neoplasms such as Warthin's tumor.[22] Retrospective analyses of patients with salivary gland carcinoma indicates a possible link between prior orthovoltage radiation given decades ago in childhood for a variety of conditions and the subsequent development of tumor.[23] Current supervoltage radiographic techniques do not confer any additional risk for salivary cancer. Malignancies of salivary gland origin caused by prior radiation exposure do not appear to demonstrate an inherent difference in biology predicting an adverse prognosis. On the other hand, if the prior exposure to radiation was extensive, as may relate to treatment of a prior cancer in the head and neck, it may be difficult to use radiotherapy in the treatment of the new cancer in the salivary gland. If this is the case, it could have implications for the outcome of the salivary gland tumor in terms of local control and/or metastatic rate or survival. Also, it may mean that function conservation, such as preservation of the facial nerve, may not be possible when radiotherapy cannot be used safely postoperatively. Therefore in the context of these outcomes, prior radiation undoubtedly has prognostic significance for some patients.

Additional exposures that have been cited as possible etiologic agents include lack of consumption of particular vegetables, exposure to silica dust, kerosene, hair dye, and other agents, but a causal role remains to be established for these and other agents.[24] Furthermore, a prognostic impact of these factors is not apparent.

CLINICAL SITUATIONS

Limiting "Unnecessary" Treatment

Tumor stage and histology may influence treatment decisions in many situations. For example, matched-pairs analysis of low-stage tumors of varying histologic grades indicate that T1 and T2 tumors treated by adequate surgical excision have a good prognosis that is not enhanced by adjuvant radiation therapy, even if the tumor proves to be a high-grade lesion. As an additional example, observation may be appropriate after excisional biopsy of a small, low-grade minor salivary gland carcinoma, provided the site is easily accessible to surveillance (e.g., palate, cheek mucosa) and careful surveillance is possible. Patients who present with a small scar after excision of a small, low-grade lesion with no gross residual tumor may be candidates for this approach. Rather than immediately perform a procedure that often yields a negative specimen, resection may be reserved for those few patients who develop a subsequent local recurrence.

Decision Making in Adenoid Cystic Carcinoma

Treatment decisions involving adenoid cystic carcinoma require that clinicians appreciate its unique biologic behavior. It is well recognized that lung metastasis is not unusual in these patients, especially after local treatment failure. On occasion, however, pulmonary metastases may become apparent despite effective locoregional control. These lung metastases are almost invariably multiple, and may show minimal change over many years. Some centers advocate pulmonary metastasectomy in this setting, but the benefit of this aggressive approach has not been established. This approach is hard to justify when dealing with adenoid cystic carcinoma, because these patients are usually asymptomatic, and survival for a decade or more with untreated lung metastases has been described for this tumor.[25,26]

Carcinoma Ex Pleomorphic Adenoma

Another clinical situation concerns carcinoma ex pleomorphic adenoma, an uncommon malignant tumor that arises from a preexisting pleomorphic adenoma, representing 2 to 5% of salivary gland neoplasms. This tumor may present as a slow-growing mass present for 10 to 15 years that suddenly increases in size, or it may evolve after multiple recurrences of what appeared to be a benign pleomorphic adenoma at initial resection. Malignant conversion should always be suspected when a pleomorphic suddenly increases in size after a prolonged, indolent growth period.[27,28] The risk of malignant degeneration increases for as long as benign pleomorphic adenomas are observed.[27,28]

■■■■■■ **APPENDIX 14A**

TNM Classification in Salivary Glands Tumors

T—Primary Tumor

TX Primary tumor cannot be assessed

T0 No evidence of primary tumor

T1 Tumor 2 cm or less in greatest dimension without extraparenchymal extension*

T2 Tumor more than 2 cm but not more than 4 cm in greatest dimension without extraparenchymal extension*

T3 Tumor having extraparenchymal extension without seventh nerve involvement and/or more than 4 cm but not more than 6 cm in greatest dimension*

T4 Tumor invades base of skull, seventh nerve, and/or exceeds 6 cm in greatest dimension

N — Regional Lymph Nodes

NX Regional lymph nodes cannot be assessed

N0 No regional lymph-node metastasis

N1 Metastasis in a single ipsilateral lymph node, 3 cm or less in greatest dimension

N2 Metastasis in a single ipsilateral lymph node, more than 3 cm but not more than 6 cm in greatest dimension, or in multiple ipsilateral lymph nodes, none more than 6 cm in greatest dimension, or in bilateral or contralateral lymph nodes, none more than 6 cm in greatest dimension

    N2a Metastasis in a single ipsilateral lymph node, more than 3 cm but not more than 6 cm in greatest dimension

    N2b Metastasis in multiple ipsilateral lymph nodes, none more than 6 cm in greatest dimension

    N2c Metastasis in bilateral or contralateral lymph nodes, none more than 6 cm in greatest dimension

N3 Metastasis in a lymph node more than 6 cm in greatest dimension

M — Distant Metastasis

MX Distant metastasis cannot be assessed

M0 No distant metastasis

M1 Distant metastasis

Stage Grouping

Stage I	T1	N0	M0
	T2	N0	M0
Stage II	T3	N0	M0
Stage III	T1	N1	M0
	T2	N1	M0
Stage IV	T4	N0	M0
	T3	N1	M0
	T4	N1	M0
	Any T	N2	M0
	Any T	N3	M0
	Any T	Any N	M1

Source: Sobin LH, Wittekind Ch (eds.): *TNM classification of malignant tumors*, 5th ed. Union Internationale Contre le Cancer Wiley-Liss, New York, 1997.

████████ **APPENDIX 14B**

Prognostic Factors in Salivary Gland Cancers

Prognostic Factors	Tumor Related	Host Related	Environment Related

Essential	TNM stage
	Tumor size
	Nodal extension
	Facial nerve
	  involvement
	Deep invasion
	Residual disease
	Histologic subtype
		Performance status
		Comorbidities
			Care supply
			Treatment support
			Prior radiotherapy may
			  affect type of surgery
			  performed

Additional	Histologic grading
	Perineural invasion
	Minor vs. major gland
	Carcinoma ex
	  pleomorphic
	  adenoma
		Compliance to
		  treatment
		Prior radiotherapy
		Young age is
		  protective
		Male gender does
		  worse
			Prior surgical
			intervention

New and promising	Molecular parameters		

REFERENCES

1. Spiro RH: Salivary neoplasms: Overview of a 35-year experience with 2,807 patients. *Head Neck Surg* 8:177–84, 1986.

2. Spiro RH, Armstrong J, Harrison L, et al.: Carcinoma of major salivary glands: Recent trends. *Arch Otolaryngol Head Neck Surg* 115:316–21, 1989.

3. Seifert G, Sobin LH: The World Health Organization's histologic classification of salivary gland tumors. *Cancer* 70:379–85, 1992.

4. Spiro RH, Huvos AG: Stage means more than grade in adenoid cystic carcinoma. *Am J Surg* 164:623–7, 1992.

5. American Joint Committee for Cancer Staging and End Results Reporting: Manual for Staging of Cancer. Chicago, American Joint Committee, 1997.

6. Spiro R, Huvos A, Strong E: Adenoid cystic carcinoma of salivary origin: A clinicopathologic study of 242 cases. *Am J Surg* 128:512–20, 1974.

7. Spiro RH, Huvos AG, Strong EW: Adenoid cystic carcinoma: Factors influencing survival. *Am J Surg* 138:579–83, 1979.

8. Eneroth CM: Facial paralysis: A criterion of malignancy in parotid tumors. *Arch Otol* 95:300–4, 1972.

9. Hicks MJ, el-Naggar AK, Flaitz CM, et al.: Histocytologic grading of mucoepidermoid carcinoma of major salivary glands in prognosis and survival: A clinicopathologic and flow cytometric investigation. *Head Neck* 17:89–95, 1995.

10. Spiro RH, Huvos AG, Strong EW: Acinic cell carcinoma of salivary origin. A clinicopathologic study of 67 cases. *Cancer* 41(3):924–5, 1978.

11. Spiro RH, Thaler HT, Hicks WF, et al.: The importance of clinical staging of minor salivary gland carcinoma. *Am J Surg* 162:330–6, 1991.

12. Garden AS, Weber RS, Morrison WH, et al.: The influence of positive margins and nerve invasion in adenoid cystic carcinoma of the head and neck treated with surgery and radiation. *Int J Rad Oncol Biol Phys* 32:619–26, 1995.

13. Perzin KH, Gullane P, Clairmont AC: Adenoid cystic carcinoma in the salivary glands: A correlation of histologic features and clinical course. *Cancer* 42:265–82, 1978.

14. Fu KK, Leibel SA, Levine ML, et al.: Carcinoma of the major and minor salivary glands: Analysis and treatment results and sites and causes of failures. *Cancer* 40:2882–90, 1997.

15. Soo KC, Carter RL, O'Brien CJ, et al.: Prognostic implication of perineural spread in squamous cell carcinomas of the head and neck. *Laryngoscope* 96:1145–8, 1986.

16. Spiro RH, Huvos AG, Strong EW: Cancer of the parotid gland: A clinicopathologic study of 288 primary cases. *Am J Surg* 130:452–9, 1975.

17. Schuller DE, McCabe BF: Salivary gland neoplasms in children. *Otolaryngol Clin North Am* 10:399–412, 1977.

18. Albeck H, Bentzen J, Ockelmann HH, et al.: Familial clusters of nasopharyngeal carcinoma and salivary gland carcinomas in Greenland natives. *Cancer* 72:196–200, 1993.

19. Chan JK, Yip TT, Tsang WY, et al.: Specific association of Epstein-Barr virus with lymphoepithelial carcinoma among tumors and tumorlike lesions of the salivary gland. *Arch Pathol Lab Med* 118:994–7, 1995.

20. Leung SY, Chung LP, Yuen ST, et al.: Lymphoepithelial carcinoma of the salivary gland: In situ detection of Epstein-Barr virus. *J Clin Pathol* 48:1022–7, 1995.

21. Land CE, Saku T, Hayashi Y, et al.: Incidence of salivary gland tumors among atom bomb survivors, 1950–1987. Evaluation of radiation-related risk. *Radiat Res* 146:28–36, 1996.

22. Spitz MR, Batsakis JG: Major salivary gland carcinoma: Descriptive epidemiology and survival of 498 patients. *Arch Otolaryngol Head Neck Surg* 110:45–9, 1984.

23. Preston-Martin S, Thomas DC, White SC, Cohen D: Prior exposure to medical and dental x-rays related to tumors of the parotid gland. *JNCI* 80:943–9, 1988.

24. Zheng W, Shu XO, Gao YT: Diet and other risk factor for cancer of the salivary glands: A population-based case-control study. *Int J Cancer* 67:194–8, 1996.

25. Pastorino U, Buyse M, Friedel G, et al.: Long-term results of lung metastasectomy: Prognostic analyses based on 5,206 cases. *J Thorac Cardiovasc Surg* 113:37–49, 1997.

26. Spiro RH: Distant metastasis in adenoid cystic carcinoma of salivary origin. *Am J Surg* 174:495–8, 1997.

27. Boles R, Johns ME, Batsakis JG: Carcinoma in pleomorphic adenomas of salivary glands. *Ann Otol Rhinol Laryngol Suppl* 82:684–90, 1973.

28. Spiro RH, Huvos AG, Strong EW: Malignant mixed tumor of salivary origin: A clinicopathologic study of 146 cases. *Cancer* 39:388–96, 1977.

CHAPTER 15

Thyroid Cancer

JAMES D. BRIERLEY and SYLVIA L. ASA

The thyroid gland is composed of follicular cells, parafollicular cells, and connective tissue with occasional lymphocytes. Each of these cell types can give rise to histologically distinct tumors that differ significantly in behavior, prognosis, and response to treatment. The commonest tumors by far are those derived from follicular epithelial cells; these tumors are classified as differentiated (papillary and follicular), poorly differentiated (insular), and undifferentiated (anaplastic). Medullary thyroid cancers are derived from parafollicular cells. Tumors derived from lymphocytes and connective tissue cells are similar to such lesions elsewhere in the body, but a detailed discussion of those entities is beyond the scope of this chapter.

In one of the earliest studies on prognostic factors in thyroid cancer, the multivariate analysis of the European Organization for Research and Treatment of Cancer (EORTC) Thyroid Cancer Co-operative Group,[1] all histologies were combined. The 5-year survival ranged from 80% in differentiated carcinoma (papillary and follicular), to 55% in medullary thyroid carcinoma (MTC), to 10% in anaplastic carcinoma. Most subsequent studies of prognostic factors in thyroid cancer were developed for individual histologic types [differentiated papillary–follicular, poorly differentiated (insular), medullary, and anaplastic thyroid carcinomas] and they will be considered separately in this review. Some studies combine papillary and follicular, while others do not. The focus of this chapter is a review of the tumor-, host- and environment-related prognostic factors in differentiated thyroid cancer, with an additional discussion of prognostic factors in other thyroid histologies.

DIFFERENTIATED PAPILLARY–FOLLICULAR CARCINOMA

Tumor-related Factors

Histopathologic Features Prognostic features in papillary and follicular tumors are often analyzed together. Prior to the recognition of the poorly

Prognostic Factors in Cancer, 2nd edition, Edited by Mary K. Gospodarowicz
ISBN 0-471-40633-3   Copyright © 2001 Wiley-Liss, Inc.

differentiated intermediate form of thyroid carcinoma, there were several reports[2-5] indicating degree of differentiation to be an independent prognostic factor for survival in papillary thyroid carcinoma. Currently, only the tall cell and columnar cell variants warrant special attention. Johnson[6] described a variant of papillary thyroid carcinoma characterized by the presence of tall columnar cells, wherein the height is at least twice the width making up at least 30% of the tumor cell mass. When matched with patients with similar tumor size and lymph-node characteristics, there was an increased incidence of local and distant relapse and reduced survival in patients with this variant. Columnar cell carcinoma was identified as a variant of tall-cell papillary carcinoma with prominent nuclear stratification.[7,8] It remains controversial whether the morphology alone predicts a worse prognosis in multivariate analysis.[9] In follicular carcinoma, the presence of vascular invasion has been reported to be an independent adverse prognostic factor.[5,10] However, in papillary carcinoma this was not confirmed in multivariate analyses.[4,5]

Extent of Disease

Size   T category is defined in the 5th Edition of the UICC TNM (International Union Against Cancer Classification of Malignant Tumors) as T1 <1 cm, T2 1–4 cm, T3 >4 cm[11] (see Appendix 15A). Although few analyses of prognostic factors use the same cutoff points, there is no doubt that increase in tumor size is associated with worse prognosis in both papillary and follicular tumors. Mazzaferri et al., in a report on 1355 patients with papillary and follicular thyroid cancer found an increased risk of both recurrence and death in patients with tumors over 1.5 cm.[12] The association between size and mortality was linear. Tumors smaller than 1.5 cm had a recurrence rate of 11% and cancer mortality of 0.4% at 30 years, compared to 33% and 7%, respectively, for tumors larger than 2.5 cm ($p < 0.001$). In a multivariate analysis, however, size was only significant for cancer death, not recurrence. In contrast, in a smaller study, size greater than 4 cm was a significant factor for both local recurrence and cancer survival in multivariate analysis.[13] Hay et al. also found in a study of papillary thyroid cancer a progressive decrease in survival with increasing tumor size.[4]

Multifocality   Mazzaferri et al. reported that 24% of cases in their study had more than one tumor and when three or more were present, there was a significant increase in cancer mortality for both follicular and papillary histologies; this was not confirmed in multivariate analysis.[12] Tsang et al. found by multivariate analysis that multifocality was associated with increased relapse rate but not mortality.[13] Not all studies have found a deleterious effect of multifocality.[5]

Extrathyroidal Extension   The presence of extrathyroidal extension (T4 category) has been found to be a poor prognostic factor in many multivariate analyses.[3-5,14] In papillary carcinoma, Hay[4] reported a 20-year cause-specific survival of 98% for tumors confined to the thyroid gland, compared to 28% for those with locally invasive tumors. Mazzaferri found that local tumor invasion was present in 8% of papillary and 12% of follicular cancers and resulted in an increase in recurrence rate at 20 years (38% vs. 25%, $p < 0.001$) and cancer mortality (20% vs. 5%, $p = 0.001$) and was significant in multivariate analysis.[12] An increase in distant as well as local regional failure has been reported in patients with differentiated thyroid cancer and extrathyroidal extension compared with those without.[15]

Lymph Node Involvement   Whereas lymph-node involvement is an indicator of poor prognosis in most cancers, the significance of this finding in thyroid cancer is controversial. Several reports suggest that lymph-node involvement does not have an adverse effect on prognosis.[3,4,16] In contrast, several multivariate analyses have identified a shorter disease-free interval and lower survival in patients with positive cervical lymph nodes.[5,12,13] The presence of extracapsular invasion of lymph-node metastasis has been reported to be a significant indicator of recurrence and poorer survival.[17]

Metastatic Disease   The presence of distant metastases at diagnosis is associated with a markedly decreased survival in patients with papillary or follicular carcinoma.[2,4,5,12,14] Nevertheless, young patients with metastatic disease have an excellent prognosis. In a series of 394 patients with differentiated thyroid cancer and lung or bone metastases, Schlumberger et al.,[18] found that age had a significant effect on prognosis. Patients aged 4–19 years had a 10-year survival of 100%, compared with 17% for patients 40 or older at time of diagnosis of metastasis ($p = 0.0001$). Although Vassilopoulou-Sellin et al. also reported a 10-year survival rate of 100% in patients less than 20 years old at time of diagnosis, with prolonged follow-up, 5% died of progressive lung and/or skeletal metastatic disease.[19] It has also been reported that female patients, papillary as compared to follicular histology, and radioiodine uptake were all associated with improved survival. Site of metastasis is also important, as the 10-year survival was 61% with lung metastasis and 13% with lung and bone metastasis.[17] Survival is longest with diffuse lung metastases that take up radioiodine and are seen on ^{131}I imaging but too small to be diagnosed by X ray.[4,18–20]

Molecular/Genetic Factors   An aneuploid DNA profile has been reported in 12% of patients with differentiated thyroid cancer, of which 47% eventually died of thyroid carcinoma. Aneuploidy was more common among male patients and older patients. In the multivariate analysis of prognostic factors age was the most important significant prognostic factor, but ploidy was an independent factor for survival.[21] In another study aneuploidy occurred in 40% of papillary thyroid cancer with extrathyroid extension, but was absent in matched controls.[22] Hay[4] found the highest mortality rate in tumors with an aneuploid pattern, and that nondiploid DNA was independently associated with increased cause-specific mortality. Joensuu et al.[23] reported that age, differentiation, and invasion through the thyroid capsule were significant poor prognostic variables in a multivariate analysis, but they found that DNA ploidy was not. This is in contrast to Kurozumi et al.[24] who reported that cause-specific survival was independently related to

DNA ploidy and S-phase fraction as well as extrathyroid invasion and distant metastasis. In follicular tumors, Grant et al.[25] found aneuploidy in benign as well as malignant lesions and were unable to demonstrate any prognostic effect of ploidy when the Hurthle cell variant was excluded, but in RET/PTC nonmetastatic tumors, DNA ploidy was the only factor that correlated significantly with reduced survival.

RET/PTC gene rearrangements are characteristic of a percentage of papillary thyroid carcinomas. When expressed at very high levels, as in an animal model where the transgene was driven by the thyroglobulin promoter, the product of these rearrangements can be oncogenic.[26] These rearrangements have been implicated as predictive of aggressive behavior in pediatric radiation-induced papillary carcinomas following the Chernobyl disaster;[27] however, in sporadic papillary carcinomas the levels of expression are highly variable.[28] It has been suggested that high levels of expression can predict a more aggressive course of lymphatic dissemination, specifically in young patients with no other adverse clinical or morphological parameters.[29] It is also recognized that RET/PTC oncogene activation defines a subset of papillary thyroid carcinomas that lack evidence of progression to poorly differentiated or undifferentiated phenotypes.[30] Ras mutations remain highly controversial as predictors of biological behavior.[31] It has been suggested that p27 downregulation[32] and p53 localization[33] are prognostically important in differentiated thyroid carcinomas.

Serum thyroglobulin has become an established marker for differentiated thyroid carcinoma in patients who have undergone total thyroidectomy and radioiodine ablation of the thyroid. Thyroglobulin levels are elevated in any thyroid disease associated with increased thyroid mass or activity, that is, goiter, Graves' disease, thyroiditis, thyroid adenoma, as well as thyroid carcinoma. Thyroglobulin therefore does not distinguish benign from malignant conditions and has no prognostic value in initial evaluation of thyroid carcinoma.[33] However, in patients with established malignancy following surgery and radioiodine ablation, the documentation of rising thyroglobulin predicts tumour recurrence or metastasis, and further investigation and treatment are required.[34]

Host-related Factors

Patient Demographics

Age As noted earlier, even patients with metastatic disease under the age of 20 have an excellent survival. Age at diagnosis has been found to be a significant variable in nearly all multivariate analyses of prognostic factors in differentiated thyroid carcinoma.[1,3,4,5,9,12-14] Survival decreases with advancing age, and age has been established as the most important prognostic factor in differentiated thyroid cancer. Although age at the time of diagnosis has been found to be a major prognostic factor in differentiated thyroid cancer, various studies use different age cutoff points. Patients less than 40 or 50 years old have been reported to have favorable prognosis. It is likely that there is no strict cutoff point at which prognosis changes suddenly, but rather the prognostic influence of age changes progressively. Whereas young age is a good factor for survival, it may be a poor prognostic factor for initial extent of disease, and recurrence.[12,19,35] Mazzaferri demonstrated that recurrence rates were highest at extremes of age, although with treatment, survival is excellent in the young.[12]

Gender   Although several univariate analyses have found a lower survival rate in male patients, this has not always been confirmed in multivariate analysis. For instance, in the (EORTC) report,[1] gender was a significant factor in the univariate but not in the multivariate analysis. In the Mayo Clinic report, male gender was associated with poorer survival in papillary carcinoma[4] but not follicular carcinoma.[10] Mazzaferri et al. reported that gender had no effect on recurrence rate but was significant for survival, with a 30-year mortality of 11% in men and 7% in women.[12] Although other investigators have documented a negative effect of male gender,[2–4] several other studies showed no effect of gender on survival.[5,13,15]

Ethnicity   The incidence of thyroid cancer shows wide racial variations that are attributed to environmental factors, primarily iodine exposure. Nevertheless, the prognosis of the tumors is determined by other factors discussed elsewhere in this chapter and there is no scientific evidence that race alone represents an independent risk-associated variable.

Heredity   A number of familial forms of thyroid carcinoma involve follicular epithelial tumors. Papillary thyroid cancer occurs at a higher frequency in patients with familial polyposis coli (Gardner's Syndrome), which is attributed to a germline mutation of the adenomatous polyposis coli (APC) gene, a tumor suppressor gene. The papillary carcinomas in these patients frequently exhibit an unusual and distinctive morphology.[36] Although the colonic neoplasms have been shown to have loss of heterozygosity involving the normal allele, resulting in lack of intact protein, this has not been confirmed in the thyroid cancers and the pathogenetic mechanisms underlying the thyroid involvement in this syndrome remain unknown.[37] Cowden's Disease is another tumor syndrome in which thyroid cancer has been found with high incidence. This disease has been attributed to germline mutations of a tumor suppressor gene on chromosome 10q23 that encode PTEN, a protein with homology to tyrosine phosphatases and tensin.[38] Somatic mutations in PTEN occur in multiple tumors, but again the role of PTEN in thyroid cancer remains unclear. Familial papillary thyroid carcinoma unassociated with other neoplastic disease remains a clinically recognized phenomenon,[39] but the molecular genetic basis of this disorder has not yet been elucidated.

Coexisting Disease   Hay[4] found 40% of papillary thyroid cancer patients had preexisting or concurrent benign thyroid conditions. Of these, 41% had benign nodular goiter and 20% had chronic lymphocytic thyroiditis. The presence of thyroiditis or benign nodular thyroid disease did not affect the outcome. Thyroid cancer in patients with Graves' disease is associated with an increased aggressive behavior with an increased incidence of multifocality, extrathyroid invasion, lymph-node involvement, and distant metastases,[40-42] although Hay found that coexisting Graves' disease had no effect on cause-specific survival.[4]

Environment Related Factors

Treatment Related Since the prognosis of young patients is excellent, the effect of treatment (extent of surgery and the use of radioiodine) on prognosis is controversial. Because of the excellent prognosis of low-risk patients (young patients with tumors smaller than 4 to 5 cm), it has been argued that limited surgery (lobectomy) is sufficient.[4,14,43] In contrast, Mazzafferri et al. reported higher recurrence and cancer deaths at 30 years in patients with tumors larger than 1.5 cm treated by lobectomy compared to subtotal thyroidectomy,[12] and that the use of radioiodine resulted in both lower recurrence and higher survival. Certainly there is good evidence that surgery greater than lobectomy and radioiodine therapy lowers recurrence rates and improves survival in patients with more advanced disease.[12,13,44,45] It remains controversial as to what group of patients should be considered at risk of relapse and to benefit from more extensive therapy. Should all patients with primaries over 1.5 cm have total/near-total thyroidectomy and iodine ablation, or can young patients with primaries less than 4–5 cm and no other poor prognostic features be treated by lobectomy alone?

Hay et al.[46] reported that incomplete resection primary papillary tumor resulted in increased mortality. Similarly, Tsang et al.[13] found that the presence of macroscopic but not microscopic postoperative residual disease resulted in an increased risk of both local recurrence and cancer-specific mortality. It has been demonstrated that delay in therapy from first manifestation of tumor increases cancer mortality; mortality more than doubles if the delay is greater than one year.[12]

Geography The mortality rates per 100,000 adjusted to the world standard population in the 1980s ranged from 0.2 in Greece and Spain to 1.2 in Iceland in males, and from 0.4 in Greece, Spain, Canada, the United States, and Australia to 2.8 in Kuwait in females. In general the mortality rates are 50% higher for females than males, but the incidence in females is more than double that of males. In areas where goiter is endemic, there appears to be a higher incidence and mortality, but this is likely because follicular and particularly anaplastic (see below) histologies are more common. In Switzerland and Paraguay, large-scale prophylactic iodinization has been followed by a relative increase in the incidence of papillary and decrease in follicular and anaplastic histologies and a fall in age-adjusted mortality.[47]

Radiation Exposure Although the association of previous radiation therapy and thyroid carcinoma is well established, the prognosis in patients who have been exposed to radiation does not appear to differ from those with no history of radiation.[3,4] As discussed earlier, RET/PTC gene rearrangements have been implicated as predictive of aggressive behavior in pediatric radiation-induced papillary carcinomas following the Chernobyl disaster.[26]

SUMMARY

Essential Factors In an attempt to stratify patients into different risk groups in terms of predicting survival, and thereby guiding therapy, a variety of prognostic indices have been formulated. They differ in the factors used and the cutoff points for various prognostic factors. Almost all, however, incorporate age, which is the most important prognostic factor in differentiated thyroid cancer. Tumor extent, T category, and the presence of metastases are major factors, especially in older patients (Table 15.1). In a review of eight different staging systems and prognostic indices, no system was superior to the UICC American Joint Committee on Cancer (AJCC) TNM staging system to predict outcome.[48] As it is the most universally known and readily applicable, it was proposed that the UICC/AJCC TNM staging system should be used in all reports of treatment and outcomes in differentiated thyroid cancer.

Additional Factors Male gender and lymph-node involvement are controversial as indicators of poor prognosis, and therefore are not incorporated in most prognostic indices used to select treatment. In patients who have metastatic disease, the site of metastases, the size of lung metastases, and the ability to take up radioiodine are important factors.

New and Promising Factors The value of novel molecular markers in determining the prognosis of differentiated thyroid cancer remains to be established.

Other Thyroid Histologies

Insular Carcinoma Langerhans originally described insular carcinoma as a pathological entity in 1907, but its significance as the manifestation of poorly differentiated carcinoma of follicular epithelial derivation has only been appreciated more recently.[49] This tumor exhibits a behavior that is intermediate between well-differentiated papillary or follicular carcinoma and the undifferentiated anaplastic carcinoma. While it remains arguable that these lesions represent an independent tumor entity, it is accepted by most investigators that thyroid carcinomas follow a stepwise progression and that insular carcinoma represents a higher tumor grade along a continuum. The identification of a component of this lesion in any thyroid carcinoma predicts more aggressive behavior and a worse response to radioactive iodine therapy.[9,50] Metastases are common, both to regional lymph nodes and to distant sites.

Anaplastic Carcinoma Anaplastic thyroid carcinoma is widely recognized to have a dismal prognosis, but the extent of anaplasia required to determine this prognosis is not entirely clear. In the analysis of the EORTC thyroid cancer study group, the presence of any element of anaplasia within a well-differentiated thyroid carcinoma was no different from anaplastic tumor throughout, with a one-year survival of 10%.[1] Nel et al.[51] have described a group of patients with better prognosis, those with small tumors (less than 5 cm), no extrathyroidal invasion,

TABLE 15.1 A Comparison of Different Prognostic Factors Used in Eight Staging Classifications of Thyroid Cancer

Classification	AGES[4]	AMES[14]	Clinical Class[44]	EORTC[1]	MACIS[46]	OHIO[12]	MSK[43]	UICC/AJCC[11]
Age	Continuous	≤40 male ≤50 female	<45	Continuous	Continuous	No	<45	<45
Gender	Yes	No	No	No	No	No	No	No
Histology	Papillary	Differentiated	Differentiated	All	Papillary	Differentiated	Differentiated	All
Grade	Yes	No	No	No	No	No	No	No
Size	Continuous	<5 / ≥5	No	No	Continuous	<1.5 / 1.5–4.4 / ≥4.4	≤1 / 1–4 / ≤4	≤1 / 1–4 / >4
Extrathyroid extension	Yes	Yes	Yes	Yes	Yes	Yes	Yes	Yes
Lymph Node	No	No	Yes	No	No	Yes	No	Yes
Residual Disease	No	No	No	No	Yes	No	No	No
Multifocal	No	No	No	No	No	Yes	No	No
Metastasis	Yes	Yes	Yes	Yes	Yes	Yes	Yes	Yes
PVE	31.15	28.1	18.5	28.0	27.3	22.9	19.2	28.5

Abbreviations: EORTC: European Organization for Research and Treatment of Cancer; AGES: Age, Grade, Extrathyroid extent and Size; AMES: Age, Metastases, Extrathyroid extension, and Size; MACIS: Metastases, Age, Completeness of resection, Invasion, and Size; UICC: International Union Against Cancer, AJCC: American Joint Committee on Cancer; PVE: Proportion of Variance Explained, which measures the ability of the classification system to predicting outcome. The higher the PVE the better the classification. The numbers in the table are derived from data from Princess Margaret Hospital, Toronto.[48]

and no lymph-node involvement. Venkatesh et al.[52] reported age and stage to be significant factors for survival in anaplastic thyroid carcinoma. Gender has not been shown to affect the outcome in these tumors. In general, patients with anaplastic thyroid carcinoma present with advanced-stage disease and invariably have a poor prognosis, although in the rare situation in which a complete surgical resection is possible with no residual disease, survival may be better, although still poor.[53,54]

Medullary Thyroid Carcinoma Familial medullary thyroid carcinoma (FMTC), with or without the association of multiple endocrine neoplasia (MEN) 2A syndrome, has a better survival than that associated with MEN 2B syndrome,[55,56] and has been associated with better survival than sporadic medullary thyroid carcinoma. However, Saaman found that in patients matched for age, extent of tumor, and lymph-node involvement, survival was similar for those with the hereditary and sporadic medullary thyroid carcinomas.[57] Any differences in survival of hereditary and sporadic cases may be due to earlier diagnosis in high-risk patients, who are screened for hereditary medullary thyroid cancers. Although presenting at an earlier age, patients with MEN 2B have more advanced disease and poorer survival than those with MEN 2A.[58] The molecular basis of this disease may explain this pattern of risk. Patients with FMTC or MEN 2A usually have activating mutations of the ret protooncogene in the extracellular domain of this tyrosine kinase receptor; in contrast, patients with MEN 2B have more potent activation of the receptor due to a specific mutation within the kinase domain that alters substrate specificity.[59] A subset of patients with sporadic tumors exhibits somatic mutations identical to those in MEN 2B. The current trend of using molecular diagnosis to identify carriers of this genetic, autosomal dominant disorder has led to the recommendation of prophylactic thyroidectomy in childhood; this will almost certainly drastically improve the prognosis of the familial forms of this malignancy. Younger age, and female gender have been reported as favorable prognostic indicators. The presence of lymph-node involvement affects survival adversely, as does extension through the thyroid capsule.[55,60-65] The most important predictive factor for survival is biochemical cure after surgery.[66] Calcitonin is a tumor marker for medullary thyroid carcinoma. The basal levels of calcitonin are proportional to the tumor burden. In a multivariate analysis of histopathological features, only calcitonin immunoreactivity and positive amyloid staining were independent prognostic factors.[67] However, a decrease in the calcitonin level may indicate progression to a poorly differentiated tumor.[68] Carcinoembryonic antigen (CEA) has also been used as a marker for disease progression in medullary thyroid carcinoma, and a short CEA doubling time is associated with rapidly progressive disease.[65]

███████ **APPENDIX 15A**

Thyroid Gland: TNM Classification

T — Primary Tumor

TX Primary tumor cannot be assessed

T0 No evidence of primary tumor

T1 Tumor 1 cm or less in greatest dimension, limited to the thyroid

T2 Tumor more than 1 cm but not more than 4 cm in greatest dimension, limited to the thyroid

T3 Tumor more than 4 cm in greatest dimension, limited to the thyroid

T4 Tumor of any size extending beyond the thyroid capsule

N — Regional Lymph Nodes

NX Regional lymph nodes cannot be assessed

N0 No regional lymph-node metastasis

N1 Regional lymph-node metastasis

    N1a Metastasis in ipsilateral cervical lymph node(s)

    N1b Metastasis in bilateral, midline, or contralateral cervical or mediastinal lymph node(s)

M — Distant Metastasis

MX Distant metastasis cannot be assessed

M0 No distant metastasis

M1 Distant metastasis

Stage Grouping

Papillary or Follicular

Under 45 years

Stage I	Any T	Any N	M0
Stage II	Any T	Any N	M1

45 years and older

Stage I	T1	N0	M0
Stage II	T2	N0	M0
	T3	N0	M0
Stage III	T4	N0	M0
	Any T	N1	M0
Stage IV	Any T	Any N	M1

Medullary

Stage I	T1	N0	M0
Stage II	T2	N0	M0
	T3	N0	M0
	T4	N0	M0
Stage III	Any T	N1	M0
Stage IV	Any T	Any N	M1

Undifferentiated

Stage IV	Any T	Any N	Any M
	(all cases are stage IV)		

Source: Sobin LH, Wittekind Ch (eds.): *TNM classification of malignant tumors*, 5th ed. Union Internationale Contre le Cancer Wiley-Liss, New York, 1997.

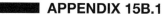 **APPENDIX 15B.1**

Prognostic Factors in Differentiated Thyroid Carcinoma

Prognostic Factors	Tumor Related	Host Related	Environment Related
Essential	T category M category	Age	Residual Disease R0, R1 vs. R2
Additional	N category Site of metastases	Gender	Extent of resection Iodine ablation
New and promising	Molecular profile		

■■■■■■■ **APPENDIX 15B.2**

Prognostic Factors in Medullary Thyroid Cancer

Prognostic Factors	Tumor Related	Host Related	Environment Related
Essential	T category N category M category		Residual disease Postoperative calcitonin
Additional		Age Gender	
New and promising	Site of mutation		

REFERENCES

1. Byar DP, Green SB, Dor P, et al.: A prognostic index for thyroid carcinoma. A study of the E.O.R.T.C. Thyroid Cancer Cooperative Group. *Eur J Cancer* 15:1033–41, 1979.

2. Akslen LA: Prognostic importance of histologic grading in papillary thyroid carcinoma. *Cancer* 72:2680–5, 1993.

3. Cunningham MP, Duda RB, Recant W, et al.: Survival discriminants for differentiated thyroid cancer. *Am J Surg* 160:344–7, 1990.

4. Hay ID: Papillary thyroid carcinoma. *Endocrinol Metab Clin North Am* 19:545–76, 1990.

5. Simpson WJ, McKinney SE, Carruthers JS, et al.: Papillary and follicular thyroid cancer. Prognostic factors in 1,578 patients. *Am J Med* 83:479–88, 1987.

6. Johnson TL, Lloyd RV, Thompson NW, et al.: Prognostic implications of the tall cell variant of papillary thyroid carcinoma. *Am J Surg Pathol* 12:22–7, 1988.

7. Evans HL: Columnar-cell carcinoma of the thyroid. A report of two cases of an aggressive variant of thyroid carcinoma. *Am J Clin Pathol* 85:77–80, 1986.

8. Sobrinho-Simoes M, Nesland JM, Johannessen JV: Columnar cell carcinoma: Another variant of poorly differentiated carcinoma of the thyroid. *Am J Clin Pathol* 89:264–7, 1988.

9. Van Den Brekel MWM, Hekkenberg RJ, Asa SL, et al.: Prognostic features in tall cell papillary carcinoma and insular thyroid carcinoma. *Laryngoscope* 107: 254–9, 1997.

10. Brennan MD, Bergstralh EJ, van Heerden JA, et al.: Follicular thyroid cancer treated at the Mayo clinic, 1946 through 1970: Initial manifestations, pathologic findings, therapy, and outcome. *Mayo Clin Proc* 66:11–22, 1991.

11. Sobin LH, Wittekind Ch (eds.). UICC. International Union Against Cancer. TNM Classification of malignant tumors. 5th edition. New York, Wiley-Liss, 1997.

12. Mazzaferri EL, Jhiang SM: Long-term impact of initial surgical and medical therapy on papillary and follicular thyroid cancer published erratum appears in *Am J Med* 98:215, 1995. *Am J Med* 97:418–428, 1994.

13. Tsang R, Brierley J, Simpson W, et al.: The effect of surgery, radioactive iodine and external radiation on the outcome of differentiated thyroid cancer. *Cancer* 82:375–88, 1998.

14. Cady B, Rossi R: An expanded view of risk-group definition in differentiated thyroid carcinoma. *Surgery* 104:947–53, 1988.

15. Anderson PE, Kinsella J, Loree TR, et al.: Differentiated carcinoma of the thyroid with extrathyroid extension. *Am J Surg* 170:467–70, 1995.

16. Sato N, Oyamatsu M, Koyama Y, et al.: Do the level of nodal disease according to the TNM Classification and the number of involved cervical nodes reflect prognosis in patients with differentiated carcinoma of the thyroid gland. *J Surg Oncol* 69:151–5, 1998.

17. Yamashita H, Nogushi S, Murakami N, et al.: Extracapsular invasion of lymph node metastasis is an indicator of distant metastasis and poor prognosis in patients with thyroid papillary carcinoma. *Cancer* 80:2268–72, 1997.

18. Schlumberger M, Challeton C, De Vathaire F, et al.: Radioactive iodine treatment and external radiotherapy for lung and bone metastases from thyroid cancer. *J Nucl Med* 37:598–605, 1996.

19. Vassilopoulou-Sellin, Goepfert H, Raney B, et al.: Differentiated thyroid cancer in children and adolescents: Clinical outcome and mortality after long-term follow-up. *Head Neck* 20:549–55, 1998.

20. Casara D, Rubello D, Saladini G, et al.: Distant metastases in differentiated thyroid cancer: Long-term results of radioiodine treatment. *Tumori* 77: 432–6, 1991.

21. Hrafnkelsson J, Stal O, Enestrom S, et al.: Cellular DNA pattern, S-phase frequency and survival in papillary thyroid cancer. *Acta Oncol* 27:329–33, 1988.

22. Stern Y, Lisnyansky I, Shpitzer T, et al.: Comparison of nuclear DNA content in locally invasive and noninvasive papillary carcinoma of the thyroid gland. *Otolaryngol Head Neck Surg* 117:501–3, 1997.

23. Joensuu H, Klemi P, Eerola E, et al.: Influence of cellular DNA content on survival in differentiated thyroid cancer. *Cancer* 58(11):2162–7, 1986.

24. Kurozumi K, Nakao K, Nishida T, et al.: Significance of biologic aggressiveness and proliferating activity in papillary thyroid carcinoma. *World J Surg* 22:1237–42, 1998.

25. Grant CS, Hay ID, Ryan JJ, et al.: Diagnostic and prognostic utility of flow cytometric DNA measurements in follicular thyroid tumors. *World J Surg* 14:283–9, 1990.

26. Jhiang SM, Sagartz JE, Tong Q, et al.: Targeted expression of the ret/PTC1 oncogene induces papillary thyroid carcinomase. *Endocrinology* 137:375–8, 1996.

27. Thomas GA, Bunnell H, Cook HA, et al.: High prevalence of RET/PTC rearrangements in Ukrainian and Belarussian post-Chernobyl thyroid papillary carcinomas: A strong correlation between RET/PTC3 and the solid-follicular variant. *J Clin Endocrinol Metab* 84:4232–8, 1999.

28. Sugg SL, Ezzat S, Rosen IB, et al.: Distinct multiple RET/PTC gene rearrangements in multifocal papillary thyroid neoplasia. *J Clin Endocrinol Metab* 83:4116–22, 1998.

29. Sugg SL, Zheng L, Rosen IB, et al.: Ret/PTC-1, -2 and -3 oncogene rearrangements in human thyroid carcinomas: Implications for metastatic potential? *J Clin Endocrinol Metab* 81: 3360–5, 1996.

30. Tallini G, Santoro M, Helie M, et al.: RET/PTC oncogene activation defines a subset of papillary thyroid carcinomas lacking evidence of progression to poorly differentiated or undifferentiated tumor phenotypes. *Clin Cancer Res* 4:287–94, 1998.

31. Ezzat S, Zheng L, Kolenda, et al.: Prevalence of activated ras mutations in morphologically characterized thyroid nodules. *Thyroid* 6:409–16, 1996.

32. Tallini G, Garcia-Rostan G, Herrero A, et al.: Downregulation of p27KIP1 and Ki67/Mib1 labeling index support the classification of thyroid carcinoma into prognostically relevant categories. *Am J Surg Pathol* 23:678–85, 1999.

33. Hosal SA, Apel RL, Freeman JL, et al.: Immunohistochemical localization of p53 in human thyroid neoplasms: Correlation with biological behavior. *Endocr Pathol* 8:21–8, 1997.

34. Refetoff S, Lever EG: The value of serum thyroglobulin measurement in clinical practice. *J Am Med Assoc* 250:2352–7, 1983.

35. Farahati J, Parlowsky T, Mader U, et al.: Differentiated thyroid cancer in children and adolescents. *Langenbeck's Arch Surg* 383:235–9, 1998.

36. Cetta F, Toti P, Petracci M, et al.: Thyroid carcinoma associated with familial adenomatous polyposis. *Histopathology* 31:231–6, 1997.

37. Soravia C, Sugg SL, Berk T, et al.: Familial adenomatous polyposis-associated thyroid cancer. A clinical, pathological, and molecular genetics study. *Am J Pathol* 154:127–35, 1999.

38. Lynch ED, Ostermeyer EA, Lee MK, et al.: Inherited mutations in PTEN that are associated with breast cancer, cowden disease, and juvenile polyposis. *Am J Hum Genet* 61:1254–60, 1997.

39. Clark OH: Thyroid cancer: Predisposing conditions, growth factors, signal transduction and oncogenes. *Aust N Z J Surg* 68:469–77, 1998.

40. Belfiore A, Garofalo MR, Giuffrida D, et al.: Increased aggressiveness of thyroid cancer in patients with Graves' Disease. *J Clin Endocrinol Metab* 70:830–5, 1990.

41. Farbota LM, Calandra DB, Lawrence AM, et al.: Thyroid carcinoma in Graves' disease. *Surgery* 98:1148–53, 1985.

42. Livadas D, Psarras A, Koutras DA: Malignant cold nodules in hyperthyroidism. *Br J Surg* 63:726–8, 1976.

43. Shaha AR, Loree TR, Shah JP: Intermediate-risk group for differentiated carcinoma of thyroid. *Surg* 116:1036–41, 1994.

44. DeGroot LJ, Kaplan EL, McCormick M, et al.: Natural history, treatment, and course of papillary thyroid carcinoma. *J Clin Endocinol Metab* 71:414–24, 1990.

45. Taylor T, Specker B, Robbins J, et al.: Multicenter prospective study of outcome following treatment of high risk papillary and non-hurtle follicular thyroid carcinoma. *Ann Intern Med* 129:622–7, 1998.

46. Hay ID, Bergstralh EJ, Goellner JR, et al.: Predicting outcome in papillary thyroid carcinoma: Development of a reliable prognostic scoring system in a cohort of

1779 patients surgically treated at one institution during 1940 through 1989. *Surgery* 114:1050–8, 1993.

47. Franceshi S, Boyle P, La Vecchia, et al.: The epidemiology of thyroid carcinoma. *Crit Rev Oncog* 4:25–52, 1993.

48. Brierley J, Tsang R, Gospodarowicz M, et al.: Comparing staging classifications using thyroid cancer as an example. *Cancer* 79:2414–23, 1997.

49. Carcangiu ML, Zampi G, Rosai J: Poorly differentiated ("insular") thyroid carcinoma. A reinterpretation of Langhans' "wuchernde Struma." *Am J Surg Pathol* 8:655–68, 1984.

50. Flynn SD, Forman BH, Stewart AF, et al.: Poorly differentiated ("insular") carcinoma of the thyroid gland: An aggressive subset of differentiated thyroid neoplasms. *Surgery* 104:963–70, 1988.

51. Nel CJ, van Heerden JA, GocEner JR, et al.: Anaplastic carcinoma of the thyroid: A clinicopathologic study of 82 cases. *Mayo Clin Proc* 60:51–8, 1985.

52. Venkatesh YS, Ordonez NG, Schultz PN, et al.: Anaplastic carcinoma of the thyroid: A clinicopathologic study of 121 cases. *Cancer* 66:321–30, 1990.

53. Passler C, Scheuba C, Prager G, et al.: Anaplastic (undifferentiated) thyroid carcinoma (ATC). *Langenbeck's Arch Surg* 384:284–93, 1999.

54. Voutilainen PE, Multanan M, Haapiainen RK, et al.: Anaplastic thyroid carcinoma survival. *World J Surg* 23:975–9, 1999

55. Kakudo K, Carney J, Sizemore GW: Medullary carcinoma of thyroid: Biologic behavior of the sporadic and familial neoplasm. *Cancer* 55:2818–21, 1985.

56. Raue F, Spdth-Roger M, Winter J, et al.: A registry of medullary thyroid cancer in West Germany. *Med Klin* 85:113–6 1990.

57. Samaan NA, Schultz PN, Hickey RC: Medullary thyroid carcinoma: Prognosis of familial versus sporadic disease and the role of radiotherapy. *J Clin Endocrinol Metab* 67:801–5, 1988.

58. O'Riordain D, O'Brien T, Weaver A, et al.: Medullary thyroid carcinoma in multiple endocrine neoplasia types 2A and 2B. *Surgery* 116:1017–23, 1994.

59. Mulligan LM, Ponder BA: Genetic basis of endocrine disease: Multiple endocrine neoplasia type 2. *J Clin Endocrinol Metab* 80:1989–95, 1995.

60. Rougier P, Pannentier C, Laplanche A, et al.: Medullary thyroid carcinoma: Prognostic factors and treatment. *Int J Radiat Oncol Biol Phys* 9:161–9, 1983.

61. Brierley J, Tsang R, Gospodarowicz M, et al.: Medullary thyroid cancer analyses of survival and prognostic factors and the role of radiation therapy. *Thyroid* 6:375–88, 1996.

62. Girelli ME, Nacamulli D, Pelizzo MR, et al.: Medullary thyroid carcinoma: Clinical features and long-term follow-up of 78 patients. *Thyroid* 8:517–22, 1998.

63. Dottorini ME, Assi A, Sironi M, et al.: Multivariate analysis of patients with medullary thyroid carcinoma. *Cancer* 77:1556–65, 1996.

64. Gharib H, McConahey WM, Tiegs RD, et al.: Medullary thyroid carcinoma: Clinicopathological and long-term follow-up of 65 patients. *Mayo Clin Proc* 67:934–40, 1992.

65. Saad MF, Orddonez NG, Rashid RK, et al.: Medullary carcinoma: Prognostic factors and treatment. *Int J Radiat Oncol Biol Phys* 9:161–9, 1984.

66. Modigliani E, Cohen R, Campos J-M et al.: Prognostic factors for survival and for biochemical cure in medullary thyroid carcinoma: Results in 899 patients. *Clin Endocrinol* 48:265–73, 1998.

67. Bergholm U, Adami HO, Auer G, et al.: Histopathologic characteristics and nuclear DNA content as prognostic factors in medullary thyroid carcinoma. A nationwide study in Sweden. The Swedish MTC Study Group. *Cancer* 64(l):135–142, 1989.

68. Trump DL, Mendelsohn G, Baylin SB: Discordance between plasma calcitonin and tumor-cell mass in medullary thyroid carcinoma. *N Engl J Med* 301:253–5, 1979.

DIGESTIVE SYSTEM TUMORS

CHAPTER 16

Cancer of the Esophagus

HUBERT J. STEIN and MARCUS FEITH

In contrast to other tumors of the gastrointestinal tract, independent prognostic factors have only recently been identified in patients with esophageal carcinoma. This is because most studies assessing the prognosis of patients with esophageal cancer were retrospective univariate analyses of small patient populations that were usually not treated according to standardized protocols. Due to interrelations between various patient- and tumor-related factors and their alterations by therapeutic strategies, the independent prognostic effect of individual parameters cannot be deducted from these analyses. This can only be achieved by multiple stepwise regression analysis applied to a sufficiently large patient population that has undergone standardized treatment and has been followed for a sufficiently long period of time. Studies that meet these criteria have become available only during the past decade. The chapter critically reviews the currently available literature on prognostic factors in patients with esophageal cancer, which are classified into the three categories: (1) tumor- or disease-related prognostic factors; (2) patient-related factors; and (3) environment- or treatment-related factors.

TUMOR-RELATED PROGNOSTIC FACTORS

A variety of tumor characteristics have been implicated as predictors of a good or poor prognosis in patients with esophageal carcinoma. These include extent of the disease, location of the primary tumor, histologic tumor type, DNA distribution pattern, and a number of molecular and other biologic factors, including growth factors, growth factor receptors, adhesion molecules, oncogenes, and tumor suppressor genes. A reliable and reproducible identification of tumor characteristics that may influence survival is only possible by an accurate

Prognostic Factors in Cancer, 2nd edition, Edited by Mary K. Gospodarowicz.
ISBN 0-471-40633-3   Copyright © 2001 Wiley-Liss, Inc.

histologic assessment of the resected specimen according to the guidelines given in the TNM classification system.[1] Only patients who had complete tumor removal together with an adequate lymph-node dissection and who survived the resection should be included in such analyses.

Disease Extent

The presence of hematogenous systemic metastases in patients with esophageal carcinoma constitutes an ominous and undisputed prognostic marker. The median survival time of these patients is below 6 months in most series. Consequently, only palliative measures improving the quality of life are usually employed in this situation.[2] In contrast, the prognostic effect of micrometastases, individual tumor cells, or tumor-cell deposits in the bone marrow detected by immunohistochemical or molecular genetic techniques remains controversial. An independent prognostic effect of this phenomenon in patients with esophageal cancer has recently been suggested by some investigators.[3,4] However, the viability of such tumor cells and their potential to form true metastases has been questioned.

With the current TNM classification of esophageal carcinoma,[1] metastasis to nonregional lymph nodes, for example, celiac axis nodes or cervical nodes, is also considered as distant tumor spread and classified as M1a or $M1_{Lymph}$. Prognostically this situation is more favorable than metastases to distant organs,[5-9] and probably does not represent true systemic disease.

On multivariate analysis, tumor length uniformly does not show any independent prognostic significance and consequently should be abandoned as a factor that influences therapeutic decisions. In contrast, in several studies the depth of invasion, that is, the pT-category, has been identified as an independent predictor of a complete tumor resectability and prognostic factor after complete tumor resection (R0-resection).[10-12] It is of particular interest that the pT-category can be predicted with a high degree of certainty by endoscopic ultrasonography.

At the time of resection, lymph-node metastases are present in the majority of patients with esophageal carcinoma.[8] Most univariate and multivariate analyses show the presence or absence of lymph-node metastases, that is, the pN-category, as the major independent predictor of survival in patients with esophageal carcinoma who had an R0-resection.[5-14] The presence of positive lymph nodes alone does not, however, lead to a sudden deterioration of the survival probability. Rather, survival decreases in a stepwise fashion with an increasing number of involved lymph nodes.[8,9,11,12,15] In patients with a limited number of involved mediastinal lymph nodes, long-term survival is still possible following a radical resection with extensive lymphadenectomy.

With the development of new sensitive immunohistochemical methods, it became possible to detect single tumor cells and cell clusters in lymph nodes that have been staged as tumor free on routine histologic examination. The prognostic role of this finding in patients with esophageal carcinoma remains controversial.[16,17]

Tumor Location

Due to the close proximity to the trachea and main-stem bronchi, extensive resection usually cannot be performed in patients with esophageal carcinoma located in the proximal part of the esophagus. The prognosis of patients with proximal esophageal tumors is therefore generally thought to be poor. The location of the primary tumor has, however, so far not been identified as an independent prognostic marker by multivariate analysis.

Histopathology

In recent years the prevalence of adenocarcinoma of the esophagus has shown a marked increase in the Western world, while the prevalence of squamous-cell esophageal carcinoma remained steady. The reasons for this change in the histologic spectrum of esophageal carcinoma are unclear. Overall, there is no prognostic difference between squamous and adenocarcinoma of the esophagus in most studies. Only patients with early adenocarcinoma, that is, pT1 tumors, appear to have a survival advantage as compared to patients with early squamous-cell tumors.[18]

Tumor differentiation is an important prognostic factor in many gastrointestinal tumors and has also been suggested as a predictor of survival in esophageal carcinoma.[19] However, an independent prognostic effect of tumor differentiation could not be shown in multivariate analyses.[11,20]

In one study venous invasion was shown to have an independent prognostic effect on survival in patients undergoing resection of esophageal carcinoma.[21] This finding requires confirmation by others.

Molecular and Other Biologic Factors

In recent years, much insight has been gained into the molecular mechanisms that underlie the process of tumor invasion and metastases. Some of these molecular and biological factors also have been related to the prognosis of the patients. These factors include ploidy and proliferation marker, mutations in oncogenes and tumor suppressor genes, and the expression of growth factors, tumor-associated proteases, protease inhibitors, and adhesion molecules. Most, if not all, of these data are still controversial.

Some authors report an independent prognostic effect of both the DNA distribution pattern and the Ki-67 labeling index on tumor recurrence and survival[22-25] in patients with esophageal cancer; however, this could not be confirmed in multivariate analyses by others.[26,27]

Mutations in the tumor suppressor gene p53 have been reported in a substantial percentage of patients with squamous and adenocarcinoma of the esophagus, and were related to a poor prognosis in some, but not all, of the studies.[15,28-33] Marked differences in the methods used to detect p53 abnormalities may account for these discrepancies. Other genetic abnormalities that have been implicated as predictors of survival include alterations of the HER-2/neu, int-2 and hst-1 oncogenes, and expression of p21.[34-36]

Amplification of the epidermal growth factor receptor gene and overexpression of the epidermal growth factor receptor, the oncoprotein c-erbB2, and the transforming growth factor alpha have been related to survival in patients with squamous cell or adenocarcinoma of the esophagus.[24,37-39] Expression of the vascular endothelial growth factor and its receptors also have been reported as prognostic markers in esophageal carcinoma.[40,41] Other biologic factors that have been related to the prognosis of patients with esophageal cancer include expression of adhesion molecule CD44 variants[42] and E-cadherin,[39] expression of cyclin D1,[39] urokinase-type plasminogen activator,[43,44] thymidine phosphorylase,[45] matrilysin,[46] microvessel density,[45] and the number of nucleolar organizer regions.[47]

In general the evaluated populations in the studies assessing the prognostic role of molecular and biologic markers were small and the clinical role of these observations is not clear at the present time. Prospective long-term follow-up studies of large patient populations are clearly required to clarify the prognostic impact of these exiting, though preliminary, observations.

Other Tumor-related Prognostic Markers

In univariate analyses the potential of cancer cells for growth in cell culture, the presence of intramural metastases, and the endoscopic growth pattern have been suggested as prognostic indicators.[48-50] These observations still need to be confirmed by other investigators.

PATIENT-RELATED PROGNOSTIC FACTORS

Age and Sex

Esophageal carcinoma is a disease that affects mostly male patients over 60 years of age. On univariate analyses patients' sex was repeatedly reported as a prognostic marker. This observation could so far not convincingly be confirmed in large multivariate analyses.

Because of an anticipated limited life expectancy a potentially curative resection is frequently not considered in patients who present with esophageal carcinoma at an advanced age. Although perioperative mortality increases with increasing age, survival following resection for esophageal carcinoma is not determined by the age of the patient.

Nutritional Status

Patients with esophageal carcinoma frequently present with a deteriorated nutritional status. So far, prospective studies cannot show the impact of nutritional status or preoperative weight loss on long-term survival.

Physiologic Status

Due to the advanced age and the factors that predispose to the development of esophageal carcinoma, the comorbidity of patients with esophageal carcinoma is high. Pulmonary, cardiac, hepatic, and renal function, general physiologic status and cooperation of the patient are the major parameters that determine postoperative mortality.[51] The preoperative physiologic status of the patient does not, however independently predict long-term survival time after a curative resection, if the patient survives the surgical procedure.

ENVIRONMENT- AND TREATMENT-RELATED PROGNOSTIC FACTORS

The tumor- and patient-related prognostic markers are given at the time of presentation and cannot be altered by therapeutic intervention. Prognostic factors associated with therapeutic measures therefore have the most important impact on the management of patients with esophageal carcinoma. Of all available therapeutic measures, esophageal resection remains the mainstay of curative therapy in patients with resectable tumors.[5] There is broad agreement that radiation, chemotherapy, combined radiochemotherapy, or local measures should be considered as primary treatment options only in patients with unresectable tumors or patients whose physiologic status does not permit major surgery.[52] Controlled studies supporting this contention are lacking.

In patients undergoing surgical resection, the prognostic impact of the residual tumor status after resection, the extent of resection, the experience of the surgeon and institution performing the resection, and the effect of perioperative adjuvant or additive therapy have been most widely assessed.

Residual Tumor Status

In most uni- and multivariate analysis the presence of residual tumor after surgical resection is the factor with the strongest independent prognostic impact.[5,10-12] The long-term survival rates for patients with squamous cell and adenocarcinoma of the esophagus who had an R0 or a R1/R2 resection at the Department of Surgery of the Technische Universität Munich are shown in Figures 16.1 and 16.2.

Surgical Approach and Extent of Lymphadenectomy

Although convincing randomized trials or multivariate analyses are still lacking, a transthoracic en bloc resection is by most experts perceived as the surgical approach of choice for patients with squamous-cell esophageal carcinoma.[5] In patients with adenocarcinoma of the distal esophagus a transthoracic

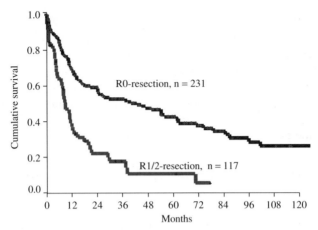

Figure 16.1 Overall 10-year survival rate of patients with resected squamous-cell esophageal cancer. Patients with complete macroscopic and microscopic tumor resection (R0 resection) versus patients with residual disease after resection (R1/R2 resection). (Data of the Chirurgische Klinik und Poliklinik, Klinikum rechts der Isar der TU München, 1982–1999).

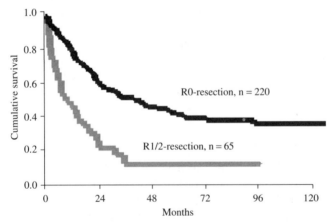

Figure 16.2 Overall 10-year survival rate of patients with resected adenocarcinoma of the distal esophagus (AEG Type I). Patients with complete macroscopic and microscopic tumor resection (R0 resection) versus patients with residual disease after resection (R1/R2 resection). (Data of the Chirurgische Klinik und Poliklinik, Klinikum rechts der Isar der TU München, 1982–1999).

esophagectomy does not appear to be associated with a substantial survival benefit as compared to a transmediastinal approach.[53]

The role of extended lymphadenectomy in patients with esophageal cancer is discussed controversially. A potential prognostic benefit of extended lymphadenectomy may be deducted from studies that show an independent prognostic effect of the so-called lymph-node ratio, that is, the ratio of invaded and removed lymph nodes.[8,11] A significant drop in the survival rate occurs when more than 20% of the removed lymph nodes are involved. Theoretically this implies that in a patient with esophageal cancer the prognosis can be improved by extending the lymph-node dissection.[5-14,54,55] So far, however, this concept has not been confirmed by prospective trials.

Combined Modality Therapy

Due to the frequently advanced tumor stages, an R0 resection is possible in only a minority of the patients presenting with esophageal carcinoma. Consequently, a variety of combined modality treatments with pre- and postoperative radiation, chemotherapy, or combined radiochemotherapy have been investigated in an effort to induce a down-staging of the primary tumor, to eliminate potential systemic micrometastasis, to treat residual tumor after surgical resection, and ultimately to prolong survival in patients with esophageal carcinoma.[56]

A number of randomized prospective trials did not show an increase in survival time with postoperative radiation in patients with or without residual tumor after surgical resection.[57] Similarly, a prognostic benefit with the use of adjuvant or additive postoperative chemotherapy currently cannot be supported by controlled trials.[56,57] Preoperative radiation, chemotherapy, or combined radiochemotherapy so far has not shown a convincing overall survival benefit in patients with potentially resectable tumors.[56,57] In contrast, preoperative chemotherapy or combined radiochemotherapy may increase the resection rate, rate of complete tumor resections, and survival time in patients with locally advanced tumors.[58] Most available studies, however, show that a prognostic benefit from multimodal therapy can be expected only in patients who have an objective response to preoperative therapy, with subsequent R0-resection or a complete histopathologic response to preoperative treatment, that is, no viable tumor in the resected specimen.[58] Unfortunately, response to preoperative treatment currently cannot predicted with a high degree of likelihood.

Other Treatment-related Prognostic Factors

Postoperative complications, for example, respiratory tract infections, anastomotic leakage, and a number of perioperative blood transfusions, have been reported as independent predictors of survival in patients with esophageal cancer.[10,52,59] These factors are clearly related to the experience of the surgeon or the institution at which the surgical procedure is performed.[60-63] Consequently, esophageal resections should only be performed in centers that have sufficient experience with the technical details of esophageal resection, reconstruction, and perioperative management.

SUMMARY

The presence of frank hematogenous distant metastases, a complete macroscopic and microscopic tumor removal, and the pT- and pN-categories after complete resection are the only undisputed independent prognostic factors in patients with esophageal carcinoma. A number of molecular and biological prognostic factors have been suggested in the recent literature and require confirmation in further studies. With the advent of new preoperative staging techniques and the currently emerging molecular and biological prognostic factors, a more selective and tailored therapeutic approach to patients with esophageal carcinoma should be possible in the near future.

■■■■■ **APPENDIX 16A**

TNM Classification

T — Primary Tumor

TX Primary tumor cannot be assessed
T0 No evidence of primary tumor
Tis Carcinoma in situ

T1 Tumor invades lamina propria or submucosa
T2 Tumor invades muscularis propria
T3 Tumor invades adventitia
T4 Tumor invades adjacent structures

N — Regional Lymph Nodes

NX Regional lymph nodes cannot be assessed
N0 No regional lymph-node metastasis
N1 Regional lymph-node metastasis

M — Distant Metastasis

MX Distant metastasis cannot be assessed
M0 No distant metastasis
M1 Distant metastasis

For Tumors of Lower Thoracic Esophagus
M1a Metastasis in celiac lymph nodes
M1b Other distant metastasis

For Tumors of Upper Thoracic Esophagus
M1a Metastasis in cervical lymph nodes
M1b Other distant metastasis

For Tumors of Midthoracic Esophagus
M1a Not applicable
M1b Nonregional lymph-node or other distant metastasis

Stage Grouping

Stage 0	Tis	N0	M0
Stage I	T1	N0	M0
Stage IIA	T2	N0	M0
	T3	N0	M0
Stage IIB	T1	N1	M0
	T2	N1	M0
Stage III	T3	N1	M0
	T4	Any N	M0
Stage IV	Any T	Any N	M1
Stage IVA	Any T	Any N	M1a
Stage IVB	Any T	Any N	M1b

Source: Sobin LH, Wittekind Ch (eds.): *TNM classification of malignant tumors*, 5th ed.: Union Internationale Contre le Cancer Wiley-Liss, New York, 1997.

████████ **APPENDIX 16b**

Prognostic Factors in Esophageal Cancer

Prognostic factors	Tumor Related	Host Related	Environment Related
Essential	Anatomic extent Histologic type R classification		Institution
Additional	Number of involved lymph nodes	Sex	
New and promising	Isolated tumor cells Molecular markers		

REFERENCES

1. Sobin LH, Wittekind, Ch (eds.): TNM classification of malignant tumors. New York, Wiley-Liss, 1997.

2. Roder JD, Stein HJ, Siewert JR: Prognostic markers in patients with carcinoma of the oesophagus. *Eur J Gastroenterol Hepatol* 6: 663–9, 1994.

3. Thorban S, Roder JD, Nekarda H, et al.: Immunocytochemical detection of disseminated tumor cells in the bone marrow of patients with esophageal carcinoma. *J Natl Cancer Inst* 88:1222–7, 1997.

4. O'Sullivan GC, Sheehan D, Clarke A, et al.: Micrometastases in esophagogastric cancer: High detection rate in resected rib segments. *Gastroenterology* 116:543–8, 1999.

5. Fumagalli U, Panel of Experts: Resective surgery for cancer of the thoracic esophagus. Results of a consensus conference. *Dis Esoph* 9:3–19, 1999.

6. Baba M, Aikou T, Yoshinaka H, et al.: Long term results of subtotal esophagectomy with three-field lymphadenectomy for carcinoma of the thoracic esophagus. *Ann Surg* 219:310–16, 1994.

7. Akiyama H, Tsurumaru M, Udagawa H, Kajiyama Y: Radical lymph node dissection for cancer of the thoracic esophagus. *Ann Surg* 220:364–72, 1994.

8. Siewert JR Stein HJ: Lymphadenectomy for esophageal cancer. *Langenbeck's Arch Surg* 384:141–8, 1999.

9. Korst RJ, Rusch VW, Venkatraman E, et al.: Proposed revision of the staging classification for esophageal cancer. *J Thorac Cardiovasc Surg* 115:660–9, 1998.

10. Sugimachi K, Matsuoka H, Ohno S, et al.: Multivariate approach for assessing the prognosis of clinical oesophageal carcinoma. *Br J Surg* 75:1115–8, 1988.

11. Roder, JD Busch R Stein HJ, Fink U, et al.: Ratio of invaded and removed lymph nodes as a predictor of survival in squamous cell carcinoma of the oesophagus. *Br J Surg* 81:410–13, 1994.

12. Hölscher AH, Bollschweiler E, Bumm R, et al.: Prognostic factors of resected adenocarcinoma of the esophagus. *Surgery* 118:845–55, 1995.

13. Tabira Y, Okuma T, Kondo K, Kitamura N: Indications for three-field dissection followed by esophagectomy for advanced carcinoma of the thoracic esophagus. *J Thorac Cardiovasc Surg* 117:239–45, 1999.

14. Tachibana M, Kinugasa S, Dhar DK, et al.: Prognostic factors after extended esophacectomy for squamous cell carcinoma of the thoracic esophagus, *J Surg Oncol* 72:88–93, 1999.

15. Wang LS, Chow KC, Chi KH, et al.: Prognosis of esophageal squamous cell carcinoma: Analysis of clinicopathological and biological factors. *Am J Gastroenterol* 94:1933–40, 1999.

16. Izbicki JR, Hosch SB, Pichlmeier U, et al.: Prognostic value of immunohistochemically identifiable tumor cells in lymph nodes of patients with completely resected esophageal cancer. *N Engl J Med* 337:1188–94, 1997.

17. Natsugoe S, Mueller J, Stein HJ, et al.: Micrometastasis and tumor cell microinvolvement of lymph nodes from esophageal squamous cell carcinoma. *Cancer* 83:858–66, 1998.

18. Hölscher AH, Bollschweiler E, Schneider PM, Siewert JR: Prognosis of early esophageal cancer. *Cancer* 76:178–86, 1995.

19. Robey-Cafferty SS, El Naggar AK, Sahin AA, et al.: Prognostic factors in esophageal squamous carcinoma. A study of histologic features, blood group expression, and DNA ploidy. *Am J Clin Pathol* 95:844–9, 1991.

20. Tachimori Y, Kato H, Watanabe H: Surgery for thoracic esophageal carcinoma with clinically positive cervical nodes. *J Thorac Cardiovasc Surg* 116:954–9, 1998.

21. Theunissen PHMH, Borchardt F, Poortvliet DCJ: Histopathological evaluation of oesophageal carcinoma: The significance of venous invasion. *Br J Surg* 78:930–2, 1991.

22. Böttger T, Störkel S, Stöckle M, et al.: DNA image cytometry. A prognostic tool in squamous cell carcinoma of the esophagus? *Cancer* 67:2290–4, 1991.

23. Tsutsui S, Kuwano H, Mori M, et al.: Flow cytometric analysis of DNA content in primary and metastatic lesions of esophageal squamous cell carcinoma. *Cancer* 70:2586–91, 1992.

24. Nakamura T, Nekarda H, Hoelscher AH, et al., Prognostic value of DNA ploidy and c-ErbB-2 oncoprotein overexpression in adenocarcinoma of Barrett's esophagus. *Cancer* 73:1785–94, 1994.

25. Ikeda G, Isaji S, Chandra B, et al.: Prognostic significance of biologic factors in squamous cell carcinoma of the esophagus. *Cancer* 86:1396–1405, 1999.

26. Patil P, Redkar A, Patel SG, et al.: Prognosis of operable squamous cell carcinoma of the esophagus. Relationship with clinico-pathologic features and DNA ploidy. *Cancer* 72:20–4, 1993.

27. Ruol A, Segalin A, Panozzo M, et al.: Flow cytometric DNA analysis of squamous cell carcinoma of the esophagus. *Cancer* 65:1185–8, 1990.

28. Shimaya K, Shiozaki H, Inuoe M, et al.: Significance of p53 expression as a prognostic factor in oesophageal squamous cell carcinoma. *Virchows Arch A Pathol Anat* 422:271–6, 1993.

29. Furihata M, Ohtsuki Y, Ogoshi S, et al.: Prognostic significance of human papillomavirus genomes (type-16, -18) and aberrant expression of p53 protein in human esophageal cancer. *Int J Cancer* 54:226–30, 1993.

30. Coggi G, Bosari S, Roncalli M, et al.: p53 protein accumulation and p53 gene mutation in esophageal carcinoma: A molecular and immunohistochemical study with clinicopathologic correlations. *Cancer* 79:425–32, 1997.

31. Casson AG, Tammemagi M, Eskandarian S, et al.: p53 alterations in oesophageal cancer: Association with clinicopathological features, risk factors, and survival. *Mol Pathol* 51:71–9, 1998.

32. Ireland AP, Shibata DK, Chandrasoma P, et al.: Clinical significance of p53 mutations in adenocarcinoma of the esophagus and cardia. *Ann Surg* 231:179–87, 2000.

33. Hashimoto N, Tachibana M, Dhar DK, et al.: Expression of p53 and RB proteins in squamous cell carcinoma of the esophagus: Their relationship with clinicopathologic characteristics. *Ann Surg Oncol* 6:489–94, 1999.

34. Kitagawa Y, Ueda M, Ando N, et al.: Significance of int2/hst-1 co-amplification as a prognostic factor in patients with esophageal squamous carcinoma. *Cancer Res* 51:1504–8, 1991.

35. Nita ME, Nagawa H, Tominaga O, et al.: p21Waf1/Cip1 expression is a prognostic marker in curatively resected esophageal squamous cell carcinoma, but not p27Kip1, p53, or Rb. *Ann Surg Oncol* 6:481–8, 1999.

36. Brien TP, Odze RD, Sheehan CE, et al.: HER-2/neu gene amplification by FISH predicts poor survival in Barrett's esophagus-associated adenocarcinoma. *Hum Pathol* 31:35–9, 2000.

37. Mukaida H, Toi M, Hirai T, et al.: Clinical significance of the expression of epidermal growth factor and its receptor in esophageal cancer. *Cancer* 68:142–8, 1991.

38. Iihara K, Shiozaki H, Tahara H, et al.: Prognostic significance of transforming growth factor-alpha in human esophageal carcinoma. Implication for the autocrine proliferation. *Cancer* 71:2902–9, 1993.

39. Shimada Y, Imamura M, Watanabe G, et al.: Prognostic factors of oesophageal squamous cell carcinoma from the perspective of molecular biology. *Br J Cancer* 80:1281–8, 1999.

40. Inoue K, Ozeki Y, Suganuma T, et al.: Vascular endothelial growth factor expression in primary esophageal squamous cell carcinoma. Association with angiogenesis and tumor progression. *Cancer* 79:206–13, 1997.

41. Koide N, Nishio A, Kono T, et al.: Histochemical study of vascular endothelial growth factor in squamous cell carcinoma of the esophagus. *Hepatogastroenterology* 46:952–8, 1999.

42. Gotoda T, Matsumura Y, Kondo H, et al.: Expression of CD44 variants and prognosis in oesophageal squamous cell carcinoma. *Gut* 46:14–9, 2000.

43. Nekarda H, Schlegel P, Schmitt M, et al.: Strong prognostic impact of tumor-associated urokinase-type plasminogen activator in completely resected adenocarcinoma of the esophagus. *Clin Cancer Res* 4:1755–63, 1998.

44. Torzewski M, Sarbia M, Verreet P, et al.: Prognostic significance of urokinase-type plasminogen activator expression in squamous cell carcinomas of the esophagus. *Clin Cancer Res* 3:2263–8, 1997.

45. Igarashi M, Dhar DK, Kubota H, et al.: The prognostic significance of microvessel density and thymidine phosphorylase expression in squamous cell carcinoma of the esophagus. *Cancer* 82:1225–32, 1998.

46. Yamamoto H, Adachi Y, Itoh F, et al.: Association of matrilysin expression with recurrence and poor prognosis in human esophageal squamous cell carcinoma. *Cancer Res* 59:3313–6, 1999.

47. Morita M, Kuwano H, Matsuda H, et al.: Prognostic significance of argyrophilic nucleolar organizer regions in esophageal carcinoma. *Cancer Res* 51:5339–41, 1991.

48. Shimada Y, Imamura M: Prognostic significance of cell culture in carcinoma of the oesophagus. *Br J Surg* 80:605–7, 1993.

49. Takubo K, Sasajima K, Yamashita K, et al.: Prognostic significance of intramural metastasis in patients with esophageal carcinoma. *Cancer* 65:1816–9, 1990.

50. Ohno S, Mori M, Tsutsui S, et al.: Growth pattern and prognosis of submucosal carcinoma of the esophagus. *Cancer* 68:335–40, 1991.

51. Bartels H, Stein HJ, Siewert JR: Preoperative risk-analysis and postoperative mortality of oesophagectomy for resectable oesophageal cancer. *Br J Surg* 85:840–4, 1998.

52. Ruol A, Panel of Experts: Multimodality treatment for non-metastatic cancer of the thoracic esophagus. Results of a consensus conference. *Dis Esoph* 9:39–54, 1996.

53. Fumagalli U, Panel of Experts: Resective surgery for adenocarcinoma of the esophagogastric junction. Results of a Consensus Conference of the International Society for Diseases of the Esophagus and International Gastric Cancer Association. *Dis Esoph* 13:2000.

54. Nishihira T, Hirayama K, Mori S: A prospective randomized trial of extended cervical and superior mediastinal lymphadenectomy for carcinoma of the thoracic esophagus. *Am J Surg* 175:47–51, 1998.

55. Hagen JA, Peters JH, DeMeester TR: Superiority of extended en bloc esophagogastrectomy for carcinoma of the lower esophagus and cardia. *J Thor Cardiovasc Surg* 106:850–9, 1994.

56. Fink U, Stein HJ, Wilke HJ, et al.: Multimodal treatment for squamous cell esophageal cancer. *World J Surg* 19:198–204, 1995.

57. Lehnert T: Multimodal therapy for squamous carcinoma of the oesophagus. *Br J Surg* 86:727–39, 1999.

58. Fink U, Stein HJ, Siewert JR: Multimodale Therapie bei Tumoren des oberen Gastrointestinaltrakts. *Chirurg* 69:349–59, 1998.

59. Tachibana M, Tabara H, Kotoh T, et al.: Prognostic significance of perioperable blood transfusions in resectable thoracic esophageal cancer. *Am J Gastroenterol* 94:757–65, 1999.

60. Mathews HR, Powell DJ, McCarley CL: Effect of surgical experience on results of resection for oesophageal carcinoma. *Br J Surg* 73:621–3, 1986.

61. Patti MG, Corvera CU, Glasgow RE, Way LW: A hospital's annual rate of esophagectomy influences the operative mortality rate. *J Gastrointest Surg* 2:186–92, 1998.

62. Miller JD, Jain MK, de Gara CJ, et al.: Effect of surgical experience on results of esophagectomy for esophageal carcinoma. *J Surg Oncol* 65:20–1, 1997.

63. Begg CB, Cramer LD, Hoskins WJ, Brennan MF: Impact of hospital volume on operative mortality for major cancer surgery. *JAMA* 280:1747–51, 1998.

CHAPTER 17

Gastric Cancer

J. HAN J.M. VAN KRIEKEN, MITSURU SASAKO and CORNELIS J.H. VAN DE VELDE

The incidence of gastric cancer is decreasing worldwide, but the prognosis is still generally poor. Insight in pathogenesis (the role of Helicobacter Pylori and Epstein-Barr virus) and molecular genetics (p53 en RAS mutations) has increased in recent years. Important new data exist on treatment: the role of local surgical treatment, extended lymphadenectomy, and chemotherapy. Outcome is clearly dependent on many factors, but complete surgical excision is still central in the treatment. This chapter deals with clinical, pathological, and genetic factors that are related to survival, especially those that can influence clinical management. An important caveat has been formulated recently: criteria to diagnose cancer of the stomach vary, clearly leading to differences in patient populations in studies. In particular, this might partially explain the higher incidence and better prognosis of gastric cancer in Japan.[1] But then, when staged similarly using the same prognostic factors, there was no difference between the prognosis for German and Japanese patients.[2] Where prior gastric surgery is concerned (gastric stump carcinoma) prognosis is very poor,[3] but dependant on stage.[4] Histology and DNA index in these cases are the same as for other upper-third stomach cancer cases.[5] In a retrospective study on 2654 patients from Japan, it was found that from the early 1960s to the early 1980s the percentage of proximally located tumors increased from 17% to 27% and signet-ring-cell carcinoma increased from 2% to 22%. Although proximally located tumors behaved more aggressive, survival was more associated with stage than with primary site in the stomach.[6]

TUMOR-RELATED FACTORS

Essential Factors

Histologic Type Histological typing is based on the Second Edition of the World Health Organization (WHO) International Histological Classification.[7] The

---

Prognostic Factors in Cancer, 2nd edition, Edited by Mary K. Gospodarowicz
ISBN 0-471-40633-3 Copyright © 2001 Wiley-Liss, Inc.

two most common types are tubular and signet-ring-cell carcinoma. In a study of 520 patients with gastric cancer, 93 were of signet-ring-cell carcinoma type, and these patients had worse survival when compared to other types of advanced cases.[8] The carcinoids (well-differentiated neuroendocrine tumors), have a much better prognosis compared to adenocarcinomas. The rare small-cell carcinoma has a very poor prognosis. This subdivision of endocrine tumors gives good prognostic information, as shown in a study on 205 cases.[9] Furthermore, outcome can be predicted by a model that includes angioinvasion, size, histological type, and proliferative index.[10]

Some rare entities have special features. Epstein-Barr virus (EBV) is associated with some cases of gastric cancer. All six lymphoepithelioma-like carcinomas (out of a series of 379 adenocarcinomas) contained EBV and occurred in the proximal stomach; these cases had a better prognosis.[11] In 99 adenocarcinomas with lymphoid stroma, EBV was detected in 82 (83%), compared to 4/42 (10%) of ordinary cases.[12] Papillary clear-cell carcinoma was diagnosed in 15/73 papillary gastric carcinomas and had poor survival.[13] Seventy-one solid carcinomas out of 2738 poorly differentiated carcinomas had poor prognosis: 5 years 37%, 44% for T1/2, and often showed venous invasion.[14] Among 1337 curative resected patients undifferentiated histology and serosal invasion predicted peritoneal recurrence. Among 477 undifferentiated cases, 5-year survival was 98% for T1/2, 83% for T3, and 48% for T4.[15] In advanced stages, adenosquamous tumors were associated with poor prognosis.[16]

Additional Factors

Histologic Classification In addition to the WHO classification there are two classification schemes based on growth patterns: the Ming (expanding and infiltrating) and the Laurén (diffuse and intestinal). More recently the Goseki classification was introduced, which gives more useful prognostic information in addition to tumors, nodules, metastases (TNM) staging when compared to the Ming and Laurén schemes.[17]

Histological typing is recommended to recognize rare types with special features. The Goseki classification scheme is a useful adjunct with good reproducibility.

Essential Factors

Stage The TNM classification remains the cornerstone in clinical management of patients with gastric cancer (see Appendix 17A). The 1997 edition[18] of the classification is quite different compared to the Fourth Edition:[19] N-categories are now based on the number of positive lymph nodes, not the location of these nodes. It can be expected that this system will be easier to apply and be more reproducible. It has been shown that with the altered N-categories and stage groupings, balanced prognostic groups with higher predictive value can be formed. Early gastric cancer has a good prognosis: in 7031 consecutive gastric cancer patients who underwent gastrectomy, patients with early carcinoma (3163) had a 5 years survival of 89%, advanced cases (3868) of 46%. In advanced cancer independent prognostic factors were age, extent of tumor, adenosquamous type, resection line involvement and lymph-node metastasis.[16] The introduction of local or mucosal resection for early gastric cancer leads to less morbidity and mortality, but N-categorization is not possible. N-Category can be predicted by a model that includes the sex, age, histology, T-category, location, and diameter of the tumor.[20] In 1196 early gastric cancer patients 3.5% had lymph-node metastasis; in the absence of lymphatic invasion, ulceration, and a tumor diameter of <0.3 cm, it was only 0.36%.[21] In a series of 100 patients with early gastric cancer (out of 195 surgically treated patients), overall 5-years survival was 82%, with 98% disease-specific survival. Mucosal cancer had no lymphatic invasion, but submucosal had such invasion in 15/41 (37%), with 5% lymph-node metastasis.[22] In an Italian study of 45 patients with early gastric cancer, out of 200 gastric cancer patients (23%), 3 out of 27 mucosal and 5 out of 18 submucosal cases had lymph-node metastasis, but only one patient died of disease (median follow up 36 months.)[23] This shows that mucosal resection might lead to understaging.

Intraoperative staging is also often not reliable: in 435 patients pre- and intraoperative staging was shown to understage 19% of patients.[24] Reliable N-staging requires proper analysis of the lymph nodes and a sufficient number, at least 15 lymph-nodes. Surgeons may retrieve more lymph nodes than pathologists do; in D1 resection an average of 15 lymph-nodes, in D2 an average of 30 was retrieved.[25] This corresponds with the occurrence of distant metastasis in 40–45%, respectively, 60–65%[26] of cases. Extended lymph-node dissection results in higher numbers of lymph-node metastasis and thus stage migration, which at least partially explains the better stage-specific survival rates after D2 resection.[27] Although the new N-staging of the TNM system relates to numbers of positive lymph-nodes only, the different levels of lymph-node involvement were associated with different 5 years survival in 240 curative resected node-positive patients: Level I ($n = 142$): 67%; Level II ($n = 71$): 35%; Level III ($n = 27$): 26%.[28] The possibilities of sentinel-node procedures have not been tested in gastric cancer surgery, although it is shown in 1931 patients that skip metastasis are rare and that metastasis are associated with T-category.[29] Currently, studies on the improvement of staging are in progress. One study shows that micrometastasis in 1368 T3 R2 patients were not of prognostic influence.[30] The detection of micrometastasis is being widely studied. It is clear that methods and results vary. At present the data are not conclusive to be of use in clinical practice, except for trials. Positive cytology from abdominal washing increased the accuracy of staging in 535 patients.[31]

The main change in the Fifth Edition (1997) of the TNM classification for gastric cancer compared to the Fourth Edition (1987) is the use of the number of involved nodes instead of the location of positive nodes. Consequently, stage grouping was also altered. A second change is the suggestion that examination of at least 15 nodes is optimal for N0 status. We studied data retrieved from our randomized trial database, which compared D1 and D2 dissection and 633 curatively operated patients.[32] According to the criteria of the Fifth Edition, 39%

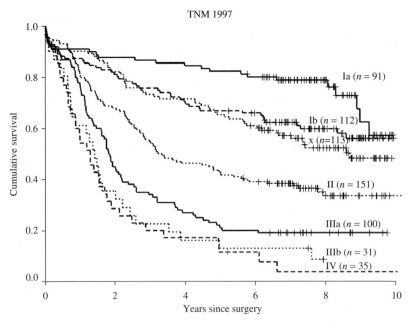

Figure 17.1   Survival in 633 patients, according to the 1987 (and 1997 TNM) stages.

of the node-positive patients had another N-category compared to the fourth Edition 21% had a lower stage and 18% had a higher stage. In the Fourth Edition, 5-year survival rates in the N0, N1, and N2 groups were, respectively, 72%, 34%, and 27%. According to the Fifth Edition, these percentages were 75%, 38%, 19%, 8%, and 65% for the N0, N1, N2, N3, and Nx groups, respectively. Significantly the 1987 N1 and N2 groups were split into three new N groups ($p < 0.01$, respectively, $p = 0.001$). The Cox regression model selected N 1997 as the most important prognostic factor, while N 1987 was not selected. In addition, the new TNM stage was also a better prognosticator (Figure 17.1 and 17.2). The recommendation to examine at least 15 nodes, however, could not be fulfilled in 38% of all node-negative patients, and we found that a minimum of five negative lymph nodes is a reliable number for staging purpose.

The new TNM classification is an improvement over the previous edition; N-category is of crucial importance and has to be based on standard analysis of 15 lymph nodes, but lower numbers also give reliable information.

New and Promising Factors

Molecular Factors   Factors associated with growth control, invasion, and metastasis are being recognized and are studied for their relation to prognosis. In general, all studies are retrospective and based on highly variable patients series. Many of the studies show conflicting data. Some of the factors are discussed in this overview but the review cannot be complete and new data are being generated rapidly.

TNM 1987

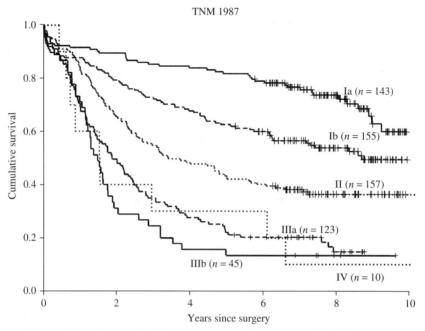

Figure 17.2   Survival in 633 patients, according to the 1997 TNM stages.

Cell Growth and Cell Death   Cells accumulate in tumors through proliferation and/or decreased cell death (apoptosis). Many studies into the growth rate of tumors have been performed. In gastric cancer, a high proliferation rate of the tumor is associated with poor prognosis and can be determined by flow cytometry, immunostaining with the monoclonal antibody Mib-1 (Ki67), or by labeling indexes. The number of apoptotic cells is higher in intestinal-type cancer with metastasis than in nonmetastatic or diffuse type.[33] Bcl-2 expression in 47/413 (11%) was associated with intestinal type, well/moderate, differentiation, and N0, but was not independently related to outcome.[34] In general, these methods require precise calibration of techniques and quantification, which has precluded their use in daily practice. In 78 cases of gastric carcinoma analysis of the expression of growth factors by reverse-transcriptase polymerase chain reaction (RT-PCR) in biopsies showed that platelet-derived growth factor A and transforming growth factor beta expression was associated with advanced stage; cyclin D1, cyclin E, urokinase-type plasminogen activator, and platelet derived growth factor A were associated with N-category.[35] In 88 British and 89 Japanese patients expression of c-erB2[n] or p53 are associated with stage of disease.[36]

Cell Adhesion   Since the process of metastasis determines the prognosis, many studies have analyzed factors that are related to decreased adhesion of tumor cells, matrix degradation, and intravascular growth. CD44, a hyaluronate receptor, is involved in cell migration through the extracellular matrix (ECM), which can be viewed as highly relevant for tumor invasion and metastasis. Several studies have indicated that CD44 isoform expression can be related to gastric tumor progression and poor prognosis for the patient.[5,6,10,11] EpCAM is an epithelial cell adhesion molecule, involved in regulation of cadherin adhesions, and possibly cell proliferation and invasion.[8,17,37] Evaluation of prognostic factors has to be based on high-quality clinical and pathological data. In The Netherlands a prospective randomized, multicenter trial was conducted on gastric cancer patients to compare the therapeutic efficacy of *extended* lymph-node dissection with *limited* lymph-node dissection. Strict quality control measures were taken to obtain optimal lymph-node retrieval and thus postoperative staging. The prospectively collected clinical and pathology data from this trial form an optimal basis to evaluate the usefulness for prognostic value of immunohistochemically determined protein expression in tumor cells. We studied 300 patients with surgically resected gastric carcinoma and could show that loss of expression of EpCAM indeed indicates more aggressive disease even in low stages; also low levels of CD44v6 expression indicate a poor prognosis.[38] Both results were independent of the TNM. There was a gradual decrease of survival rate associated with an increased loss of EpCAM. A group of the patients (19%) with excellent prognosis was detected: in these patients there was no loss at all for EpCAM staining of tumor cells and a 3-year survival rate of 73%. The 7% of patients without any staining for EpCAM had a particularly poor prognosis, with a 3-year survival rate of only 20%.

Because undergoing a curative resection is an important prognostic factor itself, we analyzed the RO resected patients separately and the results were similar. We used a Cox's regression analysis to study the prognostic value of the markers that were additional to the TNM stages. For this analysis the TNM staging was dichotomized into I + II versus III + IV. In a stepwise analysis both CD44v6 (VFF18) and EpCAM were selected as having significant prognostic value in addition to TNM (Table 17.1). Patients with Stage I or II disease without loss of EpCAM have an excellent prognosis: the 3-year survival rate is 87%. In patients with any loss the 3-year survival rate decreases to 53%, while in patients with complete loss of EpCAM expression a further decrease is seen that is down to 29%. In Stages III and IV the 3-year survival rates were 31% and

TABLE 17.1 Results of Cox's Regression Analysis Applied on the TNM stage, VFF18 and Ep-CAM Expression ($N = 251$)

		RR	95% CI	p-Value
TNM stage	I + II	1.00	2.44–4.71	<0.001
	III + IV	3.39		
VFF18	26–100%	1.00		
	0–25%	1.49	1.05–2.11	0.03
Ep-CAM	100%	1.00		
	1–99%	1.46	0.92–2.32	0.11
	0%	2.16	1.05–4.43	0.04

18%, respectively, in patients without and with any loss of EpCAM expression, while all patients with complete loss of EpCAM expression died within 3 years. Also CD44v6 (VFF18) staining had prognostic relevance in the early stages: the 3-year survival rate in patients with Stage I and II was 64% if less than 25% of the tumor cells lost expression, while this percentage decreased to 45% in patients with extensive loss of CD44v6 (VFF18) expression (>75% cells losing expression). In patients with Stage III and IV disease, 3-year survival rates were 25% and 6%, respectively.

Vascular Invasion Before tumor cells can metastasize, they have to invade vessels. Tumor cells may acquire the property to induce new vessels by producing angiogenic factors like thymidine phosphorylase. In a study of 158 R0 resected patients with gastric cancer there was a correlation between microvessel count and expression of thymidine phosphorylase; both predict poor survival and lymph-node metastasis.[39] In another study thymidine phophorylase expression in 54/72 curative resected patients was related to microvessel count and predicted better survival, especially in patients treated with fluorouracil derivates.[40] These conflicting data make it clear that the exact processes are not yet known and that these data are not of use yet.

Matrix degradation Many proteases are involved in the process of matrix degradation, which is needed for tumor cells to invade the stroma. Among the most studied examples are the plasminogen activators. Urokinase-type plasminogen activator and its receptor expression were related to poor survival in 20 patients with gastric cancer[41] and also cathepsin B and L in 25 patients.[42] High levels of urokinase-type plasminogen activator independently predicted poor survival in 160 gastric cancer patients, also lymph-node metastasis. Low t-PA and high PAI-1 levels indicate independently poor survival in 50 patients.[43] Matrix metalloproteinases MMP-2 and MMP-9, which are involved in tumor invasion and metastasis, are increased in gastric cancer tissue, and a high level predicts poor survival independently of other clinicopathological factors.[44]

Many factors have been shown to be of possible significance, but at present, none has been tested in a prognostic study. Furthermore, the data still vary from laboratory to laboratory. At present, it can be recommended to test factors in studies, but not to use the results on individual patients.

HOST-RELATED FACTORS

Many studies have been performed on the role of patient-related factors, and the results are controversial. Only factors independent of the TNM stage are of relevance. A recent study shows that 7% of patients were younger than 40 years of age and had similar stages and prognosis compared to the older patients in a retrospective study of 4608 patients.[45] In elderly patients the outcome is dependent on the possibility of performing major surgery. No conclusive data exist on the effect of gender or performance status.

ENVIRONMENT-RELATED FACTORS

Essential Factors

Surgery   It is beyond doubt that surgery is the main treatment option and the only curative one in gastric cancer patients. Cure can be obtained only when the tumor is removed completely. Resection-line involvement predicts poor survival in 22/259 patients, and only in N0 patients.[46] Resection-line involvement in 41/699 surgically treated patients was strongly associated with T- and N-categories and poor differentiation, and resulted in poor survival, independent of TNM stage.[47] Two new developments have to be mentioned: mucosal resection for early gastric cancer, and the role of extended lymphadenectomy. Several studies now show good results of limited surgery in selected patients. Endoscopic resection resulted in complete excision in 12/17 (70%) early gastric cancers and 18/23 (78%) adenomas. The success rate is dependent on the site in the stomach and the size of the tumor.[48] In another study, 102 cases of early gastric cancer were successfully resected.[49] In yet another study, 308 early gastric cancer were endoscopically resected: 89% of lesions smaller than 2cm were curatively resected, but only 50% of those larger than 2cm. No patient died of disease.[50] In the Dutch Gastric Cancer Trial (DGCT)[51,52] 80 participating centers randomized 996 patients, of which 711 (380 D1 and 331 D2) underwent the allocated treatment with curative intent and 285 patients required palliative treatment. This study was the first surgical trial ever to include a meticulous quality control protocol, instruction and supervision in the operating room, and monitoring of the pathological results. After curative resection ($N = 711$), D2 patients had significantly more complications (43% vs. 25% for D1), and postoperative deaths (10% vs. 4% for D1), and remained longer in the hospital (median 16 days vs. 14 days for D1). Five-year survival rates were not different: 45% for D1 and 47% for D2 patients. The patients of most interest for the study of the cumulative relapse risk [microscopically complete (R0) resections with postoperative deaths excluded] showed 5-year relapse risks of 43% for D1 and 37% for D2 (NS). In univariate analysis after 5 years, none of the patient subgroups resected with curative intent had significantly better survival in D2, although there was a (nonsignificant) trend toward reduced relapse risk. The authors concluded that the excess morbidity and mortality did not justify standard use of extended (D2) lymph-node dissection in Western patients with gastric cancer. D2 dissection may not be applicable for all Western gastric cancer patients, but it should not be completely discarded. Subgroup analysis in the British Medical Research Council (MRC) trial has shown that D2 dissection might offer a survival benefit for Stage II and Stage IIIA patients who have lymph-node metastases limited to the first (N1) tier. This has also been suggested in a German study.[53] Preoperative staging cannot reliably assess lymph-node involvement, although a Japanese model using various prognostic factors allowed for a reasonably correct prediction.[20] Some patients, such as females, those under 60, and those requiring partial gastrectomy, have a low risk of postoperative complications. If N1 lymph-node metastases are expected in these patients, D2 dissection can be done safely, and might even be beneficial. It is mandatory, however, to refrain from extended lymph-node dissection in patients with signs of further (locoregional) spread. Perioperative assessment of distant lymph-node involvement, peritoneal or liver seeding, and free peritoneal cancer cells should be done in all candidates for D2 dissection.[31] The possible effects of blood transfusion are probably secondary to other risk factors.[6]

Radical surgery is the most important factor that determines possible cure. Extended lymph-node dissection has effect in subgroups of patients provided that operative mortality can be kept low.

New and Promising Factors

Chemotherapy The role of chemotherapy is not established, but several clinical trials are in progress. Good responses have been described in some cases, for instance, one patient was cured of early gastric cancer by uracil and tegafur.[54] However, in a randomized trial involving 56 patients to assess the value of preoperative chemotherapy (FAMTX), there was no effect on stage or possibility for curative resection.[55] Furthermore, a meta-analysis initially did not show any effect of chemotherapy in gastric cancer,[56] though it later did.

Before recommendations can be made the results of randomized trials have to be awaited.

MULTIVARIATE ANALYSIS OF PROGNOSTIC FACTORS

Prognostic factors that related patients, tumors, and treatments were evaluated by multivariate analysis using stepwise regression analysis and/or the Cox proportional hazard model. Important prognostic factors shown by these reports are not consistent. Because these results are affected by how the authors select prognostic factors, how each factor is evaluated, and the size of the material and the treatment given. Stage comprises three factors, T, N, M, and thus shows strong correlation with them. For this reason, stage is excluded from multivariate analysis in some studies. Haugstvedt et al.[57] showed that stage, macroscopic type, hospital level, and age were the independent prognostic factors in the Norwegian multicenter study ($n = 532$). The hazard ratios (HR) of these factors are 1.81, 1.67, 1.44, and 1.27, respectively. In the German Gastric Cancer Study ($n = 1654$), Roder et al.[51] showed that nodal status, presence of residual tumor, distant metastasis, pT, preoperative risk factors (three or more), and postoperative complications were the independent prognostic factors. According to Msika et al.,[58] lymph-node involvement was the only independent prognostic factor in the French study ($n = 156$). Okajima[59] reported the results of 6540 patients treated at the National Cancer Center Tokyo between 1962 and 1991. Twenty-three factors are included in this analysis: age, sex, preoperative risk, pT, pN, liver or peritoneal metastasis, macroscopic type, tumor size, location, histological type, tumor stroma, type of invasion (infiltrative, intermediate, expansive), lymph vessel involvement, venous involvement, Japanese stage, International Union Against Cancer

(UICC) stage, type of resection, type of lymphadenectomy, combined organ resection, resection margin positivity, presence of residual disease, postoperative chemotherapy, and postoperative complications. After a correlation check, they excluded Japanese and UICC stages and presence of residual disease. By stepwise regression analysis, age, sex, pT, pN, liver or peritoneal metastasis, tumor size, location, tumor invasion, lymph vessel involvement, venous involvement, type of lymphadenectomy, and resection margin positivity were selected as independent factors. These factors were further analyzed using the Cox proportional hazard model to evaluate the importance of each factor on the prognosis. The highest HR was 4.62 shown by pT, followed by pN (HR = 3.63), age (2.07), liver or peritoneal metastasis (1.91), type of lymphadenectomy (1.58), resection margin positivity (1.55), tumor invasion (1.33), venous involvement (1.28), lymph vessel involvement (1.20), tumor size (1.18), sex (1.17), and location (1.10).

SUMMARY

In conclusion, many studies have been performed since the previous edition of this book, which contained the chapter on stomach cancer by Hermanek et al.[60] Most of the important prognostic factors still are of importance, others are less important. In the table in Appendix 17B the factors are grouped according to the present situation. It is expected that some of the new and promising factors will play a major role in the next edition of this book.

■■■■■■ **APPENDIX 17A**

TNM Classification for Stomach Cancer

T — Primary Tumor

TX Primary tumor cannot be assessed

T0 No evidence of primary tumor

Tis Carcinoma in situ: intraepithelial tumor without invasion of the lamina propria

T1 Tumor invades lamina propria or submucosa

T2 Tumor invades muscularis propria or subserosa

T3 Tumor penetrates serosa (visceral peritoneum) without invasion of adjacent structures

T4 Tumor invades adjacent structures

N — Regional Lymph Nodes

NX Regional lymph nodes cannot be assessed

N0 No regional lymph-node metastasis

N1 Metastasis in 1 to 6 regional lymph nodes

N2 Metastasis in 7 to 15 regional lymph nodes

N3 Metastasis in more than 15 regional lymph nodes

M — Distant Metastasis

MX Distant metastasis cannot be assessed

M0 No distant metastasis

M1 Distant metastasis

Stage Grouping

Stage	T	N	M
Stage 0	Tis	N0	M0
Stage IA	T1	N0	M0
Stage IB	T1	N1	M0
	T2	N0	M0
Stage II	T1	N2	M0
	T2	N1	M0
	T3	N0	M0
Stage IIIA	T2	N2	M0
	T3	N1	M0
	T4	N0	M0
Stage IIIB	T3	N2	M0
Stage IV	T4	N1, N2, N3	M0
	T1, T2, T3	N3	M0
	Any T	Any N	M1

Source: Sobin LH, Wittekind Ch (eds.): *TNM classification of malignant tumors*, 5th ed. Union Internationale Contre le Cancer Wiley-Liss, New York, 1997.

■■■■■■■ **APPENDIX 17B**

Prognostic Factors in Stomach Cancer

Prognostic Factors	Tumor Related	Host Related	Environment Related
Essential	Histologic type Anatomic extent — T-, N-, M-categories		Surgery: radical resection
Prognostic Factors	Tumor Related	Host Related	Environment Related
Additional	Goseki classification Peritumoral inflammatory reaction		D2 resection
New and promising	Isolated tumor cells in bone marrow Adhesion molecules, matrix metallo- proteinases		Chemotheraphy

REFERENCES

1. Schlemper RJ, Itabashi M, Kato Y, et al.: Differences in diagnostic criteria for gastric carcinoma between Japanese and western pathologists [published erratum appears in *Lancet* 350(9076):524, 1997]. *Lancet* 349:1725–9, 1997.

2. Bollschweiler E, Boettcher K, Hoelscher AH, et al.: Is the prognosis for Japanese and German patients with gastric cancer really different? *Cancer* 71:2918–25, 1993.

3. Kodera Y, Yamamura Y, Torii A, et al.: Gastric stump carcinoma after partial gastrectomy for benign gastric lesion: What is feasible as standard surgical treatment? *J. Surg. Oncol.* 63:119–24, 1996.

4. Kodera Y, Yamamura Y, Torii A, et al.: Gastric remnant carcinoma after partial gastrectomy for benign and malignant gastric lesions. *J. Am. Coll. Surg.* 182:1–6, 1996.

5. Ikeguchi M, Kondou A, Oka A, et al.: Flow cytometric analysis of the DNA content of tumor cells in cases of gastric cancer in the upper third of the stomach and in the remnant stomach. *Oncology* 52:116–22, 1995.

6. Kampschoer GH, Nakajima T, van de Velde CJ: Changing patterns in gastric adenocarcinoma. *Br. J. Surg.* 76:914–6, 1989.

7. Watanabe H, Jass JR, Sobin LH: Histological typing of esophageal and gastric tumors, 2nd ed. (WHO Int Histological Classification of Tumors), Berlin-New York, Springer-Verlag, 1990.

8. Yokota T, Kunii Y, Teshima S, et al.: Signet ring cell carcinoma of the stomach: A clinicopathological comparison with the other histological types. *Tohoku J. Exp. Med.* 186:121–30, 1998.

9. Rindi G, Bordi C, Rappel S, et al.: Gastric carcinoids and neuroendocrine carcinomas: Pathogenesis, pathology, and behavior. *World J. Surg.* 20:168–72, 1996.

10. Rindi G, Azzoni C, La Rosa S, et al.: ECL cell tumor and poorly differentiated endocrine carcinoma of the stomach: prognostic evaluation by pathological analysis. *Gastroenterology* 116:532–42, 1999.

11. Wang HH, Wu MS, Shun CT, et al.: Lymphoepithelioma-like carcinoma of the stomach: A subset of gastric carcinoma with distinct clinicopathological features and high prevalence of Epstein-Barr virus infection. *Hepatogastroenterology* 46:1214–9, 1999.

12. Nakamura S, Ueki T, Yao T, et al.: Epstein-Barr virus in gastric carcinoma with lymphoid stroma. Special reference to its detection by the polymerase chain reaction and in situ hybridization in 99 tumors, including a morphologic analysis. *Cancer* 73:2239–49, 1994.

13. Uefuji K, Ichikura T, Tamakuma S.: Clinical and prognostic characteristics of papillary clear carcinoma of stomach. *Surg. Today* 26:158–63, 1996.

14. Ueyama T, Tsuneyoshi M.: Poorly differentiated solid type adenocarcinomas in the stomach: A clinicopathologic study of 71 cases. *J. Surg. Oncol.* 51:81–7, 1992.

15. Ohno S, Maehara Y, Ohiwa H, et al.: Peritoneal dissemination after a curative gastrectomy in patients with undifferentiated adenocarcinoma of the stomach. *Semin. Surg. Oncol.* 10:117–20, 1994.

16. Nakamura K, Ueyama T, Yao T, et al.: Pathology and prognosis of gastric carcinoma. Findings in 10,000 patients who underwent primary gastrectomy. *Cancer* 70:1030–7, 1992.

17. Songun I, van de Velde CJ, Arends JW, et al.: Classification of gastric carcinoma using the Goseki system provides prognostic information additional to TNM staging [see comments]. *Cancer* 85:2114–8, 1999.

18. Sobin LH, Wittekind Ch: TNM classification of malignant tumors, 5th ed. Union Internationale Contre le Cancer, New York, Wiley-Liss, 1997.

19. Hermanek P, Sobin LH (eds.): TNM classification of malignant tumors, 4th ed. Heidelberg-New York, Springer-Verlag, 1987.

20. Bollschweiler E, Boettcher K, Hoelscher AH, et al. Preoperative assessment of lymph node metastases in patients with gastric cancer: Evaluation of the Maruyama computer program. *Br. J. Surg.* 79:156–60, 1992.

21. Yamao T, Shirao K, Ono H, et al.: Risk factors for lymph node metastasis from intramucosal gastric carcinoma. *Cancer* 77:602–6, 1996.

22. Tachibana M, Takemoto Y, Monden N, et al.: Clinicopathological features of early gastric cancer: Results of 100 cases from a rural general hospital. *Eur. J. Surg.* 165:319–25, 1999.

23. Sigon R, Canzonieri V, Cannizzaro R, et al.: Early gastric cancer: Diagnosis, surgical treatment and follow-up of 45 cases. *Tumori* 84:547–51, 1998.

24. Baba H, Ohshiro T, Yamamoto M, et al.: Clinicopathological characteristics of stage 1 gastric cancer: Comparison of macroscopic and microscopic findings. *Hepatogastroenterology* 44:554–8, 1997.

25. Bunt AM, Hermans J, van de Velde CJ, et al.: Lymph node retrieval in a randomized trial on western-type versus Japanese-type surgery in gastric cancer. *J. Clin. Oncol.* 14:2289–94, 1996.

26. Bunt AM, Hogendoorn PC, van de Velde CJ, et al.: Lymph node staging standards in gastric cancer. *J. Clin. Oncol.* 13:2309–16, 1995.

27. Bunt AM, Hermans J, Smit VT, et al.: Surgical/pathologic-stage migration confounds comparisons of gastric cancer survival rates between Japan and Western countries [see Comments]. *J. Clin. Oncol.* 13:19–25, 1995.

28. Adachi Y, Oshiro T, Okuyama T, et al.: A simple classification of lymph node level in gastric carcinoma. *Am. J. Surg.* 169:382–5, 1995.

29. Maruyama K, Gunven P, Okabayashi K, et al.: Lymph node metastases of gastric cancer. General pattern in 1931 patients. *Ann. Surg.* 210:596–602, 1989.

30. Gunven P, Maruyama K, Okabayashi K, et al.: Non-ominous micrometastases of gastric cancer. *Br. J. Surg.* 78:352–4, 1991.

31. Bonenkamp JJ, Songun I, Hermans J, van de Velde CJ: Prognostic value of positive cytology findings from abdominal washings in patients with gastric cancer. *Br. J. Surg.* 83:672–4, 1996.

32. Klein Krunenbarg E, Hermans J, Krieken J H J M van et al.: Evaluation of the 5th edition of the TNM classification for gastric cancer: *improved prognostic value.* Brit J Cancer Cin press.

33. Mijic A, Ferencic Z, Belicza M, et al.: Apoptosis in human gastric polyps and adenocarcinomas: A stereological analysis. *Hepatogastroenterology* 45:684–90, 1998.

34. Muller W, Schneiders A, Hommel G, Gabbert HE: Prognostic value of bcl-2 expression in gastric cancer. *Anticancer Res.* 18:4699–704, 1998.

35. Nakamura M, Katano M, Fujimoto K, Morisaki T: A new prognostic strategy for gastric carcinoma: mRNA expression of tumor growth-related factors in endoscopic biopsy specimens. *Ann. Surg.* 226:35–42, 1997.

36. McCulloch P, Taggart T, Ochiai A, et al.: c-erbB2 and p53 expression are not associated with stage progression of gastric cancer in Britain or Japan. *Eur. J. Surg. Oncol.* 23:304–9, 1997.

37. Iriyama K, Miki C, Ilunga K, et al.: Prognostic significance of histological type in gastric carcinoma with invasion confined to the stomach wall. *Br. J. Surg.* 80:890–2, 1993.

38. Songun J, Lituinov S, Velde C J H van de et al. Loss of Ep-CAM predicts survival in patients with gastric cancer, especially in early stage disease. (Submitted)

39. Takebayashi Y, Miyadera K, Akiyama S, et al.: Expression of thymidine phosphorylase in human gastric carcinoma. *Jpn. J. Cancer Res.* 87:288–95, 1996.

40. Saito H, Tsujitani S, Oka S, et al.: The expression of thymidine phosphorylase correlates with angiogenesis and the efficacy of chemotherapy using fluorouracil derivatives in advanced gastric carcinoma. *Br. J. Cancer* 81:484–9, 1999.

41. Plebani M, Herszenyi L, Carraro P, et al.: Urokinase-type plasminogen activator receptor in gastric cancer: Tissue expression and prognostic role. *Clin. Exp. Metastasis* 15:418–25, 1997.

42. Plebani M, Herszenyi L, Cardin R, et al.: Cysteine and serine proteases in gastric cancer. *Cancer* 76:367–75, 1995.

43. Ganesh S, Sier CF, Heerding MM, et al.: Prognostic value of the plasminogen activation system in patients with gastric carcinoma. *Cancer* 77:1035–43, 1996.

44. Sier CF, Kubben FJ, Ganesh S, et al.: Tissue levels of matrix metalloproteinases MMP-2 and MMP-9 are related to the overall survival of patients with gastric carcinoma. *Br. J. Cancer* 74:413–7, 1996.

45. Katai H, Sasako M, Sano T, Maruyama K: Gastric carcinoma in young adults. *Jpn. J. Clin. Oncol.* 26:139–43, 1996.

46. Cascinu S, Giordani P, Catalano V, et al. Resection-line involvement in gastric cancer patients undergoing curative resections: Implications for clinical management [see Comments]. *Jpn. J. Clin. Oncol.* 29:291–3, 1999.

47. Songun I, Bonenkamp JJ, Hermans J, et al. Prognostic value of resection-line involvement in patients undergoing curative resections for gastric cancer. *Eur. J. Cancer* 32A:433–7, 1996.

48. Suzuki Y, Hiraishi H, Kanke K, et al.: Treatment of gastric tumors by endoscopic mucosal resection with a ligating device. *Gastrointest. Endosc.* 49:192–9, 1999.

49. Inoue H: Endoscopic mucosal resection for esophageal and gastric mucosal cancers. *Can. J. Gastroenterol.* 12:355–9, 1998.

50. Takekoshi T, Baba Y, Ota H, et al.: Endoscopic resection of early gastric carcinoma: Results of a retrospective analysis of 308 cases. *Endoscopy* 26:352–8, 1994.

51. Bonenkamp JJ, Songun I, Hermans J, et al.: Randomised comparison of morbidity after D1 and D2 dissection for gastric cancer in 996 Dutch patients [see Comments]. *Lancet* 345:745–8, 1995.

52. Bonenkamp JJ, Hermans J, Sasako M, van de Velde CJ: Extended lymph-node dissection for gastric cancer. Dutch Gastric Cancer Group [see Comments]. *N. Engl. J. Med.* 340:908–14, 1999.

53. Roder JD, Bötter K, Siewert JR, et al., and the German Gastric Carcinoma Study Group. Prognostic factors in gastric carcinoma. *Cancer* 72:2089–97, 1993.

54. Akahoshi K, Chijiiwa Y, Hamada S, Hara K, Nakamura K, Nawata H et al.: Complete response of early gastric cancer to uracil and tegafur. *J.Gastroenterol.* 33:864–7, 1998.

55. Songun I, Keizer HJ, Hermans J, et al.: Chemotherapy for operable gastric cancer: Results of the Dutch randomised FAMTX trial. The Dutch Gastric Cancer Group (DGCG). *Eur. J. Cancer* 35:558–62, 1999.

56. Hermans J, Bonenkamp JJ, Boon MC, et al.: Adjuvant therapy after curative resection for gastric cancer: Meta-analysis of randomized trials [see Comments]. *J. Clin. Oncol.* 11:1441–7, 1993.

57. Haugstvedt TK, Viste A, Eide GE, Söreide O, and other members of the Norwegian Stomach Cancer Trial. Norwegian multicentre study of survival and prognostic factors in patients undergoing curative resection for gastric carcinoma. *Br J Surg* 80:475–8, 1993.

58. Msika S, Chastang C, Houry S, et al.: Lymph node involvement as the only prognostic factor in curative resected gastric carcinoma: A multivariate analysis. *World J Surg* 13:118–23, 1989.

59. Okajima K. Prognostic factors of gastric cancer patients—A study of univariate and multivariate analysis. *Jpn J Gastroenterol Surg* 30:700–11, 1997. (in Japanese with English abstract).

60. Hermanek P, Maruyama K, Sobin, LH: Prognostic factors in stomach cancer, in: Hermanek P, Gospodarowicz MK, Henson DE, Hutter RVP, Sobin, LH. (eds.): *Prognostic factors in cancer.* Berlin, Springer-Verlag, 1985.

CHAPTER 18

Colorectal Cancer

TIMOTHY J. HOBDAY and CHARLES ERLICHMAN

Colorectal cancer is the second leading cause of site-specific cancer mortality in Western nations. Over 130,000 new cases and 56,500 deaths were expected in the United States in 1998. Approximately 70–80% of patients will present with apparently localized disease that is surgically resectable.[1,2] A proportion of these patients harbor occult micrometastases and will relapse after initial therapy. Randomized, Phase III clinical trials evaluating adjuvant chemotherapy (combined with radiotherapy in rectal cancer) for patients with local/regional lymph-node involvement have clearly shown some of these patients can be cured with adjuvant therapy.[3–6]

A recent pooled analysis[7] as well as the individual prospective randomized clinical trials of adjuvant chemotherapy in patients with Stage II disease (no involvement of local/regional lymph nodes) have not clearly shown a survival benefit in these patients. Yet a significant minority of these patients will relapse and eventually die of their disease. A review by the National Surgical Adjuvant Breast and Bowel Project (NSABP) of four consecutive adjuvant chemotherapy trials in Stages II and III colorectal cancer argues that adjuvant chemotherapy does improve survival for Stage II patients.[8] The use of molecular markers that have prognostic significance in addition to pathologic and clinical factors has the potential to identify high-risk patients who may benefit from therapy. This may allow treatment of those at highest risk while sparing those with minimal risk the toxicity and expense of adjuvant chemotherapy.

Prognostic factors can also serve a useful role in advanced disease. Some factors may be predictive of response to therapy, thereby aiding in the choice of palliative treatment. In a small subset of patients with metastatic colorectal cancer, patient-and tumor-related factors impact on the potential for curative resection of metastatic disease.

Prognostic Factors in Cancer, 2nd edition, Edited by Mary K. Gospodarowicz
ISBN 0-471-40633-3 Copyright © 2001 Wiley-Liss, Inc.

Anatomic Extent of Disease

The most powerful predictor of outcome in patients with newly diagnosed colorectal cancer continues to be the pathologic stage.[3,4,7,9–14] This consists of three independent prognostic pathologic variables: the depth of tumor invasion into the bowel wall with or without extension into adjacent structures, the pathologic status of local/regional lymph nodes, and the presence or absence of metastatic disease (see Appendix 18A) In addition, review of controlled clinical trials has established that an increased number of involved lymph nodes is an independent poor prognostic factor for recurrence and survival in node-positive patients.[3,13]

Several different staging systems are used throughout the world, often inter-changeably and incorrectly. The commonly used Dukes' classification,[15] which evolved over several publications,[16] does not take into account the independent prognostic significance of tumor invasion and lymph node involvement. The Modified Astler-Coller (MAC)[17] staging system improved on Dukes' staging by separating these important pathologic variables. Currently, UICC-AJCC TNM staging system[18,19] is advocated for use in clinical trials and practice (see Appendix 18A). It accounts separately for tumor invasion and lymph-node status, but in addition stratifies for the number of lymph nodes involved with tumor. The expected 5-year survival for each TNM stage is shown in Table 18.1.

Recent investigations have attempted to further refine traditional pathologic evaluation of regional lymph nodes using immunohistochemical or polymerase chain-reaction-based methods to detect micrometastases. A worse prognosis has been reported in patients judged to be Stage II by histopathologic exam-ination where micrometastases could be identified by these more sensitive techniques.[20,21] Whether these techniques will be of prognostic utility in clinical practice remains to be determined.

In the following discussion we address prognostic factors in patients who are resected for cure (residual tumor classification R0), in patients with unresectable or metastatic colorectal cancer (R1, R2) and in patients with resectable metastatic disease as three separate settings in which the prognostic factors and outcomes may differ. The College of American Pathologists (CAP) committee on prognostic factors have developed a recent consensus statement in colorectal cancer. This consensus statement proposes criteria for prognostic factors to be considered of sufficient validity to be used in patient care.[22] In the subsequent overview we have taken into account the criteria and prognostic factors identified by the CAP.

TABLE 18.1   Survival in Colorectal Cancer by TNM Stage (without adjuvant therapy)

TNM Stage	Approximate 5-Year Disease-free Survival (%)
I	85–90
II	70–75
III	35–40
IV	<5

PROGNOSTIC FACTORS IN COLORECTAL CANCER RESECTED FOR CURE (R0)

Tumor-related Prognostic Factors

Extent of Disease In addition to the TNM stage, several other readily available pathologic features of the primary tumor have been shown to have prognostic significance independent of the pathologic stage. The presence of a positive pathologic surgical margin (R1) is a poor prognostic factor, with local failure rate in all stages increasing from 3% to 85%.[23] The presence of a positive radial margin may also carry similar prognostic significance, especially in rectal cancer. This has not been adequately studied in colon cancers with peritonealized surfaces.[22]

Histologic Grade Tumor grade has been shown in multiple large studies to correlate with recurrence and survival, with low-grade tumors being more favorable.[3,4,7,9,11] However, its utility is limited by interobserver variability. The weight of the evidence suggests that blood vessel, lymphatic, and perhaps perineural invasion by the primary tumor have a negative impact on recurrence and survival.[1,11,12,24,25]

Some reports implicate an exophytic configuration of the primary tumor as a favorable prognostic factor, independent of T status.[24] A "pushing" rather than "infiltrating" tumor border also may impart a more favorable prognosis. Colorectal cancers are predominantly adenocarcinomas (90–95%). Small-cell and signet-ring carcinomas are associated with a worse prognosis; however, this may reflect their inherent high grade, rather than an independent effect on prognosis.[22]

The use of carcinoembryonic antigen (CEA) levels in patients has been widely adopted in clinical practice for monitoring the course of patients with colorectal cancer. Studies have shown that a normal CEA prior to resection of the tumor[3] and the postoperative normalization of an elevated CEA at diagnosis[11] are prognostic for improved survival independent of stage and grade.

Molecular Prognostic Factors Several new tumor-related factors have been and continue to be investigated to further improve prognostication. This has been especially targeted to those with Stage II disease. Few have been prospectively evaluated in a rigorous way, correcting for other clinicopathologic factors and controlling laboratory techniques. Ongoing clinical trials are attempting to gather meaningful information with regard to many of these newer proposed prognostic factors. A few of the most promising are briefly discussed below. A more complete list of possible molecular prognostic factors is provided in Table 18.2.

Some colorectal cancers demonstrate increased instability of short, tandemly repeated DNA sequences, called *microsatellites*. Microsatellite instability (MSI) is a result of germline mutations in DNA mismatch repair genes such as hMSH2 and hMLH1 in 90% of families with hereditary nonpolyposis colorectal cancer (HNPCC). MSI also occurs in 15% of sporadic cases of colorectal cancer, thought to be due to hypermethylation of the hMLH1 promoter. Two recent reports have suggested an improved prognosis in sporadic colorectal cancers with high-frequency (>40% of microsatellite loci) microsatellite instability.[26,27]

TABLE 18.2   Molecular Prognostic Factors

Factor	Potential Prognostic Significance
Aneuploidy	Negative
Deletion chromosome 18q	Negative
Elevated thymidylate synthase protein	Negative
p53 deletion	Negative
Microsatellite instability (MSI)	Positive
Ras/p21 mutation	Negative
erbB2/her-2 neu	Negative
p27 expression	Negative
Expression of thymidine phosphorylase (platelet-derived endothelial growth factor)	Negative
Expression of vascular endothelial derived growth factor (VEGF)	Negative
Elevated matrix metalloproteinases	Negative
Presence of CD44	Negative
Expression of E-cadherin	Negative?
Expression of transforming growth factor (TGF) family	Negative?

The stratification of primary colorectal cancers as DNA diploid versus aneuploid appears to predict for improved survival in Stage II and Stage III patients, independent of other known prognostic factors. This has been shown in a retrospective study of 800 patients[14] and also prospective studies.[28] In patients with Stage II disease, the 5-year survival is approximately 85% for diploid tumors versus 65–70% for DNA aneuploid. Not all series have supported this finding.[25] Incorporating indicators of proliferation such as percent S-phase and G2M may add to the predictive value of ploidy.[14]

The allelic loss of chromosome 18q has been seen in many solid tumors. Multiple putative tumor suppressor genes, including the deleted-in-colon-cancer (DCC) gene mapped to 18q21.2, have been described. Three studies have independently confirmed the unfavorable prognosis of patients with loss of 18q in Stages II and III colorectal cancer. Two of these used intensive DNA analysis of allelic loss,[29,30] while one used immunohistochemistry, which is more readily accessible.[31] The 5-year disease-free survival in Stage II patients was 85–94% for DCC-positive (no allelic loss) and 61–64% for DCC-negative (allelic loss) patients. Another study suggests that loss of heterozygosity at 18q (DCC negative) is associated with a poorer prognosis in DNA diploid, but not aneuploid tumors.[32]

The tumor suppressor gene p53 is located on chromosome 17p13.1. Mutation of p53 is seen in approximately 50% of colon cancers. There are conflicting conclusions regarding the significance of p53 alterations in colorectal cancer. Some series found p53 mutation to be a poor prognostic factor, while others reported it to be a favorable prognostic factor, and yet others showed no association with survival.[33]

Thymidylate synthase (TS) is an essential enzyme needed for DNA synthesis in S-phase of the cell cycle. It is the target enzyme for 5-FU and other TS inhibitors used in the treatment of colorectal cancer. A retrospective study of 294 patients from the NSABP R-01 trial demonstrated that high levels of TS in tumor cells is a poor prognostic factor independent of stage.[34] High-level expression of TS also appears to predict resistance to fluoropyrimidine-based therapy in both the adjuvant setting and metastatic disease.[34,35] However, a recent retrospective analysis of pooled data from five prospective randomized North Central Cancer Treatment Group (NCCTG) trials of adjuvant chemotherapy in Stages II and III colorectal cancer found no difference in overall or disease-free survival with respect to TS staining (R. M. Goldberg, personal communication).

Ongoing studies are looking into the prognostic significance of many other molecular abnormalities in colorectal cancer cells. Several oncogenes (Ras, c-myc, and others); tumor suppressor genes (p27); growth factors (TGFα and β); proteins involved in apoptosis, including bcl-2 and its family of pro- and anti-apoptotic proteins; angiogenesis proteins; as well as markers of metastasis and invasion continue to be investigated for their clinical utility. A recent review of these has been published,[33] and the potential prognostic significance of these molecular markers is listed in Table 18.2.

Patient-related Prognostic Factors

The presence of tumor obstruction and/or perforation has been shown in many, though not all, large series to convey a worse prognosis in these patients stage for stage. This has been demonstrated most clearly for obstruction.[3,9,12,14,36] Location of the primary tumor in the rectum (defined as below the peritoneal reflection or within 16 cm of the anal verge as measured by a rigid proctoscope) also portends a worse prognosis independent of stage.[14,36]

Patients with several genetic syndromes are at an increased risk of colorectal cancer. These include HNPCC, chronic ulcerative colitis (CUC), and familial adenomatous polyposis (FAP), among others. HNPCC carriers have a germline defect in DNA mismatch repair genes, primarily hMLH1 and hMSH2. This leads to high-frequency MSI in these patients. Patients with HNPCC and colorectal cancer are reported to have an improved survival when corrected for stage versus sporadic colorectal cancers.[37,38] This evidence of improved prognosis is supported by similar results of studies in sporadic colorectal cancer with high-frequency MSI, as previously mentioned. There is a suggestion that colorectal cancer arising in a patient with CUC has a poorer prognosis than sporadic cases; however, this is not well demonstrated, with conflicting reports in the literature.[37,39] There is no clear effect on outcome for patients with FAP.[37]

Several other patient- and tumor-related factors at presentation have been postulated to be of prognostic relevance. However, many do not appear to be significant in multivariate analyses controlling for other known prognostic factors, especially tumor stage. These include rectal bleeding, young age, gender, tumor size, and socioeconomic status. Although a large trial by the NSABP showed the location of the primary tumor in the right colon was a negative prognostic sign,[5,36] other series have not confirmed this.[9,40]

Treatment-related Factors

The expertise of the treating surgeon can affect prognosis.[41,42] Adequate resection of primary tumor (especially if there is any invasion into adjacent structures) and the extent of regional lymphadenectomy are important. The resection of six or fewer lymph nodes was found to be a poor prognostic sign in Stage II patients.[43] Gross tumor spillage intraoperatively adversely affects prognosis.[44]

Adjuvant chemotherapy for Stage III patients clearly improves recurrence and survival rates. The relative risk of death is reduced by 30–35%, corresponding to an absolute increase in 5-year survival of 20%, from approximately 40% to 60%.[3-6] The influence of chemotherapy is less clear on the outcome of Stage II patients.[7,8]

The use of radiotherapy, either pre- or postoperatively, in addition to systemic chemotherapy decreases the local recurrence rate and improves survival in rectal cancer.[4,45]

Several papers have suggested that perioperative blood transfusion is a poor prognostic factor in resected colorectal cancer. This has not clearly been shown to be due to the transfusions and any attendant immunosuppression rather than the clinical circumstances that make transfusion necessary.[4,46,47]

PROGNOSTIC FACTORS IN UNRESECTABLE RESIDUAL AND METASTATIC DISEASE (R1 AND R2)

The prognosis for patients with unresectable metastatic disease is poor, with a median survival of 11–12 months for patients enrolled on chemotherapy protocols involving 5-flourouracil.[48] The strongest prognostic factor in these patients is performance status at the time of diagnosis of metastatic disease.[48-52] Patients with microscopic residual disease (R1) have a longer median survival than those with macroscopic residual disease (R2) or distant metastases (18.7 months vs. 10.0 months).[53] The disease-free interval between diagnosis of the primary cancer and documentation of metastatic disease is also prognostic for survival in some series. A disease-free interval of less than one year is a poor prognostic sign.[49,53]

Other poor prognostic factors reported in select series include tumor burden of metastatic disease (increased number of metastases in an organ and increased number of metastatic sites involved), high tumor grade, elevated CEA level, and the presence of symptoms. Laboratory parameters of anemia, leukocytosis, and an elevated lactate dehydrogenase (LDH) have also been found by some to portend a poor prognosis.[49-51,54,55]

RESECTABLE METASTATIC DISEASE

A subset of patients present with metastatic disease confined to one organ. Curative-intent surgery can be performed with approximately a 30% chance of cure. Poor prognostic factors for cure from salvage surgery of oligometastases include disease-free interval (less than one year portended a poor outcome, >3 years was more favorable), synchronous presentation with the primary cancer, and more than one metastatic site.[54,56]

Molecular Prognostic Factors

There is less information regarding clinical use of molecular variables in metastatic disease as opposed to completely resected disease. Low thymidylate synthase levels have been shown recently to improve the probability of response to fluorouracil-based chemotherapy. Overall survival was prolonged in patients with low TS levels.[35,57] A recent report on patients with resected hepatic metastases suggests that decreased expression of the BAX protein (a key promoter of apoptosis) is associated with a worse prognosis.[58]

SUMMARY

Although many new prognostic factors have been studied in colorectal cancer, large prospective trials will be needed to define their utility and independence from pathologic staging. Tumor stage continues to be the most useful predictor for disease recurrence and survival (see Appendix 18B). Other tumor- or patient-related prognostic factors add little to the overall risk of relapse in newly diagnosed patients with resectable disease. The recommendation of adjuvant chemotherapy in resected colorectal cancer may be further guided in the future by the validation of newer prognostic markers, especially in Stage II disease. Prognosis in metastatic disease is mainly influenced by performance status of the patient in the absence of a resectable oligometastasis. Molecular markers may help tailor the type of therapy offered to these patients in the future.

▬▬▬ APPENDIX 18A

TNM Classification for Colorectal Cancer

T—Primary Tumor

TX   Primary tumor cannot be assessed

T0   No evidence of primary tumor

Tis   Carcinoma in situ: intraepithelial or invasion of lamina propria

T1   Tumor invades submucosa

T2   Tumor invades muscularis propria

T3   Tumor invades through muscularis propria into subserosa or into nonperitonealized pericolic or perirectal tissues

T4   Tumor directly invades other organs or structures and/or perforates visceral peritoneum

N — Regional Lymph Nodes

NX Regional lymph nodes cannot be assessed

N0 No regional lymph-node metastasis

N1 Metastasis in 1 to 3 regional lymph nodes

N2 Metastasis in 4 or more regional lymph nodes

M — Distant Metastasis

MX Distant metastasis cannot be assessed

M0 No distant metastasis

M1 Distant metastasis

Stage Grouping

TNM				Dukes
Stage 0	Tis	N0	M0	
Stage I	T1	N0	M0	A
	T2	N0	M0	
Stage II	T3	N0	M0	B
	T4	N0	M0	
Stage III	Any T	N1	M0	C
	Any T	N2	M0	
Stage IV	Any T	Any N	M1	

Source: Sobin LH, Wittekind Ch (eds.): *TNM classification of malignant tumors*, 5th ed. Union Internationale Contre le Cancer Wiley-Liss, New York, 1997.

███████ **APPENDIX 18B.1**

Prognostic Factors in Colorectal Cancer Resected for Cure (R0)

Prognostic Factor	Tumor Related	Host Related	Environment Related
Essential	TNM stage Negative surgical margin Blood/lymphatic invasion CEA >5	Obstruction Perforation	Surgeon Adjuvant chemotherapy Adjuvant radiotherapy
Additional	Tumor grade Tumor border configuration Histologic type Perineal invasion		
New and promising	Microsatellite instability Deletion of 18q (DCC gene) DNA ploidy Thymidylate synthase 　expression p53 mutations Microvessel density	HNPCC family	

███████ **APPENDIX 18B.2**

Prognostic Factors in Unresectable or Metastatic Colorectal Cancer (R1,R2)

Prognostic Factors	Tumor Related	Host Related	Environment Related
Essential	Resectable metastatic disease Tumor burden Disease-free interval	Performance status	Surgeon
Additional	Tumor grade CEA level		
New and Promising	Thymidylate synthase expression BAX expression		

REFERENCES

1. Wingo PA, Ries LA, Rosenberg HM, et al.: Cancer incidence and mortality, 1973–1995: A report card for the U.S. *Cancer* 82:1197–1207, 1998.
2. Peters M, Haller DG: Therapy for early stage colorectal cancer. *Oncology* 13:307–15, 1999.
3. Moertel CG, Fleming TR, MacDonald JS, et al.: Fluorouracil plus levamisole as effective adjuvant treatment after resection of stage III colon carcinoma: A final report. *Ann Intern Med* 122:321–6, 1995.
4. O'Connell MJ, Martenson JA, Wieand HS, et al.: Improving adjuvant therapy for rectal cancer by combining protracted-infusion fluorouracil with radiation therapy after curative surgery. *N Engl J Med* 331:502–7, 1994.
5. Wolmark N, Rockette H, Fisher B, et al.: The benefit of leucovorin-modulated fluorouracil as postoperative adjuvant therapy for primary colon cancer: Results from national surgical adjuvant breast and bowel project protocol C-03. *J Clin Oncol* 11:1879–87, 1993.
6. Haller DG, Catalano PJ, MacDonald JS, et al.: Fluorouracil, leucovorin, and levamisole adjuvant therapy for colon cancer: Five year final report of INT -0089 (Abstract). *Proc Am Soc Clin Oncol* 17:256a, 1998.
7. International multicentre pooled analysis of B2 colon cancer trials (IMPACT B2) investigators. Efficacy of adjuvant fluorouracil and folinic acid in B2 colon cancer. *J Clin Oncol* 17:1356–63, 1999.
8. Mamounas E, Wieand S, Wolmark N, et al.: Comparative efficacy of adjuvant chemotherapy in patients with Dukes' B versus Dukes' C colon cancer: Results from four national surgical adjuvant breast and bowel project adjuvant studies (C-01, C-02, C-03, C-04). *J Clin Oncol* 17:1349–55, 1999.
9. Griffen MR, Bergstrahl EJ, Coffey RJ, et al.: Predictors of survival after curative resection of carcinoma of the colon and rectum. *Cancer* 60:2318–24, 1987.
10. Wolters U, Stutzer H, Keller HW, et al.: Colorectal cancer — A multivariate analysis of prognostic factors. *Eur J Surg Oncol* 22:592–7, 1996.
11. Guerra A, Borda F, Jimenez FJ, et al.: Multivariate analysis of prognostic factors in resected colorectal cancer: A new prognostic index. *Eur J Gast Hepatol* 10:51–8, 1998.
12. Ratto C, Sofo L, Ippoliti M, et al.: Prognostic factors in colorectal cancer. *Dis Colon Rectum* 41:1033–49, 1998.
13. Gastrointestinal tumor study group. Adjuvant therapy of colon cancer — Results of a prospectively randomized trial. *N Engl J Med* 310:737–43, 1984.
14. Witzig TE, Loprinzi CL, Gonchoroff NJ, et al.: DNA ploidy and cell kinetic measurements as predictors of recurrence and survival in stages B2 and C colorectal adenocarcinoma. *Cancer* 68:879–88, 1991.
15. Dukes CE: The classification of cancer of the rectum. *J Pathol Bacteriol* 35:323–32, 1932.
16. Kirklin JW, Dockerty MD, Waugh JW: The role of the peritoneal reflection in the prognosis of carcinoma of the rectum and sigmoid colon. *Surg Gynec Obstet* 88:326, 1949.

17. Astler VB, Coller FA: The prognostic significance of direct extension of carcinoma of the colon and rectum. *Ann Surg* 139:846–52, 1954.

18. American Joint Committee on Cancer. *Cancer Staging Manual*, 5th ed. Philadelphia, Lippincott, 1997.

19. Sobin LH, Wittekind Ch: (Eds.): *International Union Against Cancer. TNM classification of malignant tumors*, 5th ed. New York, Wiley-Liss, 1997.

20. Liefers GJ, Cleton-Jansen AM, van de Velde CJ, et al.: Micrometastases and survival in stage II colorectal cancer. *N Engl J Med* 339:223–8, 1998.

21. Greenson JK, Isenhart CE, Rice R, et al.: Identification of occult micrometastases in pericolic lymph nodes of Dukes' B colorectal cancer using monoclonal antibodies against cytokeratin and CC49. *Cancer* 73:563–9, 1994.

22. Compton CC, Fielding LP, Burgart LJ, et al.: Prognostic factors in colorectal cancer: College of American Pathologists Consensus Statement 1999. *Arch Path Lab Med*, 1999.

23. Quirke P, Durdy P, Dixon MF, et al.: Local recurrence of rectal adenocarcinoma due to inadequate surgical resection. Histopathological study of lateral tumor spread and surgical excision. *Lancet* 1:996–9, 1986.

24. Steinberg SM, Barwick KW, Stablein DM: Importance of tumor pathology and morphology in patients with surgically resected colon cancer. *Cancer* 58:1340–5, 1986.

25. Zarbo RJ, Nakhleh RE, Brown RD: Prognostic significance of DNA ploidy and proliferation in 309 colorectal carcinomas as determined by two-color multiparametric DNA flow cytometry. *Cancer* 79:2073–86, 1997.

26. Halling KC, French AJ, McDonnell SK, et al.: Microsatellite instability and 8p allelic imbalance in stage B2 and C colorectal cancers. *J Natl Cancer Inst* 91:1295–1303, 1999.

27. Gryfe R, Kim H, Hsieh ETK, et al.: Tumor microsatellite instability and clinical outcome in young patients with colorectal cancer. *N Engl J Med* 342:69–70, 2000.

28. Chapman MA, Hardcastle JD, Armitage NC: Five-year prospective study of DNA ploidy and colorectal cancer survival. *Cancer* 76:383–7, 1995.

29. Ogunbiyi OA, Goodfellow PJ, Herfarth K, et al.: Confirmation that 18q allelic loss in colon cancer is a prognostic indicator. *J Clin Oncol* 16:427–33, 1998.

30. Jen J, Kim H, Piantadosi S, et al.: Allelic loss of chromosome 18q and prognosis in colorectal cancer. *N Engl J Med* 331:213–21, 1994.

31. Shibata D, Reale MA, Lavin P, et al.: The DCC protein and prognosis in colorectal cancer. *N Engl J Med* 335:1727–32, 1996.

32. Sun XF, Rutten S, Zhang H, et al.: Expression of the deleted in colorectal cancer gene is related to prognosis in DNA diploid and low proliferative colorectal adenocarcinoma. *J Clin Oncol* 17:1745–50, 1999.

33. McLeod HL, Murray GI: Tumor markers of prognosis in colorectal cancer. *Br J Cancer* 79(2):191–203, 1999.

34. Johnston PG, Fisher ER, Rockette HE, et al.: The role of thymidylate synthase expression in prognosis and outcome of adjuvant therapy in patients with rectal cancer. *J Clin Oncol* 12:2640–7, 1994.

35. Aschele C, Debernardis D, Casazza S, et al.: Immunohistochemical quantitation of thymidylate synthase expression in colorectal cancer metastases predicts for clinical outcome to Fluorouracil-based chemotherapy. *J Clin Oncol* 17: 1760–70, 1999.

36. Wolmark N, Wiend HS, Rockette HE, et al.: Prognostic significance of tumor location and bowel obstruction in Dukes B and C colorectal cancer. *Ann Surg* 198:743–52, 1983.

37. Aarnio M, Mustonen H, Mecklin JP, et al.: Prognosis of colorectal cancer varies in different high-risk conditions. *Ann Med* 30:75–80, 1998.

38. Sankila R, Aaltonen L, Jarvinen HJ, et al.: Better survival rates in patients with MLH1-associated hereditary colorectal cancer. Gastroenterology 110:682–7, 1996.

39. Heimann TM, Oh SC, Martinelli G, et al.: Colorectal carcinoma associated with ulcerative colitis: A study of prognostic indicators. *Am J Surg* 164:13–7, 1992.

40. Steinberg SM, Barkin JS, Kaplan RS, et al.: Prognostic indicators of colon tumors: The gastrointestinal study group experience. *Cancer* 57:1866–70, 1986.

41. McArdle CS, Hole D: Impact of variability among surgeons on postoperative morbidity and mortality and ultimate survival. *Br Med J* 302:1501–3, 1991.

42. Hermanek P, Mansmann U, Staimmer D, et al.: The German experience. The surgeon as a prognostic factor in colon and rectal cancer surgery. *Surg Oncol Clin North Am* 9:33–49, 2000.

43. Caplin S, Cerottini JP, Bosman FT: For patients with Dukes' B (TNM stage II) colorectal carcinoma, examination of 6 or fewer lymph nodes is related to poor prognosis. *Cancer* 83(4):666–72, 1998.

44. Zirngibl H, Husemann B, Hermanek P: Intra-operative spillage of tumor cells for rectal cancer. *Dis Colon Rectum* 33:610–14, 1990.

45. Minsky BD: Adjuvant therapy for rectal cancer: Results and controversies. *Oncology* 12:1129–39, 1998.

46. Heiss MM, Mempel W, Delanoff C, et al.: Blood transfusion-modulated tumor recurrence: First results of a randomized study of autologous versus allogeneic blood transfusion in colorectal cancer surgery. *J Clin Oncol* 12:1859–67, 1994.

47. Busch OR, Hop WC, Hoynck van Papendrecht MA, et al. Blood transfusions and prognosis in colorectal cancer. *N Engl J Med* 328:1372–6, 1993.

48. Advanced Colorectal Cancer Meta-Analysis Project. Modulation of fluorouracil by leucovorin in patients with advanced colorectal cancer: Evidence in terms of response rate. *J Clin Oncol* 10:896–903, 1992.

49. Graf W, Glimelius B, Pahlman L, et al.: Determinants of prognosis in advanced colorectal cancer. *Eur J Cancer* 27:1119–23, 1991.

50. Webb A, Scott-Mackie P, Cunningham D, et al.: The prognostic value of CEA, β HCG, AFP, CA125, CA19-9, and C-erb B-2 immunohistochemistry in advanced colorectal cancer. *Ann Oncol* 6:581–7, 1995.

51. Poon MA, O'Connell MJ, Moertel CG, et al.: Biochemical modulation of fluorouracil: Evidence of significant improvement of survival and quality of life in patients with advanced colorectal carcinoma. *J Clin Oncol* 7:1407–18, 1989.

52. Nordic Gastrointestinal Tumor Adjuvant Therapy Group. Superiority of sequential methotrexate, fluorouracil and leucovorin to fluorouracil alone in advanced symptomatic colorectal carcinoma: A randomized trial. *J Clin Oncol* 7:1437–46, 1989.

53. Hermanek P, Wittekind C: Residual tumor (R) classification and prognosis. *Semin Surg Oncol* 10:12–20, 1994.

54. Goldberg RM, Fleming TR, Tangen CM, et al.: Surgery for recurrent colon cancer: Strategies for identifying resectable recurrence and success rates after resection. *Ann Intern Med* 129:27–35, 1998.

55. Yamamura T, Tsukikawa S, Akaishi O, et al.: Multivariate analysis of the prognostic factors of patients with unresectable synchronous liver metastases from colorectal cancer. *Dis Colon Rectum* 40:1425–9, 1997.

56. Fong Y, Blumgart LH: Hepatic colorectal metastasis: Current status of surgical therapy. *Oncology* 12:1489–98, 1998.

57. Leichman CG, Lenz HJ, Leichman L, et al.: Quantitation of intratumoral thymidylate synthase expression predicts for disseminated colorectal cancer response and resistance to protracted-infusion fluorouracil and weekly leucovorin. *J Clin Oncol* 15:3223–9, 1997.

58. Sturm I, Kohne C-H, Wolff G, et al.: Analysis of the p53/BAX pathway in colorectal cancer: Low BAX is a negative prognostic factor in patients with resected liver metastases. *J Clin Oncol* 17:1364–74, 1999.

CHAPTER 19

Anal Cancer

BERNARD J. CUMMINGS

The major objectives of treatment of cancers that arise in the anal canal and perianal skin are cure and preservation of anal function. The prognosis for both survival and function deteriorates as the primary tumor enlarges, and the probability of cure diminishes as cancer metastasizes to the regional lymph nodes and to extrapelvic sites. Although the incidence of anal cancer has been increasing in many countries over the past 30 years,[1] the relative rarity of such cancers (incidence about 0.5 to 1 per 100,000) has meant that there have been few large groups of patients in whom prognostic factors have been assessed by multivariate analysis or similar statistical techniques.

In the 1987[2] and 1997[3] editions of the TNM classification, the anal canal is defined as that part of the intestine that extends from the rectum to the perianal skin (to the junction with the hair-bearing skin). The extent of the perianal area is not defined in the manual, but, by common usage, is considered the skin within a 5-cm radius of the anal verge. Prior to the 1987 classification, several different conventions were used to describe the anatomy of the anal region, so that comparisons of different series are often not possible.

A significant change in the categorization system for primary anal canal cancers was also made in 1987, by basing classification on the measured size of the tumor. The T-category is determined by the largest diameter of the primary carcinoma, measured in centimeters (T1–T3-categories), except when there is direct invasion of adjacent major organs (T4-category)[3] (Appendix 19A.1). Formerly, it was necessary to estimate clinically the proportion of the length or circumference of the canal involved, and whether the external sphincter was infiltrated.[4] Perianal cancers continued to be categorized by measured size as previously (Appendix 19A.2).

The histological classification of malignancies of the anal canal and of the perianal skin has not changed substantially over the past 30 years. The

Prognostic Factors in Cancer, 2nd edition, Edited by Mary K. Gospodarowicz
ISBN 0-471-40633-3   Copyright © 2001 Wiley-Liss, Inc.

1989 edition of the World Health Organization (WHO) Classification System[5] described three major subtypes of squamous-cell cancer of the anal canal, namely large-cell keratinizing, large-cell nonkeratinizing (transitional), and basaloid. The view that all are variants of squamous-cell cancer was supported by an analysis of keratin profiles.[6,7] Many clinical investigators, agreeing that the prognostic value of histological subtyping is marginal, group all three subtypes as squamous-cell or epidermoid carcinomas of the anal canal.

The shift in treatment of anal canal cancer from radical surgery to primary radiation therapy, commonly combined with cytotoxic chemotherapy, allows preservation of function in many patients, and has affected assessment of prognostic features. Detailed gross and histopathological assessment of excised tissues, which formed the cornerstone of many earlier analyses, is no longer possible. It has not yet been established that all features of prognostic value in patients treated surgically are equally predictive of outcome following radiation with/without chemotherapy.

In the discussion that follows, cancers of the anal canal and of the perianal skin are considered separately. All comments address the patient newly diagnosed and undergoing initial treatment, except where indicated.

ANAL CANAL CANCER

About 80% of the cancers of the anal region arise in the canal. Most are variants of squamous-cell cancer.

Tumor-related Factors

Anatomic Extent The size of the primary tumor and the depth to which the tumor penetrates into and through the anal wall are strongly prognostic for both survival and local tumor control.[8,9] There is no agreement on the most useful breakpoints for division by size, particularly about the 4-cm to 5-cm range. In series in which detailed examination of excised tissues is not possible, the T-category is a surrogate for the combination of tumor size, depth of invasion, and likelihood of metastases to the pelvic lymph nodes included in many older classification systems. The risk of nodal metastases correlates reasonably well with the size of the primary tumor.[8] Imaging studies do not provide the anatomical detail available by histopathological techniques, and are more sensitive with respect to depth of penetration of cancer through the anal wall than to pelvic-node metastases.[10,11]

Overall uncorrected 5-year *survival* rates range from 35% to 80%, with an average about 55%.[12] Five-year survival rates, corrected for deaths from intercurrent disease, are typically about 65 to 70% overall, about 95 to 100% when the primary tumor is less than 2 cm in size (category-T1), and in the range of 60 to 70% for larger tumors (categories-T2 and -T3). The rate falls to about 33% or less for cancers that invade adjacent organs (category-T4). These rates include the effects of surgical salvage for local relapse after treatment with radiation-based protocols.[13,14] Some investigators consider that the depth of invasion is of greater prognostic significance than regional lymph-node metastases,[15] but this runs counter to the experience of most.[8,16] There is considerable disagreement, particularly in reports of patients treated by radiation with/without chemotherapy, as to whether invasion of adjacent organs such as the vagina or prostate (category-T4), truly has greater negative prognostic import for survival than the size of the tumor, in view of the case selection that often influences choice of treatment in patients with very advanced cancers.[13,17-20]

The negative prognostic influence on survival of regional lymph-node metastases established from series managed by radical surgery is not as clear since the emphasis changed to radiation-based protocols. This may be due to the inability of imaging modalities to identify pelvic-node metastases with the accuracy of histopathology. In surgical series, metastases in the perirectal-, superior hemorrhoidal-, pelvic- or inguinal-node groups were associated with 5-year cancer-specific survival rates of about 50%, some 20% worse than those of patients who did not have nodal metastases.[21-24] The prognosis was somewhat better when inguinal node metastases were diagnosed several months after surgical treatment of the primary cancer, provided they were the only site of recurrence.[21,22] In series treated by radiation with or without chemotherapy, only inguinal-node metastases can be diagnosed with confidence. While some investigators who use radiation-based treatment did not find a statistically significant adverse prognosis for those with inguinal-node metastases at first presentation,[25] the trend in survival rates for those patients was generally worse, and often significantly so.[13,19,26,27] The widespread practice of including clinically normal inguinal nodes electively in the volume irradiated has greatly reduced the risk of late failure in those nodes, but the effect of such elective irradiation on survival rates has not been determined.[12]

Extrapelvic metastases, to either lymph nodes or parenchymal organs such as the liver or lung, are associated with a very poor prognosis, whether these metastases are found in the course of initial evaluation or later. Survival from the time of diagnosis of metastases is in the range of 6 to 12 months.[14,22] Solitary metastases are uncommon, but have occasionally been amenable to potentially curative treatment.[28,29]

Survival rates for composite TNM stage groups have been reported infrequently,[30,31] it being much more common to classify patients by the separate tumor characteristics outlined earlier.

The probability of *local tumor control* is also related to the size of the primary tumor. While local control is not necessarily synonymous with preservation of anal function, the latter outcome of treatment has not been addressed consistently until recently and specific information on function is limited.[32-34] Three-year local control rates of 89% for tumors up to 4 cm in size and 73% for larger tumors were reported for one large series treated by radiation alone.[18] In patients treated by radiation with 5-fluorouracil and mitomycin C, local control rates for primary tumors up to 2 cm in size were in the range 95 to 100%, for 2 to 5 cm

80 to 95%, and for larger than 5 cm 65 to 80%.[13,14] The likelihood of local control and retention of effective anal function is reduced when more than about three-quarters of the anal circumference is involved by cancer, although some patients who present with extensive cancers do retain useful function following treatment.[17–19,35,36] The presence of inguinal or pelvic lymph-node metastases does not reduce the probability of control of the primary tumor in patients managed with radiation with/without chemotherapy,[13,18,37] although occasional reports dispute this.[26]

Histological Subtype　The histological subtype of squamous-cell carcinoma has generally not been found to carry independent prognostic significance for survival or local tumor control. Although the histological classification often appeared related to survival in univariate analysis, multivariate models for the most part showed that, when corrected for stage, this significance was lost. This was true whether stage was determined by the size of the primary tumor only in patients treated by radiation[13,27,38] or by surgicopathological systems that assessed tumor depth and the presence of node metastases.[8,23,38] A few rare variants, such as small-cell carcinomas and microcystic squamous-cell carcinomas, have a very poor prognosis and are characterized by early dissemination.[8,23]

Histological Grade　When independent significance for histopathological grade has been found, poorly differentiated tumors had a worse prognosis than moderately or well-differentiated cancers.[8,22,30] In a series of 235 patients managed by surgery, the 5-year survival rate was 95% for those with well-differentiated tumors, compared to 60% for those with moderately or poorly differentiated cancers.[23] Some found that histological grade lost prognostic significance when adjustment was made for stage.[8]

Histological features that did not appear to correlate with prognosis include cell size, level of keratinization, pleomorphism, invasive margin, lymphocytic infiltrate[23] and the presence of HPV RNA, and mitotic rate.[6]

Associated Intraepithelial Neoplasia　The finding of dysplasia or anal intraepithelial neoplasia (AIN) in the canal or perianal skin in addition to invasive cancer is of unknown prognostic significance. While progression from low-grade to high-grade AIN has been observed frequently,[39] the risk of progression to invasive cancer is not known.[40] Since AIN is often multicentric and frequently exhibits foci of microinvasion,[41] the presence of AIN may account for the relatively high frequency of recurrence after apparently complete local excision of small carcinomas. It has been suggested that the demonstration by immunohistochemical techniques of the accumulation of mutant p53 protein,[42] and/or overexpression of c-myc,[43] may serve as a marker of likely progression from high-grade AIN to invasive carcinoma.

Cell and Molecular Factors　In one study of flow cytometric DNA analysis of paraffin-embedded tissue from anal carcinomas managed surgically, ploidy was found by multivariate analysis to be strongly predictive of outcome, patients with diploid tumors having a 5-year survival rate of 75% compared to 55% for nondiploid tumors.[23] However, in another retrospective study of patients managed by radiation and/or surgery, in which DNA was assessed by image cytophotometry, no correlation was identified between ploidy and prognosis.[44] The prognostic significance of the recurrent chromosomal aberrations found in a small series of anal carcinomas is not known.[45]

Overexpression of p53 may be prognostic for poorer disease-free survival,[46,47] although another investigator found similar prognosis in a small number of HPV + p53+ and HPV − p53− patients.[48] Assays of vascular endothelial growth factor and vessel density, measured by Factor VIII, were not prognostic for survival.[49] Proliferation parameters, such as mitotic rate[23] and potential tumor doubling time and labeling index,[49,50] have so far not been found predictive of survival or local control.

Tumor Markers   There are no markers of established value. In one multivariate analysis, elevated serum squamous-cell carcinoma antigen (SCC Ag) was the most significant determinator of risk for survival as well as for local control, superseding even tumor size as a prognostic factor.[51] A more recent study in patients managed by radiation and chemotherapy did not confirm this observation.[52] Serum carcinoembryonic antigen (CEA) levels did not correlate with prognosis in patients treated with radiation and cytotoxic drugs.[53]

Symptoms   The duration of symptoms prior to treatment is not generally thought to be significant, although in one series it was found that those treated within a month of the onset of symptoms had a higher survival rate.[24] Small cancers found incidentally at surgery for benign anal conditions also have a good prognosis.[54]

Host Factors

The unexplained female preponderance in the incidence of anal canal cancer is not generally considered a prognostic factor, although some multivariate analyses do suggest that women have a better prognosis than men.[26,31,38] The converse has not been reported.

Age at diagnosis has been found to be of prognostic significance for survival and retention of function in some,[35] but not all, studies.[8,32,38] Since most analyses are of patients treated radically, those unfit for aggressive treatment by virtue of advanced age or poor performance status are often excluded.

Previous or coincidental benign conditions affecting the anal canal or perianal skin do not appear to have any prognostic significance.[22,55,56]

Although epidemiological studies indicate that a history of venereal disease, anoreceptive intercourse in males, cigarette smoking,[57,58] previous malignancies of the vulva, vagina, cervix or lymphoma or leukemia,[59] and immunosuppression for organ transplant[60] are each associated with a higher risk of development of anal carcinoma, these factors are not known to influence prognosis of the anal cancer directly. An association has been demonstrated between anal squamous-cell carcinomas and human papilloma virus (HPV) types 16 and 18, and herpes simplex virus (HSV).[61,62] In analyses of serum, the immunoglobulin A (IgA) response to peptide E2 : 9 (derived from HPV type-16 E2 region) had a marginally significant association with poorer survival independent of tumor size.[63] No correlation was found with antibody responses to several other antigens derived from papilloma virus.[63]

Although anal cancer is not an AIDS-defining malignancy, an increased incidence of anal cancer has been reported up to 5 years before AIDS diagnosis, and in homosexual men and, to a lesser extent, in nonhomosexual men, at and after AIDS diagnosis.[64] The prognosis in such patients is unpredictable, reflecting factors relating to both anal carcinoma and HIV infection. Patients with AIDS sometimes exhibit exaggerated acute toxicity from radiation and/or chemotherapy. It has been suggested that tumor control and acute treatment-related morbidity levels in patients with HIV infection who have CD4 counts ≥ 200 are similar to those of the general population, whereas those with lower CD4 counts are more likely to require modifications of treatment and surgery after radiation and chemotherapy to achieve local control.[65]

Treatment-related Factors

There have been no major differences apparent in the survival rates in patients managed by surgery or by radiation with or without chemotherapy. The 5-year rates range from about 35% to 80%, with an average of about 55%.[12,31] The likelihood of retaining anorectal function is much greater after radiation-based treatment, and is about 90% in those in whom the cancer is eradicated by radiation with or without chemotherapy.[12]

Randomized trials have demonstrated superior cancer-specific survival, though not overall survival, and superior local control in patients managed by radiation with concurrent 5-fluorouracil and mitomycin C compared to the same dose and schedule of radiation alone.[26,66] A further randomized trial demonstrated the superiority of the combination with radiation of both 5-fluorouracil and mitomycin C rather than 5-fluorouracil alone, in local control and cancer-specific survival rates,[67] again without significant improvement in overall survival. Some investigators have introduced cisplatin rather than mitomycin C in combined modality schedules. Although effective, this combination has not yet been demonstrated to lead to better outcomes than 5-fluorouracil and mitomycin C.[52,68]

The intensity of treatment may affect outcome. Some multivariate analyses have indicated that prognosis for local control and disease-free survival was better following higher doses of radiation,[27,38,69] but the risk of late complications was also increased by higher doses.[70,71] Opinion remains divided on whether the longer overall time in which radiation was delivered by interrupted or split-course schedules is prognostic for poorer rates of local control or survival.[27,68,72,73] The average dose intensity of the chemotherapy delivered was prognostic for disease-free survival in one series.[25]

Recent publications have suggested that failure to achieve at least partial reduction (<50% product of diameters) by 6 to 8 weeks after the initial course of radiation and chemotherapy, and prior to planned boost radiation, increased the risk of local failure.[52,71] The presence of residual carcinoma in the canal at the completion of radical radiation or radiation with chemotherapy was not predictive of eventual local control, as regression continued over many months.[13,27] Carcinoma residual or recurrent after radiation and concurrent chemotherapy was associated with poor pelvic control and survival after attempted salvage surgery in some,[74] but not all, series.[13,75,76] Just as for primary treatment by radical surgery, the likelihood of local control and survival following salvage abdominoperineal resection was affected adversely by the size of the anal cancer, extension through the anal wall into adjacent connective tissues, and tumor fixation to the pelvic wall at the time of surgery.[76] Some features of the cancer at initial presentation, such as inguinal adenopathy[75,76] and advanced T category,[75] were also found to predict poorer outcome at subsequent salvage surgery.

The extent of clinical response to chemotherapy and/or radiation in recurrent and metastatic carcinoma correlated with the duration of subsequent survival.[28]

Summary (Appendix 19B)

The most deleterious prognostic factor for survival is the presence of extrapelvic metastases. When cancer is confined to the pelvis, the size of the primary tumor is the most useful indicator for survival and for local control and preservation of anal function. After tumor size and T-category, the status of the regional lymph nodes correlates fairly well with survival, but not with control of the primary cancer. Other tumor-related features, such as DNA ploidy and expression of p53 protein, are of potential value, but their independent prognostic value has not yet been established. Most patient-related factors are of little prognostic value provided the patient is able to tolerate radical treatment of a cancer confined to the pelvis. Survival rates after radical surgery or radiation plus concurrent 5-fluorouracil and mitomycin C are similar, but the probability of retaining anal function is much greater with radiation-based treatment.

PERIANAL CANCER

About 20% of cancers in the anal region arise in the perianal skin, within a 5-cm radius of the anal verge. Most are squamous-cell cancers. The prognosis of perianal cancers is generally better than that of anal canal cancers.

Tumor-related Factors

Anatomic Extent   The size of the primary tumor is the factor most strongly predictive of local control and survival,[77,78] although, perhaps because of the excellent local control rates achieved, others have found the presence of inguinal-node metastases a stronger predictor of specific survival.[79] Visceral metastases are uncommon but carry a poor prognosis. They are usually found only in patients who have had node metastases. Overall, 5-year specific survival rates range from 70% to 80%, and local tumor control rates from 75% to 85%. In series managed by surgery, the extent of involvement of the anal canal determines whether anal function can be preserved, but this is not a factor when radiation with or without chemotherapy is used (provided continence has not already been lost irrevocably).

Histological Subtypes and Grade   Squamous-cell carcinomas of the perianal skin are usually well differentiated. Basal-cell carcinomas are uncommon, but are similar to basal-cell cancers of the skin elsewhere. Squamous-cell carcinomas, especially poorly differentiated cancers, are more likely to metastasize to the inguinal nodes, and do so in about 10% of cases, whereas metastases from basal-cell cancers are rare.

Associated Intraepithelial Neoplasia   As with anal canal cancer, the occurrence of intraepithelial neoplasia in association with perianal cancer is common but of unknown prognostic significance. The risks of multicentricity and the potential for invasive changes are those described previously for anal canal cancer.

Host Factors

The incidence of perianal cancer is about equal in men and women. Outcome depends on the extent of the cancer rather than gender. Preexisting benign conditions, including anal warts, do not appear to carry prognostic import.[77] Squamous-cell cancers of the perianal skin are increased in incidence in patients with AIDS, particularly homosexual men.[64] Prognosis is generally determined by the course of AIDS.

Treatment-related Factors

Either surgery or radiation therapy is capable of producing high local control and survival rates. Local excision is favored when an adequate margin can be achieved without compromising anal function, since this approach avoids the risk of late radiation-induced skin damage. The high local recurrence rates reported in some series[77] are likely related to failure to achieve adequate margins and/or to multicentric intraepithelial neoplasia. Many patients in whom local recurrence does occur can be salvaged by further local excision.[77] There is no convincing evidence that the combination of chemotherapy with radiation is necessary, excellent local control and survival rates being reported after radical radiation alone.[78–80] However, the United Kingdom randomized trial included patients with either anal canal or perianal cancers. Although results for these anatomical sites were not reported separately, radiation combined with 5-fluorouracil and mitomycin C gave results superior to radiation alone for both cancer-specific survival and local control.[66]

Summary

Most perianal cancers are squamous cell type. Prognosis for survival and retention of anal function depends principally on the tumor size and its location relative to the anal canal. Inguinal-node metastases are uncommon, but their presence increases the risk of death from cancer.

■■■■■■ **APPENDIX 19A.1**

Anal Canal TNM Classification

T — Primary Tumor

TX Primary tumor cannot be assessed

T0 No evidence of primary tumor

Tis Carcinoma in situ

T1 Tumor 2 cm or less in greatest dimension

T2 Tumor more than 2 cm but not more than 5 cm in greatest dimension

T3 Tumor more than 5 cm in greatest dimension

T4 Tumor of any size invades adjacent organ(s), e.g., vagina, urethra, bladder (involvement of sphincter muscle(s) *alone* is not classified as T4)

N — Regional Lymph Nodes

NX Regional lymph nodes cannot be assessed

N0 No regional lymph-node metastasis

N1 Metastasis in perirectal lymph node(s)

N2 Metastasis in unilateral internal iliac and/or inguinal lymph node(s)

N3 Metastasis in perirectal and inguinal lymph nodes and/or bilateral internal iliac and/or inguinal lymph nodes

M — Distant Metastasis

MX Distant metastasis cannot be assessed

M0 No distant metastasis

M1 Distant metastasis

Stage Grouping

Stage 0	Tis	N0	M0
Stage I	T1	N0	M0
Stage II	T2	N0	M0
	T3	N0	M0
Stage IIIA	T1	N1	M0
	T2	N1	M0
	T3	N1	M0
	T4	N0	M0
Stage IIIB	T4	N1	M0
	Any T	N2, N3	M0
Stage IV	Any T	Any N	M1

Source: Sobin LH, Wittekind Ch (eds.): *TNM classification of malignant tumors*, 5th ed. Internationale Contre le Cancer Wiley-Liss, New York, 1997.

■■■■■■■ **APPENDIX 19A.2**

Perianal Skin TNM Classification

T—Primary Tumor

TX Primary tumor cannot be assessed

T0 No evidence of primary tumor

Tis Carcinoma in situ

T1 Tumor 2 cm or less in greatest dimension

T2 Tumor more than 2 cm but not more than 5 cm in greatest dimension

T3 Tumor more than 5 cm in greatest dimension

T4 Tumor invades deep extradermal structures, i.e., cartilage, skeletal muscle, or bone

N—Regional Lymph Nodes (ipsilateral inguinal nodes)

NX Regional lymph nodes cannot be assessed

N0 No regional lymph-node metastasis

N1 Regional lymph-node metastasis

M—Distant Metastasis

MX Distant metastasis cannot be assessed

M0 No distant metastasis

M1 Distant metastasis

Stage Grouping

Stage 0	Tis		N0		M0	
Stage I	T1		N0		M0	
Stage II		T2		N0		M0
		T3		N0		M0
Stage III		T4		N0		M0
		Any T		N1		M0
Stage IV		Any T		Any N		M1

Source: Sobin LH, Wittekind Ch (eds.): *TNM classification of malignant tumors*, 5th ed. Internationale Contre le Cancer Wiley-Liss, New York, 1997.

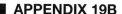 **APPENDIX 19B**

Prognostic Factors in Anal Canal Cancer

Prognostic Factors	Tumor Related	Host Related	Environment Related
Essential	Anatomic extent Histological type (squamous/other)	Performance status AIDS	Radiation and concurrent 5-fluorouracil and mito- mycin radiation dose.
Additional	Depth of invasion Histological grade		Cisplatin may be alternative to mitomycin in combined protocols Radiation time
New and promising	Ploidy Overexpression of p53		Intensity of chemotherapy Rapidity of response to radi- ation and chemotherapy

REFERENCES

1. Melbye M, Rabkin C, Frisch M, Biggar RJ: Changing patterns of anal cancer incidence in the United States, 1940–1989. *Am J Epidemiol* 139:772–80, 1994.

2. Hermanek P, Sobin H (eds.): *UICC TNM classification of malignant tumors*, 4th ed. Berlin, Springers Verlag, 1987.

3. Sobin LH, Wittekind Ch (eds.): *TNM classification of malignant tumors*, 5th ed. New York, Wiley, 1997.

4. Harmer MH (ed.): *UICC TNM classification of malignant tumors*, 3d ed. Geneva, International Union Against Cancer, 1978.

5. Jass JR, Sobin LH: *Histological typing of intestinal tumors*, 2d ed. Berlin, Springer-Verlag, 1989, pp. 41–44.

6. Williams GR, Talbot IC: Anal carcinoma—A histological review. *Histopathology* 25:507–16, 1994.

7. Williams GR, Talbot IC, Leigh IM: Keratin expression in anal carcinoma: An immunohistochemical study. *Histopathology* 30:443–50, 1997.

8. Boman BM, Moertel CG, O'Connell MJ, et al.: Carcinoma of the anal canal. A clinical and pathological study of 188 cases. *Cancer* 54:114–25, 1984.

9. Cummings BJ: The place of radiation therapy in the treatment of carcinoma of the anal canal. *Cancer Treat Rev* 9:124–47, 1982.

10. Magdeburg B, Fried M, Meyenberger C: Endoscopic ultrasonography in the diagnosis, staging and follow-up of anal carcinomas. *Endoscopy* 31:359–64, 1999.

11. Wade DS, Herrera L, Castillo NB, Petrelli NJ: Metastases to the lymph nodes in epidermoid carcinoma of the anal canal studied by a clearing technique. *Surg Gynecol Obstet* 169:238–42, 1989.

12. Cummings BJ: *Anal cancer*, in Perez CA, Brady LW (eds.): *Principles and practice of radiation oncology*, 3d ed. Philadelphia, Lippincott, 1998, pp. 1511–1524.

13. Cummings BJ, Keane TJ, O'Sullivan B, et al.: Epidermoid anal cancer: Treatment by radiation alone or by radiation and 5-fluorouracil with and without mitomycin C. *Int J Radiat Oncol Biol Phys* 21:1115–25, 1991.

14. Tanum G, Tveit K, Karlsen KO, Hauer-Jensen M: Chemotherapy and radiation therapy for anal carcinoma. Survival and late morbidity. *Cancer* 67:2462–6, 1991.

15. Dougherty BG, Evans HL: Carcinoma of the anal canal: A study of 79 cases. *Am J Clin Pathol* 83:159–164, 1985.

16. Frost DB, Richards PX, Montague ED, et al.: Epidermoid cancer of the anorectum. *Cancer* 53:1285–93, 1984.

17. Eschwege F, Lasser P, Chavy A, et al.: Squamous cell carcinoma of the anal canal: Treatment by external beam irradiation. *Radiother Oncol* 3:145–50, 1985.

18. Papillon J, Montbarbon JF: Epidermoid carcinoma of the anal canal. A series of 276 cases. *Dis Colon Rectum* 30:324–33, 1987.

19. Salmon RJ, Fenton J, Asselain B, et al.: Treatment of epidermoid anal canal cancer. *Am J Surg* 147:43–8, 1984.

20. Svensson C, Goldman S, Friberg B: Radiation treatment of epidermoid cancer of the anus. *Int J Radiat Oncol Biol Phys* 27:67–73, 1993.

21. Golden GT, Horsley JS: Surgical management of epidermoid carcinoma of the anus. *Am J Surg* 131:275–80, 1976.

22. Greenall MJ, Quan SH, Decosse JJ: Epidermoid cancer of the anus. *Br J Surg* 72(Suppl):S97–103, 1985.

23. Shepherd NA, Scholefield JH, Love SB, et al.: Prognostic factors in anal squamous carcinoma: A multivariate analysis of clinical, pathological and flow cytometric parameters in 235 cases. *Histopathology* 16:545–55, 1990.

24. Stearns MW, Urmacher C, Sternberg SS, et al.: Cancer of the anal canal. *Curr Prob Cancer* 4:1–44, 1980.

25. Ceresoli GL, Ferreri AJM, Cordio S, Villa E: Role of dose intensity in conservative treatment of anal canal carcinoma. *Oncology* 55:525–32, 1998.

26. Bartelink H, Roelofsen F, Eschwege F, et al.: Concomitant radiotherapy and chemotherapy is superior to radiotherapy alone in the treatment of locally advanced anal cancer: Results of a Phase III randomized trial of the European Organization for Research and Treatment of Cancer Radiotherapy and Gastrointestinal Co-operative Groups. *J Clin Oncol* 15:2040–9, 1997.

27. Schlienger M, Touboul E, Mauban S, et al.: Resultats du traitement de 286 cas de cancers epidermoides du canal anal dont 236 par irradiation a visée conservatrice. *Lyon Chir* 87:61–9, 1991.

28. Tanum G: Treatment of relapsing anal carcinoma. *Acta Oncol* 32:33–5, 1993.

29. Tanum G, Hannisdal E, Stenwig B: Prognostic factors in anal carcinoma. *Oncology* 51:22–4, 1994.

30. Goldman S, Glimelius B, Pahlman L, et al.: Anal epidermoid carcinoma: A population-based clinico-pathological study of 164 patients. *Int J Colorectal Dis* 3:109–18, 1988.

31. Myerson RJ, Karnell LH, Menck HR: The National Cancer Data Base report on carcinoma of the anus. *Cancer* 80:805–15, 1997.

32. Allal AS, Sprangers MAG, Laurencet F, et al.: Assessment of long-term quality of life in patients with anal carcinomas treated by radiotherapy with or without chemotherapy. *Br J Cancer* 80:1588–94, 1999.

33. Cummings BJ: Preservation of structure and function in epidermoid cancer of the anal canal, in Rosenthal CJ, Rotman M (eds.): *Infusion chemotherapy-irradiation interactions*. Amsterdam, Elsevier Science BV, 1998, pp. 165–171.

34. Vordermark D, Sailer M, Flentje M, et al.: Curative-intent radiation therapy in anal carcinoma: Quality of life and sphincter function. *Radiother Oncol* 52:239–43, 1999.

35. Chauveinc L, Buthaud X, Falcou MC, et al.: Cancer of the anal canal: A retrospective study of 346 patients (Abstract). *Int J Radiat Oncol Biol Phys* 45(Suppl):338–9, 1999.

36. Cummings BJ: Preservation of anorectal function in advanced epidermoid anal cancer (Abstract). *Dis Colon Rectum* 34:P4, 1991.

37. Friberg B, Svensson C, Goldman S, Glimelius B: The Swedish National Care Program for anal carcinoma. Implementation and overall results. *Acta Oncol* 37:25–32, 1998.

38. Goldman S, Glimelius B, Glas U, et al.: Management of anal epidermoid carcinoma — An evaluation of treatment results in two population-based series. *Int J Colorectal Dis* 4:234–43, 1989.

39. Palefsky JM, Holly EA, Hogeboom CJ, et al.: Virologic, immunologic, and clinical parameters in the incidence and progression of anal squamous epithelial lesions in HIV-positive and HIV-negative homosexual men. *J Acquired Immune Defic Syndr Hum Retrovirol* 17:314–9, 1998.

40. Lacey HB, Wilson GE, Tilston P, et al.: A study of anal epithelial neoplasia in HIV positive homosexual men. *Sex Transm Inf* 75:172–7, 1999.

41. Fenger C, Nielsen VT: Intraepithelial neoplasia in the anal canal. The appearance and relation to genital neoplasia. *Acta Pathol Microbiol Immunol Sect A* 94:343–9, 1986.

42. Ogunbiyi OA, Scholefield JH, Smith JHF, et al.: Immunohistochemical analysis of p53 expression in anal squamous neoplasia. *J Clin Pathol* 46:507–12, 1993.

43. Ogunbiyi OA, Scholefield JH, Rogers K, et al.: C-myc oncogene expression in anal squamous neoplasia. *J Clin Pathol* 46:23–7, 1993.

44. Goldman S, Auer G, Erhardt K, Seligson U: Prognostic significance of clinical stage, histologic grade, and nuclear DNA content in squamous cell carcinoma of the anus. *Dis Colon Rectum* 30:444–8, 1987.

45. Munoir S, Blegen H, Friberg B, et al.: A recurrent pattern of chromosomal aberrations and immunophenotypic appearance defines anal squamous cell carcinomas. *Br J Cancer* 76:1271–8, 1997.

46. Bonin SR, Pajak TF, Russell AH, et al.: Overexpression of p53 protein and outcome of patients treated with chemoradiation for carcinoma of the anal canal. *Cancer* 85:1226–33, 1999.

47. Wong CS, Tsao MS, Sharma V, et al.: Prognostic role of p53 protein expression in epidermoid carcinoma of the anal canal. *Int J Radiat Oncol Biol Phys* 45:309–14, 1999.

48. Indinnimeo M, Cicchini C, Stazi A, et al.: Human papillomavirus infection and p53 nuclear overexpression in anal canal carcinoma. *J Exp Clin Cancer Res* 18:47–52, 1999.

49. Wong S, Tsang R, Cummings B, Fyles A: Proliferation parameters in epidermoid carcinomas of the anal canal (Abstract). *Int J Radiat Oncol Biol Phys* 45[Suppl]:S192–3, 1999.

50. Noffsinger AE, Hui YZ, Suzuk L, et al.: The relationship of human papillomavirus to proliferation and ploidy in carcinoma of the anus. *Cancer* 75:958–67, 1995.

51. Goldman S, Svensson C, Bronnergard M, et al.: Prognostic significance of serum concentration of squamous cell carcinoma antigen in anal epidermoid carcinoma. *Int J Colorectal Dis* 8:98–102, 1993.

52. Gerard JP, Ayzac L, Hun D, et al.: Treatment of anal canal carcinoma with high dose radiation therapy and concomitant fluourouracil-cisplatinum. Long-term results in 95 patients. *Radiother Oncol* 46:249–56, 1998.

53. Tanum G, Stenwig AE, Bormer OP, Tveit KM: Carcinoembryonic antigen in anal carcinoma. *Acta Oncol* 31:333–5, 1992.

54. Grodsky L: Unsuspected anal cancer discovered after minor anorectal surgery. *Dis Colon Rectum* 10:471–8, 1967.

55. Frisch M, Glimelius B, van den Brule AJC, et al.: Benign anal lesions, inflammatory bowel disease and risk for high-risk human papilloma virus-positive and -negative anal carcinoma. *Br J Cancer* 78:1534–8, 1998.

56. Frisch M, Olsen JH, Bantz A, Melbye M: Benign anal lesions and the risk of anal cancer. *N Engl J Med* 331:300–2, 1994.

57. Daling JR, Weis NS, Hislop TG, et al.: Sexual practices, sexually transmitted diseases, and the incidence of anal cancer. *N Engl J Med* 317:973–7, 1987.

58. Frisch M, Glimelius B, van den Brule AJC, et al.: Sexually transmitted infection as a cause of anal cancer. *N Engl J Med* 337:1350–8, 1997.

59. Frisch M, Olsen JH, Melbye M: Malignancies that occur before and after anal cancer: Clues to their etiology. *Am J Epidemiol* 140:12–19, 1994.

60. Penn I: Cancer of the anogenital region in renal transplant recipients. Analysis of 65 cases. *Cancer* 58:611–16, 1986.

61. Palefsky JM, Holly EA, Gonzales J, et al.: Detection of human papillomavirus DNA in anal intraepithelial neoplasia and anal cancer. *Cancer Res* 51:1014–9, 1991.

62. Scholefield JH, McIntyre P, Palmer JG, et al.: DNA hybridization of routinely processed tissue for detecting HPV DNA in anal squamous cell carcinomas over 40 years. *J Clin Pathol* 43:133–6, 1990.

63. Heino P, Goldman S, Lagerstedt U, Dillber J: Molecular and serological studies of human papillomavirus among patients with anal epidermoid carcinoma. *Int J Cancer* 53:377–81, 1993.

64. Melbye M, Cote TR, Kessler L, Gail M, Biggar RJ, and the AIDS/Cancer Working Group: High incidence of anal cancer among AIDS patients. *Lancet* 343:636–9, 1994.

65. Hoffman R, Welton ML, Klencke B, et al.: The significance of pretreatment CD4 count on the outcome and treatment tolerance of HIV-positive patients with anal cancer. *Int J Radiat Oncol Biol Phys* 44:127–31, 1999.

66. UKCCCR Anal Canal Cancer Trial Working Party: Epidermoid anal cancer: Results from the UKCCCR randomized trial of radiotherapy alone versus radiotherapy, 5-fluorouracil and mitomycin. *Lancet* 348:1049–54, 1996.

67. Flam M, John M, Pajak TF, et al.: Role of mitomycin in combination with fluourouracil and radiotherapy, and of salvage chemoradiation in the nonsurgical treatment of epidermoid carcinoma of the anal canal: Results of a Phase III randomized intergroup study. *J Clin Oncol* 14:2527–39, 1996.

68. Martenson JA, Lipsitz SR, Wagner H, Jr, et al.: Initial results of a phase II trial of high dose radiation therapy, 5-fluorouracil, and cisplatin for patients with anal cancer (E4292): An Eastern Cooperative Oncology Group. *Int J Radiat Oncol Biol Phys* 35:745–9, 1996.

69. Constantinou EC, Daly W, Fung CY, et al.: Time-dose considerations in the treatment of anal cancer. *Int J Radiat Oncol Biol Phys* 39:651–7, 1997.

70. Allal AS, Mermillod B, Roth A, et al.: Impact of clinical and therapeutic factors on major late complications after radiotherapy with or without concomitant chemotherapy for anal carcinoma. *Int J Radiat Oncol Biol Phys* 39:1099–105, 1997.

71. Peiffert D, Bey P, Pernot M, et al.: Conservative treatment by irradiation of epidermoid cancers of the anal canal: Prognostic factors of tumoral control and complications. *Int J Radiat Oncol Biol Phys* 37:313–24, 1997.

72. Cummings BJ: Anal canal cancer — To split or not to split? *Cancer J Sci Am* 2:194–6, 1996.

73. John M, Pajak T, Flam M, et al.: Dose escalation in chemoradiation for anal cancer: preliminary results of RTOG 92–08. *Cancer J Sci Am* 4:205–8, 1996.

74. Leichman L, Nigro N, Vaitkevicius VK, et al.: Cancer of the anal canal. Model for preoperative adjuvant combined modality therapy. *Am J Med* 78:211–5, 1985.

75. Allal AS, Laurencet FM, Reymond MA, et al.: Effectiveness of surgical salvage therapy for patients with locally uncontrolled anal carcinoma after sphincter-conserving treatment. *Cancer* 86:405–9, 1999.

76. Ellenhorn JD, Enker WE, Quan SH: Salvage abdominoperineal resection following combined chemotherapy and radiotherapy for epidermoid carcinoma of the anus. *Ann Surg Oncol* 1:105–10, 1994.

77. Greenall MJ, Quan SHQ, Stearns MW, et al.: Epidermoid cancer of the anal margin. Pathologic features, treatment and clinical results. *Am J Surg* 149:95–100, 1985.

78. Touboul E, Schlienger M, Buffat L, et al.: Epidermoid carcinoma of the anal margin: 17 cases treated with curative-intent radiation therapy. *Radiother Oncol* 34:195–202, 1995.

79. Peiffert D, Bey P, Pernot M, et al.: Conservative treatment by irradiation of epidermoid carcinomas of the anal margin. *Int J Radiat Oncol Biol Phys* 39:57–66, 1997.

80. Papillon J, Chassard JL: Respective roles of radiotherapy and surgery in the management of epidermoid carcinoma of the anal margin. Series of 57 patients. *Dis Colon Rectum* 35:422–9, 1992.

CHAPTER 20

Hepatocellular Carcinoma

PHILIP J. JOHNSON

Hepatocellular carcinoma (HCC) is a common tumor that is responsible for over 5% of all cancer deaths worldwide.[1] It is highly malignant and therapy has, to date, had little impact on overall survival. Although the natural history of the disease and the essential prognostic variables are now clearly defined, we must recognize that the overall prognosis is universally poor, with most patients dying within one year of diagnosis. Part of the reason for this dismal state of affairs is that, as well as having HCC, at least 75% of patients will have an associated chronic liver disease, usually at the stage of cirrhosis.[2] The tumor and the chronic liver disease have independent natural histories and both contribute significantly to the patient's prognosis. In a disease such as HCC, where a significant proportion of patients will die within a few weeks of diagnosis, accurate prognostication is important. Information on the expected course of the disease is essential to provide a time frame in which these unfortunate patients can sort out their affairs.

In reviewing prognostic factors it is important to bear in mind that the tumor is relatively rare in the West where the incidence is only in the order of 1–2/100,000 compared to over 50/100,000 in many areas of Africa and the Far East.[3] There is therefore a tendency for patients in the West to be referred to a few specialist centers, and this process can be the source of considerable bias in reported series. For example, the figure for the rate that HCC can be resected with curative intent, an essential determinant of prognosis, has been reported to be up to 40% in series from Western surgical units. This may reflect, however, the fact that only those patients who the referring physician perceives to be good candidates for resection are referred and operated upon. The "true" rate is nearer to 10%. Another consequence of the wide geographic variation is that surgeons in high-incidence areas may have significantly more experience of operating on HCC in cirrhotic livers and may expect better results.

Prognostic Factors in Cancer, 2nd edition, Edited by Mary K. Gospodarowicz
ISBN 0-471-40633-3   Copyright © 2001 Wiley-Liss, Inc.

TUMOR-RELATED FACTORS

Histological Type

The World Health Organization (WHO) classification of HCC includes four types: trabecular, pseudoglandular, compact, or scirrhous.[4] Apart from the fibrolamellar variant (see below), none of these types, or the associated cytological variants, appears to be of any prognostic significance. Furthermore, the histological and cytological patterns often vary significantly throughout a single tumor. Early reports that the "clear cell" variant had a better prognosis have not been confirmed.[5,6] The degree of differentiation tends to correlate with tumor size, very small tumors being consistently well differentiated and larger tumors tending to be poorly differentiated.[7]

The fibrolamellar variant of HCC, which accounts for about 5% of cases in the West but less than 1% in the East, is reported to have a better prognosis than the common form of HCC. It is defined histologically by the tumor cells, deeply eosinophilic cytoplasm, and pyknotic nuclei interspersed with acellular collagen. The patients are young (mean age 26 years), the male: female ratio is 1 : 1, the nontumorous liver is not cirrhotic, and alpha-fetoprotein (AFP) is not produced in excess. Although resection rates are high, most patients will still die of their tumor, with a median overall survival of around 5 years.[8,9] Nonetheless, before attributing better survival to the biological behavior of this particular historically defined subgroup, we should note that being noncirrhotic, young, and AFP negative are all, in themselves, indicators of a relatively good prognosis in other types of HCC. For patients with nonresectable metastatic disease median survival is 14 months compared to 7 months in a matched group with the more common histological types. Poor prognostic factors in those with unresectable disease include poor performance status and large tumor.[10]

Extent of the Disease: Tumor Size and Morphology

Tumor size is an essential prognostic factor. Current imaging methods permit accurate detection and measurement of lesions down to one centimeter in diameter. Between one and 2.5 cm, the tumor does not appear to have metastatic potential. As a tumor increases in size above 3 cm, metastasis, usually intrahepatic, increases in frequency. At around 5 cm, symptoms of pain and weight loss start to develop and hepatomegaly is found. The typical size at clinical presentation is 8 cm. Survival ranges from around 3 years in those found to have "minute HCC" (<3 cm)[11] to less than 3 months for those with tumors larger than 8 cm.

The reasons why tumor size is so important are complex. Large tumors are more likely to have intra- and extrahepatic metastases, are technically more difficult to resect, and may be more likely to invade the vascular system (see below). They also tend to destroy more surrounding nontumorous liver so that liver function deteriorates. This adversely affects survival both in the untreated patient and in those considered for surgical resection, in whom there may be insufficient functional reserve to survive the operation.

It is striking that in the most widely used staging system, that of Okuda[12] (Table 20.1, Figure 20.1), the only tumor factor that is taken into account is size. In the tumors, nodules, metastases (TNM) classification and staging for primary hepatic malignancies size is, together with "vascular invasion," also an essential prognostic factor.[13] (see Appendix 20A).

The "morphology" of the tumor has also been found to be an independent risk factor, uninodular tumors having a better prognosis than multinodular ones, and this would certainly be compatible with clinical experience.[14] The definition of multinodular, however, is to some extent a function of the intensity with which

TABLE 20.1 The "Okuda" Staging System for Hepatocellular Carcinoma

Clinical Feature		Points
Tumor size (on liver scan)	>50%	1
	<50%	0
Ascites	Present	1
	Absent	0
Serum albumin (g/l)	<30	1
	>30	0
Serum bilirubin (umol/L)	>35	1
	<35	0

Total score	Stage	Median Survival (months)
0	1	28
1,2	2	8
3,4	3	1

Source: Adapted from Reference 12.

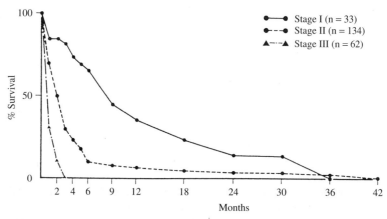

Figure 20.1 Survival of 235 untreated patients with HCC in relation to tumour stage. (See Table 20.1; from Okuda et al.[12])

the patient is investigated and the sensitivity of the techniques used. It is well recognized that at transplantation, the extent of the disease is frequently greater than that reported on radiological grounds. Specifically, multinodular disease is present more commonly than predicted by imaging procedures. Furthermore whether multifocal disease is a distinct biological entity, or simply represents intrahepatic metastasis from an initially solitary tumor, remains unclear.

Vascular Invasion

Vascular invasion signifies histological evidence that the tumor has invaded small blood vessels surrounding the tumor. The frequency of vascular invasion tends to increase with tumor size, and it is well recognized that some very large tumors can be resected with good long-term outcome if vascular invasion has not occurred.[15,16] This observation has led to "vascular invasion" being added to the TNM classification.[13] Presumably, vascular invasion is an indication of the inherent malignancy of the lesion and a channel for intrahepatic and extrahepatic metastasis. However, histological assessment of vascular invasion can only be made after tumor resection, a procedure that only a minority of patients undergoes. For this reason most clinicians will still use size as the primary prognostic criterion.

Portal vein thrombosis is detected in about 10% of cases at presentation and develops in up to 25% during the course of the disease.[17] The diagnosis can usually be accurately and noninvasively made by ultrasound examination. In most instances the thrombosis is related to invasion of the portal system by tumor and, as such, presumably represents a further indication of vascular invasion.[18,19] It is not surprising, therefore, that portal vein thrombosis has been consistently found to be an independent adverse prognostic factor in both Eastern and Western series[14,20-22] (Table 20.2).

Molecular/Genetic Factors and Tumor Markers

Serum alpha-fetoprotein (AFP) is the best and most widely used serological tumor marker. Its clinical application is mainly for diagnosis and monitoring of therapy, but the serum level does also appear to have prognostic significance. Those with a negative serum AFP appear to survive longer. At least in Western series, however, this may simply reflect the observation that AFP-negative tumors are often those arising in a noncirrhotic liver.[23] Among those who have raised serum levels, the higher the level, the worse the prognosis.[24] At first sight, it might be suspected that this simply represents increasing levels of AFP with increasing tumor size. However, it appears most likely that the adverse prognosis of a high AFP level is independent of tumor size. The rate at which the AFP rises (expressed as doubling time) may also be of prognostic significance, presumably reflecting the rate of tumor growth.[25]

Among patients who survive surgical resection, the presence of a *p53* gene mutation has been reported to be associated with a shortened overall and cancer-free survival after surgical resection.[26] Patients with a high C-erbB2 level have significantly shorter 1- and 2-year survival times.[27] The protein p73 is

TABLE 20.2   Recent Series in which Prognostic Factors in Patients with HCC have been Identified Using Multivariate Analysis

Series/Factor	Stuart et al.[22]	Chevret[20]	CLIP[14]	Calvet[21]
Liver function	Serum albumin	Serum bilirubin and serum alkaline phosphatase	Child's grade	Serum bilirubin
				Biochemistry[b]
				Ascites
Tumor factors	AFP	AFP	AFP	Tumor size
	PVT[a]	PVT[a]	PVT[a]	Metastases
			Tumor morphology[c]	
Patient factors		Karnofsky performance score		"Toxic syndrome" (see text)
				Age

[a]PVT, portal vein thrombosis.
[b]Blood urea nitrogen and gamma-GTP.
[c]Multi- or unifocal disease.

overexpressed by a subset of HCCs and has also been proposed as a useful indicator of prognosis in patients with HCC.[28] A high proliferative capacity in the tumor (as assessed by DNA flow cytometry) or the nontumorous liver [as assessed by proliferating cell nuclear antigen (PCNA) labeling] predicts a high likelihood of recurrence after resection.[29,30]

Signs and Symptoms

From a clinical point of view, these are essential prognostic factors. While they might simply reflect other factors listed elsewhere and not be independent, the simplicity with which they can be identified and the confidence with which they can be applied make them crucial. Patients who have symptoms from the tumor (pain and or hepatomegaly) have a much worse prognosis than those who do not. This is reflected in the natural history, and after treatment. Those patients detected in a surveillance program with tumor of less than 3 cm may survive for over 3 years without any treatment.[11] Furthermore, the patient undergoing liver transplantation where the tumor is detected incidentally in the explanted liver has an extremely good prognosis, indistinguishable from those transplanted for chronic liver disease without HCC, with a survival time of around 70% at 5 years.[31,32]

Once the patient develops clinical signs of liver failure — jaundice, marked ascites, encephalopathy, or recurrent variceal hemorrhage — the prognosis is extremely bleak, with a median survival of only about 3 months. It is generally accepted that no active treatment should be administered to such patients unless liver transplantation is available.

HOST-RELATED FACTORS

Under this heading, the essential (and independent) prognostic factor is liver function. In many cases the prognosis is probably related to the liver function to the extent that even if the tumor could be completely removed, the prognosis would remain very poor. As noted earlier, in the staging system that is currently most widely used, that of Okuda et al.,[12] three of the four characteristics applied reflect liver function (Table 20.1). Similarly, several recently described prognostic systems from Europe and the United States also conclude, on the basis of multivariate analyses, that liver function is of major importance as a prognostic factor.[14,20–22] (Table 20.2). The TNM staging system does not include an assessment of liver function, and for this reason it is not widely used for determining treatment options or assessing prognosis. There are three ways in which liver function can be assessed. The first is by considering individual biochemical "liver function" tests; the second by combinations of liver function tests and clinical features — typically the Child's grading[33] — and thirdly by "functional" tests such as bromsulphthalein retention. The first two are most widely used and have, in some form, been applied in most staging systems (see Tables 20.1 and 20.2).

Patient Demographics

It is widely perceived that patients from high-incidence areas, such as sub-Saharan Africa and the Far East, have tumors that run a more aggressive course, and that survival times are much shorter. In early studies from Africa, it was reported that all patients died within 4 months of the onset of symptoms,[34] and in an early staging system from Uganda the median survival of the whole group was one month.[35] The median survival time in Asia is about 10 weeks.[36] These figures are to be compared with several months in the West. For example, in a recent European study of prognostic factors in HCC, the median survival time for the entire group of 435 patients was 20 months.[14]

However, the situation is, in fact, extraordinarily complex, since the observed differences in survival may not be attributable to residence in a particular geographic area, or to the patient's race, but some other attribute of that geographical area; for example, the type of underlying cirrhosis [hepatitis B virus (HBV) related, hepatitis C virus (HCV) related, etc.], the severity of the cirrhosis at presentation, the time of presentation, and the amount of surveillance that is undertaken.

Performance Status

Performance status has received limited attention as a prognostic factor, but in one large study, it was, as would be expected, an important prognostic factor.[37] In other studies, performance status may be represented within terms such as "toxic syndrome," which refers to the combination of weight loss (defined by the presence of weight loss greater than 10% premorbid weight), malaise, and anorexia.[20] Again, by this criterion, performance status was an important prognostic factor.

ENVIRONMENT-RELATED FACTORS

Treatment-related Factors

There is no conclusive evidence that any form of treatment affects overall survival. However, circumstantial evidence suggests that surgical resection offers the only long-term chance of survival. Indeed the observation that survival curves "flatten out," after surgical resection, leading to 5-year survival rates of around 30%, whereas without treatment all patients die within 4 years,[13] supports this contention.[38,39] To this extent the "resectability" of the tumor is an essential prognostic factor. Indeed, overall those patients who undergo complete surgical resection (so-called R0 stage, no residual tumor) have the best overall prognosis. Patients are deemed "unresectable" if there are extrahepatic metastases, the main portal vein is involved, or there are serious concomitant medical illnesses. The patient must also be adjudged to have sufficient hepatic reserve to survive the operation, and the surgeon must be technically able to achieve a clear resection margin (see below). Only a minority of patients will fulfill these requirements, so that, in unselected series, only between 10% and 20% of patients will be suitable for surgical resection. The patient, offered a resection, will usually agree to the operation. The physician should make it clear to the patient, however, that the mortality rate may approach 15% for those patients with cirrhosis and that they may survive up to 3 years without the operation. Several important *scenarios* arise.

Will the Patient Survive the Operation? The major cause of postoperative death is liver failure and this, in turn, relates to the amount of hepatic reserve.[15] Clearly, those with underlying cirrhosis have a significantly greater operative mortality and can tolerate relatively smaller resections than those with a normal nontumorous liver. This is, in part, due to the decreased functional reserve of the cirrhotic liver and its limited regenerative capacity, but also technical difficulty in handling the cirrhotic liver at operation. The mortality rates will be 5–15% for those with underlying chronic liver disease and less than 5% for those with an otherwise normal liver.[38,39] A great deal of effort has gone into developing models to quantify the chance of survival after resection,[40] but the number of factors involved is considerable, so that no system has become widely accepted. Volumetric analysis of computed tomography (CT) scans and functional tests of liver reserve, including the trimethadione tolerance test and indocyanine green retention, have also been shown to be useful.[41,42] However, in practice most surgeons will only operate on patients with Child's grade A or, at worst, a good Child's grade B liver disease in whom they can obtain an adequate (1-cm) margin.[43] Preoperative treatment such as chemoembolization may effectively decrease tumor size, but may also impact adversely on liver function, thereby worsening results overall.[43] Age is not an independent risk factor, and patients over the age of 70 have similar rates of postoperative complications and long-term and disease-free survival.[44,45]

The patient should be aware that the underlying chronic liver disease will remain, and not only will there be a significant long-term morbidity and mortality associated with this condition, but also the operation will increase the likelihood of liver failure by removing some functioning liver. Furthermore, the chance of developing a "new" tumor (i.e., a second primary) or a recurrence of the original tumor remains very high (see below).

Will the Tumor Recur after Surgical Resection? Within this group (R0; no apparent residual disease after operation), gross or microscopic tumor involvement of the resection margins is an essential adverse prognostic factor and predicts almost certain "recurrence." Small tumors (<3 cm) do not appear to metastasize and have a recurrence rate of less than 5% — an essential, favorable prognostic factor. Below 5 cm the recurrence rate is around 25%, and above 5 cm it rises to 75%. Above 3 cm it appears that the presence of vascular invasion, indicated either by portal vein thrombosis or histological examination of the surrounding liver, is the major indicator of likely recurrence.[46-50] Another favorable prognostic factor that has been reported is a well-developed capsule. The presence of a p53 mutation has been associated with a shortened overall, and cancer-free, survival.[26]

Is the Patient Suitable for Liver Transplantation? Here the amount of hepatic reserve is no longer a consideration. The procedure is usually offered to patients with small tumors, as larger tumors tend to recur rapidly after transplantation. The essential prognostic factors include the number and size of the tumor nodules, the extent of vascular invasion, the presence or absence of local lymph-node metastases, and secondly whether or not the patient has symptoms.[51-55] As noted earlier, a patient undergoing liver transplantation in which a tumor is diagnosed unexpectedly for the first time in the explanted liver has a particularly good prognosis.

Chemotherapy and Locoregional Treatment for "Inoperable Disease"
Here we assume that, in consultation with a physician and experienced liver surgeon, the decision has been made that surgical resection is not feasible, or at least not with an "acceptable risk," and that liver transplantation, for whatever reason, is also not an option. This is the situation that is confronted by the majority of cases in high-incidence HCC areas, and thus the majority of patients worldwide. The prognosis is again a function of the tumor size and the status of the liver. Patients with Child's grade C liver disease, or any sign of liver failure — encephalopathy, ascites, or recurrent variceal hemorrhage — have a prognosis of less than 3 months. At least in the West, patients with underlying cirrhosis have a significantly worse overall survival than those without cirrhosis.[56] Llovet et al. have emphasized, however, that after excluding the latter group of patients (Child's grade C), there is still a considerable degree of inhomogeneity of prognosis in the absence of any treatment. The group of patients without adverse factors ("constitutional syndrome," vascular invasion, and extrahepatic spread) had 1-, 2-, and 3-year survival figures of 80%, 65%, and 50%, compared to 29%, 16%, and 8% in those with at least one adverse parameter.[37] None of

these treatments unequivocally affects overall survival, and in most cases, the treatment will adversely impact on the patient's quality of life.

Socioeconomic Factors: Geography and Access to Care

The availability of surgical resection and liver transplantation varies across the world and may be expected to have some influence on survival. This is particularly so in the case of liver transplantation. The availability varies across the Western world, where in some centers there are a significant number of deaths among those waiting. In the East and Africa the limited scope of transplantation reflects, in some cases, the cost involved, but more often the lack of donors.

Quality of Care

Two "quality of care" issues have an influence on prognosis in relation to hepatic resection. First, more experienced surgical teams seem to deliver better results.[57] Surgeons in the West have, until recently, had much less experience of operating on HCC in cirrhotic livers. Indeed it has not been uncommon in the West to hear that surgical resections cannot be undertaken in the cirrhotic liver. The second important improvement after resection has undoubtedly been in the quality of intensive care after surgical resection, and this has no doubt been responsible for the fall in postoperative mortality that has been reported in many series.[50] Finally, although difficult to quantify, there is the strong impression that surgical results are best among those who perform resection regularly and where patient care is part of a multidisciplinary team specializing in liver surgery.

The adverse prognostic implications of large tumor size make screening of high-risk populations for early detection of HCC an attractive proposition. Indeed, most of the general prerequisites for a screening program can be fulfilled by HCC. However, a clear demonstration of overall benefit in terms of public health remains elusive.[58,59] Nonetheless, ad hoc screening is widely practiced and some patients will be detected early and benefit from this strategy.

SUMMARY

The overall prognosis of patients with HCC is poor. Less than 5% will be "cured" by surgery, and for the remainder, who are unsuitable for some form of surgical resection, survival ranges from a few weeks to around 3 years. Those factors that can account for this inhomogeneity of survival experience are now well understood and relate predominately to the size of the tumor (and/or the degree of vascular invasion) and the functional reserve of the nontumorous liver (Appendix 20B). There remains an urgent need to document and understand the causes of the apparent differences in survival in different geographic areas and to identify factors that explain the intrinsic malignancy of the tumor at the molecular level.

■■■■■■ **APPENDIX 20A**

The TNM Classification of HCC

T — Primary Tumor

TX Primary tumor cannot be assessed

T0 No evidence of primary tumor

T1 Solitary tumor 2 cm or less in greatest dimension without vascular invasion

T2 Solitary tumor 2 cm or less in greatest dimension with vascular invasion; or multiple tumors limited to one lobe, none more than 2 cm in greatest dimension without vascular invasion; or solitary tumor more than 2 cm in greatest dimension without vascular invasion

T3 Solitary tumor more than 2 cm in greatest dimension with vascular invasion; or multiple tumors limited to one lobe, none more than 2 cm in greatest dimension with vascular invasion; or multiple tumors limited to one lobe, any more than 2 cm in greatest dimension with or without vascular invasion.

T4 Multiple tumors in more than one lobe; or tumor(s) involve(s) a major branch of the portal or hepatic vein(s); or tumor(s) with direct invasion of adjacent organs other than gallbladder; or tumor(s) with perforation of visceral peritoneum.

N — Regional Lymph Nodes

NX Regional lymph nodes cannot be assessed

N0 No regional lymph-node metastasis

N1 Regional lymph node metastasis

M — Distant Metastasis

MX Distant metastasis cannot be assessed

M0 No distant metastasis

M1 Distant metastasis

Stage Grouping

Stage I	T1	N0	M0
Stage II	T2	N0	M0
Stage IIIA	T3	N0	M0
Stage IIIB	T1	N1	M0
	T2	N1	M0
	T3	N1	M0
Stage IVA	T4	Any N	M0
Stage IVB	Any T	Any N	M1

Source: Sobin LH, Wittekind Ch (eds.): *TNM classification of malignant tumors*, 5th ed. Union Internationale Contre le Cancer Wiley-Liss, New York, 1997.

■■■■■ **APPENDIX 20B**

Prognostic Factors in Hepatocellular Carcinoma

Prognostic Factors	Tumor Related	Host Related	Environmental Related
Essential	Tumor size Vascular invasion Portal vein thrombosis/invasion	Liver function[a]	Birth in a high HCC incidence area
Additional	Multifocal disease	Performance status	Ready access to liver transplantation
New and promising	*p53* gene mutations		

[a]Assessed by liver-function tests, Child's classification, or clinical signs and symptoms of liver failure. Note that all the essential factors and "multifocal disease," as well as factors relating to overall survival, affect the decision as to whether or not the patient's tumor is resectable. "Resectability" is also an essential prognostic factor.

REFERENCES

1. Cancer Research for Cancer Control. International Agency for Research on Cancer. Lyon, France, WHO, 1997.

2. Johnson PJ, Williams R: Cirrhosis and the aetiology of hepatocellular carcinoma. *J Hepatol* 4:140–7, 1987.

3. Waterhouse JAH, Muir CS, Correa P, et al.: *Cancer incidence in five continents,* Vol. IV. Lyon International Agency for Research on Cancer, 1982.

4. Gibson JB, Sobin LH: Histological typing of tumours of the liver, biliary tract and pancreas, *International histological classification of tumours no. 20.* Geneva, WHO, 1978.

5. Buchannan TF, Huvos AG: Clear-cell carcinoma of the liver: A clinicopathologic study of 13 patients. *Am J Clin Pathol* 61:529–39, 1974.

6. Kishi K, Shikata T, Hirohashi S, et al.: Hepatocellular carcinoma: A clinical and pathologic analysis of 57 hepatectomy cases. *Cancer* 51:542–8, 1983.

7. Sugihara S, Nakashima O, Kojiro M, et al.: The morphologic transition in hepatocellular carcinoma: A comparison of the individual histologic features disclosed by ultrasound-guided fine-needle biopsy with those of autopsy. *Cancer* 70:1488–92, 1992.

8. Craig JR, Peters RL, Omata M: Fibrolamellar carcinoma of the liver: A tumor of adolescents and young adults with distinctive clinicopathologic features. *Cancer* 46:372–9, 1980.

9. Kane SP, Murray-Lyon IM, Paradinas FJ, et al.: High serum vitamin B$_{12}$ binding capacity as a marker of the fibrolamellar variant of hepatocellular carcinoma. *Br Med J* 285:840–2, 1982.

10. Epstein BE, Pajak TF, Haulk TL, et al.: Metastatic non resectable fibrolamellar hepatoma: Prognostic features and natural history. *Am J Clin Oncol* 22:22–8, 1999.

11. Ebara M, Ohto M, Shinagawa T, et al.: Natural history of minute hepatocellular carcinoma smaller than three centimeters complicating cirrhosis. A study in 22 patients. *Gastroenterology* 90:2207–10, 1986.

12. Okuda K, Ohtsuki T, Obata H, et al.: Natural history of hepatocellular carcinoma and prognosis in relation to treatment. *Cancer* 56:918–28, 1985.

13. Sobin LH, Wittekind Ch: *TNM classification of malignant tumors*, 5th ed. New York, Union Internationale Contre le Cancer Wiley-Liss, 1997.

14. A new prognostic system for hepatocellular carcinoma: A retrospective study of 435 patients: The Cancer of the Liver Italian Program (CLIP) investigators. *Hepatology* 28:751–5, 1998.

15. Roseman BJ, Roh MS: Prognostic factors in surgical resection for hepatocellular carcinoma, in Pollock RE (ed.): surgical oncology Dordrecht, The Netherlands, Kluwer Academic Publishers 1997, pp. 331–45.

16. Nagasue N, Uchida M, Makino Y, et al.: Incidence and factors associated with intra-hepatic recurrence following resection of hepatocellular carcinoma. *Gastroenterology* 105(2):488–94, 1993.

17. Okuda K, Ohnishi K, Kimura J, et al.: Incidence of portal vein thrombosis in liver cirrhosis. An angoiographic study in 708 patients. *Gastroenterology* 89:279–85, 1985.

18. Cedrone A, Rapaccini GL, Pompili M, et al.: Portal vein thrombosis complicating hepatocellular carcinoma. Value of ultrasound guided fine-needle biopsy of the thrombus in the therapeutic management. *Liver* 16:94–8, 1996.

19. De Sio I, Castellano L, Calandra M, et al.: Ultrasound-guided fine needle aspiration biopsy of portal vein thrombosis in liver cirrhosis: Results in 15 patients. *Jpn Gastroenterol Hepatol* 10:662–5, 1995.

20. Chevret S, Trinchet JC, Mathieu D, et al.: A new prognostic classification for predicting survival in patients with hepatocellular carcinoma. Groupe d'Etude et de Traitement du Carcinome Hepatocellulaire. *J Hepatol* 31(1):133–41, 1999.

21. Calvet X, Bruix J, Gines P, et al.: Prognostic factors of hepatocellular carcinoma in the west: A multivariate analysis in 206 patients. *Hepatology* 12:753–60, 1990.

22. Stuart KE, Anand AJ, Jenkins RL: Hepatocellular carcinoma in the United States. Prognostic features, treatment outcome, and survival. *Cancer* 77(11):2217–22, 1996.

23. Nomura F, Ohnishi K, Tanabe Y: Clinical features and prognosis of hepatocellular carcinoma with reference to serum alpha-fetoprotein levels. Analysis of 606 patients. *Cancer* 64(8):1700–7, 1989.

24. Johnson PJ, Melia WM, Palmer MK, et al.: Relationship between serum alpha-fetoprotein, cirrhosis and survival in hepatocellular carcinoma. *Br J Cancer* 44:502–5, 1981.

25. Johnson PJ, Williams R: Serum alphafetoprotein estimations in hepatocellular carcinoma: Influence of therapy and possible value in early detection. *J Natl Cancer Inst* 64:1329–32, 1980.

26. Sugo H, Takamori S, Kojima K, et al.: The significance of p53 mutations as an indicator of the biological behavior of recurrent hepatocellular carcinomas. *Surg Today* 29(9):849–55, 1999.

27. Heinze T, Jonas S, Karsten A, et al.: Determination of the oncogenes p53 and C-erb B2 in the tumour cytosols of advanced hepatocellular carcinoma (HCC) and correlation to survival time. *Anticancer Res.* 19(4A):2501–3, 1999.

28. Tannapfel A, Wasner M, Krause K, et al.: Expression of p73 and its relation to histopathology and prognosis in hepatocellular carcinoma. *J Natl Cancer Inst* 91(13):1154–8, 1999.

29. Chiu JH, Wu LH, Kao HL, et al.: Can determination of the proliferative capacity of the non tumor portion predict the risk of tumor recurrence in the liver remnant after resection of human hepatocellular carcinoma? (published erratum appears in *Hepatology* 18:1292, 1993). *Hepatology* 18:96–102, 1993.

30. Adachi E, Maeda T, Matsumata T, et al.: Risk factors for interhepatic recurrence in human small hepatocellular carcinoma. *Gastroenterology* 108:768–75, 1995.

31. Koneru B, Cassavilla A, Bowman J, et al.: Liver transplantation for malignant tumors. *Gastroenterol Clin Norm Am* 17:177–93, 1988.

32. Achkar JP, et al.: Undetected hepatocellular carcinoma: Clinical features and outcome after liver transplantation. *Liver Trans Surg* 4:477–82, 1998.

33. Pugh RHN, Murray-Lyon IM, Dawson JL, et al.: Transection of the oesophagus for bleeding oesophageal varices. *Br J Surg* 60:646–9, 1973.

34. Berman C: *Primary carcinoma of the liver*. London Lewis, 1951, pp. 46–48.

35. Primack A, Vogel CL, Kyalwazi SK, et al.: A staging system for hepatocellular carcinoma: Prognostic factors in Ugandan patients. *Cancer* 42:2149–56, 1975.

36. Shiu W, Dewar G, Leung N, et al.: Hepatocellular carcinoma in Hong Kong: A clinical study on 340 cases. *Oncology* 47:241–5, 1990.

37. Llovet JM, Bustamante J, Castells A, et al.: Natural history of untreated non-surgical hepatocellular carcinoma: Rationale for the design and evaluation of therapeutic trials. *Hepatology* 29(1):62–7, 1999.

38. Nagasue N, Kohno H, Chang YC, et al.: Liver resection for hepatocellular carcinoma. Results of 229 consecutive patients during 11 years. *Ann Surg* 217(4):375–84, 1993.

39. Fong Y, Jarnagin WR, Brennan MF, et al.: Hepatocellular carcinoma: An analysis of 412 HCC at a Western center. *Ann Surg* 229(6):790–9; discussion 799–800, 1999.

40. Yamanaka N, Okamoto E, Oriyama T, et al.: A prediction scoring system to select the surgical treatment of liver cancer. Further refinement based on 10 years of use. *Ann Surg* 219:342–6, 1994.

41. Ishikawa A, Fukao K, Tsuji K, et al.: Trimethadione tolerance tests for the assessment of feasible size of hepatic resection in patients with hepatocellular carcinoma. *J Gastroenterol Hepatol* 8:426–32, 1993.

42. Fan ST, Lai EC, Lo SM, et al.: Hospital mortality of major hepatectomy for hepatocellular carcinoma associated with cirrhosis. *Arch Surg* 130:198–203, 1995.

43. Nagasue N, Kohno H, Tachibana M, et al.: Prognostic factors after hepatic resection for hepatocellular carcinoma associated with Child-Turcotte class B and C cirrhosis. *Ann Surg* 229:84–90, 1999.

44. Takenaka K, Shimada M, Higashi H, et al.: Liver resection for hepatocellular carcinoma in the elderly. *Arch Surg* 129:846–50, 1994.

45. Nagasue N, Chang YC, Takemoto Y, et al.: Liver resection in the aged (seventy years or older) with hepatocellular carcinoma. *Surgery* 113:148–54, 1993.

46. Zhou X, Yu Y, Tang Z: Advances in surgery for hepatocellular carcinoma. *Asian J Surg* 17:34–9, 1994.

47. Lai E, Ng I, You K, et al.: Hepatectomy for large hepatocellular carcinoma: The optimal resection margin. *World J Surg* 15:141–5, 1991.

48. Lai EC, You KT, Ng IO, et al.: The pathological basis of resection margin for hepatocellular carcinoma. *World J Surg* 17:786–91, 1993.

49. Kawarda Y, Ito F, Sakurai H, et al.: Surgical treatment of hepatocellular carcinoma. *Cancer Chemother Pharmacol* 33(Suppl.); S12–7, 1994.

50. Lai EC, Fan ST, Lo CM, et al.: Hepatic resection for hepatocellular carcinoma. An audit of 343 patients. *Ann Surg* 221:291–8, 1995.

51. Iwatsuki S, Gordon RD, Shaw BJ, et al.: Role of liver transplantation in cancer therapy. *Ann Surg* 202:401–7, 1985.

52. Iwatsuki S, Starzl TE, Sheahan DG, et al.: Hepatic resection versus transplantation for hepatocellular carcinoma. *Ann Surg* 214:221–8, 1991.

53. Romani F, Belli LS, Rondinara GF, et al.: The role of transplantation in small hepatocellular carcinoma complicating cirrhosis of the liver. *J Am Coll Surg* 178:3779–84, 1994.

54. Haug CE, Jenkins RL, Rohrer RJ, et al.: Liver transplantation for primary hepatic cancer. *Transplantation* 53:376–82, 1992.

55. McPeake JR, O'Grady JG, Zaman S, et al.: Liver transplantation for primary hepatocellular carcinoma: Tumor size and number determine outcome. *J Hepatology* 18:226–34, 1993.

56. Melia WM, Wilkinson ML, Portmann BC, et al.: Hepatocellular carcinoma in the non-cirrhotic liver: A comparison with that complicating cirrhosis. *Q J Med, New Series LIII*, 211:391–400, 1984.

57. Lise M, Bacchetti S, Da Pian P, et al.: Prognostic factors affecting long term outcome after liver resection for hepatocellular carcinoma: Results in a series of 100 Italian patients. *Cancer* 15:82:1028–36, 1998.

58. Collier J, Sherman M: Screening for hepatocellular carcinoma. *Hepatology* 27:273–8, 1998.

59. Blakey J: Screening for hepatitis B carriers: Evidence and policy developments in New Zealand. *N Z Med J* 112: 4321–3, 1999.

CHAPTER 21

Extrahepatic Biliary Tract and the Ampulla of Vater Cancers

DONALD EARL HENSON, LYNN G. RIES and JORGE ALBORES-SAAVEDRA

This chapter reviews the most useful prognostic factors that are available for carcinomas arising in the gallbladder, extrahepatic bile ducts, or the ampulla of Vater. In considering these prognostic indicators, the complex anatomy of the extrahepatic biliary system and its relation to adjacent structures becomes critical. For this reason, the prognostic factors are described separately for the gallbladder, extrahepatic bile ducts, and ampulla. For all three sites, however, the single most important factor having the greatest effect on survival is the extent of tumor at the time of diagnosis. In preparing this chapter, data were reviewed from the Surveillance, Epidemiology, and End Results (SEER) program of the National Cancer Institute for the years 1973–1995. In the SEER Program, the extent of disease can be classified as "localized," regional, and "distant" or by the standard TNM classification. A "localized" tumor is confined to the organ of origin without nodal involvement; "regional," denotes regional lymph-node involvement or direct extension to adjacent organs; and "distant" indicates that distant metastases have been found. The prognostic factors are presented as tumor-related, host-related, and environment-related.

CANCER OF THE GALLBLADDER

Carcinoma of the gallbladder is a relatively uncommon but a highly lethal disease that often causes death in less than one year after diagnosis. For all stages combined, the relative 5-year survival is only about 15%.[1] In this section, we review the reliable prognostic factors that are available to plan therapy and estimate outcome. These factors apply primarily to carcinomas, which comprise

Prognostic Factors in Cancer, 2nd edition, Edited by Mary K. Gospodarowicz
ISBN 0-471-40633-3 Copyright © 2001 Wiley-Liss, Inc.

more than 90% of all cancers found in the gallbladder.[2] Gallbladder cancer often presents as benign lithic disease, which may cause delays in diagnosis.

Tumor-Related Factors

Clinical Observations Presenting signs and symptoms, such as weight loss, nausea and vomiting, jaundice, or right upper quadrant pain, are unfavorable prognostic signs and usually indicate extension of tumor to the liver or to the extrahepatic bile ducts. Jaundice usually indicates unresectable liver involvement or bile-duct obstruction. Laboratory findings in cases of jaundice include hyperbilirubinemia, bilirubinuria, and increased levels of serum alkaline phosphatase and lactic acid dehydrogenase. While these clinical findings are considered poor prognostic signs, they have not been integrated into any clinical or laboratory prognostic system.

Serum markers have not proven useful for estimating outcome. Although tumor cells produce carcinoembryonic antigen (CEA), serum levels of CEA cannot be used to estimate tumor bulk, since serum levels also increase as a result of bile-duct obstruction from any cause. Other serum tumor markers, such as CA19-9, have been found in patients with carcinoma of the gallbladder, but have not proven to be prognostic.

Seeding of the abdominal cavity can occur. Ascites secondary to intra-abdominal tumor dissemination invariably indicates a poor outcome. As with cancers arising in other sites, performance status can be used to assess prognosis.

Extent of Tumor The extent of tumor at time of diagnosis, usually expressed by the TNM classification,[3] is one of the most reliable prognostic factors.[2,4–9] The TNM can be assessed clinically at time of diagnosis or pathologically if the primary tumor is resected. As expected, in situ carcinomas (Stage 0) are associated with excellent outcome. The 5-year relative survival for patients with carcinoma in situ is 90% (Table 21.1).

Stage I and stage II cancers, that is, those confined to the gallbladder, have the most favorable outcome (Table 21.1). These cancers can be subdivided histologically by the depth of invasion into the wall of the gallbladder

TABLE 21.1 Relative Survival of Patients with Gallbladder Cancer by Stage

Stage of Disease	Number of Cases	2-Year Survival (%)	5-Year Survival(%)
Stage 0	64	99	90
Stage I	186	61	49
Stage II	79	65	42
Stage III	312	26	15
Stage IV	939	3	0
Unstaged	534	31	20
All stages	2,114	24	16

Source: Data from SEER (1988–1995); cases staged according to the *AJCC Manual*.[3]

TABLE 21.2   **Staging for Gallbladder Cancer as Defined by Depth of Invasion**

Stage	% of Cases	Description	5-Year Survival (%)
I	8	Confined to mucosa	86
II	18	Extension into muscularis	57
III	19	Extension into subserosal connective tissue	15
IV	11	Confined to wall with cystic-duct lymph-node involved	13
V	44	Liver involvement or distant metastasis	5

Source: Data from Reference 10.

(Table 21.2).[10] In general, the deeper the invasion, the shorter the survival. Even the frequency of regional lymph-node spread is determined by the depth of tumor invasion.[11] The size of the primary tumor does not seem to be a useful prognostic factor, since small tumors can invade through the wall and large ones remain in the gallbladder. For patients with stage III disease, the 5-year survival is less than 20%. Liver extension is found in almost 70% of cases at the time of surgical evaluation. For patients with distant metastasis, the 5-year survival is virtually 0%. Most in situ and localized carcinomas are found incidentally in gallbladders removed for benign disease.[12–14] Histological examination of laparoscopic cholecystectomy specimens will occasionally reveal a localized unsuspected cancer.[15,16] It has been reported that only 10% of patients have cancer limited to the gallbladder at time of diagnosis.[17] In SEER, 15% of patients had their cancer limited to the gallbladder (Table 21.1).

Residual Tumor   Macroscopic or microscopic residual tumor is an adverse prognostic factor. In one study, the median survival for patients with no evidence of residual disease was 67 months, whereas the median survival rates for patients with microscopic or macroscopic residual tumor were 8.9 and 3.8 months, respectively.[18] Residual tumor often depends on the extent of disease at the time of diagnosis.

Histological Type   Of all histological types,[19] papillary carcinomas have the most favorable prognosis. The 2-year relative survival rate, all stages combined, is 53% and the 5-year rate is 43%. For adenocarcinomas, on the other hand, the 2-year relative survival is 17% and the 5-year survival is 11%. There is no compelling evidence that adenocarcinomas showing focal endocrine differentiation have a prognosis different from tumors without such differentiation. No patient with small-cell carcinoma of the gallbladder has survived 5 years.[20] Undifferentiated spindle and giant-cell tumors also have a less favorable outcome compared to better-differentiated carcinomas.[21] In SEER, the 2-year relative survival of undifferentiated tumors was 1%.

Histological Grade   As with carcinomas arising in other sites, the histological grade (that is, extent of tumor differentiation) has been associated with survival

TABLE 21.3 Relation of Tumor Differentiation to Survival in Patients with Gall-bladder Carcinoma

Differentiation	Number of Cases	Percent	Mean Survival (Months)
Well-differentiated	6	11.3	17.5
Moderately-differentiation	12	22.6	9.4
Poorly-differentiated	24	45.3	4.3
Unclassified	11	20.8	2.2
Total	53	100	

Source: Data taken from Reference 24.

(Table 21.3). An inverse relation between increasing grade and outcome has been observed by many investigators.[22–24] The cumulative survival rate was 33% for poorly differentiated carcinomas at one year compared to 79% for well-differentiated carcinomas.[25] However, the histological grade has not been integrated into the TNM or in any prognostic system for carcinomas of the gallbladder.

The SEER program also revealed a relation between histological grade and stage. For localized disease, 33% of cases were listed as Grade 1, but for distant disease, only 12% were recorded as Grade 1. Others have made similar observations.[24]

Vascular Invasion Vascular or lymphatic invasion is a significant prognostic factor, since it reduces survival according to data recorded in SEER. For localized disease, the 5-year survival for patients with vascular invasion was 13% compared to 31% for patients without known vascular invasion. The median survival for patients with vascular invasion was 10 months, and for those without vascular invasion it was 18 months.[22]

Molecular Factors There was no association observed between expression of *ras* p21 protein and outcome nor between amplification of c-erb-2 and outcome.[26] Similarly, no relation was observed between p53 protein expression and outcome.[27,28] DNA ploidy seems to provide no additional prognostic information than that provided by traditional tumor staging.[29] Expression of vascular endothelial growth factor correlated with tumor progression, but it was less reliable as a prognostic factor than extent of disease.[30] Further, the extent of neovascularization has not proven to be an independent prognostic factor.[31] Overexpression of cyclin E does not correlate with stage.[32]

Host Factors

Host factors include age, since the disease is usually found in the elderly, and comorbid conditions. These factors often preclude adequate or extensive therapy. For patients with residual tumor, host prognostic factors such as performance status become significant.

Environment-Related Factors

Treatment   The primary treatment of gallbladder cancer is surgery. It provides the only opportunity for long-term survival if complete resection of the tumor is possible.[8] Liver involvement usually precludes complete resection, although some patients with limited direct liver extension may be salvaged by a major hepatic resection. Liver or lymph-node involvement usually indicates future recurrence. A simple cholecystectomy may suffice for patients with T1aN0M0 disease. Chemotherapy and radiation therapy have been studied, but their effectiveness seems limited.

Table 21.4 shows survival according to no surgery or to cancer-directed surgery. No surgery includes palliative or other procedures that may have been performed, but were not specifically directed at the cancer. Cancer-directed surgery includes specific cancer-directed treatment. Presumably most patients who did not have cancer-directed surgery had residual tumor and should be classified R1. For all stages, cancer-directed surgery is a significant prognostic factor judging by the 2-year and 5-year survival rates.

Summary   With current information, the extent of disease, histologic type (papillary or nonpapillary), and histologic grade are the most reliable prognostic factors available for carcinoma of the gallbladder. Numerous authors have commented on the association that exists between survival and extent of disease at time of diagnosis. Patients with regional or metastatic disease have shorter survival than patients with localized disease, an observation made by all investigators. Carcinomas of the gallbladder are insidious in their spread, often metastasizing before a diagnosis is made. Because of the location of the

TABLE 21.4   Relative Survival According to No Surgery or Cancer-directed Surgery for Patients with Cancer of the Gallbladder

Procedure	Stage	Number of Cases	2-Year Survival (%)	5-Year Survival (%)
No Surgery	Stage 0	0		
	Stage I	1		
	Stage II	0		
	Stage III	37	3	
	Stage IV	480	2	0.3
	Unstaged	145	5	3
	All stages	663	3	0.8
Surgery	Stage 0	64	97	90
	Stage I	185	61	49
	Stage II	79	65	42
	Stage III	275	29	17
	Stage IV	459	4	0.6
	Unstaged	389	40	25
	All stages	1,451	33	23

Source: Data from SEER (1988–1995).

gallbladder, tumors can spread by several routes: direct extension to adjacent organs, through lymphatic and vascular channels, transcoelomically, and along small nerve trunks. Vascular invasion can serve as an additional prognostic finding, but the presence or absence of vascular invasion is not reported in the majority of cases. Based on our estimation, overt vascular invasion reduces survival to the next lower stage of disease.[22] Molecular markers, such as p53, appear to have a minimal role in guiding treatment or in estimating outcome. Of all histological types, papillary carcinomas have the most favorable outcome.[33,34] Papillary carcinomas are associated with localized disease more than any other histologic type. In SEER, 64% of patients with papillary carcinoma had localized disease at diagnosis. This association should not be surprising, since papillary carcinomas are exophytic in growth. For comparison, only 25% of patients with adenocarcinoma had localized disease at diagnosis. Noninvasive papillary carcinomas of the gallbladder and extrahepatic bile ducts have the same behavior as carcinoma in situ. Unfortunately, papillary carcinomas are found in less than 10% of patients.[1]

For practical purposes the extent of disease is the most powerful predictor of outcome and should be reported in all cases using the TNM.[3,35] If the tumor is limited to the gallbladder wall, then its depth of penetration should be recorded. Short survival can safely be predicted if the tumor has invaded deep into the liver or into the abdominal cavity. The extent of disease seems to overpower the importance of all cellular and molecular characteristics of the primary tumor in the determination of outcome. Perhaps, some of the nonanatomic-based prognostic factors can take on more importance if the treatment of gallbladder cancer improves.

EXTRAHEPATIC BILE DUCTS CANCER

Compared to malignant tumors of the gallbladder, malignant tumors of the extrahepatic bile ducts are less common, occur more frequently in men than in women, are usually not associated with lithiasis, and have an entirely different epidemiologic distribution. Because malignant tumors of the extrahepatic bile ducts are uncommon, there has been no systematic approach to the evaluation of the prognostic factors. More than 98% of all malignant tumors of the extrahepatic bile ducts are carcinomas.

Tumor-Related Factors

Clinical Observations Cholestatic jaundice is the presenting sign in the majority of patients. Other findings, such as abdominal pain, weight loss, pruritus, and a right upper quadrant mass, are frequently encountered. A palpable mass usually indicates advanced disease, which precludes complete resection of the tumor. Laboratory findings are usually compatible with bile-duct obstruction. They include elevated levels of serum bilirubin and alkaline phosphatase. Serum CEA and CA 19-9 are often elevated. These markers can be used to detect recurrence. Because these clinical observations are found in almost all patients, they have not been classified in any prognostic system. Initially, the jaundice can be intermittent. Jaundice often develops while the tumor is relatively small, before it has had the opportunity to metastasize.

Tumor Location   The location of the primary tumor within the biliary tree is prognostic largely because of therapeutic considerations. Tumors located in the distal third of the extrahepatic bile duct are easier to resect than those arising in the proximal one-third.[36–38] Unfortunately, most tumors originate within the upper third of the extrahepatic bile duct, above the junction of the cystic and hepatic ducts. Less than 50% of carcinomas arising in the upper segment of the extrahepatic bile duct, including the hepatic ducts, can be resected.[39,40] Tumors that spread diffusely within the wall of the extrahepatic bile duct or arise from multiple foci are more difficult to resect than those that are unifocal in origin.

Extent of Tumor   The extent of tumor is an important prognostic indicator.[9] The overall relative 5-year survival, all histological types combined, was 22% for stage I disease, 11% for stage II disease, 2% for stage III disease, and 8% for stage IV disease (Table 21.5). The difference in survival between stage III and stage IV is not significant. Proximal tumors usually spread directly to the liver, while distal tumors usually initially spread into the pancreas. Patients with insitu carcinoma (stage 0) have only a 62% 5-year relative survival, presumably because tumors can arise from more than a single focus or an area of invasion may not have been visible during histological examination.

The depth of tumor invasion into the wall of the extrahepatic bile duct is also a prognostic factor.[41,42] In most cases, however, the tumor has extended through the wall by the time the diagnosis is made. Perineural invasion has also been considered an adverse prognostic factor.[43] It probably has the greatest significance for localized tumors. Although data are limited, perineural invasion seems less frequent in papillary carcinomas.[43] Perineural invasion does not exclude long-term survival. It is found in most tumors if careful search is made.

TABLE 21.5   Relative Survival of Patients with Cancer of the Extrahepatic Bile Ducts by Stage

Stage	Number of Cases	2-Year Survival (%)	5-Year Survival (%)
Stage 0	10	70	62
Stage I	225	38	22
Stage II	65	30	11
Stage III	46	22	2
Stage IV	571	17	8
Unstaged	316	16	6
All stages	1,233	22	10

Source: Data from SEER (1988–1995); cases staged according to the *AJCC Manual*.[3]

Tumors can be staged clinically by imaging,[44] or pathologically after resection. The presence of peripheral hepatic metastasis or extrahepatic disease usually precludes curative resection. The extent of disease is usually recorded according to the TNM.[3,35]

Residual Tumor   Macroscopic or microscopic residual tumor is a strong predictor of an unfavorable outcome.[45,46] Local recurrence is usually related to residual tumor located at the proximal or distal surgical margins of the bile duct or along the dissected soft tissue margin in the portal area.[46] In one study, the 5-year survival was 40% in cases with tumor-free margins and 18% in cases with tumor found at the margin.[47]

Histological Type   The histologic type influences outcome. Of all histologic types, papillary carcinomas, which comprise only 5.5% of all invasive cancers, have the highest 5-year relative survival rate (24%), all stages combined. For adenocarcinomas, the 5-year survival is only 7%. In 48% of cases of papillary carcinoma, the tumor was localized at diagnosis, while it was localized in 23% of the cases of adenocarcinoma. Only 11% of papillary carcinomas were associated with distant metastasis at diagnosis, while 26% of adenocarcinomas were associated with distant metastasis. For localized disease, the 2-year relative survival for adenocarcinomas was 33%, but for papillary carcinomas, it was 53%. The 5-year survival for adenocarcinomas, localized stage, was 16%, and for papillary carcinomas, it was 33%. Other investigators have also observed higher survival for papillary carcinomas.[3,48,49] In fact, non-invasive and minimally invasive papillary carcinomas behave as in situ carcinomas.[55]

Histological Grade   As a group, the carcinomas arising in the extrahepatic bile ducts are better differentiated than carcinomas arising in the gallbladder, perhaps because they are found earlier as a result of obstruction. The 2-year and 5-year survival by histologic grade is shown in Table 21.6. For all stages combined, there is a correlation between histological grade and outcome. Median survival times also declined with advancing histologic grade. Within each stage, there was decreasing survival with increasing grade.

Molecular Markers   There are data indicating that proliferating cell nuclear antigen (PCNA) is prognostic.[50] However, none of the molecular markers

TABLE 21.6   Relative Survival of Patients with Cancer of the Extrahepatic Bile Ducts According to Histologic Grade

Histologic Grade	Number of Cases	2-Year Survival (%)	5-Year Survival (%)
Grade 1	500	33	16
Grade 2	619	24	10
Grade 3	472	12	4
Grade 4	51	12	1

Source: Data from SEER (1973–1995).

that have been reported have proven a substitute for extent of disease as a prognostic factor.[51,52] High immunohistochemical expression of mucin core protein-1 (MUC1) correlates with hepatic metastasis and short survival.[53]

Host Factors

The host factors include age, comorbid conditions, and predisposing diseases such as chronic sclerosing cholangitis. Advanced age may prevent extensive surgical resection.

Environmental Factors

Treatment Surgical resection is the only curative approach.[54] However, despite the fact that most of these tumors are small, well-differentiated, and localized, the results of surgical treatment have been disappointing. Locoregional recurrences are frequent. Resection of extrahepatic bile-duct tumors is complicated by their anatomic location, as indicated earlier. Patients with tumors in the proximal ductal system are the most difficult to treat and often require major hepatic resections. Although computed tomography, ultrasonography, cholangiography, and cytological examination of cholangiography specimens have led to earlier diagnosis, survival rates have essentially remained unchanged.[1,39] Often treatment is only palliative to remove the obstruction in the extrahepatic bile duct.

Table 21.7 shows survival according to no surgery or cancer-directed surgery. No surgery includes palliative or other procedures that were not directed specifically at the cancer. Cancer-directed surgery is defined as specific cancer-directed treatment. Most patients who did not have cancer-directed surgery

TABLE 21.7 Relative Survival According to No Surgery or Cancer-directed Surgery for Patients with Cancer of the Extrahepatic Bile Ducts

Procedure	Stage	Number of Cases	2-Year Survival (%)	5-Year Survival (%)
No Surgery	Stage 0	2		
	Stage I	108	15	1
	Stage II	13	10	
	Stage III	11	10	0
	Stage IV	333	6	2
	Unstaged	292	16	3
	All stages	759	11	3
Surgery	Stage 0	8		
	Stage I	117	58	39
	Stage II	52	35	15
	Stage III	35	26	3
	Stage IV	238	32	16
	Unstaged	18	31	29
	All stages	468	39	22

Source: Data from SEER (1988–1995).

presumably had residual tumor and should be classified R1. Survival of patients not specifically treated was significantly reduced compared to those who had cancer-directed surgery.

Summary Because carcinoma of the extrahepatic bile ducts is relatively rare, there are only a limited number of reports that deal specifically with its prognostic factors. The most reliable factors include the extent of disease, histologic type (papillary versus nonpapillary), histological grade, and location of the primary tumor within the biliary tree. Data suggest that vascular invasion is also an important prognostic factor, especially in the proximal segments of the extrahepatic bile duct.[48] As a group, carcinomas of the extrahepatic bile ducts are detected at an earlier stage than carcinomas of the gallbladder, largely because obstructive symptoms appear while the tumor is relatively small. Nonetheless, the overall 5-year relative survival for malignant tumors of the extrahepatic bile duct is only 10%. Of all histological types, papillary carcinomas have been consistently associated with a favorable prognosis. Such a favorable outcome is probably related to the extent of tumor, since papillary carcinomas are less likely to penetrate the wall of the extrahepatic bile duct.[42,55] For example, in the SEER Program, 48% of patients with papillary carcinoma had localized disease (that is, confined to the extrahepatic bile duct), while only 15% of patients with mucinous carcinoma had localized disease. Because papillary carcinomas behave as insitu carcinomas, a conservative surgical approach such as segmental resection with frozen section of the surgical margins should be considered. Perhaps the most important prognostic factor is resectability of the primary tumor.[54] Proximal tumors are more difficult to resect because of their location in the hepatic hilum. Furthermore, carcinomas that arise in the hilum frequently invade adjacent structures, including the hepatic artery and portal vein. Better treatment results are observed in patients with tumors originating in the distal third of the common bile duct for which a pancreatoduodenectomy is possible.

In summary, the extent of tumor, histologic type, histologic grade, and location of the primary tumor are dependable prognostic factors for carcinoma of the extrahepatic bile duct. Other prognostic factors, such as performance status, clinical findings, DNA ploidy, and molecular changes, may be useful in many cases. For uniform reporting the extent of disease is usually recorded by the TNM staging system.[3,35] Residual tumor, which is often found at the margins of resection, is a powerful prognostic factor, for which additional treatment approaches are being explored.

CANCER OF THE AMPULLA OF VATER

Because cancers of the ampulla are relatively rare, research into the identification of useful prognostic factors has been limited. Carcinomas occurring in the ampulla are less common than those occurring in the gallbladder, in the extrahepatic bile ducts, or in the head of the pancreas. Clinically and pathologically, carcinomas arising in the ampulla may be difficult to separate from those arising in the head of the pancreas, or in the distal common bile duct, or even in the second part of the duodenum. Separation is especially difficult for large tumors. In some cases, it may even be difficult to establish a diagnosis, since large adenomas can conceal a small underlying carcinoma. Approximately 30% of ampullary carcinomas arise from preexisting adenomas.[56] Most of the malignant tumors in the ampulla are adenocarcinomas of the intestinal type, but undifferentiated and small-cell carcinomas have also been reported. Furthermore, the prevalence of ampullary carcinomas in patients with familial adenomatosis polyposis is higher than the prevalence of sporadic ampullary carcinomas.[2] The increased risk for carcinoma in these patients has been estimated to be 100–200 times greater than for sporadic cases.

Tumor-Related Factors

Clinical Observations Clinical findings are usually similar to those seen in cases of carcinoma of the extrahepatic bile ducts. There is often a sudden onset of jaundice due to bile-duct obstruction, weight loss, abdominal pain, and pancreatitis. Because of early obstruction, many tumors of the ampulla are detected while relatively small. About 70% of cases are found in stage I,[57,58] although some authors have reported lower figures. In SEER, 17% are confined to the ampulla at diagnosis. Usually weight loss and abdominal pain indicate more advanced-stage disease. With progression of the disease, performance status becomes a prognostic factor. Patients with ampullary carcinomas that arise in familial adenomatous polyposis are younger than those with sporadic carcinoma, probably related in part to earlier detection because of screening endoscopy.

Extent of Disease Extent of disease at diagnosis is the most reliable prognostic factor.[59,60] Carcinomas confined to the ampulla have the most favorable outcome. Direct extension is usually into the head of the pancreas and/or into the duodenum. Survival is also compromised if regional lymph nodes are involved.[56,61,62] In cases of negative nodes, the 5-year survival is 45%, but in patients with positive nodes, the 5-year survival drops to 10%.[61] The extent of disease is usually recorded using the TNM,[2,35] although a number of staging systems have been proposed.[63] Tumors are usually staged clinically by endoscopic ultrasonography or computed tomography before resection and pathologically after resection.[64] Table 21.8 shows the relative survival according to the TNM staging system. Host factors, such as anemia, may adversely impact on survival.

For endocrine tumors arising in the ampulla, liver metastasis is a major prognostic factor.[65]

Residual Tumor As in other anatomic sites, residual tumor is a significant prognostic factor. Factors associated with long survival include complete resection of tumor, negative surgical margins, and no lymph-node involvement.[66]

TABLE 21.8   Relative Survival of Patients with Cancer of the Ampulla of Vater According to Stage

Stage	Number of Cases	2-Year Survival (%)	5-Year Survival (%)
Stage 0	16	77	60
Stage I	121	72	49
Stage II	207	67	45
Stage III	140	49	22
Stage IV	100	21	15
Unstaged	197	35	14
All stages	781	51	31

Source: Data from SEER (1988–1995); cases staged according to the *AJCC Manual*.[3]

TABLE 21.9   Relative Survival of Ampullary Cancer According to Histologic Grade

Histologic Grade	Number of Cases	2-Year Survival (%)	5-Year Survival (%)
Grade 1	346	61	45
Grade 2	495	50	27
Grade 3	271	40	17
Grade 4	33	39	11

Source: Data from SEER (1973–1995).

Histological Type   Careful histological review is imperative because many tumors that arise in this region are carcinoids or functional endocrine tumors, which have a different outcome and clinical management than carcinomas. Of the carcinomas, the papillary types have the most favorable outcome. These types have a 2-year relative survival of 65% and a 5-year relative survival of 44%. Adenocarcinomas, in contrast, have a 2-year survival of 47% and a 5-year survival of 25%. Adenocarcinomas arising under a villous adenoma have a 2-year survival of 82% and a 5-year survival of 66%. Carcinoids, which constitute less than 2% of all tumors reported in the ampulla, have a 2-year survival of 60% and a 5-year survival of 55%.[1]

Histological Grade   The histological grade has been reported to be a determinant of outcome,[67,68] although this factor is much less useful than extent of disease. SEER data revealed a correlation between histological grade and outcome (Table 21.9).

Molecular Factors   Although K-*ras* mutations are commonly found in carcinomas of the ampulla, their occurrence has not correlated with survival.[69] There is evidence that the MIB-1 index and DNA ploidy, which assess cell proliferation rate, are important prognostic factors for resectable cases,[70] although further evaluation is needed.

Host Factors

Host prognostic factors can include predisposing conditions, such as familial adenomatosis polyposis, age, and comorbid diseases. Comorbid conditions may prevent complete resection of tumor.

Environmental Factors

Treatment Treatment is usually a pancreatoduodenectomy, since it offers the best chance for long-term survival. Overall, the 5-year relative survival, all stages combined, is about 30% (Table 21.8). Some authors advocate a localized resection for T1N0M0 tumors, especially in older patients, and for patients with advanced cancers. Treatment is usually based on the clinical evaluation of extent of disease.

Table 21.10 shows survival according to no surgery or to cancer-directed surgery for each stage of disease. No surgery means that the patient had no specific cancer-directed surgery, but may have had palliative surgery. Usually, these patients had metastatic disease or comorbid conditions. Cancer-directed surgery is defined as specific cancer-directed treatment. Most likely, patients who did not have cancer-directed surgery presumably had residual tumor and should be classified R1. For all stages, patients who did not have cancer-directed surgery had a significantly less favorable outcome that those who did.

Summary The most useful prognostic factor is the extent of tumor, which should be recorded according to the standard TNM staging system.[2,35] All investigators have observed a correlation between tumor extent and survival.

TABLE 21.10 Relative Survival According to No Surgery or Cancer-directed Surgery for Patients with Carcinoma of the Ampulla of Vater

Procedure	Stage	Number of Cases	2-Year Survival (%)	5-Year Survival (%)
No Surgery	Stage 0	6		
	Stage I	32	39	
	Stage II	36	16	6
	Stage III	13	22	12
	Stage IV	62	1	
	Unstaged	161	26	10
	All stages	310	21	7
Surgery	Stage 0	10	100	91
	Stage I	89	83	60
	Stage II	171	76	51
	Stage III	127	52	23
	Stage IV	38	55	36
	Unstaged	36	67	25
	All stages	471	69	43

Source: Data from SEER (1988–1995).

Initially, tumor seems to spread directly, extending into the pancreas, duodenum, and/or soft tissue adjacent to the ampulla, but lymph-node involvement eventually follows. Separation of primary tumors arising in the ampulla, head of pancreas, and distal common duct may be difficult. Papillary carcinomas have the best survival. However, these tumors constitute only 11% of all primary tumors arising in the ampulla. It should be noted that 38% of papillary tumors are found localized, while 30% of all adenocarcinomas are localized at diagnosis. Other authors have also observed better survival in the presence of papillary tumors.[71]

▬▬▬ APPENDIX 21A.1

TNM Classification: Gall Bladder

T — Primary Tumour

TX Primary tumor cannot be assessed

T0 No evidence of primary tumor

Tis Carcinoma in situ

T1 Tumor invades lamina propria or muscle layer

T1a Tumor invades lamina propria

T1b Tumor invades muscle layer

T2 Tumor invades perimuscular connective tissue, no extension beyond serosa or into liver

T3 Tumor perforates serosa (visceral peritoneum) or directly invades into one adjacent organ or both (extension 2 cm or less into liver)

T4 Tumor extends more than 2 cm into liver and/or into two or more adjacent organs (stomach, duodenum, colon, pancreas, omentum, extrahepatic bile ducts, any involvement of liver)

N — Regional Lymph Nodes

NX Regional lymph nodes cannot be assessed

N0 No regional lymph-node metastasis

N1 Metastasis in cystic duct, pericholedochal, and/or hilar lymph nodes (i.e., in the hepatoduodenal ligament)

N2 Metastasis in peripancreatic (head only), periduodenal, periportal, coeliac, and/or superior mesenteric lymph nodes

M — Distant Metastasis

MX Distant metastasis, cannot be assessed

M0 No distant metastasis

M1 Distant metastasis

Stage Grouping

Stage 0	Tis	N0	M0
Stage I	T1	N0	M0
Stage II	T2	N0	M0
Stage III	T1	N1	M0
	T2	N1	M0
	T3	N0, 1	M0
Stage IVA	T4	N0, 1	M0
Stage IVB	Any T	N2	M0
	Any T	Any N	M1

Source: Sobin LH, Wittekind Ch (eds.): *TNM Classification of Malignant Tumors*, 5th ed. New York, Union Internationale Centre le Cancer Wiley-Liss, 1997.

■■■■ **APPENDIX 21A.2**

TNM Classification: Extrahepatic Bile Duct

T — Primary Tumour

TX Primary tumor cannot be assessed

T0 No evidence of primary tumor

Tis Carcinoma in situ

T1 Tumor invades subepithelial connective tissue or fibromuscular layer

T1a Tumor invades subepithelial connective tissue

T1b Tumor invades fibromuscular layer

T2 Tumor invades perifibromuscular connective tissue

T3 Tumor invades adjacent structures: liver, pancreas, duodenum, gallbladder, colon, stomach

N — Regional Lymph Nodes

NX Regional lymph nodes cannot be assessed

N0 No regional lymph-node metastasis

N1 Metastasis in cystic duct, pericholedochal, and/or hilar lymph nodes (i.e., in the hepatoduodenal ligament)

N2 Metastasis in peripancreatic (head only), periduodenal, periportal, coeliac, superior mesenteric, posterior peripancreatico–duodenal lymph nodes

M — Distant Metastasis

MX Distant metastasis, cannot be assessed

M0 No distant metastasis

M1 Distant metastasis

Stage Grouping

Stage 0	Tis	N0	M0
Stage I	T1	N0	M0
Stage II	T2	N0	M0
Stage III	T1	N1, N2	M0
	T2	N1, N2	M0
Stage IVA	T3	Any N	M0
Stage IVB	Any T	Any N	M1

Source: Sobin LH, Wittekind Ch (eds.): *TNM Classification of Malignant Tumors*, 5th ed. New York. Union Internationale Centre le Cancer Wiley-Liss, 1997.

■■■■■■ **APPENDIX 21A.3**

TNM Classification: Ampulla of Vater

T — Primary Tumor

TX Primary tumor cannot be assessed

T0 No evidence of primary tumor

Tis Carcinoma in situ

T1 Tumor limited to ampulla of Vater or sphincter of Oddi

T2 Tumor invades duodenal wall

T3 Tumor invades 2 cm or less into pancreas

T4 Tumor invades more than 2 cm into pancreas and/or into other adjacent organs

N — Regional Lymph Nodes

NX Regional lymph nodes cannot be assessed

N0 No regional lymph-node metastasis

N1 Regional lymph-node metastasis

M — Distant Metastasis

MX Distant metastasis, cannot be assessed

M0 No distant metastasis

M1 Distant metastasis

Stage Grouping

Stage 0	Tis	N0	M0
Stage I	T1	N0	M0
Stage II	T2	N0	M0
	T3	N0	M0
Stage III	T1	N1	M0
	T2	N1	M0
	T3	N1	M0
Stage IV	T4	Any N M0	
	Any T	Any N M1	

Source: Sobin LH, Wittekind Ch (eds.): *TNM classification of malignant tumors*, 5th ed. New York, Union Internationale Centre le Cancer Wiley-Liss, 1997.

■■■■■■ **APPENDIX 21B.1**

Prognostic Factors Related to Survival for Cancers of the Gallbladder

	Tumor Related	Host Related	Environmental Related
Essential	TNM stage Clinical observations	Age Performance status	Treatment
Additional	Histological grade Histological type Vascular invasion Residual tumor		
New and promising			

■■■■■■ **APPENDIX 21B.2**

Prognostic Factors Related to Survival for Cancers of the Extrahepatic Bile Ducts

	Tumor Related	Host Related	Environmental Related
Essential	TNM stage	Age	Treatment
	Tumor location Clinical observations	Performance status	
Additional	Histological grade Residual tumor Histological type Perineural invasion		
New and promising			

■■■■■■ **APPENDIX 21B.3**

Prognostic Factors Related to Survival for Cancers of the Ampulla of Vater

	Tumor Related	Host Related	Environmental Related
Essential	TNM stage Clinical observations	Age Performance status Comorbidity	Treatment
Additional	Histological grade Histological type Residual tumor		
New and promising			

REFERENCES

1. SEER*Stat.: *SEER Cancer Incidence Public-Use Database, 1973-1996*, Bethesda, MD, National Cancer Institute, 1999.
2. Albores-Saavedra J, Henson DE, Klimstra D: *Tumors of the gallbladder, extrahepatic bile ducts, and ampulla of Vater 3rd ser.* Washington, DC, Armed Forces Institute of Pathology, 2000.

3. Fleming ID, Cooper JS, Henson DE, et al.: *AJCC cancer staging manual*, 5th ed, Philadelphia, Lippincott-Raven, 1997.

4. Benoist S, Panis Y, Fagniez PL: Long-term results after curative resection for carcinoma of the gallbladder. *Am J Surg* 175:118–22, 1990.

5. Pradeep R, Kaushik SP, Sikora SS, et al.: Predictors of survival in patients with carcinoma of the gallbladder. *Cancer* 76:1145–9, 1995.

6. Frezza EE, Mezghebe H: Gallbladder Carcinoma: A 28 year experience. *Int Surg* 82:295–300, 1997.

7. White K, Kraybill WG, Lopez MJ: Primary carcinoma of the gallbladder: TNM staging and prognosis. *J Surg Oncol* 39:251–5, 1988.

8. Donohue JH, Stewart AK, Menck HR: The National Cancer Data Base report on carcinoma of the gallbladder, 1989-1995. *Cancer* 83:2618–28, 1998.

9. Lee RG, Emond J: Prognostic factors and management of carcinomas of the gallbladder and extrahepatic bile ducts. *Surg Oncol Clinics North Am* 6:639–59, 1997.

10. Nevin JE, Moran TJ, Kay S, King R: Carcinoma of the gallbladder; Staging, treatment, and prognosis. *Cancer* 37:141–8, 1976.

11. Tsukada K, Kurosaki I, Uchida K, et al.: Lymph node spread from carcinoma of the gallbladder. *Cancer* 80:661-7, 1997.

12. Bergdahl L: Gallbladder carcinoma first diagnosed at microscopic examination of gallbladders removed for presumed benign disease. *Ann Surg* 191:19–22, 1980.

13. Kwon SY, Chang HJ: A clinicopathological study of unsuspected carcinoma of the gallbladder *J Korean Med Sci* 12:519–22, 1997.

14. Piehler JM, Crichlow RW: Primary carcinomas of the gallbladder. *Surg Gyn Obstet* 147:929–42, 1978.

15. Mori T, Souda S, Hashimoto J, et al.: Unsuspected gallbladder cancer diagnosed by laparoscopic cholecystectomy: A clinicopathological study. *Surg Today* 27:710–3, 1997.

16. Box JC, Edge SB: Laparoscopic cholecystectomy and unsuspected gallbladder carcinoma. *Semin Surg Oncol* 16:327–31, 1999.

17. Nagorney DM, McPherson GAD: Carcinoma of the gallbladder and extrahepatic bile ducts. *Semin Oncol* 15:106, 1988.

18. North JH, Jr, Pack MS, Hong C, Rivera DE: Prognostic factors for adenocarcinoma of the gallbladder: An analysis of 162 cases. *Am Surg* 64:437–40, 1998.

19. Albores-Saavedra J, Henson DE, Sobin LH: *Histological typing of tumors of the gallbladder and extrahepatic bile ducts.* Geneva, World Health Organization, 1991.

20. Albores-Saavedra J, Molberg K, Henson DE: Unusual malignant epithelial tumors of the gallbladder. *Semin Diagn Pathol* 13:326–38, 1996.

21. Nishihara K, Tsuneyoshi M: Undifferentiated spindle cell carcinoma of the gallbladder: A clinicopathologic, immunohistochemical, and flow cytometric study of 11 cases. *Hum Pathol* 24:1298–1305, 1993.

22. Henson DE, Albores-Saavedra J, Corle D: Carcinoma of the gallbladder: Histologic types, stage of disease, grade and survival rates. *Cancer* 70:1493–7, 1992.

23. Guo KJ, Yamaguchi K, Enjoji M: Undifferentiated carcinoma of the gallbladder: A clinicopathologic, histochemical, and immunohistochemical study of 21 patients with a poor prognosis. *Cancer* 61:1872–9, 1988.

24. White K, Kraybill WG, Lopez MJ: Primary carcinoma of the gallbladder; TNM staging and prognosis. *J Surg Oncol* 39:251–5, 1988.

25. Yamaguchi K, Enjoji M: Carcinoma of the gallbladder; A clinicopathology of 103 patients and newly proposed staging. *Cancer* 62:1425–32, 1988.

26. Suzuki T, Takano Y, Kakita A, Okudaira M: An immunohistochemical and molecular biological study of c-erb-2 amplification and prognostic relevance in gallbladder cancer. *Pathol Res Pract* 189:283–92, 1993.

27. Ajiki T, Onoyama H, Yamamoto M, et al.: p53 protein expression and prognosis in gallbladder carcinoma and premalignant lesions. *Hepatogastroenterology* 43:521–6, 1996.

28. Shrestha ML, Miyake H, Kikutsuji T, Tashiro S: Prognostic significance of Ki 67 and p53 antigen expression in carcinoma of the bile duct and gallbladder. *J Med Invest* 45:95–102, 1998.

29. Baretton G, Blasenbreu S, Vogt T, et al.: DNA ploidy in carcinoma of the gallbladder: Prognostic significance and comparison of flow and image cytometry in archival tumor material. *Pathol Res Pract* 190:584–92, 1994.

30. Okita S, Kondoh S, Shiraishi K, et al.: Expression of vascular endothelial growth factor correlates with tumor progression in gallbladder cancer. *Int J Oncol* 12:1013–8, 1998.

31. Sugawara Y, Makuuchi M, Harihara Y, et al.: Tumor angiogenesis in gallbladder carcinoma. *Hepatogastroenterology*, 46:1682–6, 1999.

32. Eguchi N, Fujii K, Tsuchida A, et al.: Cyclin E overexpression in human gallbladder carcinoma. *Oncol Rep* 6:93–6, 1999.

33. Hisatomi K, Haratake J, Horie A, Ohsato K: Relation of histopathological features to prognosis of gallbladder cancer. *Am J Gastroenterol* 85:567–72, 1990.

34. Sumiyoshi K, Nagai E, Chijiwa K, Nakayama F.: Pathology of carcinoma of the gallbladder. *World J Surg* 15:315–21, 1992.

35. Sobin LH, Wittekind C: *TNM classification of malignant tumors.* 5th ed New York, Wiley-Liss, 1997.

36. Chung C, Bautista N, O'Connell TX: Prognosis and treatment of bile duct carcinoma. *Am Surg* 64:921–5, 1998.

37. Alexander F, Rossi RL, O'Bryan M, et al.: Biliary Carcinoma; A review of 109 cases. *Am J Surg* 147:503–9, 1984.

38. Alden ME, Waterman FM, Topham AK, et al.: Cholangiocarcinoma: Clinical significance of tumor location along the extrahepatic bile duct. *Radiology* 197:511–6, 1995.

39. Tompkins RK, Thomas D, Wile A, Longmire WP: Prognostic factors in bile duct carcinoma; Analysis of 96 cases. *Ann Surg* 194:447–57, 1981.

40. Evander A, Fredlund P, Hoevels J, et al.: Evaluation of aggressive surgery for carcinoma of the extrahepatic bile ducts. *Ann Surg* 191:23–9, 1980.

41. Henson DE, Albores-Saavedra J, Corle D: Carcinoma of the extrahepatic bile ducts: histologic types, stage of disease, grade and survival rates. *Cancer* 70:1498, 1992.

42. Kozuka S, Tsubone M, Hachisuka K: Evolution of carcinoma in the extrahepatic bile ducts. *Cancer* 54:65–72, 1984.

43. Bhuiya MMR, Nimura Y, Kamiya J, et al.: Clinicpathologic studies on perineural invasion of bile duct carcinoma. *Ann Surg* 215:344–9, 1992.

44. Van Delden OM, de Wit LT, Nieveen van Dijkum EJ, et al.: Value of laparoscopic ultrasonography in staging of proximal bile duct tumors. *J Ultrasound Med* 16:7–12, 1997.

45. Yamaguchi K, Chijiiwa K, Saiki S, et al.: Carcinoma of the extrahepatic bile duct: Mode of spread and its prognostic implications. *Hepatogastroenterology* 44:1256–61, 1997.

46. Ogura Y, Takahashi K, Tabata M, Mizumoto R: Clinicopathological study on carcinoma of the extrahepatic bile-duct with special focus on cancer invasion on the surgical margins. *World J Surg* 18:778–84, 1994.

47. Kurosaki I, Tsukada K, Watanabe H, Hatakeyama K: Prognostic determinants in extrahepatic bile duct cancer. *Hepato-Gastroenterology* 45:905–9, 1998.

48. Ouchi K, Suzuki M, Hashimoto L, Sato T: Histologic findings and prognostic factors in carcinoma of the upper bile duct. *Am J Surg* 157:552–6, 1989.

49. Todoroki T, Okamura T, Fukao K, et al.: Gross appearance of carcinoma of the main hepatic duct and its prognosis. *Surg Gynecol Obstet* 150:33–40, 1980.

50. Nishida T, Nakao K, Hamaji M, et al.: Prognostic significance of proliferative cell nuclear antigen in carcinoma of the extrahepatic bile duct. *World J Surg* 21:634–9, 1997.

51. Rijken AM, van Gulik TM, Polak MM, et al.: Diagnostic and prognostic value of incidence of K-*ras* codon 12 mutations in resected distal bile duct carcinoma. *J Surg Oncol* 68:187–92, 1998.

52. Rijken AM, Umezawa A, van Gulik TM, et al.: Prognostic value of cell proliferation (Ki-67 antigen) and nuclear DNA content in clinically resectable, distal bile duct carcinoma. *Ann Surg Oncol* 5:699–705, 1998.

53. Takao S, Uchikura K, Yonezawa S, et al.: Mucin core protein expression in extrahepatic bile duct carcinoma is associated with metastases to the liver and poor prognosis. *Cancer* 86:1966–77, 1999.

54. Klempnauer J, Ridder GJ, von Wasielewski R, et al.: Resectional surgery of hilar cholangiocarcinoma: A multivariate analysis of prognostic factors. *J Clin Oncol* 15:947–54, 1997.

55. Albores-Saavedra, J, Murakata L, Krueger JE, Henson DE.: Non-invasive and minimally invasive papillary carcinomas of the extrahepatic bile ducts. *Cancer* 89:508–15, 2000.

56. Berger HG, Treitschke F, Gansauge F, et al.: Tumor of the ampulla of Vater: Experience with local or radical resections in 171 consecutively treated patients. *Arch Surg* 134:526–532, 1999.

57. Bakkevold KE, Arnesjo B, Kambestad B: Carcinoma of the pancreas and papilla of Vater; Presenting symptoms, signs, and diagnosis related to stage and tumor site. *Scand J Gastroenterol* 27:317–25, 1992.

58. Schlippert W, Lucke D, Anuras S, Christensen J: Carcinoma of the papilla of Vater: A review of fifty-seven cases. *Am J Surg* 135:763–70, 1978.

59. Yamaguchi K, Enjoji M: Carcinoma of the ampulla of Vater. A clincopathologic study and pathologic staging of 109 cases of carcinoma and 5 cases of adenoma. *Cancer* 59:506–15, 1987.

60. Barton RM, Copeland EM, III: Carcinoma of the ampulla of Vater. *Surg Gynecol Obstet* 156:297–301, 1983.

61. Su CH, Shyr YM, Lui WY, P'eng FK: Factors affecting morbidity, mortality and survival after pancreaticoduodenectomy for carcinoma of the ampulla of Vater. *Hepatogastroenterol* 46:1973–9, 1999.

62. Bakkevold KE, Kambestad B: Staging of carcinoma of the pancreas and ampulla of Vater. *Int J Pancreas* 17:249–59, 1995.

63. Talbot IC, Neoptolemos JP, Shaw DE, Carr-Locke D: The histopathology and staging of carcinoma of the ampulla of Vater. *Histopathology* 12:155–65, 1988.

64. Mukai H, Yasuda K, Nakajima M: Tumors of the papilla and distal common bile duct. *Gastrointest Endos(c) Clin North Am* 5:763–72, 1995.

65. Madeira I, Terris B, Voss M, et al.: Prognostic factors in patients with endocrine tumors of the duodenopancreatic area. *Gut* 43:422–7, 1998.

66. Howe JR, Klimstra DS, Moccia RD, et al.: Factors predictive of survival in ampullary carcinoma. *Ann Surg* 228:87–94, 1998.

67. Monge JJ, Judd ES, Gage RP: Radical pancreatoduodenectomy: A 22-year experience with the complications, mortality rate and survival rate. *Ann Surg* 160:711–22, 1964.

68. Neoptolemos JP, Talbot IC, Shaw DC, Carr-Locke DL: Long-term survival after resection of ampullary carcinoma is associated independently with tumor grade and a new staging classification that assesses local invasiveness. *Cancer* 61:1403–7, 1988.

69. Howe JR, Klimstra DS, Cordon-Cardo C, et al.: K-ras mutation in adenomas and carcinomas of the ampulla of Vater. *Clin Cancer Res* 3:129–33, 1997.

70. Shyr YM, Su CH, Wu LH, et al.: Prognostic value of MIB-1 index and DNA ploidy in resectable ampulla of Vater carcinoma. *Ann Surg* 229:523–7, 1999.

71. Makipour H, Cooperman A, Danzi JT, Farmer RG: Carcinoma of the ampulla of Vater. *Ann Surg* 183:341–4, 1976.

CHAPTER 22

Cancer of the Pancreas

JÜRGEN D. RODER and KATJA OTT

Pancreatic cancer remains an important cause of death in many nations. In most patients pancreatic adenocarcinoma is diagnosed at a stage of disease that is not curable by surgery and can only be little affected by multimodality treatment options (chemotherapy, radiotherapy, immunotherapy). Surgery is the only curative approach, but success with resection is low and the prognosis remains extremely poor, for example, patients with completely resected tumors have a 5-year survival rate of 15–28%.[1,2] The overall 5-year survival remains extremely low despite a slight improvement during the last few years: figures of 1–3% for all,[3] and 5–25% for resected patients[3–5] are reported.

More than 90–95% of carcinomas of the pancreas are exocrine tumors. Over 90% of these tumors, as referred to in the World Health Organization (WHO) classification,[6] are ductal adenocarcinomas, including rare types, such as mucinous noncystic, adenosquamous, anaplastic, and osteoblast-like giant-cell carcinoma. The mucinous cystadenocarcinoma (about 1% of all cases or 5% of resected cases) had a relatively good prognosis[7–9] and a 5-year survival rate of 54.3% in a Japanese study. Also, the uncommon intraductal papillary mucinous adenocarcinoma has a better prognosis than the common ductal adenocarcinoma.[7,8] These two tumor types, as well as the carcinoma in situ, are excluded in the following review of prognostic factors.

The most important prognostic factor is the possibility of curative resection.[5] The outcome of patients who undergo resection is definitely superior to those not undergoing resection. In the literature the resection rates for exocrine pancreatic carcinoma range from 2.6% to 30%.[5,10,11] In contrast to patients without resection, who practically never show a long-term survival rate, in specialized centers resected patients show a 5-year survival rate of 20–25%.[10,11] The median survival time for resected patients is 10–20 months.[11,12] Therefore, the prognostic factors for those patients who have not been resected will be discussed separately in the section on treatment-related prognostic factors.

Prognostic Factors in Cancer, 2nd edition, Edited by Mary K. Gospodarowicz
ISBN 0-471-40633-3   Copyright © 2001 Wiley-Liss, Inc.

Due to the small number of resected patients and the poor prognosis, the importance of several prognostic factors still remains unclear, because most studies are based on univariate analysis. Only a few studies with more than 100 resected patients analyzed by multivariate analysis have been published.[11,13,14]

In the following analysis of prognostic factors, the relevant international literature will be considered. Problems in reviewing the actual literature are that often carcinomas of the head of the pancreas are not separated from those of the ampulla of Vater and the distal bile duct, which have a better prognosis. Furthermore, in 1997 the new International Union Against Cancer Tumors, Nodules, Metastases (UICC TNM) classification (5th ed.)[15] was published this manual relates better to prognosis than does the old classification (4th ed.).[16,17] Also, in the interpretation of prognostic factors, the reduction of perioperative mortality to less than 5% also has to be considered.[5,18]

TUMOR-RELATED FACTORS

Essential Factors

The prognosis of a patient with pancreatic ductal adenocarcinoma depends primarily on the anatomic extent defined by the TNM classification and stage grouping (see Appendix 22A). The 5th Edition of TNM (1997)[15] contains some changes for exocrine pancreatic carcinoma, which is now comparable to the other gastrointestinal (GI) tumors that are divided into four categories. T1 (tumor size ≤ 2 cm) and T2 (tumor size >2 cm) tumors are limited to the pancreas; T3 invades directly any of the following tissues: duodenum, bile duct, or peripancreatic tissue; T4 involves one or more adjacent organs: stomach, spleen, colon, or adjacent large vessels. Infiltration of the vessels of the spleen is classified as T3.[15] Univariate analysis revealed that survival rates for patients with a tumor limited to the pancreas (former T1 and now T1/2) are better than with more advanced tumor stages[17,19] (Figure 22.1). According to clinical experience, only a few tumors were observed in the pT1 or pT2 categories, while 87–97% presented as pT3 or pT4 tumors.[17,20]

The inclusion of a pT4 category equivalent to the other GI tumors made a new stage grouping necessary. There was a significant improvement in the patients' distribution to the new stage grouping, because of the homogenous groups. In comparison to the 1987/92 classification, the prognostic relevance of the new stage II is improved[17,21] (Figure 22.1).

Lymph-node metastases showed a definitive influence on the prognosis of ductal pancreatic adenocarcinoma. The weakening of prognosis by lymph-node metastasis in univariate analysis is described by Klempauer et al.[13] and Kayahara et al.,[22] as well as by Magistrelli et al.[23] for multivariate analysis. In some studies, however, lymph-node involvement is not of statistical significance.[24] Most of the former studies were based only on the differentiation between node-positive and node-negative patients. To improve the prognostic relevance of lymph-node staging, differentiation between single- and multiple-lymph-node metastases was established.[25–27] Hermanek showed that if two or more lymph nodes were

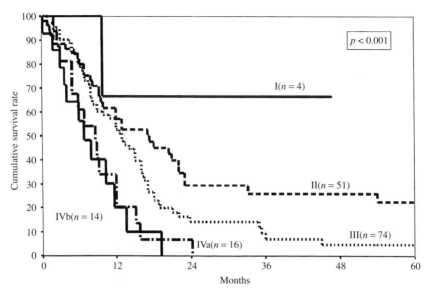

Figure 22.1   Prognostic factors in ductal adenocarcinoma: UICC stage.[17]

involved, a dramatic worsening of prognosis following resection for cure was observed.[26] Cohen[25] reported a 0% 5-year survival rate if only one lymph node was involved. This fact was considered in the new TNM 5th Edition of 1997, and the division in pN1a and pN1b was introduced. The prognosis between pN0 and pN1a/b was significantly different in several studies.[13,22,23,28] The significant difference between pN1a and pN1b in 5-year survival as shown by Compton[29] cannot be proven by other investigators.[17] (Figure 22.2).

No significant correlation could be noted between tumor size and nodal involvement.[20,24,30] Forty-two percent of patients with tumors smaller than 2.5 cm in diameter showed lymph-node metastases that resulted in a bad prognosis.[24,31,32]

In earlier studies, lymph-node involvement was caused a worse prognosis than did involvement of adjacent large vessels.[27] Today, lymph-node involvement results in stage III, while infiltration of adjacent organs and vessels, correlating with the definitive deterioration of prognosis, results in stage IV. This change may be based on the extended standard lymph-node dissection with respect to the complex lymphatic drainage of the head of the pancreas improving prognosis in recent years.[20,27,33]

Direct extension of the tumor into adjacent peripancreatic tissue as well as into peripancreatic organs was found to significantly influence survival. Tumor infiltration in lymphatic vessels was present in up to 74% of the resected carcinomas and significantly correlated with shorter survival time. It had been suggested that the frequency of tumor invasion relates strongly with tumor size. For example, retroperitoneal invasion was found in 19.3% of tumors 2 cm or less in size, and in 89.5% in tumors greater than 6 cm in size. In some publications multivariate analysis has shown that tumor size is the strongest determinant of

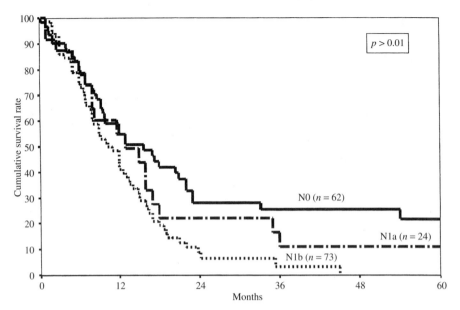

Figure 22.2   Prognostic factors in ductal adenocarcinoma: lymph-node metastases.[17]

prognosis, even more so than lymph-node metastasis and tumor stage. Tumors larger than 2.5 cm had a lower survival rate than smaller tumors (33% 5-year survival versus 12%).[13,24] In other series, tumor diameter had no influence on survival.[23] Therefore, tumor size per se seems not to be an independent determinant of prognosis, but relates to invasion of lymphatic vessels, large vessels, peripancreatic tissues, and adjacent organs.

There are conflicting reports on the prognostic influence of histological grade. In the analyses of Klempnauer et al.,[13] Geer and Brennan,[11] and Giulianotti et al.,[34] tumor grade was an independent prognostic factor. Geer's 5-year survival for poorly differentiated tumors was 10% compared to nearly 50% for well-differentiated tumors. No differences in survival rates were reported by other investigators.[23]

In the multivariate analysis carried out by Geer and Brennan,[11] tumor localization had no influence on prognosis. According to most studies the prognosis for tumors of the head of the pancreas seems to be more favorable than other sites, but this still has not been established.[35,36] Generally, tumors of the body and tail of the pancreas are diagnosed at more advanced stages due to a lack of symptoms.[37,38] A 5-year survival of up to 14% is reported for tumors of the body and tail treated by resection.[35,36]

Additional Factors

Recent publications demonstrated that the detection of cytokeratin-positive cells in bone marrow and peritoneal lavage in the case of gastric and colorectal cancer could serve as a new prognostic factor.[39] Up to now, there has been no conclusive data concerning the clinical implication of such minimal residual disease in pancreatic cancer. Few studies investigating peritoneal lavage and bone marrow samples to determine the predictive value of detected disseminated tumor cells have been performed. Univariate analysis revealed that when disseminated tumor cells were present in the bone marrow detection by immunocytochemical methods was predictive of reduced overall survival.[40] Furthermore, the detection of tumor cells in the peritoneal cavity correlated significantly with the survival time of the patients. All of the patients showing minimal residual disease in at least one compartment (52%) died within 18 months, whereas the negative patients showed a 5-year survival rate of 30%.[41] These results show potential for determining prognosis of pancreatic cancer.

New and Promising Factors

It has been reported that pancreatic carcinoma-cell DNA content influences overall prognosis. Allison et al. found that patients with diploid tumors survived significantly longer than did aneuploid patients (median of 25 months versus 10.5 months). In multivariate analysis, DNA content was a strong independent prognostic factor.[2,19,42]

In general, pancreatic tumors seem a high degree of global genetic instability.[43,44] Recent molecular biological analysis generated the hypothesis that abnormalities in tumor suppressor genes and oncogenes can be loosely correlated with prognosis. Tumors with a mutation of the tumor suppressor gene p53 seem to have a shorter survival.[45] Evaluation of the three tumor suppressor genes p16, p53, and DPC4 showed that the inactivation of all three genes served as a risk factor for death from disease.[46] Positive immunohistochemical staining for p53 and/or Bcl-2 overexpression were, on univariate and multivariate analysis, to be independent predictors of survival.[47] In multivariate analysis weak expression of the proto-oncogene Ki-67 was the most important determinant for long-term survival.[48] The evaluation of pancreatic carcinoma patients with a mutant-type K-ras oncogene in plasma DNA showed a significantly shorter survival time compared to patients with the wild-type gene, and plasma K-ras mutations were identified as the only prognostic factors in this study.[49]

The expression of various growth factors have been analyzed immunohisto-chemically and related to prognosis. By multivariate analysis expression of vascular endothelial growth factor (VEGF) was shown to be an independent prognostic factor[50] and correlated with a significantly shorter survival. In contrast, Ellis et al.[51] reported that neither VEGF expression nor vessel count are predictors of survival.

The positive coexpression of epidermal growth factor (EGF) and its receptor (EGFR) were strongly associated with poor prognosis,[52] while TGF-beta expression seemed to be a stage-independent predictor of patients' survival.[53]

FDG-PET was also considered for identifying patients with good prognosis by determining the degree of FDG-integration. The patients with low standardized uptake value (SUV) had a significantly longer survival time (14 months versus 5 months).[54]

Further progress will be necessary for understanding the value of various molecular genetic abnormalities in determining the prognosis in patients with pancreatic cancer.

HOST-RELATED FACTORS

There are no proven host-related factors related to the demographics that influence a patient's prognosis. Neither age, gender, race, nor presenting symptoms demonstrated an independent influence on prognosis.[55,56] However, some authors reported a better prognosis for patients with a good performance status.[57]

ENVIRONMENT-RELATED FACTORS

Essential Factors

The most important treatment-related factor is the possibility of resection.[3,58] A comparison of annual crude survival rates according to the treatment received (resection versus bypass versus laparotomy alone versus supportive care) showed highly significant survival differences between treatment groups (1-year survival: resection, 30.6%; supportive care, 2%).[5] Therefore, for patients without resection due to the poor prognosis, we can expect to see only a limited number of prognostic factors. The only independent negative prognostic factor for unresected patients in multivariate analysis was jaundice on presentation. In patients with palliative surgical treatment, such as bypass surgery or laparotomy, only infiltration of the superior mesenteric vein, regional lymph-node metastasis, and weight loss led to a reduction in the prognosis. In this study surgical procedure (laparotomy, biliary bypass, or double bypass) did not influence survival.[55,56] In a retrospective study on 13,560 patients in the West Midlands of Great Britain, made between 1977 and 1986, 1-year survival with resection was 30.6%, with bypass surgery 15.1%, with diagnostic laparotomy 4.4% and with supportive care 2.0%. The percentage receiving only supportive care increased to 47.8% in the period 1977–1986, compared to the period 1957–1976. The overall resection rate was only 2.6% during both periods.[5]

For long-term survival, a complete resection is essential. For resected patients the strongest predictor of outcome is the presence of residual tumor (R).[59] The most valuable prognostic factor was curative resection, as shown by univariate and multivariate analysis.[13,19] In contrast, in some studies negative resection margins did not improve prognosis significantly (5-year survival: 12% vs. 7%).[23] In R1 resections (microscopic residual tumor), residual tumor was located in most of the cases at the retroperitoneal resection margin, 73%[60] and 88%.[61]

Radical resection to cure pancreatic carcinoma (partial, subtotal, or total duodenopancreatectomy, subtotal left pancreatectomy) includes en bloc dissection of the regional lymph nodes and the surrounding connective tissue with its lymphatic and perineural spaces. Improvements in surgical technique and postoperative patient care have led to an impressive decrease in the high morbidity and mortality after pancreatic resection. If the tumor can be resected at an early stage, and the regional lymph nodes are not involved, median 5-year survival rates of 20–40% are commonly reported. Further approaches include more radical surgery with dissection of the entire pancreatic region and resection of the upper abdominal blood vessels.[62] However, portal vein resection performed on 31 patients did not prolong survival in patients undergoing partial pancreatoduodenectomy for carcinoma of the pancreas or bile duct.[33]

Furthermore there is some evidence, especially from clinical experience in Japan, that wider lymphatic resection (i.e., wider than those commonly done with the standard Whipple resection) may prolong survival.[63] For prognosis, the ratio of metastatic lymph nodes to resected lymph nodes also indicates that an extensive lymph-node dissection can increase long-term survival.[20] Reported results of these extended procedures have varied considerably and concomitant morbidity has often exceeded that of standard resection.[64]

There are three important studies concerning the wide dissection of lymph nodes and connective tissue that demonstrate an improvement in survival, but with perioperative mortality ranging from 5–17%.[65–67] On the basis of these results, wide dissection of lymph nodes and connective tissue is not indicated in an advanced tumor stage.[68] Most of the data available are retrospective and are not randomized between the standard and radical operation. Therefore, before any modification of the standard pancreaticoduodenectomy is adopted, appropriately designed studies should test its efficacy.

Patient volume of a hospital is a strong prognostic indicator. Gordon et al.[69] and Sosa et al.[70] reported that hospital mortality after pancreaticoduodenectomy was up to six times lower in high-volume centers compared to smaller hospitals.

Additional Factors Application of postoperative adjuvant therapy is still controversial. In some studies, the survival of patients treated with radical surgery alone was significantly poorer than that of patients who received adjuvant radiation therapy. In the study by Dobelbowers et al.,[71] patients treated with all three modalities (surgery, intraoperative radiation therapy, and external beam radiation therapy) displayed the best median survival (17.5 months median).[71] Also DiCarlos' investigation showed that, according to univariate and multivariate analysis, adjuvant treated patients had a survival rate comparable to that of patients without adjuvant therapy. Similarly, patients treated with a combination of intraoperative radiotherapy, chemotherapy, and radiotherapy had significantly better survival outcome.[72] In contrast, Geer and Brennan could not prove longer survival for adjuvant treated patients.[11] Also, indications are that the use of radiotherapy alone or chemotherapy alone improves postoperative survival.[73,74]

Studies in this area often are hampered by being nonrandomized and with too few patients. Overall, there is now no adjuvant treatment model that can be suggested for routine use.[75]

New and promising factors To increase resectablity and the rate of complete resections of pancreatic cancer, neoadjuvant concepts, consisting mostly of combined radio and chemotherapy similar to other GI tumors, have been established.[76,77] Available data for neoadjuvant treatment approaches are not based on randomized studies. Promising therapeutic innovations include cytokine-secreting pancreatic adenocarcinoma vaccine made from primary pancreatic adenocarcinoma, which was used in human trials.[78] In addition, the inhibition of tumor-associated angiogenesis and related processes could conceivably form the foundation upon which the treatment of aggressive malignancies such as pancreatic cancer is based.[79]

SCENARIOS

At the moment, surgical resection remains the only chance for cure for pancreatic cancer. The main clinical issue in patients with a malignant tumor is to identify the ones who would benefit from surgical treatment. Resection of pancreatic cancer bares the only, albeit small, chance of cure, and the possible advantages in terms of prognosis and quality of life should be balanced with surgical mortality and morbidity. The decision to perform a palliative resection in patients with a ductal adenocarcinoma of the pancreas should be made by an experienced surgeon, who is capable of performing an intraoperative risk benefit analysis for the individual patient.[80] For this reason, the management of this disease involves a multidisciplinary approach, and the surgeon should join with the other specialists in oncologic centers.

At the time of diagnosis, the most important prognostic factors are a correct clinical staging and evaluation of resectability. To avoid incomplete resections, extensive clinical staging to exclude distant metastases and unresectability has to be performed.

For patients with curatively resected tumors, anatomic extent (TNM classification) is the main accepted prognostic factor. In the future, tumor biology with molecular markers might become more important for prediction of survival.

Improvement in noninvasive imaging techniques may enhance the possibility of early diagnosis and less invasive staging. In the future, molecular genetics might allow earlier detection of pancreatic cancer. Probably improvement in adjuvant therapy, perhaps combined modality (radiation/chemotherapy) or immunotherapy, will be able to increase disease-free and overall survival. Potentially genetic mapping of tumors could make early response prediction to neoadjuvant or adjuvant treatment concepts.

■■■■■■■ **APPENDIX 22A**

TNM Classification for Pancreatic Cancer

T — Primary Tumor

TX Primary tumor cannot be assessed

T0 No evidence of primary tumor

Tis Carcinoma in situ

T1 Tumor limited to the pancreas, 2 cm or less in greatest dimension

T2 Tumor limited to the pancreas, more than 2 cm in greatest dimension

T3 Tumor extends directly into any of the following: duodenum, bile duct, peripancreatic tissues

T4 Tumor extends directly into any of the following: stomach, spleen, colon, adjacent large vessels

N — Regional Lymph Nodes

NX Regional lymph nodes cannot be assessed

N0 No regional lymph-node metastasis

N1 Regional lymph-node metastasis

    N1a Metastasis in a single regional lymph node

    N1b Metastasis in multiple regional lymph nodes

M — Distant Metastasis

MX Distant metastasis cannot be assessed

M0 No distant metastasis

M1 Distant metastasis

Stage Grouping

Stage 0	Tis	N0	M0
Stage I	T1	N0	M0
	T2	N0	M0
Stage II	T3	N0	M0
Stage III	T1	N1	M0
	T2	N1	M0
	T3	N1	M0
Stage IVA	T4	Any N	M0
Stage IVB	Any T	Any N	M1

Source: Sobin LH, Wittekind Ch (eds.): *TNM classification of malignant tumors*, 5th ed. New York, Union Internationale Contre le Cancer Wiley-Liss, 1997.

■■■■■■■ **APPENDIX 22B**

Prognostic Factors in Pancreatic Cancer

Prognostic Factors	Tumor Related	Host Related	Environment Related
Essential	TNM classification *Lymph-node metastasis* Infiltration of peripancreatic tissue and organs Lymphatic vessel invasion *Tumor size* *Curative resection (R0)*		Possibility of resection High volume centers
Additional	Disseminated tumor cells in the bone marrow Disseminated tumor cells in the peritoneal cavity	Performance status	*Adjuvant therapy*
New and promising	DNA content Genetic instability Tumor suppressor genes *p53*, p16, DPC4, Bcl-2 Protooncogenes: Ki-67 Oncogenes *K-ras* Growth factors *VEGF* EGF/EGFR TGF-beta FDG-PET		Neoadjuvant concepts Antiangiogenesis Cytokine-secreting pancreatic adeno-carcinoma vaccine

REFERENCES

1. Beger HG: Prognosefaktoren beim Pankreaskarzinom. *Langenbecks Arch Chir* 380:131–2, 1995.
2. Yeo CJ, Cameron JL, Lillemoe KD, et al.: Pancreaticoduodenectomy for cancer of the head of the pancreas: 201 patients. *Ann Surg* 221:721–33, 1995.
3. Carr JA, Ajlouni M, Wollner I, et al.: Adenocarcinoma of the head of the pancreas: Effects of surgical and non surgical therapy on survival-a ten-year experience. *Am Surg* 65:1143–9, 1999.

4. Yeo CJ, Sohn TA, Cameron JL, et al.: Periampullary adenocarcinoma: Analysis of 5-year survivors. *Ann Surg* 227:821–31, 1998.

5. Bramhall SR, Allum WH, Jones AG, et al.: Treatment and survival in 13560 patients with pancreatic cancer, and incidence of the disease, in the West Midlands: An epidemiological study. *Br J Surg* 82:111–5, 1995.

6. Kloppel G, Solcia E, Longnecker DS, et al.: Histological typing of tumors of the exocrine pancreas, 2nd ed., in WHO International Histological Classification of Tumors. Berlin-New York, Springer-Verlag, 1996.

7. Yeo CJ, Cameron JL, Sohn TA, et al.: Six hundred fifty consecutive pancreatico-duodenectomies in the 1990s: Pathology, complications, and outcomes. *Ann Surg* 226:248–57, 1997.

8. Le Borgne J, de Calan L, Partensky C: Cystadenomas and cystadenocarcinomas of the pancreas: A multiinstitutional retrospective study of 398 cases. French Surgical Association. *Ann Surg* 230:152–61, 1999.

9. Rosewicz S, Wiedenmann B: Pancreatic carcinoma. *Lancet* 349:485–9, 1997.

10. Sener SF, Fremgen A, Menck HR, Winchester DP: Pancreatic cancer: A report of treatment and survival trends for 100,313 patients diagnosed from 1985–1995, using the National Cancer Database. *J Am Coll Surg* 189:1–7, 1999.

11. Geer RJ, Brennan MF: Prognostic indicators for survival after resection of pancreatic adenocarcinoma. *Am J Surg* 165:68–73, 1993.

12. Millikan KW, Deziel DJ, Silverstein JC, et al.: Prognostic factors associated with resectable adenocarcinoma of the head of the pancreas. *Am Surg* 65:618–23, 1999.

13. Klempnauer J, Ridder GJ, Bektas H, Pichlmayr R: Multivariate analysis of prognostic factors after resection of ductal pancreatic carcinomas. *Langenbecks Arch Chir* 380:133–8, 1995.

14. Schwarz RE, Harrison LE, Conlon KC, et al.: The impact of splenectomy on outcomes after resection of pancreatic adenocarcinoma. *J Am Coll Surg* 188:516–21, 1999.

15. Sobin LH, Wittekind Ch (ed.): *UICC: TNM Classification of malignant tumours*, 5th ed. New York, Wiley-Liss, 1997.

16. Hermanek P, Sobin LH (ed.): *TNM Classification of malignant tumors*, 4th ed. Heidelberg-New York, Springer-Verlag, 1987; (rev.) 1992.

17. Ott K, Böttcher K, Werner M, et al.: Erlaubt die neue UICC-Klassifikation eine bessere Prognoseabschätzung für das duktale Pankreaskarzinom? *Chirurg*, 71:189–95, 2000.

18. Yeo CJ, Cameron JL: Improving results for pancreaticoduodenectomy for pancreatic cancer. *World J Surg*, 23:907–12, 1999.

19. Takada T, Yasuda H: A search for prognostic factors in cancer of the pancreatic head: The significance of the DNA ploidy pattern. *Surg Oncol* 4:237–43, 1995.

20. Böttger T, Boddin J, Küchle R, Junginger T: Hat das Ausmaß der Lymphknotendis-sektion einen Einfluß auf die Morbidität und Prognose nach Pankreaskopfresektion wegen eines duktalen oder periampullären Panpreaskarzinoms? *Langenbecks Arch Chir* 382:209–15, 1997.

21. Tsunoda T, Toshifumi E, Tsuchiya R: Clinical comparison of UICC and Japanese Classifications Japanese experience. *Int J Pancreatol* 16:105, 1994.

22. Kayahara M, Nagakawa T, Ueno K, et al.: Surgical strategy for carcinoma of the pancreas head area based on clinicopathologic analysis of nodal involvement and plexus invasion. *Surgery* 117:616–23, 1995.

23. Magistrelli P, Antinori A, Crucitti A, et al.: Surgical resection of pancreatic cancer. *Tumori* 85:22–6, 1999.

24. Fortner J, Klimstra D, Senie R, Maclean B: Tumor size is the primary prognosticator for pancreatic cancer after regional pancreatectomy. *Ann Surg* 223:147–53, 1996.

25. Cohen JR, Kuchta N, Geller N, et al.: Pancreatduodenectomy: A 40-year experience. *Ann Surg* 195:608–17, 1982.

26. Hermanek P: Chirurgische Pathologie des Pankreaskarzinoms, in Trede M, Saeger HD (eds.): *Aktuelle Pankreaschirurgie*. Berlin, Springer-Verlag, 1990, p. 3.

27. Ishikawa O, Ohigashi H, Sasaki Y, et al.: Practical grouping of positive lymph nodes in pancreatic head cancer treated by an extended pancreatectomy. *Surgery* 121:244–9, 1997.

28. Yeo CJ, Cameron JL: Prognostic factors in ductal pancreatic cancer. *Langenbeck's Arch Surg* 383:129–33, 1998.

29. Compton C, Henson D: Protocol for the examination of specimens removed from patients with carcinoma of the exocrine pancreas. *Arch Pathol Lab Med* 121:1129–36, 1997.

30. Kayahara M, Nagakawa T, Futagami F, et al.: Lymphatic flow and neural plexus invasion associated with carcinoma of the body and tail of the pancreas. *Cancer* 78:2485–91, 1996.

31. Hermanek P: Pathology and biology of pancreatic ductal adenocarcinoma. *Langenbeck's Arch Surg* 383:116–20, 1998.

32. Warshaw AL: Prevalence and patterns of spread in early pancreatic adenocarcinoma. *Int J Pancreatol* 16:225, 1994.

33. Roder JD, Stein HJ, Siewert JR: Carcinoma of the periampullary region: Who benefits from portal vein resection? *Am J Surg* 171:170–4, 1996.

34. Giulianotti PC, Boggi U, Fornaciari G, et al.: Prognostic value of histological grading in ductal adenocarcinoma of the pancreas. Kloppel vs TNM grading. *Int J Pancreatol* 17:279–89, 1995.

35. Brennan MF, Moccia RD, Klimstra D: Management of adenocarcinoma of the body and tail of the pancreas. *Ann Surg* 223:506–11, 1996.

36. Sperti C, Pasquali C, Pedrazzoli S: Ductal adenocarcinoma of the body and tail of the pancreas. *J Am Coll Surg* 185:255–9, 1997.

37. DiMagno: Pancreatic cancer: Clinical presentation, pitfalls and early clues. *Ann Oncol* 4:140–2, 1999.

38. Nakao A, Harada A, Nonami T, et al.: Lymph node metastases in carcinoma of the body and tail of the pancreas. *Br J Surg* 84:1090–2, 1997.

39. Nekarda H, Gess C, Stark M, et al.: Immunocytochemically detected free peritoneal tumor cells (FPTC) are strong prognostic factor in gastric carcinoma. *Br J Cancer* 79:611–9, 1999.

40. Roder JD, Thorban S, Pantel K, Siewert JR: Micrometastases in bone marrow: Prognostic indicators for pancreatic cancer. *World J Surg* 23:888–91, 1999.

41. Vogel I, Kruger U, Marxsen J, et al.: Disseminated tumor cells in pancreatic cancer patients detected by immunocytology: A new prognostic factor. *Clin Cancer Res* 5:593–9, 1999.

42. Allison DC, Bose KK, Hruban RH et al.: Pancreatic cancer cell DNA content correlates with long term survival after pancreaticoduodenectomy. *Ann Surg* 214:648–56, 1991.

43. Seymour AB, Hruban RH, Redston M, et al.: Allelotype of pancreatic adenocarcinoma. *Cancer Res* 54:2761–4, 1994.

44. Brat DJ, Hahn SA, Griffin CA, et al.: The structural basis of molecular genetic deletions: An integration of classical cytogenetic and molecular analysis of pancreatic adenocarcinoma. *Am J Pathol* 150:383–91, 1997.

45. DiGiuseppe JA, Yeo CJ, Hruban RH: Molecular biology and the diagnosis and treatment of adenocarcinoma of the pancreas. *Adv Anat Pathol* 3:139–55, 1996.

46. Rozenblum E, Schutte M, Goggins M, et al.: Tumor suppressive pathways in pancreatic carcinoma. *Cancer Res* 57:1731–4, 1997.

47. Ferrara C, Tessari G, Poletti A, et al.: Ki-67 and c-jun expression in pancreatic cacner: A prognostic marker? *Oncol Rep* 6:1117–22, 1999.

48. Bold RJ, Hess KR, Pearson AS, et al.: Prognostic factors in resectable pancreatic cancer: p53 and Bcl-2. *J Gastrointest Surg* 3:263–77, 1999.

49. Castells A, Puig P, Mora J, et al.: K-ras mutations in DANN extracted from the plasma of patients with pancreatic carcinoma: Diagnostic utility and prognostic significance. *J Clin Oncol* 17:578–84, 1999.

50. Ikeda N, Adachi M, Taki T, et al.: Prognostic significance of angiogenesis in human pancreatic cancer. *Br J Surg* 79:1553–63, 1999.

51. Ellis LM, Takahashi Y, Fenoglio CJ, et al.: Vessel counts and vascular endothelial growth factor expression in pancreatic adenocarcinoma. *Eur J Cancer* 34:337–40, 1998.

52. Dong M, Nio Y, Guo KJ, et al.: Epidermal growth factor and its receptor as prognostic indicators in Chinese patients with pancreatic cancer. *Anticancer Res* 18:4613–9, 1998.

53. Coppola D, Lu L, Fruehauf JP, et al.: Analysis of p53, p21WAF1 and TGF-beta1 in human ductal adenocarcinoma of the pancreas: TGF-beta1 protein expression predicts longer survival. *Am J Clin Pathol* 110:16–23, 1998.

54. Nakata B, Chung YS, Nishimura S, et al.: 18F-fluorodeoxyglucose positron emission tomography and the prognosis of patients with pancreatic adenocarcinoma. *Cancer* 79:695–9, 1997.

55. Bakkevold KE, Kambestad B: Long-term survival following radical and palliative treatment of patients with carcinoma of the pancreas and papilla of Vater—The prognostic factors influencing the long-term results. *Eur J Surg Oncol* 19:147–61, 1993.

56. Levin DL, Connelly RR, Devesa SS: Demographic characteristics of cancer of the pancreas: Mortality, incidence, and survival. *Cancer* 47:1456–68, 1981.

57. Ishii H, Okada S, Nose H, et al.: Prognostic factors in patients with advanced pancreatic cancer treated with systemic chemotherapy. *Pancreas* 12:267–71, 1996.

58. Kayahara M, Nagakawa T, Ueno K, et al.: Distal pancreatectomy—does it have a role for pancreatic body and tail cancer? *Hepatogastroenterology* 45:827–32, 1998.

59. Hermanek P: Tumors of the gastrointestinal tract and the pancreas: histopathology, staging and prognosis. *Anticancer Res* 19:2393–6, 1999.

60. Willet CG, Lewanbrowski K, Warshaw AI, et al.: Resection margins in carcinoma of the head of the pancreas. Implications for radical therapy. *Ann Surg* 217:144–8, 1993.

61. Wittekind C: Bedeutung von Tumorwachstum und — Ausbreitung für die chirurgische Radikalität. *Zentralbl Chir* 118:500–7, 1993.

62. Friess H, Isenmann R, Berberat P, et al.: Die Prognose des Pankreaskarzinom. *Ther Umsch* 53:401–7, 1996.

63. Reber HA, Ashley SW, McFadden D: Curative treatment for pancreatic neoplasms. Radical resection. *Surg Clin North Am* 75:905–12, 1995.

64. Schumpelick V, Kasperk R: Principles and value of lymph node excision in tumors of the pancreatobiliary system. *Chirurg* 67:900–9, 1996.

65. Ishikawa O: Surgical technique, curability and postoperative quality of life in an extended pacreatectomy for adenocarcinoma of the pancreas. *Hepato-Gastroenterology* 43:320–5, 1996.

66. Nagakawa T, Nagamori M, Futakami F, et al.: Results of extensive surgery for pancreatic carcinoma. *Cancer* 77:640–5, 1996.

67. Henne-Bruns D, Kremer B, Meyer-Pannwitt U, et al.: Partial duodenopancreatectomy with radical lymphadenectomy in patients with pancreatic and periampullary carcinomas: Initial results. *Hepato-Gastroenterology* 40:145–9, 1993.

68. Roder JD: Stellenwert der Lymphknoten — Und Bindegewebsdissektion beim Pankreaskarzinom. *Chir Gastroenterol*, 13(Suppl):33–5, 1997.

69. Gordon TA, Burleyson GP, Tielsch JM, Cameron JL: The effects of regionalisation on cost and outcome for one general high-risk surgical procedure. *Ann Surg* 221:43–9, 1995.

70. Sosa JA, Bowman HM, Bass EB, et al.: Importance of hospital volume in the surgical management of pancreatic cancer. *Surg Forum* 48:584–6, 1997.

71. Dobelbower RR, Merrick HW, Khuder S, et al.: Adjuvant radiation therapy for pancreatic cancer: A 15 year experience. *Int J Radiat Oncol Biol Phys* 39:31–7, 1997.

72. DiCarlo V, Zerbi A, Balzano G, Villa E: Intraoperative and postoperative radiotherapy in pancreatic cancer. *Int J Pancreatol* 21:53–8, 1997.

73. Bosset J, Pay JJ, Giblet M, et al.: Conventional external irradiation alone as adjuvant treatment in respectable pancreatic cancer: Results of a prospective study. *Radiother Oncol* 24:191–4, 1992.

74. Bakkevold KE, Arnesjo B, Dahl O, Kambestad B: Adjuvant combined chemotherapy (AMF) following radical resection of carcinoma of the pancreas and papilla of Vater — Results of a controlled, prospective, randomized multicenter trial. *Eur J Cancer* 29:698–703, 1993.

75. Ihse I, Andersson R, Axelson J, Hansson L: Combination therapy in oncology (multimodal treatment) in pancreatic tumors. *Chirurg* 69:366–70, 1998.

76. Pister PW, Abbruzzese JL, Janjan NA, et al.: Rapid-fractionation preoperative chemoradiation, pancreaticoduodenectomy, and intraoperative radiation therapy for resectable pancreatic adenocarcinoma. *J Clin Oncol* 16:3843–50, 1998.

77. Poen JC, Collins HL, Niederhuber JE, et al.: Chemo-radiotherapy for localized pancreatic cancer: Increased dose intensitiy and reduced acute toxicity with concomitant radiotherapy and protracted venous infusion 5-fluorouracil. *Int J Radiat Oncol Biol Phys* 40:93–9, 1998.

78. Jaffe EM, Schutte M, Gossett J, et al.: Development and characterization of cytokine-secreting pancreatic adenocarcinoma vaccine from primary tumor for use in clinical trials. *Cancer J Sci Am* 4:194–203; 1998.

79. Pluda JM, Parkinson DR: Clinical implications of tumor-associated neovascularisation and current antiangiogenic strategies for the treatment of malignancies of pancreas. *Cancer* 78:680–7, 1996.

80. Roder JD, Siewert JR: Ist die palliative Resektion beim Pankreaskarzinom sinnvoll? *Acta Chir* Austrica 5:278–80, 1997.

LUNG AND PLUNAL TUMORS

CHAPTER 23

Lung Cancer

MICHAEL D. BRUNDAGE and WILLIAM J. MACKILLOP

Lung cancer is best conceptualized as a group of heterogeneous clinical entities with common molecular and cellular origins, but with different clinical behaviors, and hence, different prognoses. Lung cancer has a major impact on population health; taken together, lung cancers are the most common cause of cancer death in both males and females in North America.[1,2] Overall, only 13% of patients survive more than 5 years after being diagnosed.[1]

Determining the prognosis for an individual patient with lung cancer is difficult, in part, because the clinical course of the disease in the individual case can evolve along a seemingly infinite combination of branching pathways. Over 90% of lung cancer patients present with signs or symptoms of disease, and since no symptoms or signs are pathognomonic for lung cancer, the disease has a capacity clinically to mimic other cancers and other nonmalignant diseases with a constellation of possible presenting symptoms. These varying presentations, and potential clinical evolutions, are in turn due to the multiple potential manifestations of the primary tumor, metastatic sites of involvement, and paraneoplastic syndromes.

Despite the heterogeneity of the clinical manifestations of lung cancer, the prognosis for a population of patients with lung cancer is remarkably predictable. The overall mortality rates for lung cancer in North America over the last 15 years have remained unchanged.[1] A population-based study of over 12,000 patients with unresected non-small-cell lung cancer registered in seven Ontario Regional Cancer Centers (1982–1991) demonstrated no significant differences in patient survival either between Centers or over time.[3] The predictability of population survival outcomes is of limited usefulness, however, due to the marked heterogeneity of patients making up the overall population. Prognostic factors are thus used to divide the overall population of lung cancer patients into subgroups in order to realize the benefits of prognostic stratification (see Chapters 1 and 2). A number of studies have addressed the identification and application of such factors.

Prognostic Factors in Cancer, 2nd edition, Edited by Mary K. Gospodarowicz
ISBN 0-471-40633-3 Copyright © 2001 Wiley-Liss, Inc.

THE EXTENT OF THE LITERATURE

A substantial amount of clinical and basic science research has focused on prognostic factors in patients with lung cancer. Early investigation of prognostic factors in lung cancer patients concerned clinical characteristics of the tumor and of the patient, such as extent of the disease and of weight loss, respectively.[4] A number of clinical laboratory tests, such as the serum lactate dehydrogenase level, were subsequently identified as relevant,[5] followed most recently by the investigation of a plethora of new factors arising out of an increased understanding of the cellular and molecular biology of lung cancer.[4,6,7] The literature continues to grow rapidly. A search of the Medline database from 1985 to 1999, combining the Mesh subject heading "prognosis" with "carcinoma, non-small cell lung," and with "carcinoma, small cell," respectively, together identified nearly 1500 indexed entries. Figure 23.1 shows the pattern of this indexed research, and illustrates that the literature regarding prognostic issues in non-small-cell carcinoma seems to have grown at a faster rate than that pertaining to small-cell lung carcinoma. Indexed publications addressing the prognosis of patients with small-cell carcinoma continue to be published at

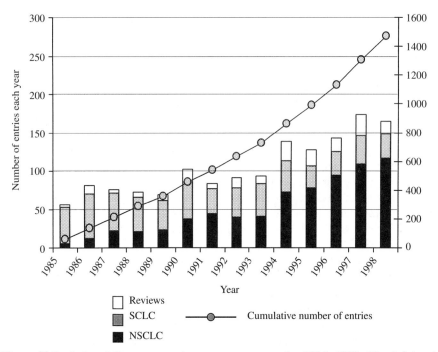

Figure 23.1 Indexed literature on lung cancer prognosis: 1985–1998. The left-hand ordinate indicates the number of indexed entries by year, according to study type. The right-hand ordinate indicates the cumulative number of all entries. The index criteria are found in the text.

a relatively constant rate, as do reviews of the literature (Figure 23.1). Over 100 prognostic factors pertaining to the tumor, the patient, or the environment have been reported. Given the extent and heterogeneity of the literature, many review papers addressing prognosis in lung cancer patients have attempted to identify clinically important and/or promising new prognostic factors in patients with lung cancer (for example, Buccheri[4]). International consensus workshops aimed at achieving similar goals have been conducted.[5] This chapter provides an overview of the literature, updating previous reviews with information from recently published studies.

THE IMPORTANCE OF HISTOLOGY AND STAGE OF DISEASE

The recognized heterogeneity among lung cancer patients has led to the definition of major clinical subgroups that are seen as clinically dissimilar from one another. The most important distinction is between small-cell lung carcinoma (SCLC) and non-small-cell lung carcinoma (NSCLC). Early studies of prognostic factors, including a relatively large study of the M.D. Anderson Cancer Center experience published in 1977, considered NSCLC and SCLC within the same statistical models of analyses.[8] The two entities are, however, generally considered to be so dissimilar that the principles governing their respective clinical management are discussed and evaluated entirely separately.[1] While, strictly speaking, the use of tumor histology to define these two entities is itself an application of a prognostic factor, the distinction between groups is so widely accepted that the analysis and application of prognostic factors generally now occurs within each group. A second major prognostic factor that defines distinct clinical entities is that of disease extent, or stage.[10] One staging system used to classify patients with lung cancer is that developed by the Veterans Administration Lung Cancer Study Group (VALCSG).[8] The VALCSG divides patients into those with limited or extensive disease based on the definition of limited stage as: disease confined to one hemithorax and those regional lymph nodes that can be encompassed within a tolerable radiotherapy port. As such, the classification considers both the anatomical extent of disease and the pathophysiological status of the patient. This staging system is now considered the standard for the staging of patients with SCLC,[1] and also has been utilized in the classification of unresectable NSCLC,[8] given the predominantly nonsurgical management of these clinical entities. NSCLC, however, is generally staged using the (TNM) staging system[10] (see Appendix A). The TNM staging system for lung cancer was last revised in 1997.[10] The derivation of the staging criteria was based on the analysis of a composite database representing clinical, surgical-pathologic, and follow-up information for 5319 patients treated for primary lung cancer, predominantly NSCLC patients treated at the M.D. Anderson Cancer Center from 1975 to 1988. In both SCLC and NSCLC, anatomic stage of disease has been consistently shown to be the most powerful prognostic factor predicting the survival of lung cancer patients overall.[10,11] Table 23.1 summarizes the influence of stage on survival outcomes, where stage is defined by the VALCSG system for SCLC and the TNM system for NSCLC.

TABLE 23.1   The Prognostic Importance of Stage in Lung Cancer

Stage	Median Survival (weeks)	Percent Surviving 3 Years	Percent Surviving 5 Years
SCLC[12]			
Limited	15.5		
Extensive	7.2		
NSCLC			
Clinical Stage[10]			
IA (*n* = 687)		71	61
IB (*n* = 1189)		46	38
II A (*n* = 29)		38	34
IIB (*n* = 357)		33	24
IIIA (*n* = 511)		18	13
IIIB (*n* = 1030)		7	5
IV (*n* = 1427)		2	1
Pathological Stage[10]			
IA (*n* = 511)		80	67
IB (*n* = 549)		67	57
IIA (*n* = 76)		66	55
IIB (*n* = 375)		46	39
IIIA (*n* = 399)		32	23

Given the overarching importance of disease stage in NSCLC, many authors evaluating prognosis distinguish between surgically resected and surgically unresectable disease. Accordingly, the remainder of this chapter divides the discussion of prognostic factors first as they apply to NSCLC, and second as they apply to SCLC. Within NSCLC, the discussion separates three common presentations: resectable, locally advanced, and advanced disease. The focus of the chapter is on factors predictive of patient survival, given the magnitude of the literature. Moreover, we focus on patient and tumor factors, and refer to oncologic reference textbooks with regard to treatment factors. Finally, a comprehensive review of all patient and tumor factors examined to date is beyond the scope of this discussion — rather we will focus on those factors that have established clinical importance, as well as some "new and promising" factors, which we arbitrarily define as those shown to be independently predictive of a salient clinical endpoint in at least one study.

PROGNOSTIC FACTORS IN NON-SMALL-CELL LUNG CARCINOMA

Clinical Presentations of Disease

Figure 23.2 illustrates common clinical presentations relevant to the prognosis for patients with NSCLC. As represented in the shaded area at the left of Figure 23.2, patients may initially present with apparently resectable disease, with locally advanced (unresectable) disease, or with metastatic disease. On the basis of

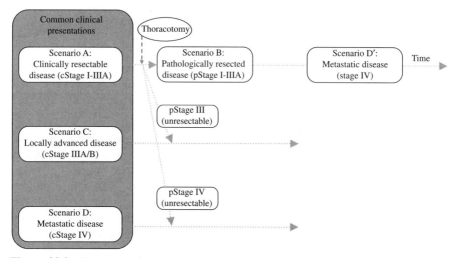

Figure 23.2 Prognosis for non-small cell lung cancer patients: Common clinical presentations. The figure illustrates three common presentations in patients with NSCLC. Potential subsequent presentations for patients with clinically resectable disease are also shown.

the pretreatment clinical assessment, patients are classified according to clinical stage (cTNM).[10] The horizontal arrows in Figure 23.2 represent the clinical course of disease, over time, for each presentation. Those patients presenting with apparently resectable disease may indeed undergo successful complete resection, or may be found at surgical exploration to have unresectable or metastatic disease, as illustrated. In any case, patients who undergo a thoracotomy are staged according to the pathological extent of disease. The top line in Figure 23.2 illustrates the clinical course of a patient who develops recurrent metastatic disease following initial resection. Although many permutations of disease progression not shown in Figure 23.2 are known to occur, the illustrated examples are sufficient for a discussion of prognosis in NSCLC. The following sections discuss each of these common clinical presentations.

Prognostic Factors in Clinically Resectable Disease

Few studies have systematically addressed the prognosis of patients with early-stage disease solely on the basis of clinically available information (including clinical stage). Since surgery is considered the standard management of patients who are medically fit for thoracotomy,[12] clinical decision making in this situation generally focuses on patient-related factors that estimate the patient's likelihood of surviving a pulmonary resection, and tumor-related factors that estimate the likelihood of complete resection. Textbooks of surgical principles typically address patients' prognoses with respect to surgical morbidity and mortality (for example, predictors of postoperative pulmonary function), or with respect to competing surgical options (for example, wedge resection versus lobectomy),[12] rather than the utility of surgery over other therapeutic options. An exception occurs in patients with more advanced clinical stages of uncertain operability (for example, cN2 or cT4 disease), in whom the extent of disease can be considered as a contraindication to thoracotomy. These patients can be classified as having inoperable disease, as is discussed below.

One notable departure from the trend to assess prognosis based on pathological rather than clinical features is the work of Feinstein and colleagues,[13] who have proposed, developed, and validated a "clinical-severity" staging system. Feinstein has pointed out that the anatomical and morphologic descriptors of lung cancer are classifiable according to widely accepted criteria, but the clinical manifestations of disease, while also widely accepted to have important prognostic value, are not systematically classified in a standard taxonomy. Through a process of sequential sequestration of prognostic strata and subsequent consolidation of clinical indicators, five clinical severity stages have been defined based on the presence and severity of clinical manifestations and functional effects of the tumor and/or patient comorbidity. Pfister and Feinstein have demonstrated that this system is more robust and reliable than indicators such as patients' performance status or weight loss applied in isolation.[13]

A special case of prognosis in the setting of clinically resectable disease occurs in patients who have disease amenable to resection but who are inoperable for medical reasons. Primary radiotherapy with curative intent is generally recommended in this situation, and although no modern randomized trials have directly compared surgery to radiotherapy, radiotherapy is generally believed to afford results that are inferior to surgical resection, both in terms of local disease control and overall survival.[1] Nonetheless, substantial cure rates have been reported in patients receiving primary radiotherapy, and prognostic factors predicting patient survival have been studied retrospectively. Wigren and colleagues,[14] for example, recently reported a multivariate model derived from a study of over 500 patients demonstrating that tumor size was the most powerful predictor of survival. Other significant factors included tumor stage and patient symptoms, performance status, and hemoglobin.

Prognostic Factors in Patients with Resected NSCLC

Perhaps somewhat surprisingly, the vast majority of studies addressing the prognosis of patients with NSCLC do so in patients who have already undergone surgical resection of the primary disease — a minority of NSCLC patients[10] — rather than in patients who are treatment naïve. Patients are thus selected in these studies as those who are well enough to undergo successful resection, who have disease that is amenable to complete (or, in some cases, attempted) resection, and who are staged by the pTNM criteria (Figure 23.2).

The rationale for the study of prognostic factors in this situation lies in the recognition that even with complete resection, recurrence rates are substantial (20–85%, depending on stage[10]), thus making the determination of prognosis clinically relevant. Moreover, the strategy allows sufficient access to fresh or archived pathologic specimens to allow multiple biochemical or molecular evaluations of tumor factors. Appendix 23B.1 lists prognostic factors that have been identified as independently predictive of patient survival in resected NSCLC.

Tumor-related Factors in Patients with Resected NSCLC   As discussed earlier, and as shown in Table 23.1, tumor stage is generally considered to be the most important prognostic factor identified in patients with resected NSCLC.[10,16] Revisions to the TNM system were made in 1997 in order to provide greater specificity for identifying patient subgroups with similar prognoses and treatment options. For example, patients with pTIN0 disease have been consistently shown to have significantly better survival outcomes than those with pT2N0 (3-year survival 80% vs. 67%; 5-year survival 67% vs. 57%). These and parallel observations in clinically staged patients led to revision of stage I into stage IA (T1N0) and stage IB (T2N0). Similarly, pT1N1M0 disease is now designated as stage IIA, whereas pT2N1M0 and pT3N0M0 are grouped as stage IIB. Stage IIIA has been revised to include pT3N1M0, and pT1-3N2M0 tumors, reflecting the superior survival results in patients with Stage III disease that are amenable to definitive surgical resection. Intrapulmonary ipsilateral satellite tumor metastases (not in lymph nodes) involving lobes other than that containing the primary tumor are now classified as M1. As discussed earlier, an assessment of clinical stage is essential in determining the appropriateness of attempted surgical resection, while in the setting of resected disease, the designation of pTNM stage is more important for estimating prognosis.

One important circumstance of prognostic importance is that of incomplete resection, either with gross tumor remaining, or with positive microscopic resection margins, in which postoperative therapy (radiotherapy or chemoradiotherapy) is usually recommended.[1] The majority of studies confirm that microscopically involved margins are a strong negative predictor of survival, even when additional therapy is offered, suggesting that the biological characteristics of the tumor that are associated with microscopic residual disease are also associated with systemic spread of disease.

As shown in Appendix 23B.1, additional tumor-related prognostic factors include other elements of the anatomical extent of disease, and conventional histologic parameters, that are clinically useful in estimating prognosis. For example, the T factor has been shown to have independent significance within Stage I, and tumor size and volume have been shown to provide additional information beyond the T factor. With regard to histologic parameters, the prognostic significance of tumor cell type (large-cell undifferentiated, adenocarcinoma, or squamous cell) has been studied extensively. Many of these studies conclude that adenocarcinoma has an independent negative impact on survival prognosis (Appendix 23B.1), whereas other studies of comparable design have not shown cell type to have independent prognostic value.[17,18] Bronchioalveolar carcinoma[19] and carcinoid tumors[20] constitute notable exceptions, as they are each considered distinct clinical entities with natural histories that differ from the more common NSCLC tumor types.

Many other tumor factors have been shown in at least one study to have independent prognostic significance,[4] but these factors are not typically reported in routine clinical assessment. A detailed discussion of each factor is beyond the scope of this chapter; Appendix 23B.1 provides an overview, and excellent reviews are available.[4,20,21] These factors are briefly summarized as (1) histological features; (2) clinical chemistry and serum tumor markers; (3) markers of tumor proliferation; (4) markers of cellular adhesion; (5) other molecular biological markers, including regulators of cellular growth (kRAS, RB, EGFr, erb-b2, MRP-1, HGF), of the metastatic cascade (TPA, Cyclin D-1, cathepsin), of apoptosis (p53, bcl-2), and others. The potential clinical application of these factors is discussed below.

Host-related Factors in Patients with Resected NSCLC   Many studies of prognostic factors have addressed patient characteristics as predictors of survival after complete surgical resection. In general, these factors have been found to be less powerful predictors of outcome than in the advanced-disease setting, particularly in Stage I disease. Thus, this group of factors is not generally considered important for clinical decision making in this situation. One promising molecular factor related to the host is the patient's CYPIA-1 status. This gene is responsible for the metabolic activation of benzopyrene found in cigarette smoke, and high susceptibility to smoking-related lung cancer has been associated with polymorphism of the CYP1A-1 gene. In addition, the susceptible genotype has been found to be associated with higher disease recurrence rates and lower survival in multivariate analyses.[22]

Environment-related Factors in Patients with Resected NSCLC   A full description of therapeutic options and the impact of therapy on patients' prognosis is beyond the scope of this chapter, but general principles are considered here. Incomplete resection of disease, as discussed earlier, is considered a treatment-related factor by some authors.[1] Given the recognition of poor prognosis groups after resection, adjuvant radiotherapy or chemotherapy (or both) have been advised for selected patients by various authors.[1] Adjuvant radiotherapy has been studied in clinical trials enrolling pN0, pN1, and pN2 stage patients, alone or in combination, in an effort to treat potential occult residual disease in the mediastinum, there by decreasing postresection recurrence rates. While there is general agreement that radiotherapy offers no clear benefit in pN0 patients, and reduces the probability of regional recurrence in some pN2 patients, its use has not been consistently associated with improved overall patient survival in any patient group.

Postoperative chemotherapy has been advocated by some authors for selected patients following resection, although no consistent benefit has been demonstrated in clinical trials thus far. In contrast, some randomized trials have shown improvement in patient survival with preoperatively administered chemotherapy.[1] Some authors have challenged these findings on the basis that prognostic factors were not equally balanced between groups, leading to spurious results. The use of prognostic factors to select patients for adjuvant treatment is discussed below.

Locally Advanced NSCLC

The majority of patients with unresectable disease will have significant symptoms or other general manifestations of illness, such as weight loss or poor performance status. Accordingly, most studies of prognostic factors consider locally advanced and metastatic NSCLC under the general rubric of "advanced" disease, as is addressed in the next section. The distinction between the two entities, however, is important for the consideration of particular subgroups of patients due to treatment decision-making implications.

Patients without systemic manifestations of illness — generally defined as those patients with high performance status and no substantial weight loss — have been shown in a number of clinical trials to have higher survival rates when they receive induction chemotherapy followed by radiotherapy, or concurrent chemoradiotherapy.[23] The same subgroup of patients have been shown to experience higher survival rates when treated with continuous hyperfractionated and accelerated radiotherapy (CHART) as compared to conventional fractionation, and when treated with higher doses of conventional radiation as compared to lower doses.[24] The role of surgery in relation to induction chemotherapy and radiotherapy is currently being investigated, as is the role of combination chemoradiotherapy in more symptomatic patients.[1]

A second notable subgroup of patients is those with cT3N0M0 disease, particularly when located in the superior pulmonary sulcus (Pancoast's tumor). A number of recent reviews highlight the role of prognostic factors such as neurologic involvement and vertebral body involvement in this particular clinical setting.[25-28]

Advanced NSCLC

Tumor, host, and environment factors pertaining to the prognosis of patients with advanced NSCLC are listed in Appendix 23B.2. As shown in this appendix, and as noted earlier, factors essential to decision making are the stage of disease, weight loss, and performance status, as indicators of potential success with combined-modality locoregional therapy. Even in the setting of Stage IV disease, markers of functional impact (weight loss, performance status, symptom burden, and pretreatment quality of life) predict the length of median survival with systemic therapy. Chemotherapy itself, as an environment-related factor, is known to improve patients' median survival over best-supportive care alone in patients without substantial systemic manifestations of illness. More recent clinical trials research has been directed at finding chemotherapy regimens with higher response rates and/or lower toxicity.[1]

Additional factors that can be used to refine the accuracy of prognosis are listed in Appendix 23B.2. These include markers relating to the extent of clinically detectable disease, hematological or biochemical markers associated with disease extent, and the "intangible" factor inherent in the opinion of the physician. In a large study of 2531 patients enrolled on a variety of clinical trials, Albain and colleagues[29] identified good performance status, female sex, and age <70 years as the most important factors predictive of favorable survival overall. The study also identified three prognostic subgroups with significantly distinct survival expectations — based on performance status, age, hemoglobin, and serum LDH levels — in patients receiving cisplatin chemotherapy. Others studies employing secondary analysis of clinical-trial information have reached similar conclusions,[30] as have retrospective studies of patients not enrolled in clinical-trial protocols.[31,32]

New and promising prognostic factors are also listed in Appendix 23B.2. In contrast to the setting of resected disease, only a few studies have investigated the impact of molecular markers in the setting of advanced disease, and most of these do so only in the context of evaluating all patients in whom tissue is available, rather than specifically addressing the advanced-disease cohort. Thus, determining the most appropriate way to integrate new knowledge regarding these factors with more readily available tumor- and patient-based indicators requires further study.

An increasing amount of research has addressed the use of patient-reported parameters, such as quality of life scores and/or anxiety and depression measures as prognostic factors. These pretreatment parameters may be markers of disease impact, and hence, may be seen as providing information complementary to performance status and weight loss assessments. However, these parameters can also reflect constructs such as the patients' inherent characteristics, or the level of their emotional support, that can independently predict better disease outcomes, possibly through psychophysiologic mechanisms. Further research is required to clarify the nature of the observed association between favorable scores on these assessments and superior clinical outcomes.

Prognostic Factors in Small-cell Lung Carcinoma

The main factors known to influence the prognosis of patients with small-cell lung carcinoma are listed in Appendix 23B.3. As noted earlier, the stage of disease is the most powerful predictor of survival outcomes. The designation of stage is considered an "essential" factor since patients with limited disease generally receive locoregional radiotherapy and prophylactic cranial radiotherapy in addition to chemotherapy.[1] The use of prophylactic cranial radiotherapy predicts for fewer central nervous system (CNS) recurrences compared to untreated patients, but has not been consistently shown to increase patients' median survival. In contrast, the use of locoregional radiotherapy, has been clearly demonstrated to improve survival of limited stage patients. In addition, the timing of thoracic radiotherapy (early versus late in relation to chemotherapy treatment), and the use of altered fractionation strategies and/or higher doses of radiotherapy have been shown in some studies to increase patient survival. These issues, in addition to novel systemic therapeutic strategies, continue to be investigated in clinical trials.[1]

In a large study of over 2500 patients with SCLC treated on clinical trial protocols,[11] Albain and colleagues calculated Cox multivariate analyses in localized and extensive disease subgroups, respectively. Survival outcomes for patients with localized disease were best predicted by good performance status, female sex, age <70 years, white race, normal serum lactate dehydrogenase (LDH), and concurrent chemoradiotherapy. Survival outcomes for patients with extensive disease were best predicted by a normal serum LDH, multidrug chemotherapy, and a single metastatic lesion. Subsequent recursive partitioning and amalgamation showed that four distinct subgroups could be identified using a subset of these factors. Other authors have investigated recursive partitioning models in patients with SCLC and have reported similar findings. Sagman and colleagues,[33] for example, also identified four distinct patient groups, although eight attributes were factored into their model (disease extent, performance status, serum alkaline phosphatase (ALP) and LDH, white-cell counts, mediastinal spread, sex, and liver metastases). The interactions among factors resulted in "reassignment" of patients across conventional staging distinctions into alternate prognostic groups.

Additional tumor factors that have been shown to affect prognosis are listed in Appendix 23B.3. While application of these factors may refine estimates of patients' survival outcomes, they are not generally applied to treatment decision making.

Integration and Clinical Application of Prognostic Factors

In the context of a very large literature reporting putative prognostic factors in lung cancer patients, many authors have highlighted methodological issues in the interpretation and integration of existing studies.[4,7] In this section, we address the integration and clinical application of research knowledge pertaining to prognostic factors by discussing a number of our observations and their implications.

First, existing reports of prognostic factors make up a body of literature that is markedly heterogeneous on a number of criteria, as has been noted by others.[4] The interstudy variations include: variation in the study population(s); variation in the diagnostic and staging criteria used to identify the study patients; variation in the type of statistical analyses applied in the studies; variation in the prognostic factors included in the analyses; variation in the methods used to define, measure, or classify the factors; variation in the treatments received by the study patients; and variation in the appropriate statistical correction for analysis of posttreatment factors. These variations result in the potential problems of patient selection bias, leading to spurious results; low statistical power, leading to false negative results; differences in laboratory techniques used to determine the presence of specific factors, leading to conflicting results between studies; limited opportunity to integrate studies, leading to failure of meta-analytic approaches; inability to define the true influence of prognostic factors due to uncontrolled treatment effects or inappropriate patient selection criteria, among others.[4]

Second, the quality of published reports varies. While fully described studies can be seen to differ from one another, some studies are described in insufficient detail to determine the study methods and/or identify variations.[34] Thus, interpretation of the literature is further complicated by missing information. This problem is germane to studies of molecular markers, where differences in laboratory techniques have been shown to have a marked impact on the study results,[35] and is also relevant to the increased interest in psychosocial and other patient-based factors, where valid methods for measuring and evaluating psychosocial and behavioral outcomes are required.

Third, the breadth of prognostic factors studied in the literature is extensive, and growing, whereas the scope of prognostic factors evaluated in individual studies is inappropriately narrow.[4] Most individual studies have addressed only a few prognostic factors, typically controlling for patient stage and readily available patient and tumor characteristics such as age, sex, cell type, and/or tumor grade. Few studies attempt to integrate the significant factors identified in earlier studies, and even fewer studies are prospectively designed efforts to validate the predictive models identified in earlier patient cohorts.

Fourth, with the exception of a few predictive factors, the literature demonstrates conflicting evidence of each factor's prognostic power. In the great majority of studies, at least one representation of pTNM stage is significantly associated with survival, the exceptions typically being studies that focus on a stage-specific cohort (for example, pT I patients). In contrast, tumor-cell type, patient sex, and patient age are generally found to be not significantly associated with survival outcome, and when statistically significant, are of weak predictive power.[36] Given the number of studies investigating these patient attributes, some positive associations may also represent Type I statistical errors. Some factors are now generally accepted as having prognostic significance, such as molecular markers for *ras* and p53,[37] but interstudy differences in the predictive power of these factors are not well explained by statistical power considerations, or by technical differences between study methods, and require further elucidation.[34] Other prognostic factors, such as measures of tumor proliferation, have seemingly balanced evidence for and against an independent prognostic effect, and their clinical value thus remains controversial. As mentioned earlier, attempts to evaluate this literature using meta-analytical techniques can be compromised by study heterogeneity.

Fifth, the multidimensional nature of prognosis is underinvestigated, the focus of the majority of research being on predictors of survival. Further investigation of factors predictive of survival is clearly required, given the limitations in existing studies outlined thus far. Of concern, however, is that the prognostic factors predicting the many other clinical endpoints that are of potential interest to patients and their physicians are investigated to a limited extent, or not at all. Research investigating the information needs of patients with lung cancer has shown that patients are interested in a broad spectrum of endpoints other than survival, such as the chances of symptom relief, chances of response to therapy, likely impact on quality of life, and likely patterns of disease recurrence.[38] Prognosis regarding these outcomes may be pertinent to treatment decision making, or may be important to the patient for purposes of personal decision making, understanding the nature of the illness, or for other reasons.[38] A minority of studies of lung cancer treatment, for example, have examined the impact of treatment on patterns of disease recurrence, or on symptom relief, and fewer still have examined what factors predict these important clinical endpoints. Since it has been demonstrated that many cancer patients in general, and many lung cancer patients specifically,[38,39] wish to participate in treatment decision making, enhanced understanding of these predictors will be necessary to improve the quality of information that clinicians are able to provide to individual patients.

Sixth, comparatively little research has focused on patients at points beyond their initial presentation. For example, returning to Figure 23.2, patients presenting with metastatic disease are not distinguished from those whose initial presentation is with Stage IV disease. Although some studies have considered the prognosis of patients with recurrent disease, prognostic factors relevant to the internal frame of reference for a given patient have been rarely elucidated.

Finally, more comprehensive research is required to fully realize the benefits of prognosis in lung cancer patients. New studies are needed to better evaluate how factors that are already established to have prognostic value are best combined in clinically useful stratification models, and to validate these models. At the level of the specific patient, medical and personal decision making will be enhanced by more accurate predictors of outcomes germane to the individual patients. At the level of patient populations, further research is necessary to establish the risks and benefits of competing treatment approaches as they apply to patient strata that have distinct prognoses. For example, ongoing randomized clinical trials, designed to determine the risks and benefits of adjuvant chemotherapy after complete surgical resection, are also evaluating if the k-*ras* status of the tumor is associated with the efficacy of chemotherapy. At the level of the disease, better integration of prognostic factors in individual studies may reveal unanticipated associations that, in turn, may lead to new insights into opportunities for therapeutic intervention.

ACKNOWLEDGMENT

Supported in part by a grant from the National Cancer Institute of Canada.

▬ APPENDIX 23A

TNM Classification: Lung

T — Primary Tumor

TX Primary tumor cannot be assessed, *or* tumor proven by the presence of malignant cells in sputum or bronchial washings but not visualized by imaging or bronchoscopy

T0 No evidence of primary tumor

Tis Carcinoma in situ

T1 Tumor 3 cm or less in greatest dimension, surrounded by lung or visceral pleura, without bronchoscopic evidence of invasion more proximal than the lobar bronchus (i.e., not in the main bronchus)

T2 Tumor with *any* of the following features of size or extent: more than 3 cm in greatest dimension, involves main bronchus 2 cm or more distal to the carina, invades visceral pleura, is associated with atelectasis or obstructive pneumonitis that extends to the hilar region but does not involve the entire lung

T3 Tumor of any size that directly invades any of the following: chest wall (including superior sulcus tumors), diaphragm, mediastinal pleura, parietal pericardium; *or* tumor in the main bronchus less than 2 cm distal to the carina[1] but without involvement of the carina; *or* associated atelectasis or obstructive pneumonitis of the entire lung

T4 Tumor of any size that invades any of the following: mediastinum, heart, great vessels, trachea, oesophagus, vertebral body, carina; separate tumor nodule(s) in the same lobe; tumor with malignant pleural effusion

N — Regional Lymph Nodes

NX Regional lymph nodes cannot be assessed

N0 No regional lymph-node metastasis

N1 Metastasis in ipsilateral peribronchial and/or ipsilateral hilar lymph nodes and intrapulmonary nodes, including involvement by direct extension

N2 Metastasis in ipsilateral mediastinal and/or subcarinal lymph node(s)

N3 Metastasis in contralateral mediastinal, contralateral hilar, ipsilateral or contralateral scalene, or supraclavicular lymph node(s)

M — Distant Metastasis

MX Distant metastasis cannot be assessed

M0 No distant metastasis

M1 Distant metastasis, includes separate tumor nodule(s) in a different lobe (ipsilateral or contralateral)

Stage Grouping

Occult carcinoma	TX	N0	M0
Stage 0	Tis	N0	M0
Stage IA	T1	N0	M0
Stage IB	T2	N0	M0
Stage IIA	T1	N1	M0
Stage IIB	T2	N1	M0
	T3	N0	M0
Stage IIIA	T1	N2	M0
	T2	N2	M0
	T3	N1, N2	M0
Stage IIIB	Any T	N3	M0
	T4	Any N	M0
Stage IV	Any T	Any N	M1

Source: Sobin LH, Wittekind Ch (eds).: *TNM classification of malignant tumors*, 5th ed. New York, Union Internationale Contre le Cancer Wiley-Liss, 1997.

■■■■■■■ **APPENDIX 23B.1**

Prognostic Factors in Patients with Surgically Resected NSCLC

Prognostic Factors	Tumor Related		Host Related	Environment Related
Essential	Stage Hypercalcemia	"N" category	Weight loss Performance status	Resection margin

Additional	*Anatomic*
	"T" category
	Nodal level
	
	Intrapulmonary
	  metastasis
	Histologic
	Grade
	Vessel invasion
		Tumor size
		Pleural
		  cytology
		
		Cell Type
			Sex
			Age	

New and promising	*Histologic*
	Cells in mitosis
	Lymphoid infiltration
	
	Clinical chemistry
	Blood group Ag
	
	NSE
	CA-125
	TPA
	Proliferation markers
	DNA ploidy and/or
	  % S-phase
	PCNA
	Thymidine labeling
	Cellular adhesion markers
	CD44
	Other molecular biologic
	markers
	k RAS
	RB gene
	bcl-2
	c-jun
	MRP-1
	EGFr (c-erbB-1)
	HGF
	TPA
	Cyclin D-1
		Angiogenesis
		
		Coagulation
		  factors
		Proteinuria
		CEA
		
		Ki67
		
		AgNOR
		
		Plankoglobin
		
		P53
		P21
		c-fos
		CYFRA 21-1
		KAI-1
		c-erbB-2
		VEGF
		sIL-2R
		Cathepsin B
			Smoking habit
			Quality of life
			Marital status
			Depressed
			  mood
			
			CYPIA-1
				Adjuvant
				  radiotherapy
				Adjuvant
				  chemotherapy

Prognostic Factors in Patients with Advanced NSCLC

Prognostic Factors	Tumor Related	Host Related	Environment Related
Essential	Stage (III vs. IV) Hypercalcemia SVCO	Weight loss Performance status	Chemoradiotherapy (selected Stage III) Chemotherapy (selected Stage IV)
Additional	*Anatomic* "T" category "N" category Stage IIIA vs. IIIB Number of sites involved Pleural effusion Liver metastases *Clinical chemistry/ hematology* Hemoglobin LDH Albumin	Sex Symptoms Age	Physician opinion
New or Promising	*Clinical chemistry/ hematology* Coagulation factors Proteinuria *Proliferation markers* DNA ploidy and/or % S-phase Ki-67 *Other molecular biologic markers* Replication errors 2p/3p K ras P53 c-erbB-1 TPA NSE *Other radiology* Thalium-201 uptake	Quality of life Marital status Depressed mood CYPIA-1	In vitro drug assay

■■■■■■ **APPENDIX 23B.3**

Prognostic Factors in Patients with SCLC

Prognostic Factors	Tumor Related	Host Related	Environment Related
Essential	Stage	Performance Status	Chemotherapy Thoracic radiotherapy
Additional	Histologic subtype Serum LDH Serum alkaline phosphatase Cushing's syndrome Limited disease: mediastinal involvement Extensive disease: number of sites involved Bone or brain involved WBC count Platelet count	Weight loss Sex	Completion of chemotherapy
New or promising	MDR1 Serum VEGF Interleukin-2 NSE Blood coagulation Successful establishment of cell lines		

REFERENCES

1. Anonymous: Cancer of the lung, in DeVita VT, Hellman S, Rosenberg SA (eds.): *Cancer: Principles and practice of oncology*. Philidelphia, Lippincott-Raven, 1999.

2. Anonymous: *National Cancer Institute of Canada: Canadian Cancer Statistics 1998*. Toronto, Canada, 1998.

3. Mackillop WJ, Zhou Y, Dixon P, et al.: Variation in the management and outcome of non-small cell lung cancer in Ontario. *Radiother Oncol*. 32:106–15, 1994.

4. Buccheri G, Ferrigno D: Prognostic factors in lung cancer: Tables and comments. *Eur Respir J* 7:1350–64, 1994.

5. Feld R, Borges M, Giner V, et al.: Prognostic factors in non-small cell lung cancer. *Lung Cancer* 11(Suppl. 3):S19–23, 1994.

6. Smit EF, Groen HJ, Splinter TA, et al.: New prognostic factors in resectable non-small cell lung cancer. *Thorax* 51:638–46, 1996.

7. Mountain CF: New prognostic factors in lung cancer. Biologic prophets of cancer cell aggression. *Chest* 108:246–54, 1995.

8. Lanzotti VJ, Thomas DR, Boyle LE, et al.: Survival with inoperable lung cancer: An integration of prognostic variables based on simple clinical criteria. *Cancer* 39:303–13, 1977.

9. Sobin LH, Fleming ID: *TNM classification of malignant tumors, fifth edition (1997). Union Internationale Contre le Cancer and the American Joint Committee on Cancer. Cancer* 80:1803–4, 1997.

10. Mountain CF. Revisions in the international system for staging lung cancer, *Chest,* 111:1710–7, 1997.

11. Albain KS, Crowley JJ, LeBlanc M, Livingston RB: Determinants of improved outcome in small-cell lung cancer: An analysis of the 2,580-patient Southwest Oncology Group database. *J Clin Oncol* 8:1563–74, 1990.

12. Sabiston DCJ, Spencer FC: *Surgery of the chest*, 6th ed. Philadelphia, Saunders, 1995.

13. Pfister DG, Wells CK, Chan CK, Feinstein AR: Classifying clinical severity to help solve problems of stage migration in nonconcurrent comparisons of lung cancer therapy. *Cancer Res.* 50:4664–9, 1990.

14. Wigren T, Oksanen H, Kellokumpu-Lehtinen P: A practical prognostic index for inoperable non-small-cell lung cancer. *J Cancer Res Clin Oncol* 123:259–66, 1997.

15. Mountain CF, Dresler CM: Regional lymph node classification for lung cancer staging. *Chest* 111:1718–23, 1997.

16. Mori M, Kohli A, Baker SP, et al.: Laminin and cathepsin B as prognostic factors in stage I non-small cell lung cancer: Are they useful? *Mod Pathol* 10:572–7, 1997.

17. Fontanini G, Lucchi M, Vignati S, et al.: Angiogenesis as a prognostic indicator of survival in non-small-cell lung carcinoma: A prospective study. *J Natl Cancer Inst* 89:881–6, 1997.

18. Clayton F: The spectrum and significance of bronchioloalveolar carcinomas. *Pathol Annu*
23(Pt 2):361–94, 1988.

19. Kayser K, Kayser C, Rahn W, et al.: Carcinoid tumors of the lung: Immuno- and ligandohistochemistry, analysis of integrated optical density, syntactic structure analysis, clinical data, and prognosis of patients treated surgically. *J Surg Oncol* 63:99–106, 1996.

20. D'Amico TA, Massey M, Herndon JE, et al.: A biologic risk model for stage I lung cancer: Immunohistochemical analysis of 408 patients with the use of ten molecular markers. *J Thorac Cardiovasc Surg* 117:736–43, 1999.

21. Johnson BE: Biologic and molecular prognostic factors — impact on treatment of patients with non-small cell lung cancer. *Chest* 107:287S–90S, 1995.

22. Goto I, Yoneda S, Yamamoto M, Kawajiri K: Prognostic significance of germ line polymorphisms of the CYP1A1 and glutathione S-transferase genes in patients with non-small cell lung cancer. *Cancer Res* 56:3725–30, 1996.

23. Stewart LA, Pignon JP: Chemotherapy in non-small cell lung cancer: A meta-analysis using updated data on individual patients from 52 randomized clinical trials. *BMJ* 311:899–909, 1995.

24. Emami B, Perez CA: Lung, in Perez CA (ed.): *Radiation oncology*, 2d ed. Philadelphia, Lippincott, 1993, pp. 806–36.

25. Anderson TM, Moy PM, Holmes EC: Factors affecting survival in superior sulcus tumors. *J Clin Oncol* 4:1598–603, 1986.

26. Beyer DC, Weisenburger T: Superior sulcus tumors. *Am J Clin Oncol* 9:156–61, 1986.

27. Detterbeck FC: Pancoast (superior sulcus) tumors. *Ann Thorac Surg* 63:1810–8, 1997.

28. Shaw RR: Pancoast's tumor. *Ann Thorac Surg* 37:343–5, 1984.

29. Albain KS, Crowley JJ, LeBlanc M, Livingston RB: Survival determinants in extensive-stage non-small-cell lung cancer: The Southwest Oncology Group experience. *J Clin Oncol.* 9:1618–26, 1991.

30. Paesmans M, Sculier JP, Libert P, et al.: Prognostic factors for survival in advanced non-small-cell lung cancer: Univariate and multivariate analyses including recursive partitioning and amalgamation algorithms in 1,052 patients. The European Lung Cancer Working Party. *J Clin Oncol* 1995; 13:1221–1230.

31. Hespanhol V, Queiroga H, Magalhaes A, et al.: Survival predictors in advanced non-small cell lung cancer. *Lung Cancer* 13:253–67, 1995.

32. Takigawa N, Segawa Y, Okahara M, et al.: Prognostic factors for patients with advanced non-small cell lung cancer: Univariate and multivariate analyses including recursive partitioning and amalgamation. *Lung Cancer* 15:67–77, 1996.

33. Sagman U, Maki E, Evans WK, et al.: Small-cell carcinoma of the lung: Derivation of a prognostic staging system. *J Clin Oncol* 9:1639–49, 1991.

34. Watine J: Further comments on "A practical prognostic index for inoperable non-small-cell lung cancer": A clinical biologist's point of view. *J Cancer Res Clin Oncol* 124:581–3, 1998.

35. Jacobson DR: *ras* mutations in lung cancer, in Brambilla C, Brambilla E (eds.): *Lung tumors: Fundamental biology and clinical management*. New York, Marcel Dekker, 1999, pp. 139–156.

36. Feinstein AR, Wells CK: A clinical-severity staging system for patients with lung cancer. *Medicine* 69:1–33, 1990.

37. Michalides RJ: Deregulation of the cell cycle in lung cancer, in Brambilla C, Brambilla E (eds.): *Lung tumors: Fundamental biology and clinical management*. New York, Marcel Dekker, 1999, pp. 211–223.

38. Davidson JR, Brundage MD, Feldman-Stewart D: Cancer treatment decisions: patients' desires for participation and information. *Psycho-Oncology* 8(6)511–20, 1999.

39. Brundage MD, Davidson JR, Mackillop W, et al.: Using a treatment-tradeoff methods to elicit preferences for the treatment of locally advanced non-small cell lung cancer. *Med Decis Making* 18:256–67, 1998.

CHAPTER 24

Malignant Pleural Mesothelioma

HENG-NUNG KOONG, RICHARD J. BATTAFARANO,
and ROBERT J. GINSBERG

Malignant pleural mesothelioma (MPM) is an uncommon tumor with approximately 2000 to 3000 new cases diagnosed in United States each year.[1] The incidence varies from 13 to 33 to 66 per million per year in the United States, South Africa, and Western Australia, respectively.[2] Between 1940 and 1970, there has been a steady increase in the incidence due to occupational exposure to asbestos,[2] and is expected to peak somewhere between 1990 and 2010.[3] However, additional factors are likely to contribute to the development of this malignancy, since approximately 20% of patients who develop MPM have no history of asbestos exposure.[4-6] Regardless of its cause, the natural history of MPM is one of locoregional progression of disease with the ultimate development of distant metastases.[7,8] Despite aggressive multimodality therapy, the median survival of patients diagnosed with this disease ranges from 9 months to 20 months.[7,9-14]

The association of asbestos with MPM was first recognized by Wagner et al.[15] and confirmed by others.[16,17] Asbestos fibers lodged in the respiratory bronchioles and alveoli promote alveolar inflammation, interstitial pneumonitis, and eventual fibrosis, resulting in the clinical syndrome of asbestosis. The fibers are also conveyed to the pleural space by subpleural lymphatics where chronic inflammation and subsequent fibrosis form parietal pleural plaques. Such plaques can transform into malignant mesothelioma. Initially manifesting as small nodules, they coalesce and ultimately invade adjacent structures such as the visceral pleura, mediastinum, pericardium, and diaphragm.[2]

The tumor is notorious for its nonspecific presentation and extensive local infiltration. Diagnosis is often delayed by 2 months and even beyond 6 months in a quarter of patients.[7,18] Overall median survival of unresected patients ranges from 7 to 11 months,[7,18] with more than 80% of patients succumbing to local disease rather than metastatic spread.[19] While the natural history of

Prognostic Factors in Cancer, 2nd edition, Edited by Mary K. Gospodarowicz
ISBN 0-471-40633-3 Copyright © 2001 Wiley-Liss, Inc.

this debilitating disease is well recognized, treatment options are limited and controversial. In addition, there is no "standard" therapy in the management of patients with this disease. Surgery, radiation therapy, chemotherapy, and immunotherapy have all been used with varying success. More recently, multimodality treatment regimens have combined surgery with adjuvant radiation therapy and chemotherapy. However, most patients with this disease have been treated in an individualized manner, and this has hampered the ability to accurately identify factors of prognostic significance.

Despite the limitations just described, earlier retrospective[7,10,20] and recent prospective studies[18,21-24] have identified prognostic variables using univariate and multivariate analyses of large groups of patients with MPM. These factors can be broadly grouped into clinical and pathologic factors. Clinical factors associated with a favorable prognosis include: (1) age less than 65, (2) absence of chest pain, (3) long duration of symptoms, (4) weight loss of less than 5% at presentation, (5) good performance status, and (6) a normal platelet count. Surgical–pathologic factors include (1) epithelial histology, (2) absence of nodal metastases, (3) early surgical–pathologic stage, and (4) complete resection. Although some of the clinical factors identified by univariate analysis lose their statistical significance when evaluated by multivariate analysis, they remain important because they often serve to identify patients with advanced disease who are unlikely to benefit from aggressive multimodality therapy.

TUMOR-RELATED FACTORS

Histologic Types

Malignant mesotheliomas are classified into epithelial, sarcomatoid, mixed, or biphasic (both epithelial and sarcomatoid cells) and undifferentiated types.[25] Epithelial type is the most common (50–57%), followed by mixed (24–34%) and sarcomatoid types (16–19%).[7,26] The epithelial type has been shown to be associated with better survival.[7,18,21-24] In a series of 136 patients in which the majority (68%) received chemotherapy and 30% underwent pleuropneumonectomy, the overall median survival of patients with epithelial mesothelioma was 17 months, mixed histology 12 months, and sarcomatoid mesothelioma 6 months.[21] Sugarbaker et al. reported that the epithelial type ($n = 67$) was associated with a 5-year survival of 27% versus 0% in the sarcomatoid or mixed ($n = 47$) tumors after pleuropneumonectomy.[23] Recent papers utilizing larger prospective databases continue to verify the prognostic significance of this histologic classification.[14,24]

The dismal outcome of sarcomatoid mesotheliomas has been well documented. Boutin et al., in a predominantly nonresected series (93%), reported a median survival of 5 months,[22] while Sugarbaker and coworkers noted that despite pleuropneumonectomy, no patient with sarcomatoid type lived longer than 25 months.[27] Desmoplastic mesothelioma, in which more than 50% of the tumor consists of dense hypocellular collagen tissue irrespective of epithelial or sarcomatoid cells, has similar poor prognosis, with a mean survival of 6 months.[28,29] No prognostic distinction has been described for the various epithelial (which include tubular, papillary, glandular, myxoid, adenoid cystic, large-, and small-cell mesothelioma) or sarcomatoid (osteogenic and lymphohistiocytoid) subtypes.

Extent of Disease

Mesotheliomas arise in the parietal pleura, then extend into the visceral and diaphragmatic pleura. Visceral pleura involvement appears to impact prognosis.[22] In a series of 188 patients in which the majority (93%) who were treated nonsurgically, the mean survival was 8 months compared to 22 months for those with or without invasion of the visceral pleura. This difference was further highlighted in the subgroup of Stage I patients (Butchart's staging system; Table 24.1) where the median survival was 7 months versus 33 months in patients with ($n = 43$) and without ($n = 23$) invasion of the visceral pleura.[20] Invasion through the diaphragm is related to poor survival (median of 11 months), irrespective of histology or nodal status.[23] Although known to frequently invade adjacent structures such as the mediastinum (63%), pericardium (49%), peritoneum (39%), and bowel (33%),[7] there is no tissue-specific prognostic information. A recent paper suggested that three-dimensional computed tomographic measurements of pre- (less than 100 milliliters) and postresection tumor volume (less than 9 milliliters) may be associated with improved survival.[30]

Lymph-node Involvement

With up to 50% of surgically resected patients having one or more sites of metastatic mediastinal nodes, the prognostic impact of nodal disease is crucial.[31] In a series of 52 resected patients who had systematic lymph-node dissection, the 1- and 2-year survival rates for patients without regional lymph-node involvement were 71 and 46%, respectively, in contrast to 41% and 0% with nodal involvement ($p < 0.05$).[27] This was further substantiated by a later report on patients who underwent extrapleural pneumonectomy in which node-negative patients had better survival at 2 and 5 years (50 and 25%, respectively; $n = 66$) than did the group with nodal involvement (35 and 0%; $n = 48$; $p = 0.02$).[23] In another series, an analysis of 109 patients indicated that patients with less than four involved nodes had statistically better survival than those with four or more metastatic lymph nodes.[24]

Staging Classifications

One of the difficulties associated with identifying prognostic risk factors in patients with MPM is the lack of an accurate, universally accepted staging system. Earlier staging systems by Butchart and Chahinian (Tables 24.1 and 24.2) inadequately described the extent of pleural and nodal disease and were

TABLE 24.1   Staging Proposed by Butchart et al.

Stage	Description
I	Tumor confined within the "capsule" of the parietal pleura, i.e., involving only the ipsilateral pleura, lung, pericardium, and diaphragm
II	Tumor invading chest wall or involving mediastinal structures, e.g., esophagus, heart, opposite pleura. Lymph-node involvement within the chest
III	Tumor penetrating diaphragm to involve peritoneum; involvement of the opposite pleura. Lymph-node involvement outside the chest
IV	Distant blood-borne metastases

Source: Reference 20.

TABLE 24.2   Staging Proposed by Chahinian et al.

Stage	Description
I	T1N0M0
II	T1–2N1M0
	T2N0M0
III	T3, any N, M0
IV	T4, and N, M0, any M1

Source: Reference 18.
T1 = Limited to ipsilateral pleura only (parietal and visceral pleura); T2 = superficial local invasion (diaphragm, endothoracic fascia, ipsilateral lung, fissures); T3 = deep local invasion (chest wall beyond endothoracic fascia); T4 = extensive direct invasion (opposite pleura, peritoneum, retroperitoneum); N0 = no positive lymph nodes; N1 = positive ipsilateral hilar lymph nodes; N2 = positive mediastinal lymph nodes; N3 = positive contralateral hilar lymph nodes; M0 = no metastases; M1 = metastases, blood-borne or lymphatics.

TABLE 24.3   Staging Proposed by Sugarbaker et al.

Stage	Description
I	Disease confined to within capsule of the parietal pleura: ipsilateral pleura, lung, pericardium, diaphragm, or chest-wall disease limited to previous biopsy sites
II	All of Stage I with positive intrathoracic (N1 or N2) lymph nodes
III	Local extension of disease into chest wall or mediastinum; heart, or through diaphragm, peritoneum; with or without extrathoracic or contralateral (N3) lymph-node involvement
IV	Distant metastatic disease

Source: Reference 27.

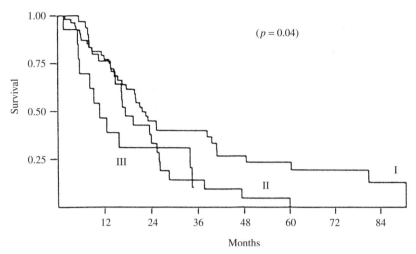

Figure 24.1 Overall survival of patients stratified by the proposed Brigham's staging system.[23]

not validated by survival data.[18,20] More recent staging systems appear to show significant survival differences among the various stages. The Brigham system (Table 24.3), a Butchart modification based on 120 patients, demonstrated a median survival of 22 months for Stage I, 17 months for Stage II, and 11 months for Stage III (Figure 24.1), but fails to utilize (TNM).[23] The International Union Against Cancer (UICC) recognized the discrepancies among the various proposed staging systems, and initiated a consensus based TNM classification in 1990 to promote more uniform staging of the disease and better comparison of treatment outcomes.[32] The TNM system is the universally accepted method of classifying the anatomic disease extent (see Appendix 24A). A more recent staging system by the International Mesothelioma Interest Group (IMIG) (Table 24.4) proposed modifications to the UICC staging system using more specific descriptors. Using the IMIG staging, Rusch et al. reported a series of 231 patients with median survivals of 30, 19, 10, and 8 months for Stage I ($n = 21$), II ($n = 38$), III ($n = 102$), and IV ($n = 70$), respectively (Figure 24.2).[24] However, these three latter systems have not been validated in any prospective multicenter analyses and will continue to be modified as more data are obtained.

Molecular and Biologic Markers

There are limited data on the usefulness of such markers in MPM. High S-phase fraction has been suggested to be associated with a shorter survival, but not aneuploidy.[33,34] Codeletion of the tumor suppressors p15 and p16 has been identified in 72% of patients with malignant mesotheliomas.[35] However, correlation between the presence of such genetic alterations and survival has not been described. Similarly, the simian virus 40 (SV40) DNA sequences

TABLE 24.4 Staging System Proposed by International Mesothelioma Interest Group

T1 T1a Tumor limited to the ipsilateral parietal pleura, including mediastinal and diaphragmatic pleura

No involvement of the visceral pleura

T1b Tumor involving the ipsilateral parietal pleura, including mediastinal and diaphragmatic pleura

Scattered foci of tumor also involving the visceral pleura

T2 Tumor involving each of the ipsilateral pleural surfaces (parietal, mediastinal, diaphragmatic, and visceral pleura) with at least one of the following features:
- involvement of diaphragmatic muscle
- confluent visceral pleural tumor (including the fissures) or extension of tumor from visceral pleura into the underlying pulmonary parenchyma

T3 Describes locally advanced but potentially resectable tumor

Tumor involving all of the ipsilateral pleural surfaces (parietal, mediastinal, diaphragmatic, and visceral pleura) with at least one of the following features:
- involvement of the endothoracic fascia
- extension into the mediastinal fat
- solitary, completely resectable focus of tumor extending into the soft tissues of the chest wall
- nontransmural involvement of the pericardium

T4 Describes locally advanced technically unresectable tumor

Tumor involving all of the ipsilateral pleural surfaces (parietal, mediastinal, diaphragmatic, and visceral) with at least one of the following features:
- diffuse extension or multifocal masses of tumor in the chest wall, with or without associated rib destruction
- direct transdiaphragmatic extension of tumor to the peritoneum
- direct extension of tumor to the contralateral pleura
- direct extension of tumor to one or more mediastinal organs
- direct extension of tumor into the spine
- tumor extending through to the internal surface of the pericardium with or without a pericardial effusion; or tumor involving the myocardium

N–Lymph nodes

NX Regional lymph nodes cannot be assessed

N0 No regional lymph-node metastases

N1 Metastases in the ipsilateral bronchopulmonary or hilar lymph nodes

N2 Metastases in the subcarinal or the ipsilateral mediastinal lymph nodes, including the ipsilateral internal mammary nodes

N3 Metastases in the contralateral mediastinal, contralateral internal mammary, ipsilateral, or contralateral supraclavicular lymph nodes

M–Metastases

MX Presence of distant metastases cannot be assessed

M0 No distant metastasis

M1 Distant metastases present

Stage Grouping

Stage Ia	T1a	N0	M0
Ib	T1b	N0	M0
Stage II	T2	N0	M0
Stage III	Any T3		M0
	Any	N1	M0
	Any	N2	M0
Stage IV	Any T4		
	Any N3		
	Any M1		

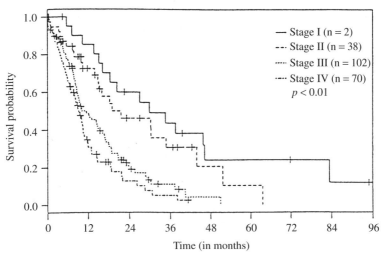

Figure 24.2 Overall survival of patients stratified by the proposed IMIG staging system.[32]

and SV40 large T-antigen expression have been identified in up to 83% of cases,[4,36] but, the diagnostic and prognostic value of these findings remains to be proven. Other cellular markers that have been examined include the oncogene Wilms tumor 1 (WT1), the tumor suppressor gene p53, the cell proliferation markers proliferating-cell nuclear antigen (PCNA) and Ki-67, and markers for angiogenesis such as thrombospondin 1 (TSP-1). Although these markers may give insight into the cellular processes associated with the development of MPM, they do not serve as independent prognostic indicators in this disease.[37–42]

Thrombocytosis

Thrombocytosis (platelet count >400,000/μL) as a negative prognostic variable in MPM has been demonstrated in multiple series. Ruffie et al. and Herndon et al. found that patients with a platelet count greater than 400,000 had a significantly shorter median survival compared to patients whose platelet count was less than 400,000.[7,43] These differences were highly statistically significant by both univariate and multivariate analysis. Pass et al. found that the median survival after surgical treatment correlated with the preoperative platelet count.[44] Patients with platelet counts greater than 462,000/μL had a significantly shorter median survival compared to patients with counts less than 462,000/μL. Patients with normal platelet counts (179,000–295,000) had the longest median survival. The Lung Cancer Study Group Trial identified a platelet count greater than 400,000 as a significant prognostic factor in the univariate analysis, although it did not retain statistical significance in the multivariate analysis.[12] The prognostic significance of thrombocytosis remains controversial. While its negative predictive value was shown in earlier reports,[7,45] association with poorer survival was not seen in a larger multivariate analysis of surgically resected patients.[24]

HOST-RELATED FACTORS

Age and Gender

Multiple studies have demonstrated that patients less than or equal to 65 years of age with MPM have a longer median survival compared to patients who are older than 65 years of age. Ruffie et al. found that patients aged 65 or younger had a median survival of 10 months compared to 6 months in patients older than 65.[7] This difference was significant in both univariate and multivariate analyses. In a review of 167 patients with diffuse MPM, Van Gelder et al. noted a similar finding with median survival of 12 months versus 8 months, respectively.[46] Importantly, this latter study found a significantly worse prognosis in patients older than 74 (median survival 4.0 months), a finding also noted by other investigators.[43]

Two smaller series also suggested a better prognosis in younger patients. Chahinian et al. found a median survival of 15 months in 46 patients younger than 65, compared to 10 months in 11 patients aged 65 or older.[18] In a review of 80 patients with MPM, De Pangher Manzini et al. noted a median survival of 19 months in patients less than age 65 versus 11 months for patients age 65 or older.[47] However, this trend did not achieve statistical significance in the multivariate analysis. A recent multivariate analysis of a larger series of 231 surgically treated patients demonstrated a significantly longer survival among females.[24]

Symptoms and Signs

Although symptoms tend to be nonspecific, the indolent epithelial mesothelioma is more often associated with dyspnea and pleural effusion, while the sarcomatoid tumor is more frequently accompanied by chest pain and a mass lesion on chest X ray.[7] The lack of chest pain and presence of symptoms for more than 6 months have been reported to be favorable prognostic factors.[21]

Chest Pain   The presence of chest pain in patients with pleural mesothelioma often suggests progression of disease through the parietal pleura and into the endothoracic fascia. In both univariate and multivariate analysis, Antman et al. found that patients with chest pain at the time of presentation had a shorter median survival than those patients who presented without chest pain (10 months versus 17 months).[21] This finding was also noted in the review of patients treated on protocols sponsored by the Cancer and Leukemia Group B (CALGB).[43]

Duration of Symptoms   In contrast to many other malignancies, a long interval (>6 months) from the onset of symptoms to the time of diagnosis of MPM has been associated with a longer median survival. This most likely reflects a less aggressive biology of the individual patient's tumor. Alberts et al. found that patients with symptoms greater than 6 months was associated with a median survival of 12 months versus 8.7 months in patients with symptoms less than 6 months.[48] This difference was significant in both univariate and multivariate analysis. Antman et al. also found in their multivariate analysis that an interval of greater than 6 months was associated with a longer median survival.[21] However, this is not a universal finding. In a retrospective review of 332 patients with diffuse MPM, Ruffie et al. found no statistical difference in median survival between patients with symptoms of greater or less than 6 months (10.4 months versus 8.4 months, respectively).[7]

Weight Loss

Weight loss of more than 5% at diagnosis appears to be an important negative prognostic factor. Ruffie et al. observed a statistically significant difference in the median survival of patients with and without weight loss (5 months versus 11 months) in a univariate analysis.[7] This was confirmed by a multivariate analysis in which the mean survival of patients without weight loss was 20 months, compared to 5 months in those with more than 5% weight loss.[22]

Performance Status

Many studies have observed that patients with a performance status of less than or equal to 1 utilizing the Eastern Cooperative Oncology Group scale at presentation have longer median survival compared to patients with scores greater than 1.[18,21,47–49] Antman et al. observed a median survival of 16 months for patients with ECOG performance values of 0, 10 months for ECOG score of 1, compared to 5 months in patients with ECOG performance values of 2 or more.[21] Similarly, a retrospective review of 337 patients with mesothelioma treated on investigational protocols sponsored by the CALGB found that ECOG performance score at diagnosis was an independent predictor of outcome in both univariate and multivariate analyses. In this study, patients with an ECOG performance score of 0 had a median and 2-year survival of 14 months and 38%, respectively. In patients with a performance score of 1 or more, the median and 2-year survival dropped to 9.5 months and 21%, respectively.[43]

ENVIRONMENT-RELATED PROGNOSTIC FACTORS

Treatment

Early Diagnosis   It has been suggested that early diagnosis may affect survival. Boutin et al. demonstrated by univariate studies that small nodules, which appear like nonspecific inflammatory lesions on thoracoscopy, represent early disease and were associated with a mean survival of 28 months.[22] Larger nodules or tumor-like thickening were associated with a poorer mean survival of 10 months. This may suggest lead-time bias rather than response to therapy.

Extent of Surgical Resection   The extent of surgical resection does not predict survival. An earlier prospective study by Rusch et al. demonstrated no survival difference between extrapleural pneumonectomy and more limited operations.[12] This was confirmed by a subsequent report on a larger group of patients following extrapleural pneumonectomy ($n = 115$) or pleurectomy/decortication ($n = 59$).[24] The presence of residual tumor at surgical resection margins impacts survival. In many series, complete resection is defined as no gross residual tumor at the completion of the operation.[30,50] Sugarbaker et al. performed an analysis of each extrapleural pneumonectomy specimen to determine the prognostic significance of microscopically positive margins involving the chest wall, bronchus, pericardium, and diaphragm.[14] In this series, univariate analysis demonstrated patients with negative resection margins had prolonged 2-year and 5-year survivals (44%, 25%) compared with patients who had positive resection margins (33%, 9%). Negative surgical margins remained statistically significant in the multivariate analysis.

Adjuvant Therapy   Response to chemotherapy has not been shown to be of any prognostic value, although an average response of only 20% with single-agent treatment[51] and more than 50% response with combination therapy have been reported.[52] Multimodality therapy comprising surgery, chemotherapy, and radiation appears to confer survival advantage.[14,24] When Rusch et al. compared the overall survival between patients who did not receive adjuvant external beam radiation ($n = 24$) with patients who received it ($n = 106$), the latter had significantly better survival.[24]

Asbestos and Smoking Exposure

Although one group reported that exposure to asbestos was a strong prognostic factor,[7] others have found no association between this risk factor and survival.[14,21–23] Similarly, cigarette smoking has not been shown to impact the prognosis of MPM.[7,14,21,23] However, it significantly increases the risk of lung cancer in the asbestos-exposed worker.[53]

SUMMARY

Carefully collected prospective data have contributed to our current knowledge on the determinants of survival for malignant mesothelioma (see Appendix 24B). Histological type is the most consistent predictor. While host-related factors, such as chest pain, weight loss, and performance status, appear to influence prognosis, age, gender, and thrombocytosis remain controversial. Stage of disease, stratified by the tumor, node, and metastasis status, appears to prognosticate, but several staging classifications continue to evolve as more information becomes available. Perhaps employment of a universally accepted staging system will enable a more accurate analysis of controversial factors. In addition, given the paucity of randomized data, this will facilitate better comparison of different patient populations and treatment regimes. The trend toward multimodality therapy, molecular, and genetic analysis may identify new prognostic factors. Ultimately, this may help us better stage and select patients for the appropriate therapy and hopefully improve the survival of this dreaded disease.

■■■■■■■ APPENDIX 24A

TNM Classification: Pleural Mesothelioma

T — Primary Tumor

TX Primary tumor cannot be assessed

T0 No evidence of primary tumor

T1 Tumor limited to ipsilateral parietal and/or visceral pleura

T2 Tumor invades any of the following: ipsilateral lung, endothoracic fascia, diaphragm, pericardium

T3 Tumor invades any of the following: ipsilateral chest-wall muscle, ribs, mediastinal organs or tissues

T4 Tumor directly extends to any of the following: contralateral pleura, contralateral lung, peritoneum, intra-abdominal organs, cervical tissues

N — Regional Lymph Nodes

NX Regional lymph nodes cannot be assessed

N0 No regional lymph-node metastasis

N1 Metastasis in ipsilateral peribronchial and/or ipsilateral hilar lymph nodes, including involvement by direct extension

N2 Metastasis in ipsilateral mediastinal and/or subcarinal lymph node(s)

N3 Metastasis in contralateral mediastinal, contralateral hilar, ipsilateral or contralateral scalene, or supraclavicular lymph node(s)

M — Distant Metastasis

MX Distant metastasis cannot be assessed

M0 No distant metastasis

M1 Distant metastasis

	Stage Grouping		
Stage I	T1	N0	M0
	T2	N0	M0
Stage II	T1	N1	M0
	T2	N1	M0
Stage III	T1	N2	M0
	T2	N2	M0
	T3	N0, N1, N2	M0
Stage IV	Any T	N3	M0
	T4	Any N	M0
	Any T	Any N	M1

Source: Sobin LH, Wittekind Ch (eds.): *TNM classification of malignant tumors*, 5th ed. New York, Union Internationale Contre le Cancer Wiley-Liss, 1997.

███████ **APPENDIX 24B**

Prognostic Factors in Mesothelioma

Prognostic Factors	Tumor Related	Host Related	Environment Related
Essential	Stage of disease (TNM status) Histologic type	Age Weight loss >5% ECOG performance status	Completeness of resection
Additional	Symptoms	Gender	
New and promising	S-phase fraction		Early diagnosis Multimodality therapy

REFERENCES

1. Walker AM, Loughlin JE, Freidlander ER, et al.: Projections of asbestos-related disease 1980–2009. *J Occup Med* 25:409–25, 1983.
2. Rom WM: Asbestos-related lung disease, in Fishman AP, Elias JA, Fishman JA, et al. (eds.): *Fishman's pulmonary diseases and disorders*. New York, McGraw-Hill, 1998, pp. 877–891.
3. Nicholson WJ, Perkel G, Selikoff IJ: Occupational exposure to asbestos: Population at risk and projected mortality 1980–2030. *Am J Indust Med* 3:259–311, 1982.
4. Pass HI, Donington JS, Wu P, et al.: Human mesotheliomas contain the simian virus-40 regulatory region and large tumor antigen DNA sequences. *J Thorac Cardiovasc Surg* 116:854–9, 1998.

5. Carbone M, Rizzo P, Grimley PM, et al.: Simian virus-40 large-T antigen binds p53 in human mesotheliomas. *Nat Med* 3:908–12, 1997.

6. Carbone M, Fisher S, Powers A, et al.: New molecular and epidemiological issues in mesothelioma: Role of SV40. *J Cell Physiol* 180:167–72, 1999.

7. Ruffie P, Feld R, Minkin S, et al.: Diffuse malignant mesothelioma of the pleura in Ontario and Quebec: A retrospective study of 332 patients. *J Clin Oncol* 7:1157–68, 1989.

8. Baldini EH, Recht A, Strauss GM, et al.: Patterns of failure after trimodality therapy for malignant pleural mesothelioma. *Ann Thorac Surg* 63:334–8, 1997.

9. McCormack PM, Nagasaki F, Hilaris BS, et al.: Surgical treatment of pleural mesothelioma. *J Thorac Cardiovasc Surg* 84:834–42, 1982.

10. DaValle MJ, Faber LP, Kittle CF, et al.: Extrapleural pneumonectomy for diffuse, malignant mesothelioma. *Ann Thorac Surg* 42:612–8, 1986.

11. Martini N, McCormack PM, Bains MS, et al.: Pleural mesothelioma. *Ann Thorac Surg* 43:113–20, 1987.

12. Rusch VW, Piantadosi S, Holmes EC: The role of extrapleural pneumonectomy in malignant pleural mesothelioma. A Lung Cancer Study Group trial. *J Thorac Cardiovasc Surg* 102:1–9, 1991.

13. Huncharek M, Kelsey K, Mark EJ, et al.: Treatment and survival in diffuse malignant pleural mesothelioma; A study of 83 cases from the Massachusetts General Hospital. *Anticancer Res* 16:1265–8, 1996.

14. Sugarbaker DJ, Flores RM, Jaklitsch MT, et al.: Resection margins, extrapleural nodal status, and cell type determine postoperative long-term survival in trimodality therapy of malignant pleural mesothelioma: results in 183 patients. *J Thorac Cardiovasc Surg* 117:54–63, 1999.

15. Wagner JC, Sleggs EA, Marchand P: Diffuse pleural mesothelioma and asbestosis in the Northern Western Cape Province. *Br J Indust Med* 7:260, 1960.

16. Selikoff IJ, Churg J, Hammond EC: Asbestos exposure and neoplasia. *JAMA* 188:22–6, 1964.

17. Newhouse ML, Berry G, Wagner JC: Mortality of factory workers in East London, 1933–980. *Br J Indust Med* 42: 4–11, 1980.

18. Chahinian AP, Pajak TF, Holland JF, et al.: Diffuse malignant mesothelioma: Prospective evaluation of 69 patients. *Ann Intern Med* 96:746–55, 1982.

19. Antman KH, Blum RH, Greenberger JS, et al.: Multimodality therapy for malignant mesothelioma based on a study of natural history. *Am J Med* 68:356–62, 1980.

20. Butchart EG, Ashort T, Barnsley WC, et al.: Pleuropneumonectomy in the management of diffuse malignant mesothelioma of the pleura. Experience with 29 patients. *Thorax* 31:15–24, 1976.

21. Antman K, Shemin R, Ryan L, et al.: Malignant mesothelioma: Prognostic variables in a registry of 180 patients, the Dana-Farber Cancer Institute and Brigham and Women's Hospital experience over two decades, 1965–1985. *J Clin Oncol* 6:147–53, 1988.

22. Boutin C, Rey F, Gouvernet J, et al.: Thoracoscopy in pleural malignant mesothelioma: A prospective study of 188 consecutive patients. Part 2: Prognosis and staging. *Cancer* 72:394–404, 1993.

23. Sugarbaker DJ, Gracia JP, Richards WG, et al.: Extrapleural pneumonectomy in the multimodality therapy of malignant pleural mesothelioma. Results in 120 consecutive patients. *Ann Surg* 224:288–96, 1996.

24. Rusch VW, Venkatraman ES: Important prognostic factors in patients with malignant pleural mesothelioma, managed surgically. *Ann Thorac Surg* 68:1799–1804, 1999.

25. Churg J, Rosen SH, Moolten S: Histological characteristics of mesothelioma associated with asbestos. *Ann NY Acad Sci* 132:614–22, 1965.

26. Hillerdal G: Malignant mesothelioma 1982: Review of 4710 published cases. *Br J Dis Chest* 77:321–43, 1983.

27. Sugarbaker DL, Strauss GM, Lynch TJ, et al.: Node status has prognostic significance in the multimodality therapy of diffuse, malignant mesothelioma. *J Clin Oncol* 11:1172–8, 1993.

28. Cantin R, Al-Jabi M, McCaughey WTE: Desmoplastic diffuse mesothelioma. *Am J Surg Pathol* 6:215–22, 1982.

29. Wilson GE, Hasleton PS, Charterjee AK: Desmoplastic malignant mesothelioma: A review of 17 cases. *J Clin Pathol* 45:295–8, 1992.

30. Pass HI, Temeck BK, Kranda K, et al.: Preoperative tumor volume is associated with outcome in malignant pleural mesothelioma. *J Thorac Cardiovasc Surg* 115:310–8, 1998.

31. Rusch V, Saltz L, Venkatraman E, et al.: A phase II trial of pleurectomy/decortication followed by intrapleural and systemic chemotherapy for malignant pleural mesothelioma. *J Clin Oncol* 12:1156–63, 1994.

32. Rusch VW, Ginsberg RJ: New concepts in the staging of mesothelioma, in Deslauriers J, Lacquet LK (eds.): *Thoracic surgery: Surgical management of pleural diseases*. St Louis, MO, Mosby, 1990, pp. 336–43.

33. Dazzi H, Thatcher N, Hasleton PS, et al.: DNA analysis by flow cytometry in malignant pleural mesothelioma: Relationship to histology and survival. *J Pathol* 162:51–5, 1990.

34. Pyrhonen S, Laasonen A, Tammilehto L, et al.: Diploid predominance and prognostic significance of S-phase cells in malignant mesothelioma. *Eur J Cancer* 27:197–200, 1991.

35. Xio S, Li D, Vijg J, et al.: Codeletion of p15 and p16 in primary malignant mesothelioma. *Oncogene* 3:511–5, 1995.

36. Testa JR, Carbone M, Hirvonen A, et al.: A multi-institutional study confirms the presence and expression of simian virus 40 in human malignant mesothelioma. *Cancer Res* 58:4505–9, 1998.

37. Kumar-Singh S, Segers K, Rodeck U, et al.: WT1 mutation in malignant mesothelioma and WT1 immunoreactivity in relation to p53 and growth factor receptor expression, cell-type transition, and prognosis. *J Pathol* 181:67–74, 1997.

38. Kumar-Singh S, Vermeulen PB, Weyler J, et al.: Evaluation of tumor angiogenesis as a prognostic marker in malignant mesothelioma. *J Pathol* 182:211–6, 1997.

39. Esposito V, Baldi A, De Luca A, et al.: Role of PCNA in differentiating between malignant mesothelioma and mesothelial hyperplasia: Prognostic considerations. *Anticancer Res* 17:601–4, 1997.

40. Ohta Y, Shridhar V, Kalemkerian GP, et al.: Thrombospondin-1 expression and clinical implications in malignant pleural mesothelioma. *Cancer* 85:2570–6, 1999.

41. Beer TW, Buchanan R, Matthews AW, et al.: Prognosis in malignant mesothelioma related to MIB 1 proliferation index and histological subtype. *Hum Pathol* 29:246–51, 1998.

42. Kumar-Singh S, Jacobs W, Dhaene K, et al.: Syndecan-1 expression in malignant mesothelioma: Correlation with cell differentiation, WT1 expression, and clinical outcome. *J Pathol* 186:300–5, 1998.

43. Herndon JE, Green MR, Chahinian AP, et al.: Factors predictive of survival among 337 patients with mesothelioma treated between 1984 and 1994 by the Cancer and Leukemia Group B. *Chest* 113:723–31, 1998.

44. Pass HI, Kranda K, Temeck BK, et al.: Surgically debulked malignant pleural mesothelioma: Results and prognostic factors. *Ann Surg Oncol* 4:215–22, 1997.

45. Olesen LL, Thorshauge H: Thrombocytosis in patients with malignant pleura mesothelioma. *Cancer* 62:1194–6, 1988.

46. Van Gelder T, Damhuis RA, Hoogsteden HC: Prognostic factors and survival in malignant pleural mesothelioma. *Eur Respir J* 7:1035–8, 1994.

47. De Pangher Manzini V, Brollo A, Franceschi S, et al.: Prognostic factors of malignant mesothelioma of the pleura. *Cancer* 72:410–7, 1993.

48. Alberts AS, Falkson G, Goedhals L, et al.: Malignant pleural mesothelioma: A disease unaffected by current therapeutic maneuvers. *J Clin Oncol* 6:527–35, 1988.

49. Curran D, Sahmoud T, Therasse P, et al.: Prognostic factors in patients with pleural mesothelioma: The European Organization for Research and Treatment of Cancer experience. *J Clin Oncol* 16:145–52, 1998.

50. Rusch VW, Venkatraman E: The importance of surgical staging in the treatment of malignant pleural mesothelioma. *J Thorac Cardiovasc Surg* 111:815–25, 1996.

51. Sterman DH, Kaiser LR, Albelda SM: Advances in the treatment of malignant pleural mesothelioma. *Chest* 116: 504–20, 1999.

52. Byrne ME, Davidson JA, Musk AW, et al.: Cisplatin and gemcitabine treatment for malignant mesothelioma: A phase II study (abstract). Paper presented at the 34th Annual Meeting of the American Society of Clinical Oncology, Los Angeles, CA, 1998.

53. Selikoff IJ, Seidman H: Asbestos-associated deaths among workers in the United States and Canada, 1967–1987. *Ann NY Acad Sci* 643:1–14, 1991.

CHAPTER 25

Malignant Thymoma

DAVID G. PAYNE

The thymus gland, located in the anterior mediastinum, plays a crucial role in the development of immunological competence during fetal development and infancy. It is composed of both thymic epithelial cells and lymphoid cells, many originating in the bone marrow. During the development period, the complex system of T lymphocytes evolves, underpinning functions of foreign antigen processing and self-recognition of the organism's histocompatibility complex. The gland undergoes significant involution in childhood, resulting in a twin-lobed organ composed of fibrous, lymphatic, and epithelial elements. Its function in the adult is unknown; however, evidence for its immunologic role is seen in the involution associated with various disorders, including autoimmune diseases and AIDS, and conversely in the immunodeficiency associated with primary thymic aplasia. Tumors of the thymus are unusual, but account for about 15% of mediastinal tumors (or over 50% of masses in the anterior mediastinum). These neoplasms contain varying proportions of lymphocytes and of thymic epithelial cells, with a generally benign appearance. However, all thymomas are considered to be malignant tumors possessing differing degrees of aggressivity, or invasiveness. When frank cytologic features of malignancy are seen in epithelial cells, the tumor is regarded as a thymic carcinoma.

Clinical features typically relate to the size of the mass and proximity to other organs. The introduction of the Masaoka classification,[1] based on the extent of local invasion by malignant cells, was an important advance in the addressing the need for comparative studies. However, the association of thymoma with various autoimmune disorders is distinctive and possibly prognostic. These conditions include myasthenia gravis, hypogammaglobulinemia, and red-cell aplasia. Interestingly these syndromes are not associated with thymectomy in another context. A variety of other paraneoplastic syndromes are seen; about 40% of thymoma patients have one, and many suffer from multiple such disorders.

Prognostic Factors in Cancer, 2nd edition, Edited by Mary K. Gospodarowicz.
ISBN 0-471-40633-3   Copyright © 2001 Wiley-Liss, Inc.

For the purpose of this discussion these will be considered to be tumor-related factors. Note that in accordance with the guidelines for this text, only factors that are required for clinical decision making are considered "essential."

TUMOR-RELATED PROGNOSTIC FACTORS

Many factors have been assessed in various reports on this unusual tumor. The current UICC manual for anatomic TNM staging (5th edition, 1997) has no classification for tumors of the thymus.

Histopathologic Features

Cell Type   The American classification proposed by Bernatz in 1961, based on an analysis of 181 patients,[2,3] is generally considered the "classic" one. The malignancy is regarded as arising from the epithelial component from which the so-called spindle cell is thought to derive. A better long-term survival of these (surgically) treated patients was correlated with the predominance of the spindle and/or lymphocytic cell type, whereas those patients classified with epithelial or mixed cell types experienced an inferior rate of survival. The authors noted, however, that the cell type was strongly related to the presence of local invasion by the tumor. A more recent "European" classification of Muller-Hermelink[4,5] is based on the degree of differentiation of the malignant cell toward a pattern corresponding to the thymic cortex or medulla. The medullary type lacks squamous differentiation and is relatively noninvasive. Cortical thymomas show large epithelial cells and may resemble the outer cortex. A morphometric formulation was described by Nomori.[6] In this scheme, the well-differentiated thymic carcinoma emerges at the invasive end of the spectrum of cortical thymoma. This scheme has been slow to gain acceptance because of perceived difficulties in applying its use in a standard fashion. An Italian series[7] reported on 83 operated patients with a multivariate analysis of multiple factors. They found that both the Marino cortical-medullary classification and the Masaoka staging scheme were significant and independent prognostic factors for survival, and could be combined into a prognostic index. Blumberg[8] reached the same conclusions with a similar analysis, but using the traditional classification for cell type. However, there are no large series making a direct comparison between the Bernatz and Marino cell type classifications (Table 25.1). It should be noted that

TABLE 25.1   Histopathologic Classification

Classic	European
Spindle cell	Medullary
Predominately lymphocytic	Mixed
Mixed lymphoepithelial	Predominantly cortical
Predominantly epithelial	Cortical
Thymic carcinoma	Thymic carcinoma

the well-differentiated thymic carcinoma is not part of the traditional (Bernatz) classification. It can be included, however, as a tumor of epithelial thymic cells showing malignant cytologic features — it may, however, be difficult to distinguish from lung cancer. Many reports prior to 1990 have included cases of invasive thymoma that later would have been classified as thymic carcinoma.[9] These classifications are subject to observer variation, and the "mixed groups" account for about 35–40% of cases in typical series.

In summary, cell type is an accepted prognostic factor, in which tumor with primarily "spindle" or "medullary" features have low invasiveness and good prognosis, while those with predominately "epithelial" or "cortical" makeup have a poor outlook. A new histological classification of thymic epithelial tumors has recently appeared in the World Health Organization (WHO) tumor classification series.[10] It brings together the cytological, histological, and behavioral elements of the previous classifications (Table 25.2). The precise usage may depend importantly on the training and experience of the pathologist.

Cytologic and Genetic Features

Efforts have been made to identify thymomas at risk for recurrence despite relatively favorable staging, benign histologic appearance, and complete resection. Analysis by flow cytometry to assess DNA content has indicated an increased risk of relapse associated with aneuploidy.[11] This finding was not confirmed in two studies[12,13] in which p53 overexpression in a series of noninvasive thymomas was predictive of poor survival. Other immunohistochemical and genetic factors have been studied, but there are no established cell markers supported by well-done correlative studies.

Other Histologic Features

Histologic features, which could be prognostic, include multifocality and vascular invasion. These features have not been studied in detail, or distinguished from the diagnosis of microscopic invasiveness. The histologic diagnosis of extrathymic extension, or local invasion, however, is extremely important. This is incorporated into the standard clinical staging systems as discussed below. Similarly, the histologic identification of pleural or other sites of metastatic spread is essential to establishing the clinical stage.

Paraneoplastic Syndromes

Thymomas are commonly associated with autoimmune or neuromuscular syndromes. Most are rare; myasthenia gravis (30%) is the most common, and others, such as pure red-cell aplasia and hypogammaglobulinemia, are considered classic. About 15% of patients with myasthenia will have thymoma, though more will simply have a thymic hyperplasia. Three large trials with multivariate analysis[8,14,15] found that while nonmyasthenia autoimmune disorders, notably hallmark conditions such as red-cell aplasia and hypogammaglobulinemia, conferred a poor prognosis for survival, myasthenia gravis did not. This

TABLE 25.2 WHO Histological Classification of Tumors of the Thymus

1		Epithelial Tumors	
	1.1	Thymoma	8580/1
	1.1.1	Type A (spindle cell: medullary)	8581/1
	1.1.2	Type AB (mixed)	8582/1
	1.1.3	Type B1 (lymphocyte-rich; lymphocytic; predominantly cortical; organoid)	8583/1
	1.1.4	Type B2 (cortical)	8584/1
	1.1.5	Type B3 (epithelial; atypical; squamoid; well-differentiated thymic carcinoma)	8585/1
	1.2	Thymic carcinoma (Type C thymoma)	8586/3
	1.2.1	Epidermoid keratinizing (squamous cell) carcinoma	8071/3
	1.2.2	Epidermoid nonkeratinizing carcinoma	8072/3
	1.2.3	Lymphoepithelioma-like carcinoma	8082/3
	1.2.4	Sarcomatoid carcinoma (carcinosarcoma)	8980/3
	1.2.5	Clear-cell carcinoma	8310/3
	1.2.6	Basaloid carcinoma	8123/3
	1.2.7	Mucoepidermoid carcinoma	8430/3
	1.2.8	Papillary carcinoma	8050/3
	1.2.9	Undifferentiated carcinoma	8020/3
2		Neuroendocrine tumors	
3		Germ-cell tumors	
4		Lymphoid tumors	
5		Stromal tumors	
6		Tumor-like lesions	
7		Neck tumors of thymic or related branchial pouch derivation	
8		Metastatic tumors	
9		Unclassified tumors	

Source: Morphology code of the International Classification of Diseases for Oncology (ICD-O) and the Systematized Nomenclature of Medicine (SNOMED).

Note: Behavior is coded /0 for benign tumors; /3 for malignant tumors, and /1 for unspecified, borderline or uncertain behavior. Tumors in the thymoma group may be benign or malignant, depending on whether they are encapsulated or invasive; when this is unspecified, they are coded /1.

is in accordance with the modern view that current preoperative management of myasthenia gravis has abolished the adverse prognostic impact of this disorder reported in the older literature. Conversely, two studies[16,17] demonstrated that for myasthenia, the presence of an associated thymoma has adverse prognostic import. Other syndromes described, such as various cytopenias, vasculitides, neuropathies, collagen vascular disorders, and nephrotic syndrome, are much less common, and not of proven prognostic significance. The presence of a paraneoplastic syndrome is considered to be an essential prognostic factor because it affects clinical decision making and treatment of the patient.

Anatomic Disease Extent

Size Large retrospective studies have included tumor size as a factor for multivariate analysis.[8,14] The two series cited defined thresholds of 11–15 cm for the adverse prognostic effect on survival; an independent effect on local relapse rate was not observed. One study showed mediastinal compression at presentation to be a significant adverse sign in a multivariate analysis.[15]

Regional Spread   Thymomas spread primarily by direct infiltration of contiguous organs, though cells may contaminate the pleural surface, giving rise to nodules or plaques. Metastasis to mediastinal or supraclavicular lymph nodes is unusual. Both forms of spread carry a poor prognosis for survival and are accounted for in the clinical staging system.

Distant Metastasis   Distant metastatic deposits are quite rare, even when the primary disease has relapsed. Its presence signifies an advanced clinical stage.[18]

Clinical Stage

The inference that invasiveness was the crucial prognostic factor, and was probably not independent of cell type, has formed the basis of most subsequent developments in this field. Following this, clinical staging systems expressing the role of local invasions were proposed by Bergh[19] and Wilkins.[20] These principles were extended by Masaoka in 1981, who reported on 96 cases analyzed according to the degree of local invasion as determined from histopathological examination of the resected specimen. The authors proposed four clinical "stages," which have been widely adopted. A variant, that of the Groupe d'Etudes de Tumeurs Thymiques (GETT),[21,22] adds a parameter describing the extent, or completeness, of surgical resection. In a series of 149 cases in which both systems were used, this French group found stage agreement in 88%, though definitions differed slightly[15] (Table 25.3). These classifications depend on a histopathological assessment of the degree of tumor infiltration into the capsule

TABLE 25.3   Clinical Staging of Thymoma

	Masaoka		GETT
1	Macroscopically completely encapsulated; Microscopically no capsular invasion	1a	Encapsulated tumor, totally resected
		1b	Macroscopically encapsulated tumor, totally resected, surgeon suspects mediastinal adhesions and potential capsular invasion
2	Macroscopic invasion into surrounding fatty tissue or mediastinal pleura; Microscopic invasion into capsule	2	Invasive tumor, totally resected
3	Macroscopic invasion into neighboring organ; i.e., pericardium, great vessels, lung	3a	Invasive tumor, subtotally resected
		3b	Invasive tumor, biopsy
4a	Pleural or pericardial dissemination	4a	Supraclavicular metastasis or distant pleural implant
4b	Lymphogenous or hematogenous metastasis	4b	Distant metastasis

or associated neighboring tissues. Both systems have the disadvantage that they require a resected specimen. With the application of modern imaging techniques, however, most Masaoka Stage III or IV tumors can be identified nonsurgically. Major uncertainty remains in the Stage II subgroup (about 10%), but most of these go on to be resected and examined histopathologically anyway.

HOST-RELATED FACTORS

Demographic Factors

Patients with thymoma are typically between the ages of 20 years and 75 years, with equal representation of the sexes. The larger series using multivariate analyses have not demonstrated patient age or sex to be prognostic. An exception is that of the Mayo series,[14] in which the patients under age 30 (less than 10% of the total) had an unfavorable prognosis. There is no established hereditary or racial predilection, or impact on prognosis.

Coexisting Disease

Thymoma in general presents with the insidious onset of thoracic or paraneoplastic symptoms, is not associated with adverse lifestyle choices, and affects a relatively young population (median age 45 years). For these reasons, performance status indicators are usually generally good, and not often analyzed. An exception is a German series[28] of 70 patients in which only 11% had Karnofsky performance status ≤70, but this low level of function was unfavorable for overall survival (though not for disease-free survival) by multivariate analysis. It is probable that patients with poor performance status are more likely to be elderly and/or suffering from a paraneoplastic syndrome. On the other hand, for reasons stated above, thymoma patients tend not to suffer from significant comorbid conditions, in contrast to those with lung cancer, for example.

ENVIRONMENT-RELATED PROGNOSTIC FACTORS

Extent of Surgical Resection

This important parameter is evidently not independent of treatment. That is, it is not a prognostic factor a priori, since it can usually be determined only at and after surgery. Rather it is a practical surrogate for the degree of local invasion manifested by the degree of local invasion manifested by the untreated tumor. Thus incompletely resected tumors may have an unfavorable prognosis for several reasons. First, there is demonstrable tumor remaining in the patient, which may be hard to control; second, the inability to resect may indicate an intrinsic aggressive biology in the tumor, and third, this inability may simply reflect the availability of less than optimal medical care to the patient. Nonetheless, the extent of resection is a readily identifiable surgical pathological endpoint. It has been shown in numerous multivariate retrospective analyses to carry prognostic weight[7,8,14,15] This observation may be over interpreted if used to justify high-risk attempts to obtain complete resections. This is an unavoidable risk when treatment parameters are included in prognostic analysis. The extent of surgical staging forms a part of the clinical-pathologic anatomic staging systems, as discussed below.

Postoperative Therapy

The use of these therapies is not considered to be prognostic, though they may influence the outcome. A review of their role is beyond the scope of this discussion. They are included here for completeness, since surgery plays an important role in the clinical staging system. The indications for postoperative radiotherapy are reasonably well established.[15,24–26] Radiotherapy is recommended for completely resected invasive disease, provided it shows invasive features (at least Masaoka stage II). In addition, almost all patients with subtotal resection, or only a biopsy, will receive radiotherapy.[27] Chemotherapy has been used mainly with advanced or relapsed disease.[24,28] Interestingly, the French multivariate analysis found a survival benefit for chemotherapy in the subset presenting with mediastinal compression.

There are no known etiologic associations, indicators, or markers for thymoma, and no identified geographic clusters. A role for the Epstein-Barr virus has been postulated,[29] but never demonstrated. The impact of socioeconomic, geographic, or ethnic factors is probably limited to consideration of patient access to modern medical techniques for diagnosis, evaluation, and treatment.

SUMMARY

The factors discussed in this chapter are summarized in the Appendix. Factors considered essential are those that are required for clinical decision making. Choice of therapy, for example, to use surgery or not, is not considered to be a prognostic factor. For reasons discussed earlier, however, the factor representing clinical stage is somewhat dependent on therapy. It must be emphasized that our understanding is continually evolving, and that this classification of factors may change with time. It is inevitable that the study of a rare disease may suffer from a lack of large prospective or well-controlled clinical trials. Caution should be exercised in interpreting these data, since conclusions may be influenced by the retrospective nature of the data sets, small subset populations, and the associated low statistical power of many studies. Nonetheless, Table 25.4 represents as close as possible our present knowledge of prognostic factors in thymoma and malignant thymic tumors.

████ **APPENDIX**

Summary of Prognostic Factors in Thymoma

	Tumor Related	Host Related	Environment Related

Essential	Cell type
	Clinical Stage:
	  Invasiveness
	  Size
	  Extent of resection
	  Metastases:
	    Lymph-node
	    Pleural
	    Distant
	  Paraneoplastic syndrome		

Additional		Performance status Age	Access to care
New and promising	Aneuploidy p53		

REFERENCES

1. Masaoka A, Monden Y, Nakahara A, et al.: Follow-up study of thymomas with special reference to their clinical stages. *Cancer* 48:2485–92, 1981.

2. Bernatz P, Khonsari S, Harrison E, et al.: Thymoma: Factors influencing prognosis. *Surg Clin North Am.* 53:885–92, 1973.

3. Verley J, Hollmann K: Thymoma. A comparative study of clinical stages, histologic features, and survival in 200 cases. *Cancer* 55:1074–86, 1985.

4. Marino M, Muller-Hermelink H: Thymoma and thymic carcinoma: Relation of thymoma epithelial cells to the cortical and medullary differentiation of thymus. *Virchows Arch A Pathol Anat Histopathol* 407:119–149, 1985.

5. Kirchner T, Schalke B, Marx A, et al.: Evaluation of prognostic features in thymic epithelial tumors. *Thymus* 14:195–203. 1989.

6. Nomori H, Ishihara T, Torikata C: Malignant grading of cortical and medullary differentiated thymoma by morphometric analysis. *Cancer* 64:1694–9, 1989.

7. Pescarmona E, Rendina E, Venuta F, et al.: Analysis of prognostic factors and clinicopathological staging of thymoma. *Ann Thorac Surg* 50:534–8, 1990.

8. Blumberg D, Port J, Weksler B, et al.: Thymoma: A multivariate analysis of factors predicting survival. *Ann Thorac Surg* 60:908–13; Discussion 914, 1995.

9. Arriagada R, Bretel J, Caillaud J, et al.: Invasive carcinoma of the thymus. A multicenter retrospective review of 56 cases. *Eur J Cancer Clin Oncol* 20:69–74, 1984.

10. Rosai J: *Histological typing of tumors of the thymus. WHO International Histological Classification of Tumors.* Berlin-New York, Springer-Verlag, 1999.

11. Pollack A, El-Naggar A, Cox J, et al.: Thymoma. The prognostic significance of flow cytometric DNA analysis. *Cancer* 69:1702–9, 1992.

12. Sauter E, Sardi A, Hollier L, et al.: Prognostic value of DNA flow cytometry in thymomas and thymic carcinomas. *South Med J* 83:656–9, 1990.

13. Pich A, Chiarle R, Chiusa L, et al.: p53 expression and proliferative activity predict survival in non-invasive thymomas. *Int J Cancer Predict Oncol* 69:180–3, 1996.

14. Lewis J, Wick M, Scheithauer B, et al.: Thymoma. A clinicopathologic review. *Cancer* 60:2727–43, 1987.

15. Cowen D, Richaud P, Mornex F, et al.: Thymoma: Results of a multicentric retrospective analysis of 149 non-metastatic irradiated patients and review of the literature. *Radiother Oncol* 34:9–16, 1995.

16. Bril V, Kojic J, Dhanani A: The long-term clinical outcome of myasthenia gravis in patients with thymoma. *Neurology* 51:1198–1200. *Review*, 1998.

17. Christensen P, Jensen T, Tsiropoulos I, et al.: Mortality and survival in myasthenia gravis: A Danish population based study. *J Neurol Neurosurg Psychiatry* 64:78–83, 1998.

18. Jose B, Yu A, Morgan T, et al.: Malignant thymoma with extrathoracic metastasis: A case report and review of the literature. *J Surg Oncol* 15:259–263, 1980.

19. Bergh N, Gatzinsky P, Larsson S, et al.: Tumors of the thymus and thymic region: I. Clinicopathological studies on thymomas. *Ann Thorac Surg* 25:91–8, 1978.

20. Wilkins EW, Jr., Castleman B.: Thymoma: A continuing survey at the Massachusetts General Hospital. *Ann Thorac Surg* 28:252–6, 1979.

21. Guerin R, Malhaire J, Touboul E, et al.: Radiotherapy of lymphoepithelial thymomas. Results in 29 cases. *J Eur Radiother* 5, 1984.

22. Resbeut M, Mornex F, Richaud P, et al.: Radiotherapie des thymomes. Etude de la literature a propos d'une serie retrospective et multicentrique de 149 cas. *Bull Cancer/Radiother* 82:9–19, 1995.

23. Gripp S, Hilgers K, Wurm R, et al.: Thymoma: Prognostic factors and treatment outcomes. *Cancer* 83:1495–503, 1998.

24. Thomas C, Jr., Cameron D, Loehrer P, Sr.: Thymoma: State of the art. *J Clin Oncol* 17:2280–9, 1999.

25. Curran W, Jr., Kornstein M, Brooks J, et al.: Invasive thymoma: The role of mediastinal irradiation following complete or incomplete surgical resection. *J Clin Oncol* 6:1722–7, 1988.

26. Mornex F, Resbeut M, Richaud P, et al.: Radiotherapy and chemotherapy for invasive thymomas: A multicentric retrospective review of 90 cases. The FNCLCC trialists. Federation Nationale des Centres de Lutte Contre le Cancer. *Int J Radiat Oncol Biol Phys* 32:651–9, 1995.

27. Pollack A, Komaki R, Cox J, et al.: Thymoma: Treatment and prognosis. *Int J Radiat Oncol Biol Phys* 23:1037–43, 1992.

28. Tomiak E, Evans W: The role of chemotherapy in invasive thymoma: A review of the literature and considerations for future clinical trials. *Crit Rev Oncol Hematol* 15:113–24. 1993. (Review available.)

29. McGuire L, Huang D, Teogh R, et al.: Epstein-Barr virus genome in thymoma and thymic lymphoid hyperplasia. *Am J Pathol* 131:385–90, 1988.

TUMORS OF BONE AND SOFT TISSUES

CHAPTER 26

Osteosarcoma

AILEEN M. DAVIS, JAY S. WUNDER, and ROBERT S. BELL

Primary bone tumors are rare with an incidence of 2 to 3 per million,[1] and of these, high-grade osteosarcoma is the most common, representing 35% of all bone sarcomas.[2] The typical patient diagnosed with osteosarcoma is male, between the ages of 10 and 20 years, and complains of pain for one to three months.[3-5] The tumor is most commonly at the metaphysis of a long bone, with a predilection to the knee region.[4,5] Dramatic improvements in disease-free (DFS) and overall survival (OS) were demonstrated with the advent of doxorubicin and methotrexate chemotherapy regimes.[6,7] The current standard of treatment for the patient with osteosarcoma is chemotherapy and resection of the primary tumor, most commonly preserving the limb.[8] Despite the advances in radiological imaging, chemotherapy and surgery, 40 to 50% of patients will develop distant metastases and die of their disease.[9,10]

This chapter discusses the prognostic factors of disease outcome for osteosarcoma patients, specifically disease- or tumor-related factors, host-related factors, and environment- or treatment-related factors.

TUMOR-RELATED FACTORS

Tumor Grade

Classic osteosarcoma is a high-grade, intramedullary tumor that frequently erodes through bone such that there is a tumorous soft tissue mass.[3,5] Low-grade intramedullary tumors rarely metastasize,[11] and local recurrence is prevented by wide surgical excision.[12] Parosteal and periosteal osteosarcoma are rare variants of this osteoid-producing tumor, are usually low grade, and have excellent prognosis.[3] High-grade parosteal and periosteal tumors have disease relapse and survival risks similar to classic osteosarcoma.[13-17]

Prognostic Factors in Cancer, 2nd edition, Edited by Mary K. Gospodarowicz.
ISBN 0-471-40633-3 Copyright © 2001 Wiley-Liss, Inc.

Disease Extent at Presentation

In patients with high-grade osteosarcoma, the extent of disease at initial diagnosis is the most powerful predictor of patient outcome. Only 20 to 30% of osteosarcoma patients with detectable metastatic disease at diagnosis have long-term survival, despite chemotherapy and surgical removal of the primary and metastatic tumor.[18-21] The presence of multifocal disease, including skip metastases, has similarly adverse effects on disease outcome. For the patient who develops metastases, the most important prognostic factors for survival were the number of metastases,[22,23] complete metastatectomy,[22] administration of salvage chemotherapy,[22] and greater than 1.5–2 years to development of metastases.[22]

Histopathological Subtype

The prognostic significance of histopathological subtyping of osteosarcoma is undetermined, as there are conflicting reports in the literature. Some studies[24-28] found that subtyping was of no prognostic significance. Other authors suggest that osteoblastic subtype is an adverse predictor,[29,30] while Petrelli et al.[31] found patients with osteoblastic tumors to have a more favorable outcome. The study by Bentzen et al.[32] found patients with fibroblastic tumors to have improved outcome.

Anatomical Site

The proximal tibia is the most favorable anatomic site in relation to disease outcome.[10,25,26,33] Meyers et al.[33] found the proximal humerus as well as the tibia to be a favorable site. Patients with osteosarcoma of the pelvis and axial skeleton have the worst prognosis.[32-35] Pelvic tumors tend to be large and, as with axial lesions, can be difficult to resect completely.[35] A number of authors have not found anatomical location of the tumor to be a significant predictor of disease outcome.[24,27,29,31,36-38]

Tumor Size

Tumor size has been shown to be an adverse predictor of disease outcome, with patients with large tumors having a greater risk of disease relapse. The predictive value of tumor size has been demonstrated in both univariate[10,26,36,39] and multivariate[30,31,40] analyses. The cutpoint at which tumor size is a significant adverse predictor is undetermined. Based on maximum tumor diameter, Taylor et al.[30] and Petrelli et al.[31] found that patients with tumors greater than 15 cm had worse outcome. Spanier[36] found the cutpoint was 10 cm; Krailo et al.[37] suggested 8 cm; and, Link et al.[10] found the cutpoint was 5 cm. Hudson et al.[27] based size on two dimensions and found greater than 35 cm^2 to be an adverse predictor. Bieling and colleagues[40] found tumor volume with an approximate cutpoint of 124 cm^3 to be the most accurate predictor of outcome. In a more recent study, Lidner et al.[28] found tumor volume greater than 400 cc to be an adverse factor.

Local Tumor Extension

Tumor extent within the bone and into surrounding tissues has also been evaluated as a predictor of disease relapse. Bacci et al.[24] did not find the percent of the bone involved with tumor to be predictive. Tumors that had a soft tissue component were not prognostic in the study of Hudson et al.[27] or Goorin et al.[29] Studies by Wuisman et al.[26] and Spanier et al.[36], however, found that tumor extent, independent of size, was a significant predictor of disease relapse. Specifically, Wuisman et al.[26] found that tumors of the distal femur or proximal tibia that were extracompartmental and spanned the full mediolateral aspect of the bone were adverse features. Spanier et al.[36] found that tumors that invaded two or more of tendon, ligament, space such as the axilla or popliteal fossa, or were intra-articular had worse outcome. Vascular invasion by the tumor was not prognostic.[29]

Symptoms

Short symptom duration, that is less than six months, was found to be an adverse prognostic factor by Bentzen et al.[32] and Taylor et al.[30] Hudson et al.[27] did not find this factor to be statistically significant.

Serum Markers

Increased levels of plasma alkaline phosphatase[33,34,41] and serum lactate dehydrogenase[10,33,41] at the time of diagnosis have been associated with increased risk of disease relapse. However, some studies did not find plasma alkaline phosphatase[10,24] or serum lactate dehydrogenase[24] to be a significant predictor of disease relapse.

Tumor Biology

Ploidy   As most osteosarcomas are nondiploid,[42] DNA analysis has provided minimal prognostic information. However, Look et al.[43] found near-diploid variants to protect against disease relapse using flow cytometry. In cell–cycle analysis, Bauer[44] reported that tumors with less than 15% of cells in S-phase had a better prognosis.

p53 Mutation   Certain genetic abnormalities are associated with increased frequency of tumor occurrence, and it is possible that specific genetic alterations carry prognostic significance for osteosarcoma patients.[45] The tumor cells of patients with primary sarcoma have abnormalities in the p53 gene in approximately 30% of patients.[46] The Li-Fraumeni familial cancer syndrome is associated with a high incidence of sarcoma, and p53 mutations are frequent with this syndrome.[46,47] However, a high incidence of p53 mutations has also been reported in osteosarcoma patients with a strong family history of cancer[46] without the Li-Fraumeni syndrome and in patients in which osteosarcoma is a second primary malignancy.[48] The p53 gene has an important role in controlling cell growth and in programmed cell death,[49] including apoptosis induced by chemotherapy.[50-54] Mutations of the p53 gene may lead to chemotherapy resistance.[49,51]

Retinoblastoma Gene   Over 50% of osteosarcomas have a loss of heterozygosity in the retinoblastoma gene, and Wadayama et al.[55] found this genetic alteration to be correlated with poor outcome. Feugeas et al.[56] found similar results in a small sample of nonmetastatic osteosarcoma patients.

MDM2 Gene   Amplification of the proto-oncogene MDM2 was associated with disease relapse in the studies of Oliner et al.[57] and Ladanyi et al.[58] However, the studies of Lonardo et al.[59] and Nakayama et al.[60] did not find this association.

c-erb B-2/neu/HER2 Proto-Oncogenes   The *c-erb* B-2/neu/HER2 proto-oncogenes are expressed in a high frequency in osteosarcomas, and Onda et al.[61] and Gorlick et al.[62] reported a high correlation with early systemic relapse and poor survival in patients with osteosarcoma.

Multiple–Drug Resistance   One of the main causes of disease failure in osteosarcoma is thought to result from resistance to chemotherapeutic agents. Overexpression of P-glycoprotein, the product of the multidrug resistance gene (MDR1), may be one mechanism by which multidrug resistance occurs and has been identified as a potential prognostic marker for osteosarcoma. Overexpression of P-glycoprotein at diagnosis or at the time of disease relapse has been identified in osteosarcoma,[63-65] however, the relationship of P-glycoprotein overexpression to disease outcome is unclear. In a study of 92 nonmetastatic extremity osteosarcoma patients, Baldini et al.[66] found that increased levels of P-glycoprotein based on immunohistochemistry were associated with a high probability of disease relapse in both univariate and multivariate analyses. Although an additional study[67] identified a similar relationship between P-glycoprotein expression and outcome, two immunohistochemical studies of P-glycoprotein[62,68] and a prospective analysis of MDR1 mRNA expression did not confirm these results.[69] Ongoing evaluation of genetic abnormalities is required to determine their clinical relevance in diagnosis, treatment, and prognosis of osteosarcoma.

HOST-RELATED FACTORS

Age

Age is a frequently evaluated factor, and there is a suggestion that the very young and the older patient have poorer prognosis. Spanier et al.[36] found that patients under 10 years of age had decreased DFS in univariate analysis. Age less than 15 years was the most significant independent predictor of the development of metastatic disease in the study reported by the French Bone Tumor Study

Group.[70] Taylor et al.[30] also found that younger patients (<20 years) had a worse prognosis (recognizing that bias was introduced by a disproportionately large sample of patients over 20 years in the later study era when survival improved). Bentzen et al.[32] found that patients between the ages of 25 and 30 had the best prognosis, with prognosis worsening with advancing age. The 5- and 10-year survival estimates reported by Huvos et al.[71] were 18 and 7%, respectively, in patients older than 60 years. The poor prognosis in older patients has been attributed to the development of osteosarcoma in Pagetic lesions or in previously irradiated tissues, as well as to the difficulty administering high doses of chemotherapeutic agents in this population.[71–75] Individuals with Paget's disease who develop primary bone sarcoma have a dismal outcome, with less than 8% surviving their disease and most dying within two years of diagnosis.[72] In contrast to the preceding authors, a number of studies have not found age to have prognostic significance in osteosarcoma.[10,24–27,31,37,39] Four studies[29,31,38,39] found male gender to be an adverse prognostic factor; however, gender was only an independent predictor in multivariate analysis in the work of Petrelli et al.[31] and Saeter et al.[38] Many studies did not find gender to be prognostic.[10,24–27,30,33,36,37]

Ethnicity

Ethnicity has been infrequently evaluated, but neither Meyers et al.[33] nor Glasser et al.[25] found race to be an independent prognostic factor in multivariate analysis. Blacks tended to have a worse prognosis (1.9 increased risk) when evaluated in a univariate statistical model as compared to whites or Hispanics.[33]

ENVIRONMENT-RELATED FACTORS

Cancer Center Care

Individuals with osteosarcoma are routinely treated in a cancer center in the Western world. This practice has occurred due to the rarity of the disease and the use of chemotherapy as standard care in high-grade osteosarcoma. Although there are no specific data comparing disease outcomes for patients treated in a specialized cancer center as compared to nonspecialized centers, data from the EUROCARE Working Group[76] showed substantially lower 5-year survival rates for bone cancer (20–40%) in eastern Europe, where specialized cancer care is uncommon, as compared to western European countries with cancer centers, where 5-year survival rates ranged from 50% to 70%.[76]

Chemotherapy

The dramatic increases in DFS and OS in patients with osteosarcoma occurred in the 1970s with the introduction of effective multiagent chemotherapy regimes, including high-dose methotrexate and doxorubicin.[6,7,77] Cortes et al.[77] reported regression of pulmonary metastases in 41% of those treated with doxorubicin, and Jaffe et al.[7] reported similar results using high-dose methotrexate. Rosen et al.[6] introduced a prolonged chemotherapy regime with a combination of drugs and achieved regression of metastatic disease in 54% of patients. These initial studies in patients with metastatic disease led to the administration of chemotherapy in nonmetastatic patients in an attempt to prevent the development of systemic disease. Adjuvant, and more recently, neoadjuvant chemotherapy using high-dose methotrexate-based chemotherapy, or a doxorubicin/cisplatin drug combination is considered standard practice in treating patients with high-grade osteosarcoma. Five-year DFS and OS rates of 60% and 60 to 80%, respectively, are generally reported[10,29,70,78] with this practice.

The methotrexate-based Rosen protocol 5-year DFS rate was 80%[79] based on a single institution study, but results were inferior in other settings.[80] Because this multiagent regime has a high level of toxicity, the effects of shorter regimes were evaluated. In 1997, the European Osteosarcoma Intergroup published comparable survival in a multicentered randomized trial of the 12-month, methotrexate multiagent regime and the six–course, combination doxorubicin/cisplatin regime.[81] Criticism of the results of this trial include poor compliance with the multiagent regime and a lower survival (55%) than in previous studies.

The Pediatric Oncology Group has recently initiated a randomized trial to determine if intensified chemotherapy, including high-dose ifosfamide, will improve DFS and OS rates. Intensification of chemotherapy is enhanced by the use of hematopoietic growth factors such as granulocyte stimulating factor (G-CSF).[82]

Chemotherapy Dose Intensity

Chemotherapy dose intensity based on serum methotrexate levels or dose reduction has been evaluated as a prognostic factor.[33,38,70,83] The French Bone Tumor Group[70] found that patients who had dose reduction, particularly if there was a delay of treatment for more than two cycles, had a worse outcome. Bacci et al.[83] found that patients who received 80% or more of their prescribed dose had significantly improved survival. However, neither Saeter et al.[38] nor Meyers et al.[33] found that dose intensity was prognostic. These four studies utilized multiagent, high-dose methotrexate-based chemotherapy. Smith et al.[84] reported that dose intensity of doxorubicin is correlated with tumor response to preoperative chemotherapy and DFS.

Chemotherapy Response

Histological tumor response to neoadjuvant chemotherapy appears to be the most important independent prognostic factor for DFS in osteosarcoma.[38,85,86] Huvos[87] described a method for evaluating tumor necrosis following neoadjuvant chemotherapy, and a "good" response to chemotherapy has been defined as greater than 90% necrosis. With the exception of the study by Bacci et al.,[24] in which there was a trend toward increased DFS with good chemotherapy response, all authors[25-28,31,33,34,38-40] found a DFS advantage. Tumor necrosis was not only a univariate predictor but remained a very strong independent predictor when included in a multivariate analysis.[25-27,33,34,39,40,85]

Chemotherapy Administration

The administration of chemotherapy intra-arterially versus intravenous administration has been evaluated.[31,88-90] Intravenously administered chemotherapy provides both a local and system effect, and while intra-arterial chemotherapy may provide a superior local tumor effect compared to intravenous administration,[89] the systemic effect is unknown. Data from a randomized trial comparing the two methods of chemotherapy administration did not demonstrate a disease outcome benefit for the intra-arterial treatment group.[91]

Limb Preservation versus Amputation

Neoadjuvant chemotherapy and improved imaging and staging techniques have allowed limb-preservation surgery rather than amputation for the vast majority of patients with extremity osteosarcoma.[8,92,93] Initial concerns that limb preservation might result in increased rates of local tumor recurrence and poorer disease outcomes were unfounded, as there was no difference in disease outcomes for the two surgical approaches.[10,24,30,31,93] Specifically, the 2- and 5-year survival for patients treated by hip disarticulation, above-knee amputation, and limb preservation for high grade osteogenic sarcoma, (OSA) of the distal femur were equivalent for all three groups at 65% and 55%, respectively.[93] Complete resection of the tumor with negative margins on pathological review is most important in preventing local tumor recurrence.[93] Patients presenting with pathological fracture, which theoretically allows tumor spread via hematoma, is not necessarily an indication for amputation, and a pathological fracture has not been shown to have an impact on DFS.[25,27,29,94] The main indications for amputation in the patient with osteosarcoma are encasement of the neurovascular structures such that a functional limb cannot be preserved, and the inability to completely remove the tumor with a cuff of normal tissue around the tumor.

Complete removal of the tumor obtaining negative pathological resection margins is critical to preventing local tumor recurrence. Three factors were found to be significant in preventing local recurrence following limb preservation: chemotherapy-induced tumor necrosis, surgical margin, and older age.[95] The prognosis of patients who develop local recurrence is poor, as most will develop systemic disease.[25,28,70,92,95]

SUMMARY

The current knowledge regarding the prognostic factors for patients with high-grade osteosarcoma is summarized in Table 26.1 and Appendix 26B. While a number of studies have evaluated these prognostic factors, a variety of study methodologies have been utilized and candidate predictor variables have not been defined or measured in a consistent manner.[85] Consequently, there are inconsistent results among studies as to specific criteria for stratifying osteosarcoma patients into low- and high-risk groups prior to initiation of treatment.[85,96] It is well accepted that patients presenting with metastatic disease at the time of diagnosis have a very poor prognosis. Chemotherapy-induced tumor necrosis of greater than 90% is consistently reported to predict more favorable DFS for the patient presenting with localized disease. Unfortunately, tumor necrosis cannot be determined at the time of diagnosis. Additional techniques are required to identify high-risk patients at the time of diagnosis such that novel therapies can be developed to improve disease outcomes in this patient group.

TABLE 26.1   Prognostic Factors in High-grade Osteosarcoma

Factor	Prognostic Implication	Comments
Tumor-related factors		
Disease extent at diagnosis	Metastases and multifocal disease have poor prognosis	Long-term survival of 20%
Histopathological typing	Inconsistent reports in the literature	Unlikely of prognostic significance
Anatomical site	Proximal tibia most favorable; axial and pelvic sites have worst prognosis	
Tumor size	Large tumors have poorer prognosis	Critical cutpoint of maximum diameter unclear; volume may be a superior predictor
Local tumor extension	Inconsistent reports in the literature	Unlikely of significance
Symptom duration	<6 months has poor prognosis	Infrequently evaluated
Alkaline phosphatase and LDH	Increased levels at diagnosis have worse prognosis	
p53 gene	Unknown	Investigation continues
Retinoblastoma gene	Loss of heterozygosity correlates with poor outcome	Small samples; requires confirmation
MDM2 gene amplification	Inconsistent results	Requires further study
P-glycoprotein	High expression may be unfavorable, but results inconsistent	Requires standardization of methods and further evaluation
c-erb B-2/neu/HER2 proto-oncogenes	Expression is associated with poor prognosis	Small samples, and requires further study

(*continued*)

TABLE 26.1   (*continued*)

Factor	Prognostic Implication	Comments
Host-related factors		
Age	Very young (<20 years) and older patients (>50–60 years) have unfavorable outcome	Difficulty delivering chemotherapy; Paget's disease and radiation–induced tumor may account for poor outcome in older patients
Gender	Male unfavorable prognosis	Many studies found gender to be insignificant; unlikely of prognostic importance
Environment-related factors		
Cancer center treatment	Suggestion of improved survival based on EUROCARE study	Standard care in the Westernized world is in a cancer center
Multiagent vs. short-course chemotherapy	DFS and OS results are comparable	Intensified chemotherapy protocols with growth factor support are in progress
Dose intensity	Less than 80% of planned dose has adverse outcomes; however, results are inconsistent	
Tumor necrosis	>90% chemotherapy-induced necrosis is favorable	Currently the most important independent predictor of DFS in patients nonmetastatic at diagnosis

LDH = serum lactate dehydrogenase;
DFS = disease-free survival.

■■■■■■■ **APPENDIX 26A**

TNM Classification: Bone

T — Primary Tumor

TX Primary tumor cannot be assessed

T0 No evidence of primary tumor

T1 Tumor confined within the cortex

T2 Tumor invades beyond the cortex

N — Regional Lymph Nodes

NX Regional lymph nodes cannot be assessed

N0 No regional lymph-node metastasis

N1 Regional lymph-node metastasis

M — Distant Metastasis

MX Distant metastasis cannot be assessed

M0 No distant metastasis

M1 Distant metastasis

G — Histopathological Grading

GX Grade of differentiation cannot be assessed

G1 Well differentiated

G2 Moderately differentiated

G3 Poorly differentiated

G4 Undifferentiated

Stage Grouping

Stage IA	G1, 2	T1	N0	M0
Stage IB	G1, 2	T2	N0	M0
Stage IIA	G3, 4	T1	N0	M0
Stage IIB	G3, 4	T2	N0	M0
Stage III	Not defined			
Stage IVA	Any G	Any T	N1	M0
Stage IVB	Any G	Any T	Any N	M1

Source: Sobin LH, Wittekind Ch (eds.): *TNM classification of malignant tumors*, 5th ed. New York, Union Internationale Contre le Cancer Wiley-Liss, 1997.

■■■■■■ **APPENDIX 26B**

Prognostic Factors in High-grade Osteosarcoma as They Influence Treatment Decisions

Prognostic Factors	Tumor Related	Host Related	Environment Related
Essential	Anatomic disease extent Anatomic site Tumor size	Age	Cancer center care Chemotherapy-induced tumor necrosis
Additional	Histopathologic type Local tumor extension Symptom duration Serum markers	Gender	
New and promising	p53 Retinoblastoma gene MDM2 gene amplification P-glycoprotein *c-erb* B-2/neu/HER2 proto-oncogenes		Multiagent vs. short-course chemotherapy Chemotherapy dose intensity

Note: Essential = factors that influence treatment decisions; Additive = additional information that may provide prognostic information, but that does affect treatment decisions; New and Promising = factors that may affect prognosis and influence treatment planning; however, there is insufficient knowledge about these factors at the present time

REFERENCES

1. Malawar MM, Link MP, Donaldson SS: Sarcomas of the soft tissues and bone, in DeVita VT, Hellman SH, Rosenberg ST (eds.): *Cancer principles and practice of oncology*, 5th ed. Philadelphia; Lippincott-Raven, 1997, p. 1789.

2. Dorfman HD, Czerniak B: Bone cancers. *Cancer* 75:203–10, 1995.

3. Dahlin DC, Unni KK: Osteosarcoma of bone and its important recognizable varieties. *Am J Surg Pathol* 1:61–72, 1977.

4. Campanacci MC: Classic osteosarcoma, in Campanacci MC (ed.): *Bone and soft tissue tumours*. Vienna, Springer-Verlag, 1990, pp. 455–505.

5. Simon MA: Causes of increased survival of patients with osteosarcoma: Current controversies. *J Bone Joint Surg* 72A:643–54, 1990.

6. Rosen G, Suwansirikul S, Kwon C, et al.: High-dose methotrexate with citrovorum factor rescue and doxorubicin in childhood osteogenic sarcoma. *Cancer* 33:1151–63, 1974.

7. Jaffe N, Frei E, Traggis D, et al.: Adjuvant methotrexate and citrovorum-factor treatment of osteogenic sarcoma. *NEJM* 292:994–7, 1974.

8. Aboulafia A, Malawar M: Surgical management of pelvic and extremity osteosarcoma. *Cancer* 71:3358–66, 1993.

9. Eilber F, Guiliano A, Eckardt J, et al.: Adjuvant chemotherapy for osteosarcoma: A randomized prospective trial. *J Clin Oncol* 5:21–8, 1987.

10. Link MP, Goorin AM, Horowitz M, et al.: Adjuvant chemotherapy of high grade osteosarcoma of the extremity: Update results of the Multi-Institutional Osteosarcoma Study. *Clin Orthop* 270:8–14, 1991.

11. Unni KK: Osteosarcoma, in Unni KK (ed.): *Dahlin's bone tumours. General aspects and data on 12,087 cases*, 5th ed. Philadelphia, Lippincott-Raven, 1996, pp. 143–83.

12. Kurt AM, Unni KK, McLeod RA, et al.: Low-grade intraosseous osteosarcoma. *Cancer* 65:1418–28, 1990.

13. Unni KK: Parosteal osteosarcoma (juxtacortical osteosarcoma), in Unni KK (ed.): *Dahlin's bone tumours. General aspects and data on 12,087 cases*, 5th ed. Philadelphia, Lippincott-Raven, 1996, pp. 185–96.

14. Sheth DS, Yasko AW, Raymond AK, et al.: Conventional and dedifferentiated parosteal osteosarcoma. Diagnosis, treatment, and outcome. *Cancer* 78:2136–45, 1996.

15. Schajowicz F, McGuire MH, Santini AE, et al.: Osteosarcoma arising on the surfaces of long bones. *J Bone Joint Surg (Am)* 70:555–64, 1988.

16. Raymond AK: Surface osteosarcoma. *Clin Orthop* 270:140–8, 1991.

17. Okada K, Frassica FS, Sim FH, et al.: Parosteal osteosarcoma: A clinicopathological study. *J Bone Joint Surg* 76:366–78, 1994.

18. Bacci G, Picci P, Briccoli A, et al.: Osteosarcoma of the extremity metastatic at presentation: Results achieved in 26 patients treated with combined therapy (primary chemotherapy followed by simultaneous resection of the primary and metastatic lesions). *Tumori* 78:200–6, 1992.

19. Ward WG, Mikaelian K, Dorey F, et al.: Pulmonary metastases of stage IIB extremity osteosarcoma and subsequent pulmonary metastases. *J Clin Oncol* 12:1849–58, 1994.

20. Beattie EJ, Havey JC, Marcove R, et al.: Results of multiple pulmonary resections for metastatic osteogenic sarcoma after two decades. *J Surg Oncol* 46:154–5, 1991.

21. Morgan E, Baum E, Bleyer WA, et al.: Treatment of patients with metastatic osteogenic sarcoma: A report from the Children's Cancer Study Group. *Cancer Treat Rep* 68:661–4, 1984.

22. Saeter GA, Hoie J, Stenwig AE, et al.: Systemic relapse of patients with osteogenic sarcoma. *Cancer* 75:1084–93, 1995.

23. Meyer WH, Schell MJ, Kumar APM, et al.: Thoracotomy for pulmonary metastatic osteosarcoma. An analysis of prognostic indicators of survival. *Cancer* 59:374–9, 1987.

24. Bacci G, Picci P, Ferrar S, et al.: Primary chemotherapy and delayed surgery for nonmetastatic osteosarcoma of the extremities. Results in 164 patients preoperatively

treated with high doses of methotrexate followed by cisplatin and doxorubicin. *Cancer* 72:3227–38, 1993.

25. Glasser DB, Lane JM, Huvos AG, et al.: Survival, prognosis and therapeutic response in osteogenic sarcoma. *Cancer* 69:698–708, 1992.

26. Wiusman P, Enneking WF, Roesner A: Local growth and the prognosis of osteosarcoma. *Internat Orthop* 16:55–8, 1992.

27. Hudson M, Jaffe MR, Jaffe N, et al.: Pediatric osteosarcoma: Therapeutic strategies, results, and prognostic factors derived from a 10-year experience. *J Clin Oncol* 8:1988–97, 1990.

28. Lidner NJ, Ramm O, Hillmann A, et al.: Limb salvage and outcome of osteosarcoma. *Clin Orthop* 358:83–9, 1999.

29. Goorin AM, Perez-Atayde A, Gebhardt M, et al.: Weekly high-dose methotrexate and doxorubicin for osteosarcoma: The Dana-Faber Cancer Institute/The Children's Hospital-Study III. *J Clin Oncol* 5:1178–84, 1987.

30. Taylor WF, Ivins JC, Pritchad DJ, et al.: Trends and variability in survival among patients with osteosarcoma: A 7-year update. *Mayo Clin Proc* 60:91–104, 1985.

31. Petrelli S, Penna V, Lopes A, et al.: IIB osteosarcoma current management, local control, and survival statistics-Sao Paulo, Brazil. *Clin Ortho* 270:60–6, 1991.

32. Bentzen SM, Poulsen HS, Kaae S, et al.: Prognostic factors in osteosarcomas. A regression analysis. *Cancer* 62:194–202, 1988.

33. Meyers PA, Heller G, Healey J, et al.: Chemotherapy for nonmetastatic osteogenic sarcoma: The Memorial Sloan-Kettering experience. *J Clin Oncol* 10:5–15, 1992.

34. Provisor AJ, Ettinger LJ, Nachman JB, et al.: Treatment of nonmetastatic osteosarcoma of the extremity with preoperative and postoperative chemotherapy: A report for the Children's Cancer Group. *J Clin Oncol* 15:76–84, 1997.

35. Abudu A, Grimer RJ, Cannon SR, et al.: Reconstruction of the hemipelvis after the excision of malignant tumours. Complications and functional outcome of prostheses. *J Bone Joint Surg* 79:773–9, 1997.

36. Spanier SS, Shuster JJ, Vander Griend RA: The effect of local extent of the tumour on prognosis in osteosarcoma. *J Bone Joint Surg* 72:643–53, 1990.

37. Krailo M, Erte I, Makley J, et al.: A randomized study comparing high-dose methotrexate with moderate-dose methotrexate as components of adjuvant chemotherapy in childhood nonmetastatic osteosarcoma: A report from the Children's Cancer Study Group. *Med Pediatr Oncol* 15:69–77, 1987.

38. Saeter G, Wiebe T, Wiklund T, et al.: Chemotherapy in osteosarcoma the Scandinavian Sarcoma Group experience. *Acta Orthop Scand* 70(Suppl 285):74–82, 1999.

39. Raymond AD, Chawla SP, Carrasco H, et al.: Osteosarcoma chemotherapy effect: A prognostic factor. *Sem Diagn Pathol* 4:212–36, 1987.

40. Bieling P, Rehan N, Winkler P, et al.: Tumor size and prognosis in aggressively treated osteosarcoma. *J Clin Oncol* 14:848–58, 1996.

41. Bacci G, Ferrari S, Sangiorgi L, et al.: Prognostic significance of serum lactate dehydrogenase in patients with osteosarcoma of the extremities. *J Chemotherapy* 6:204–10, 1994.

42. Bauer HCF: Current status of DNA cytometry in osteosarcoma, in Bennett Humphrey G, Schraffordt Koops H, Molenaar WM, Postman A (eds.). *Osteosarcoma*

in children and young adults: new developments and controversies. Dordrecht, The Netherlands, Kluwer, 1993, pp. 151–161.

43. Look AT, Douglass EC, Meyer WH: Clinical importance of near-diploid tumour stem lines in patients with osteosarcoma of an extremity. *N Engl J Med* 318:1567–72, 1988.

44. Bauer HCF: DNA cytometry of osteosarcoma. *Acta Orthop Scand* 59(Suppl 228):1–39, 1988.

45. Bell RS, Wunder JS: Molecular alterations in sarcoma management. *Curr Opin Orthop* 8:66–70, 1997.

46. Toguchida J, Yamaguchi T, Dayton S, et al.: Prevalence and spectrum of germline mutations of the p53 gene among patients with sarcoma. *N Engl J Med* 326:1301–8, 1992.

47. Malkin D, Li FP, Strong LC, et al.: Germ line p53 mutations in a familial syndrome of breast cancer, sarcomas, and other neoplasms. *Science* 250:1233–4, 1990.

48. Malkin D, Jolly KW, Barbier N, et al.: Germline mutations of the p53 tumour-suppressor gene in children and young adolescents with second malignant neoplasms. *N Engl J Med* 326:1309–15, 1992.

49. Levine AJ, Momand J, Finlay CA: The p53 suppressor gene. *Nature* 351:453–6, 1991.

50. Vogelstein B, Kinzler KW: p53 functions, mutations and sarcomas. *Acta Orthop Scand* 68(Suppl 273):68–73, 1992.

51. Hollstein M, Sidransky D, Vogelstein B, et al.: p53 mutations in human cancers. *Science* 253:49–53, 1991.

52. Lowe SE, Ruley EH, Jacks T, et al.: p53-dependent apoptosis modulates the cytotoxicity of anticancer agents. *Cell* 74:957–67, 1993.

53. Graeber TG, Osmanian C, Jacks T, et al.: Hypoxia-mediated selection of cells with diminished apoptotic potential in solid tumours. *Nature* 379:88–91, 1996.

54. Kinzler KW, Vogelstein B: Life (and death) in a malignant tumour. *Nature* 379:19–20, 1996.

55. Wadayama B, Toguchida J, Shimizu T, et al.: Mutation spectrum of the retinoblastoma gene in osteosarcomas. *Cancer Res* 54:3042–8, 1994.

56. Feugeas O, Curiec N, Babin-Boilletot A, et al.: Loss of heterozygosity of the RB gene is a poor prognostic factor in patients with osteosarcoma. *J Clin Oncol* 14:467–72, 1996.

57. Oliner JD, Kinzler KW, Meltzer PS, et al.: Amplification of a gene encoding a p53-associated protein in human sarcomas. *Nature* 358:80–3, 1992.

58. Ladanyi M, Cha C, Lewis R, et al.: MDM2 gene amplification in metastatic osteosarcoma. *Cancer Res* 53:16–8, 1993.

59. Lonardo F, Ueda T, Huvos AG, et al.: p53 and MDM2 alterations in osteosarcomas. Correlation with clinicopathologic features and proliferative rate. *Cancer* 79:1541–7, 1997.

60. Nakayama T, Toguchida J, Wadayama B, et al.: MDM2 gene amplification in bone and soft tissue tumours: Association with tumour progression in dedifferentiated adipose tissue tumours. *Int J Cancer* 64:342–6, 1993.

61. Onda M, Matsuda S, Higaki S, et al.: ErbB-2 expression is correlated with poor prognosis for patients with osteosarcoma. *Cancer* 77:71–8, 1996.

62. Gorlick R, Huvos AG, Heller G, et al.: Expression of HER2/erbB-2 correlates with survival in osteosarcoma. *J Clin Oncol* 17(9):2781, 1999.

63. Ling V: Multidrug resistance: Molecular mechanisms and clinical relevance. *Cancer Chemother Pharmacol* 40(Suppl):S3–8, 1999.

64. Noonan KE, Beck C, Holzmayer TA, et al.: Quantitative analysis of MDR1 (multidrug resistance) gene expression in human tumors by polymerase chain reaction. *Proc Natl Acad Sci USA* 87:7160–4, 1990.

65. Wunder JS, Bell RS, Wold L, et al.: Expression of the multidrug resistance gene in osteosarcoma: A pilot study. *J Orthop Res* 11:396–403, 1993.

66. Baldini N, Scotlandi K, Barbanti-Brodano G, et al.: Expression of P-glycoprotein in high grade osteosarcomas in relation to clinical outcome. *N Engl J Med* 333:1380–5, 1995.

67. Chan HS, Grogan TM, Haddad G, et al.: P-glycoprotein expression: Critical determinant in the response to osteosarcoma chemotherapy. *J Natl Cancer Inst* 89:1706–15, 1997.

68. Radig K, Hackel C, Herting J, et al.: Expression of P-glycoprotein in high grade osteosarcomas with special emphasis on chondroblastic subtype. *Gen Diagn Pathol* 142:139–45, 1997.

69. Wunder JS, Bull SB, Aneliunas V, et al.: MDR1 gene expression and outcome in osteosarcoma: A prospective, multicenter study. *J Clin Oncol* 18:2685–94, 2000.

70. French Bone Tumour Study Group: Age and the dose of chemotherapy as major prognostic factors in a trial of adjuvant therapy of osteosarcoma combining two alternating drug combinations and early prophylactic lung irradiation. *Cancer* 61:1304–11, 1988.

71. Huvos AG: Osteogenic sarcoma of bones and soft tissues in older patients. A clinicopathologic analysis of 117 patients older than 60 years. *Cancer* 57:1442–9, 1986.

72. Huvos AG, Butler A, Bretsky SS: Osteogenic sarcoma associated with Paget's disease of bone. A clinicopathological study of 65 patients. *Cancer* 52:1489–95, 1983.

73. Huvos AG, Woodard HQ, Cahan WG, et al.: Postradiation osteogenic sarcoma of bone and soft tissues. A clinicopathological study of 66 patients. *Cancer* 55:1244–55, 1982.

74. Healey JH, Buss D: Radiation and Pagetic osteogenic sarcomas. *Clin Orthop* 270:128–34, 1991.

75. Frassica FJ, Sim FH, Grassica DA, et al.: Survival and management considerations in postirradiation osteosarcoma and Paget's osteosarcoma. *Clin Orthop* 270:120–7, 1991.

76. Storm HH and the EUROCARE Working Group: Survival of adult patients with cancer of soft tissues or bone in Europe. *Eur J Cancer* 34:2212–17, 1998.

77. Cortes EP, Halland JF, Wang JJ, et al.: Doxorubicin in disseminated osteosarcoma. *JAMA* 221:1132–8, 1972.

78. Goorin AM, Andersen JW: Experience with multi-agent chemotherapy for osteosarcoma. Improved outcome. *Clin Orthop* 270:22–8, 1991.

79. Rosen G, Marcove RC, Caparros B, et al.: Primary osteogenic sarcoma. The rationale for preoperative chemotherapy and delayed surgery. *Cancer* 43:2163–77, 1979.

80. Bramwell VHC: The role of chemotherapy in the management of non-metastatic operable extremity osteosarcoma. *Semin Oncol* 24:561–71, 1997.

81. Souhami RL, Craft AW, van der Eijke JS, et al.: Randomised trial of two regimens of chemotherapy in operable osteosarcoma: A study of the European Osteosarcoma Intergroup. *Lancet* 350:911–17, 1997.

82. Ornadel D, Souhami RL, Whelan J, et al.: Doxorubicin and cisplatin with granulocyte colony-stimulating factor as adjuvant chemotherapy for osteosarcoma. Phase II trial of the European Osteosarcoma Intergroup. *J Clin Oncol* 12:1842–8, 1994.

83. Bacci G, Picci P, Avella M, et al.: The importance of dose-intensity in neoadjuvant chemotherapy of osteosarcoma: A retrospective analysis of high-dose methotrexate, cisplatinum and doxorubicin used preoperatively. *J Chemother* 2:127–35, 1990.

84. Smith MA, Ungerleider RS, Horowitz ME, et al.: Influence of doxorubicin dose intensity on response and outcome for patients with osteogenic sarcoma and Ewing's sarcoma. *J Natl Cancer Inst* 83:1460–70, 1991.

85. Davis AM, Bell RS, Goodwin PJ: Prognostic factors in osteosarcoma: A critical review. *J Clin Oncol* 12:423–31, 1994.

86. Dome JS, Schwatz CL: Osteosarcoma, in Walterhouse DO and Cohn SL (eds.): *Diagnostic and therapeutic advances in pediatric oncology.* Boston, Kluwer, 1997, pp. 215–51.

87. Huvos AG, Rosen G, Marcove RC: Primary osteogenic sarcoma: Pathologic aspects in 20 patients after treatment with chemotherapy, en bloc resection, and prosthetic bone replacement. *Arch Pathol Lab Med* 101:14–8, 1977.

88. Malawar M, Buch R, Reaman G, et al.: Impact of two cycles of preoperative chemotherapy with intraarterial cisplatin and intravenous doxorubicin on the choice of surgical procedure for high-grade bone sarcomas of the extremities. *Clin Orthop* 270:214–22, 1991.

89. Yasko AW, Lane JM: Chemotherapy for bone and soft-tissue sarcomas of the extremities. *J Bone Joint Surg* 73:1263–71, 1991.

90. Jaffe N, Robertson R, Ayal A, et al.: Comparison of intra-arterial cis-diammine-dichloroplatinum-II with high dose methotrexate and citrovorum factor rescue in the treatment of primary osteosarcoma. *J Clin Oncol* 3(Suppl 2):3–6, 1985.

91. Winkler K, Bielack S, Delling G, et al.: Effect of intraarterial versus intravenous cisplatin in addition to systemic doxorubicin, high-dose methotrexate, and ifosfamide on histologic tumour response in osteosarcoma (Study COSS-86). *Cancer* 66:1703–10, 1990.

92. Simon MA, Aschliman MA, Thomas N, et al.: Limb-salvage treatment versus amputation for osteosarcoma of the distal end of the femur. *J Bone Joint Surg* 68:1331–7, 1986.

93. Simon MA: Limb salvage for osteosarcoma. *J Bone Joint Surg* 70:307–10, 1988.

94. Abudu A, Sferopoulos NK, Tillman RM, et al.: The surgical treatment and outcome of pathological fractures in localised osteosarcoma. *J Bone Joint Surg* 78(5):694–8, 1996.

95. Picci P, Sangiogi L, Rougraff BT, et al.: Relations of chemotherapy-induced necrosis and surgical margins to local recurrence in osteosarcoma. *J Clin Oncol* 12:2699–705, 1994.

96. Saeter G, Elomaa I, Wahlqvist Y, et al.: Prognostic factors in bone sarcomas. *Acta Orthop Scand* 68(Suppl 273):156–60, 1997.

CHAPTER 27

Soft Tissue Sarcoma

PETER W.T. PISTERS, BRIAN O'SULLIVAN, and RAPHAEL E. POLLOCK

Significant advances have been made over the past decade in the understanding of clinicopathologic prognostic factors for soft tissue sarcoma. Foremost among these advances is an improved ability to recognize the subset of patients at high risk for recurrent disease and tumor-related death based on clinicopathologic data available at the time of initial presentation. Recent advances have also helped to elucidate specific molecular factors that have independent prognostic significance. This review summarizes the available data on traditional clinicopathologic, medical, and molecular prognostic factors for adult soft tissue sarcoma. Expected outcomes will be provided, drawing in particular from the results of a large series of patients managed at one center. Although there are many potential outcomes that could be assessed, the discussion will focus almost entirely on the traditional oncology outcomes of local control, metastatic risk, and survival. Other important outcomes, such as limb preservation; function, and quality of life will not be emphasized because of space limitations.

The factors will be discussed in a framework that focuses on the *tumor-related, host-related* (or patient associated), and *environment-related* background for these factors. The review will conclude with a summary tabulation identifying strata of the importance of factors to everyday clinical practice using the principles outlined in Chapter 2. These include *essential* factors (needed for treatment decision-making), *additional* factors (of benefit for describing a cohort of patients), and *new and promising* factors that may of benefit in the future to exploit new treatment or diagnostic strategies.

TUMOR-RELATED FACTORS

Conventional Clinicopathologic Factors

Anatomic Prognostic Factors (including grade)   A thorough understanding of the clinicopathologic factors known to impact outcome is essential in formulating

Prognostic Factors in Cancer, 2nd edition, Edited by Mary K. Gospodarowicz
ISBN 0-471-40633-3   Copyright © 2001 Wiley-Liss, Inc.

a treatment plan for a patient with soft tissue sarcoma. Over the past decade, more than a dozen multivariate analyses of prognostic factors for patients with localized sarcoma have been reported.[1–19] With few exceptions,[1,7,16,18,19] however, most studies have analyzed fewer than 300 patients (range, 82–297 patients).

Three detailed analyses of prognostic factors in soft tissue sarcoma merit comment.[1,18,19] The initial study of prognostic factors in extremity sarcoma from Memorial Sloan-Kettering Cancer Center evaluated clinicopathologic prognostic factors in a series of 423 patients with localized extremity soft tissue sarcoma seen from 1968 to 1978.[1] This analysis, among the first to discriminate between specific clinical endpoints of local recurrence, distant recurrence, and disease-specific survival, clearly established the clinical profile of what is now accepted as the high-risk patient with extremity soft tissue sarcoma: the patient with a large (>5 cm), high-grade, deep lesion. In that series, the authors noted that these three variables were not significantly different from each other, using the Cox model coefficients. Consequently, they felt it reasonable to create prognostic groups according to the number of unfavorable characteristics that the patient possesses: 0, 1, 2, or 3. These four groups provided Kaplan-Meier estimates (±1 SE) of the probability of remaining free of distant metastasis at 12 years to be 85% ± 8.7%, 69.3% ± 7.3%, 57.1% ± 6.2%, and 24.8 ± 4.0% respectively[1] (see Figure 27.1).

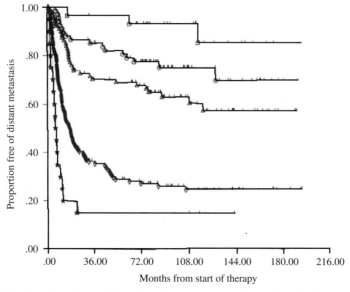

Figure 27.1 Freedom from distant metastases curves according to the number of unfavorable characteristics in the final Cox model. □ — none (28 patients, 25 censored); ○ — one (67 patients, 60 censored); △ — two (88 patients, 55 censored); or ◇ — three (138 patients, 42 censored). A freedom from extranodal metastasis curve ★ for 20 patients (3 censored) who presented with nodal metastasis is also included to illustrate the unfavorable outcome of lymph-node metastasis is soft tissue sarcoma. (Reproduced with permission of the *Journal of Clinical Oncology.*[1])

The rate of distant metastasis also mirrored the survival probability.[1] In fact, the principles derived from this analysis and confirmatory studies[18,19] with other data sets outlined below, were used International Union Against Cancer American Joint Committee on Cancer to develop the revised 5th Edition TNM stage classification for soft tissue sarcoma (see Appendices). (See Appendix 27.A).

The adverse prognostic implications of a high tumor grade, deep tumor location, and tumor size greater than 5 cm were also independently confirmed in the recent report of the French Federation of Cancer Centers study of 546 patients with sarcomas of the extremities, head and neck, trunk wall, retroperitoneum, and pelvis.[19] In a follow-up report from Memorial Sloan-Kettering of prospectively documented clinicopathologic prognostic factors in 1041 patients with extremity soft tissue sarcoma,[18] the endpoints were local recurrence at presentation, distant recurrence (metastasis), and disease-specific survival. Results of the regression analyses for each of these endpoints are summarized in Table 27.1 In Table 27.2 we provide the 5-year rates for freedom from local relapse and for disease-specific survival for the presence or absence of the adverse prognostic factors observed to be significant in the final regression model.[18] These also confirmed the initial observations made at the same institution.[1] In addition, the previously unappreciated prognostic significance of specific histologic subtypes and the

TABLE 27.1   Multivariate Analysis of Prognostic Factors in Patients with Extremity Soft Tissue Sarcoma

Endpoint	Adverse Prognostic Factor	Relative Risk
Local recurrence	Age >50 years	1.6
	Local recurrence at presentation	2.0
	Microscopically positive margin	1.8
	Fibrosarcoma	2.5
	Malignant peripheral nerve-sheath tumor	1.8
Distant recurrence	Size 5.0–9.9 cm	1.9
	Size ≥10.0 cm	1.5
	High grade	4.3
	Deep location	2.5
	Local recurrence at presentation	1.5
	Leiomyosarcoma	1.7
	Nonliposarcoma histology	1.6
Disease-specific survival	High grade	4.0
	Size ≥10.0 cm	2.1
	Deep location	2.8
	Local recurrence at presentation	1.5
	Leiomyosarcoma	1.9
	Malignant peripheral nerve-sheath tumor	1.9
	Microscopically positive margin	1.7
	Lower extremity site	1.6

Source: Modified from Reference 18 with permission.
Note: Adverse prognostic factors identified are independent by Cox regression analysis.

TABLE 27.2 Five-year Local Relapse-free Rates and Disease-Specific Survival Rates in 1041 Patients with Extremity Soft Tissue Sarcoma Treated at MSKCC from 1982 to 1994 for Prognostic Factors Observed to be Independently Significant for These Endpoints

Endpoint	Adverse Prognostic Factor	Variable Categories	Rate (%)
Local relapse-free rate	Crude overall local rate[a]	181/1041	83
	Age	>50 years	79.9
		≤50 years	70.7
	Local recurrence at presentation	Primary	79.2
		Recurrent	60.3
	Surgical/pathologic margins	Negative	80.0
		Mic positive	59.9
	Histology[c]	MPNST	68.7
		Fibrosarcoma	60.1
Disease-specific survival	Crude overall survival rate[b]	250/1041	76
	High grade	Low	94.7
		High	65.7
	Size	>10.0 cm	84.8
		5–10 cm	81.5
		<5 cm	60.5
	Depth	Superficial	91.7
		Deep	69.4
	Local recurrence at presentation	Primary	75.1
		Recurrent	74.7
	Histology[c]	Leiomyosarcoma	71.0
		MPNST	50.5
	Surgical/pathologic margins	Negative	77.6
		Mic positive	68.6
	Location in limb	Proximal	72.7
		Distal	79.9

Source: Data from Reference 18 for independently significant prognostic factors shown in Table 27.1.

[a]Kaplan-Meier 5-year local relapse-free rate for overall population not available.

[b]Kaplan-Meier rate not provided. Two hundred and fifty patients (24%) died during follow-up. Of these, 199 died of sarcoma, 42 of other cause, and 9 of unknown causes.

[c]Only the adverse histologic subtypes following Cox regression[16] are shown.

Abbreviations: MPNST: malignant peripheral nerve-sheath tumor; Mic positive: microscopic positive;

increased risk for adverse outcome associated with a microscopically positive surgical margin or locally recurrent disease at presentation were noted.

Unlike for many other solid tumors, the adverse prognostic factors for local recurrence of a soft tissue sarcoma are different from those that predict distant metastasis and/or tumor-related mortality (Table 27.1).[18] In other words, patients with a constellation of adverse prognostic factors for local recurrence are not necessarily at increased risk for distant metastasis or tumor-related death. Therefore, prognostic factors and anatomic staging systems that are designed to stratify patients for risk of distant metastasis and tumor-related mortality (such as the present TNM classification; see Appendix 27A) will not necessarily stratify patients for risk of local recurrence. It is also noteworthy that certain prognostic factors may have a direct bearing on the treatment approach, but may not independently influence survival. An example is envelopment or invasion of neurovascular structures ± bone that would have a direct influence on the requirement of an amputation, and therefore would be *essential* factors for an endpoint like limb preservation. In fact, the literature is conflicting with respect to these factors, which formally were included in TNM as the additional T3 category and based on multivariate assessment.[5,20] More recently some authors have suggested these are prognostic.[16,21] Others have found they are not independently significant.[18] It is possible that differences in definitions and in the ability to determine the presence of such invasion precisely in a clinical staging system may account for the discrepancies in reported results.

It should be emphasized that the prognostic factors identified have been derived from studies of patients with localized extremity sarcomas, which make up the majority of sarcomas. These prognostic factors therefore may not be generalizable to the greater population of soft tissue sarcoma patients. Separate reviews of prognostic factors for sarcomas of the retroperitoneum,[17,22,23] head and neck,[24-28] gastrointestinal tract,[29,30] colon and rectum,[31] and uterus,[32] and for synovial sarcomas,[33,34] malignant fibrous histiocytomas,[35-37] have been conducted. In general, most of these studies have suggested that tumor size and histologic grade are the primary determinants of overall survival, but there is little doubt that the different anatomic subsites add their own challenges to treatment and cause patients to present in different ways and with variable tumor size, local extension, or metastasis. Consequently, outcome and pattern of recurrence differ for the different anatomic sites.[16]

Prognostic Significance of Local Recurrence   Whether local recurrence impacts overall survival for patients with soft tissue sarcoma remains unclear and highly controversial.[14,38-41] Solving the answer to this question is problematic because a given cohort of patients undoubtedly comprises a mixture of heterogeneous cases: (1) potentially curable cases that may or may not be managed successfully at the local site but with little predisposition to develop metastases; (2) a putative potentially curable group that may or may not be managed successfully at the local site but possesses the ability to develop metastases from disseminated seeding from a primary that recurs; (3) biologically condemned cases destined for both local recurrence and metastasis despite standard local treatment approaches; and (4) similarly condemned cases destined for metastasis alone if local treatment is aggressive. Therefore the true consequence of a local recurrence on the risk of distant metastasis can probably only be evaluated when comparing similarly derived cohorts of patients from which no cases have been excluded. This is very difficult to achieve in a rare disease like soft tissue sarcoma.

Population-based comparisons provide an opportunity (see environment-related factors below), but have shortcomings due to the inability to readily control for important factors such as stage of disease and comorbidity when making comparisons, since they may differ in different populations due to health care access and education in the population. Comparisons between sequential or concurrent cohorts accrued in identical ways provides an additional opportunity, assuming that potential sources of bias in assembling and describing the cohorts can be controlled for. The method of comparing the outcome of cases presenting at an institution with local recurrence but without metastases compared to those with primary presentations has also been performed.[16,18] The weakness of this method is that those patients with local recurrence at the time of referral to the index institution are unlikely to be representative of the full spectrum of the sarcoma population. The very fact that metastases have not yet developed at the time of referral, despite a local recurrence, sets them apart from the remainder of the cases referred with recurrence, who have metastases. In turn it probably also indicates they are not completely comparable to the general population of patients referred primarily, some of whom will have biologically unfavorable disease that can metastasize early. This is discussed elsewhere.[16]

Ideally a prospective randomized trial could assess the precise nature of a relationship between local recurrence and overall survival. Three major Phase III trials have evaluated local tumor control and survival in the context of defining treatment approaches for soft tissue sarcoma. In a randomized trial of amputation versus limb-sparing surgery plus radiation conducted by the National Cancer Institute, local recurrence rates were 19% in the limb-sparing group versus 6% in the amputation group ($p = 0.022$).[42,43] Despite this, overall survival rates were equal: 70% for patients who had limb-sparing surgery versus 71% for those who had amputation ($p = 0.97$). In addition, in randomized trials of postoperative radiotherapy[44,45] the improvement in local control noted in patients treated with surgery plus radiotherapy versus surgery alone did not translate into any detectable survival advantage. Thus, none of the currently available prospective randomized data support the hypothesis that better local control enhances survival in patients with sarcoma. Furthermore, data from nonrandomized studies support the concept that there is little, if any, relationship between local control and survival. In a recent series from Sweden, the outcome of patients treated with an inadequate excision was compared with those who had an adequate operation.[40] Local recurrence was 3.5 times more common after inadequate excision, but there was no difference in the incidence or timing of distant metastases.

Notwithstanding the available data, it is important to note that the power of the reported randomized trials to detect a difference in survival related to local control is relatively small and the available trials have had modest numbers and relatively few events. A large number of patients may be required to determine whether prevention of local recurrence impacts survival.[38] Stotter et al. have argued that local recurrence is a time-dependent variable and should be considered as such in multivariate studies.[14] Analyzing their nonrandomized data in this fashion, Stotter et al. demonstrated a statistically significant relationship between local control and survival in patients with extremity soft tissue sarcoma. Other retrospective analyses have yielded similar conclusions.[6,13] These methods of considering or adjusting for a variable after treatment allocation has been the focus of critical comment recently. Gelman and Harris argue that it is problematic to compare groups of patients by an event (such as local recurrence) that occurs at some variable time after primary treatment.[46] They argue that there is a statistical bias in analyzing patients with such a delayed event that cannot be eliminated by the use of time-varying covariates with Cox modeling.[46]

It is clearly important to distinguish between the well-defined adverse prognostic impact of subsequent local recurrence on the survival of a given patient.[18,41] What is much less clear is whether amelioration of the risk of distant metastasis by improving local control is possible (i.e., prevention of local recurrence with improved local therapy) and can improve survival. As noted earlier, the former may be nothing more than a manifestation of more aggressive tumor biology, that is, biologically more aggressive lesions may recur locally and metastasize more frequently.

Potential Nonanatomic Prognostic Factors

Molecular Prognostic Factors Attention has recently been focused on the evaluation of molecular pathologic prognostic factors. Specific molecular parameters evaluated for prognostic significance have included mutations in *p53*,[47–49] and *mdm2*,[50] Ki-67 status,[50] altered expression of the retinoblastoma gene product (pRb)[51,52] in high-grade sarcomas, and the presence of SYT-SSX fusion transcripts in synovial sarcoma.[53]

A preliminary report from Memorial Sloan-Kettering evaluating the prognostic role of pRb expression in 44 primary and 12 metastatic high-grade human sarcomas by immunohistochemical methods and Western blotting demonstrated that alterations in pRb expression are more commonly associated with high-grade tumors, metastatic lesions, and decreased survival rates.[51] However, a subsequent report from the same group in an expanded population of 174 adult patients with soft tissue sarcoma revealed that pRb alterations were frequently observed in both low- and high-grade lesions and that altered pRb expression did not correlate with known predictors of survival and was not an independent predictor of long-term outcome.[52] These studies and the now well-documented phenomenon of late (>5 years posttreatment) recurrence of soft tissue sarcoma[54] underscore the importance of long-term follow-up and relatively large sample size in these types of analyses.

Somatic mutations in the *p53* tumor suppressor gene have been reported in 4–65% of patients with soft tissue sarcoma.[47,55–58] Detection of *p53* mutations in paraffin-embedded soft tissue sarcomas also has been correlated with reduced overall survival rates. However, data on the underlying prognostic significance of *p53* status are conflicting. Some investigators report no independent adverse prognostic significance by regression analysis,[50,59] whereas others report a highly significant correlation between *p53/mdm2* status and outcome.[60]

Ki-67, an antigen expressed throughout the majority of the cell cycle, is utilized as a measure of cell proliferation.[61] Preliminary studies of series of heterogeneous sarcomas in adults have suggested that the proliferative index, as measured by Ki-67 nuclear staining, is correlated with histologic grade, but is not of independent prognostic significance when histologic grade is taken into account.[48,59] However, other studies of larger numbers of sarcomas have demonstrated that Ki-67 status is an independent prognostic factor.[50,62,63] Immunohistochemical analysis of an initial cohort of 65 soft tissue sarcomas and a subsequent cohort of 132 soft tissue sarcomas from the French Federation of Cancer Centers Sarcoma Group demonstrated that increased Ki-67 activity has adverse prognostic significance.[62,63]

Recently, Heslin and colleagues evaluated by immunohistochemical techniques the potential prognostic significance of pRb, *p53, mdm2*, and Ki-67 status in a population of 121 patients with primary, high-grade extremity sarcomas and compared these factors to conventional clinicopathologic prognostic factors (median follow-up, 64 months).[50] Clinicopathologic and molecular factors found to be statistically significant adverse prognostic factors in both univariate and multivariate analyses for the separate endpoints of distant metastasis and tumor-related mortality included tumor size of more than 5 cm, microscopically positive surgical margin, and a Ki-67 score of greater than 20 (>20% nuclear staining). Overexpression of *p53* or *mdm2* or deletion of Rb did not correlate with an increased risk of distant metastasis or tumor-related mortality. In contrast to the findings of Wurl and colleagues,[60] Heslin et al.[50] did not find that *p53* or *mdm2* co-overexpression had adverse prognostic significance. This discrepancy underscores the uncertainty in interpreting the data on the prognostic significance of *p53* and *mdm2* status.

Synovial sarcoma is characterized by a specific chromosomal translocation [t(X;18) (p11;q11)] that is seen in more than 90% of these tumors.[64,65] This had led to studies evaluating the potential prognostic significance of SYT-SSX fusion transcripts, which arise from this translocation.[53] The t(X;18)(p11;q11) translocation fuses the *SYT* gene from chromosome 18 to either of two homologous genes at Xp11, *SSX1* or *SSX2*. The fusion transcripts SYT-SSX1 and SYT-SSX2 are believed to function as aberrant transcriptional regulators. The prognostic significance of these alternative forms of the *SYT-SSX* fusion gene and the relationship between these fusion transcripts and synovial sarcoma tumor morphology (monophasic versus biphasic subtype) were examined in 45 patients with synovial sarcoma.[53] There was a significant correlation ($p = 0.003$) between histologic subtype and fusion transcript type; all 12 biphasic synovial sarcomas (100%) had an SYT-SSX1 fusion transcript, whereas 17 (52%) of 33 monophasic tumors were positive for SYT-SSX1. Moreover, the presence of the SYT-SSX1 transcript was an independent adverse prognostic factor for metastasis-free survival. Thus, SYT-SSX fusion transcripts may be used as a diagnostic marker for synovial sarcoma, although the independent prognostic value of transcript subtype needs to be confirmed.

Although specific cellular and molecular parameters have been identified as having independent prognostic significance, there is currently no consensus on how such factors should be utilized in clinical practice. Developing meaningful cellular and molecular markers of prognosis for soft tissue sarcoma is hampered by the relative rarity of this disease. Only a few centers, for whom resected tumor specimens and autologous normal tissues are available for molecular analysis will be able to accrue a statistically robust number of patients with known clinical outcome. Moreover, standardization of immunohistochemistry techniques, such as establishing threshold levels for staining positivity, standardizing densitometry readings for interpretation of Western blot data, and standardizing polymerase chain reaction probes and numbers of cycles of amplification, will all require consensus development. These technical problems notwithstanding, the potential applications are extremely powerful, particularly as molecular aberrations also become the target for therapy itself.

The Significance of Tumor Hypoxia   Recently the microenvironment of soft tissue sarcomas has been studied using polarographic pO_2 measurements. The data from these studies suggest that hypoxia may influence the risk of development of distant metastasis in an adverse way.[66–70] Some therapeutic strategies are being developed to exploit these findings, although the data are preliminary.[71]

HOST-RELATED FACTORS

Intrinsic Host-related Factors

Patients with soft tissue sarcomas are usually free of significant patient or host-related comorbidities, which would impact adversely on the outcome of their disease. Frequently these patients, who are of younger age and without a predisposing cause for the sarcoma, are generally fit for most treatments. Nevertheless depending on the endpoint chosen, patient age >50 years may influence outcome, as shown for local control (Tables 27.1 and 27.2).[18]

In addition, one of the more adverse histologic subtypes for all endpoints, the peripheral nerve-sheath tumor, may have a strong link to an adverse host factor in a subset of the disease. This is because patients with neurofibromatosis 1 (NF1) are at significant risk of developing neurogenic sarcomas. A recent report from the Princess Margaret Hospital described 18 cases of neurogenic sarcoma, of which 7 had NF1.[72] Of the 7 with NF1, 6 developed distant metastases compared to 4 of 11 for patients without NF1. In addition, patients with NF1 may be difficult to evaluate, independent of the features of the tumor itself. Staging and follow-up assessments are confounded by the detection of other nodules and masses which, although generally representing benign neurofibromas in that patient, need to be distinguished from recurrent local or metastatic disease or a second neurogenic sarcoma presenting in the patient.

Acquired Host-related Factors

Another potential host-related prognostic factor is seen in the patient who develops an irradiation-induced soft tissue sarcoma.[73–75] The prognosis of these lesions is poor.[75] Frequently adjacent to prior radiotherapy fields administered for a different tumor in the remote past, these sarcomas are more difficult to treat because the host's capacity to tolerate additional adjuvant radiotherapy is usually severely compromised. This is unrelated to the tumor-related characteristics of the new sarcoma. Wider surgical resection compared to usual presentations, including amputation, may be required. Alternatively, radiation can be used with success in soft tissue sarcomas within prior radiotherapy fields,[76,77] but a higher rate of complications and morbidity may be expected.[76] This topic has recently been discussed in the context of the local management of recurrent sarcoma, which shares similarities of approach to the irradiation-induced tumor because of compromised host factors.[78]

ENVIRONMENT-RELATED FACTORS

Prognostic Significance of Treatment at Multidisciplinary Sarcoma Centers

Recent data on other tumor types have demonstrated that outcomes for patients who require complex treatment are improved if they are treated at experienced centers with high case loads.[79,80] Similar data confirm the same phenomenon in soft tissue sarcoma.[81,82] Gustafson and colleagues analyzed the outcome of treatment in a population-based series of 375 patients with primary soft tissue sarcomas arising in the extremities ($n = 329$) or the trunk ($n = 46$).[81] Comparison was made between patients referred to a specialty soft tissue tumor center prior to surgery ($n = 195$), those referred to a specialty center after surgery ($n = 102$), and those not referred to a specialty center for treatment of the primary tumor ($n = 78$). The total number of operations for the primary tumor was 1.4 times higher in patients not referred and 1.7 times higher in patients referred after surgery than in patients referred prior to surgery. Of greatest significance, however, was the finding that the local recurrence rate was 2.4 times higher in patients not referred and 1.3 times higher in patients referred after surgery than in patients referred to a specialty soft tissue tumor center prior to any manipulation of their tumors. Similar observations were noted in a recent population-based study from the South-East Thames Region in the United Kingdom.[82] In another UK study, disappointing results were obtained in a region during a period of time devoid of a dedicated sarcoma unit, which prompted recommendation to introduce multidisciplinary care.[83] Such a recommendation has also been suggested by others.[84–86]

These findings support the principle of centralizing treatment of these rare tumors, which frequently require complex multimodality therapy. Referral of soft tissue sarcoma patients to a specialty center with a multidisciplinary sarcoma group facilitates optimal treatment and participation in clinical trials and provides the best chance for a favorable outcome.

The "Unplanned Excision" Prior to Specialty Referral

Giuliano and Eilber originally coined the term "unplanned resection" for the environment-related prognostic adverse factor where an operation is performed for gross removal of a sarcoma without regard for preoperative imaging or the necessity of removing a margin of normal tissue covering the cancer.[87] These procedures are generally undertaken prior to referral for specialty care, and the patient thus arrives having undergone an unsatisfactory operation related almost exclusively to the pattern of the initial referral. About one-third of new patients referred to a specialized center have undergone such an "unplanned" excision and residual microscopic sarcoma can be detected in the wound at re-resection in 40 to 80% of cases.[88,89] Therefore in the unplanned resection, there is likely to be a substantial amount of residual tumor in the wound, and potentially widespread local seeding of cancer cells, although this is rarely detectable by computerized tomography scan or magnetic resonance imaging. This differs from the positive microscopic resection margin following a planned attempt at complete resection preceded by careful local staging.[89] In patients referred to Princess Margaret Hospital following unplanned resection, if adjuvant radiation without further surgery was the only management undertaken, 50% recurred locally.[12]

The management of the unplanned excision should include reexcision of the tumor bed. Detailed knowledge of the first surgical approach and the potentially contaminated structures should be obtained. Where possible, all contaminated tissues should be removed without sacrificing critical structures. If microscopic evidence of sarcoma is identified in the reexcision specimen, radiotherapy should be considered, unless particularly wide surgery has been undertaken.[90]

Intercountry Differences in Survival

The influence of the environment of the patient has been further studied by comparison of outcome in different countries using population-based registries. The recent EUROCARE project examined the outcome of the 5845 patients with soft issue sarcoma treated across Europe from 1985 to 1989.[91] The study also looked at bone sarcomas where the 5-year survival rates tended to be highest in northern Europe and were lowest in eastern European countries. A similar but less variable pattern was present for soft tissue sarcomas, but the eastern countries again had the lowest rates.[91] One is left to speculate about the reasons for these findings, but it is presumed that access to diagnostic and treatment facilities plays a role. Controlling for covariates such as stage was not possible in the study. However, even if tumor-related variables did demonstrate larger and more extensive tumors in the countries with the lowest rates of survival, this again focuses on an environment cause, including education of the population and medical and other health care workers, or timely access to assessment and diagnosis.

SUMMARY

Over the past decade, there has been significant emphasis on the elucidation of clinicopathologic prognostic factors in sarcoma (see Appendix 27B). This has allowed for identification of the "high-risk" patient at presentation. Even with current clinicopathologic prognostic factors, however, we can identify only patients who have a 50% or greater risk of distant failure (i.e., the patient with a TNM Stage III lesion). The current challenge is to extend our ability to identify the high-risk subset of patients to facilitate more judicious use of costly therapies, many of which have substantial toxicity. Molecular staging may be one important tool in the quest to identify high-risk patients with an accuracy greater than 50%. Even while such research is ongoing, however, environmental-related factors appear amenable to intervention immediately and patients should be referred for specialty consultation prior to treatment so that they can benefit from optimal diagnostic, therapeutic, and multidisciplinary approaches. This includes novel investigative protocols in situations where there is uncertainty about correct management.

■■■■■ **APPENDIX 27A**

TNM Classification: Soft Tissue Sarcoma

T — Primary Tumor

TX Primary tumor cannot be assessed

T0 No evidence of primary tumor

T1 Tumor 5 cm or less in greatest dimension

    T1a Superficial tumor

    T1b Deep tumor

T2 Tumor more than 5 cm in greatest dimension

    T2a Superficial tumor

    T2b Deep tumor

N — Regional Lymph Nodes

NX Regional lymph nodes cannot be assessed

N0 No regional lymph-node metastasis

N1 Regional lymph-node metastasis

M — Distant Metastasis

MX Distant metastasis cannot be assessed

M0 No distant metastasis

M1 Distant metastasis

G — Histopathological Grading

GX Grade of differentiation cannot be assessed

G1 Well differentiated

G2 Moderately differentiated

G3 Poorly differentiated

G4 Undifferentiated

Stage Grouping

Stage IA	G1, 2	T1a	N0	M0
	G1, 2	T1b	N0	M0
Stage IB	G1, 2	T2a	N0	M0
Stage IIA	G1, 2	T2b	N0	M0
Stage IIB	G3, 4	T1a	N0	M0
	G3, 4	T1b	N0	M0
Stage IIC	G3, 4	T2a	N0	M0
Stage III	G3, 4	T2b	N0	M0
Stage IV	Any G	Any T	N1	M0
	Any G	Any T	Any N	M1

Source: Sobin LH, Wittekind Ch (eds.): *TNM classification of malignant tumors*, 5th ed. New York, Union Internationale Contre le Cancer Wiley-Liss, 1997.

███████ **APPENDIX 27B**

Prognostic Factors in Soft Tissue Sarcoma

Prognostic Factors	Tumor Related	Host Related	Environment Related
Essential	Anatomic site Size Histologic grade Depth Presence of metastases		Treatment center (sarcoma referral center vs. community care) Unplanned excision at presentation
Additional	Histologic subtype Microscopic margin	Neurofibromatosis 1 (NF-1) Prior radiotherapy	Presentation (primary vs. locally recurrent) Adverse geographic location
New and promising	Ki-67 *p53* SYT-SSX fusion transcript (synovial sarcoma) EWS-FL11 fusion transcript (Ewing's sarcoma) Tumor hypoxia		

Note: The factors tabulated generally reflect survival outcome. Other endpoints may have direct bearing on the treatment to be given for alternative endpoints, but may not independently influence survival. An example is envelopment or invasion of neurovascular structures ± bone, and which would have a direct influence on the requirement of an amputation, and therefore would be *essential factors* for an endpoint like limb preservation

REFERENCES

1. Gaynor JJ, Tan CC, Casper ES, et al.: Refinement of clinicopathologic staging for localized soft tissue sarcoma of the extremity: A study of 423 adults. *J Clin Oncol* 10(8):1317–29, 1992.
2. Sears HF, Hopson R, Inouye W, et al.: Analysis of staging and management of patients with sarcoma: A ten-year experience. *Ann Surg* 191:488–93, 1980.
3. Trojani M, Contesso G, Coindre JM, et al.: Soft-tissue sarcomas of adults; Study of pathological prognostic variables and definition of a histopathological grading system. *Int J Cancer* 33(1):37–42, 1984.

4. Rydholm A, Berg NO, Gullberg B, et al.: Prognosis for soft-tissue sarcoma in the locomotor system. A retrospective population-based follow-up study of 237 patients. *Acta Pathol Microbiol Immunol Scand [A]* 92:375–86, 1984.

5. Heise HW, Myers MH, Russell WO, et al.: Recurrence-free survival time for surgically treated soft tissue sarcoma patients. Multivariate analysis of five prognostic factors. *Cancer* 57:172–7, 1986.

6. Rooser B, Attewell R, Berg NO, Rydholm A: Survival in soft tissue sarcoma. Prognostic variables identified by multivariate analysis. *Acta Orthop Scand* 58:516–22, 1987.

7. Collin CF, Godbold J, Hajdu SI, Brennan MF: Localized extremity soft tissue sarcoma: An analysis of factors affecting survival. *J Clin Oncol* 5:601–12, 1987.

8. Tsujimoto M, Aozasa K, Ueda T, et al.: Multivariate analysis for histologic prognostic factors in soft tissue sarcomas. *Cancer* 62:994–8, 1988.

9. Ueda T, Aozasa K, Tsujimoto M, et al.: Multivariate analysis for clinical prognostic factors in 163 patients. *Cancer* 62:1444–50, 1988.

10. Rooser B, Attewell R, Berg NO, Rydholm A: Prognostication in soft tissue sarcoma. A model with four risk factors. *Cancer* 61:817–23, 1988.

11. Mandard AM, Petiot JF, Marnay J, et al.: Prognostic factors in soft tissue sarcomas. A multivariate analysis of 109 cases. *Cancer* 63:1437–51, 1989.

12. Bell RS, O'Sullivan B, Liu FF, et al.: The surgical margin in soft-tissue sarcoma. *J Bone Joint Surg [Am]* 71(3):370–5, 1989.

13. Emrich LJ, Ruka W, Driscoll DL, Karakousis CP: The effect of local recurrence on survival time in adult high-grade soft tissue sarcomas. *J Clin Epidemiol* 42:105–10, 1989.

14. Stotter AT, A'Hern RP, Fisher C, et al.: The influence of local recurrence of extremity soft tissue sarcoma on metastasis and survival. *Cancer* 65(5):1119–29, 1990.

15. Alvegard TA, Berg NO, Baldetorp B, et al.: Cellular DNA content and prognosis of high-grade soft tissue sarcoma: The Scandinavian Sarcoma Group experience. *J Clin Oncol* 8:538–47, 1990.

16. Le Vay J, O'Sullivan B, Catton C, et al.: Outcome and prognostic factors in soft tissue sarcoma in the adult. *Int J Radiat Oncol Biol Phys* 27(5):1091–9, 1993.

17. Catton CN, O'Sullivan B, Kotwall C, et al.: Outcome and prognosis in retroperitoneal soft tissue sarcoma. *Int J Radiat Oncol Biol Phys* 29(5):1005–10, 1994.

18. Pister PWT, Leung DHY, Woodruff J, et al.: Analysis of prognostic factors in 1041 patients with localized soft tissue sarcomas of the extremities. *J Clin Oncol* 14(5):1679–89, 1996.

19. Coindre JM, Terrier P, Bui NB, et al.: Prognostic factors in adult patients with locally controlled soft tissue sarcoma. A study of 546 patients from the French Federation of Cancer Centers Sarcoma Group. *J Clin Oncol* 14(3):869–77, 1996.

20. Russell WO, Cohen J, Enzinger F, et al.: A clinical and pathologic staging system for soft tissue sarcomas. *Cancer* 40:1562–70, 1977.

21. Ruka W, Emrich LJ, Driscoll DL, Karakousis CP: Prognostic significance of lymph node metastasis and bone, major vessel, or nerve involvement in adults with high-grade soft tissue sarcomas. *Cancer* 62:999–1006, 1988.

22. Bevilacqua RG, Rogatko A, Hajdu SI, Brennan MF: Prognostic factors in primary retroperitoneal soft-tissue sarcomas. *Arch Surg* 126:328–34, 1991.

23. Heslin MJ, Lewis JJ, Nadler E, et al.: Prognostic factors associated with long-term survival for retroperitoneal sarcoma: Implications for management. *J Clin Oncol* 15(8):2832–9, 1997.

24. Tran LM, Mark R, Meier R, et al.: Sarcomas of the head and neck. *Cancer* 70(1):169–77, 1992.

25. Le Vay J, O'Sullivan B, Catton C, et al.: An assessment of prognostic factors in soft-tissue sarcoma of the head and neck. *Arch Otolaryngol Head Neck Surg* 120(9):981–6, 1994.

26. Kowalski LP, San CI: Prognostic factors in head and neck soft tissue sarcomas: Analysis of 128 cases. *J Surg Oncol* 56(2):83–8, 1994.

27. Kraus DH, Dubner S, Harrison LB, et al.: Prognostic factors for recurrence and survival in head and neck soft tissue sarcomas. *Cancer* 74(2):697–702, 1994.

28. Le QT, Fu KK, Kroll S, et al.: Prognostic factors in adult soft-tissue sarcomas of the head and neck. *Int J Radiat Oncol Biol Phys* 37(5):975–84, 1997.

29. McGrath PC, Neifeld JP, Lawrence W, Jr., et al.: Gastrointestinal sarcomas. Analysis of prognostic factors. *Ann Surg* 206:706–10, 1987.

30. Ng EH, Pollock RE, Munsell MF, et al.: Prognostic factors influencing survival in gastrointestinal leiomyosarcomas. implications for surgical management and staging. *Ann Surg* 215(1):68–77, 1992.

31. Meijer S, Peretz T, Gaynor JJ, et al.: Primary colorectal sarcoma. A retrospective review and prognostic factor study of 50 consecutive patients. *Arch Surg* 125:1163–8, 1990.

32. Olah KS, Dunn JA, Gee H: Leiomyosarcomas have a poorer prognosis than mixed mesodermal tumours when adjusting for known prognostic factors: The result of a retrospective study of 423 cases of uterine sarcoma. *Br J Obstet Gynaecol* 99:590–4, 1992.

33. Rooser B, Willen H, Hugoson A, Rydholm A: Prognostic factors in synovial sarcoma. *Cancer* 63:2182–5, 1989.

34. Singer S, Baldini EH, Demetri GD, et al.: Synovial sarcoma: Prognostic significance of tumor size, margin of resection, and mitotic activity for survival. *J Clin Oncol* 14(4):1201–8, 1996.

35. Le Doussal V, Coindre JM, Leroux A, et al.: Prognostic factors for patients with localized primary malignant fibrous histiocytoma: A multicenter study of 216 patients with multivariate analysis. *Cancer* 77(9):1823–30, 1996.

36. Pezzi CM, Rawlings MS, Jr., Esgro JJ, et al.: Prognostic factors in 227 patients with malignant fibrous histiocytoma. *Cancer* 69(8):2098–2103, 1992.

37. Rooser B, Willen H, Gustafson P, et al.: Malignant fibrous histiocytoma of soft tissue. A population-based epidemiologic and prognostic study of 137 patients. *Cancer* 67(2):499–505, 1991.

38. Barr LC, Stotter AT, A'Hern RP: Influence of local recurrence on survival: A controversy reviewed from the perspective of soft tissue sarcoma. *Br J Surg* 78:648–50, 1991.

39. Rooser B, Gustafson P, Rydholm A: Is there no influence of local control on the rate of metastases in high-grade soft tissue sarcoma? *Cancer* 65(8):1727–9, 1990.

40. Gustafson P, Rooser B, Rydholm A: Is local recurrence of minor importance for metastases in soft tissue sarcoma? *Cancer* 67:2083–6, 1991.

41. Lewis JJ, Leung DHY, Heslin MJ, et al.: Association of local recurrence with subsequent survival in extremity soft tissue sarcoma. *J Clin Oncol* 15:646–52, 1997.

42. Rosenberg SA, Tepper J, Glatstein E, et al.: The treatment of soft-tissue sarcomas of the extremities: Prospective randomized evaluations of (1) limb-sparing surgery plus radiation therapy compared with amputation and (2) the role of adjuvant chemotherapy. *Ann Surg* 196(3):305–15, 1982.

43. Yang JC, Rosenberg SA: Surgery for adult patients with soft tissue sarcomas. *Semin Oncol* 16:289–96, 1989.

44. Pisters PW, Harrison LB, Leung DH, et al.: Long-term results of a prospective randomized trial of adjuvant brachytherapy in soft tissue sarcoma. *J Clin Oncol* 14(3):859–68, 1996.

45. Yang JC, Chang AE, Baker AR, et al.: Randomized prospective study of the benefit of adjuvant radiation therapy in the treatment of soft tissue sarcomas of the extremity. *J Clin Oncol* 16(1):197–203, 1998.

46. Gelman R, Harris JR: Editorial comment on "The link between local recurrence and distant metastasis in human breast cancer" by Serge Koscielny and Maurice Tubiana. *Int J Radiation Oncol Biol Phys* 43(1):7–9, 1999.

47. Andreassen A, Oyjord T, Hovig E, et al.: p53 abnormalities in different subtypes of human sarcomas. *Cancer Res* 53(3):468–71, 1993.

48. Drobnjak M, Latres E, Pollack D, et al.: Prognostic implications of p53 nuclear overexpression and high proliferation index of Ki-67 in adult soft-tissue sarcomas. *J Natl Cancer Inst* 86(7):549–54, 1994.

49. Kawai A, Noguchi M, Beppu Y, et al.: Nuclear immunoreaction of p53 protein in soft tissue sarcomas. A possible prognostic factor. 73(10):2499–2505, 1994.

50. Heslin MJ, Cordon-Cardo C, Lewis JJ, et al.: Ki-67 detected by MIB-1 predicts distant metastasis and tumor mortality in primary, high grade extremity soft tissue sarcoma. *Cancer* 83:490–7, 1998.

51. Cance WG, Brennan MF, Dudas ME, et al.: Altered expression of the retinoblastoma gene product in human sarcomas. *N Eng J Med* 323:1457–62, 1990.

52. Karpeh MS, Brennan MF, Cance WG, et al.: Altered patterns of retinoblastoma gene product expression in adult soft-tissue sarcomas. *Br J Cancer* 72(4):986–91, 1995.

53. Kawai A, Woodruff J, Healey JH, et al.: SYT-SSX gene fusion as a determinant of morphology and prognosis in synovial sarcoma (see Comments). *N Engl J Med* 338(3):153–60, 1998.

54. Lewis JJ, Leung DHY, Casper ES, et al.: Multifactorial analysis of long-term follow-up (more than 5 years) of primary extremity sarcoma. *Arch Surg* 134:199–4, 1999.

55. Toguchida J, Yamaguchi T, Dayton SH, et al.: Prevalence and spectrum of germline mutations of the p53 gene among patients with sarcoma. *N Eng J Med* 326(20):1301–8, 1992.

56. Toguchida J, Yamaguchi T, Ritchie B, et al.: Mutation spectrum of the p53 gene in bone and soft tissue sarcomas. *Cancer Res* 52:6194–9, 1992.

57. Wadayama B, Toguchida J, Yamaguchi T, et al.: p53 expression and its relationship to DNA alterations in bone and soft tissue sarcomas. *Br J Cancer* 68(6):1134–9, 1993.

58. Stratton MR, Moss S, Warren W, et al.: Mutation of the p53 gene in human soft tissue sarcomas: Association with abnormalities of the RB1 gene. *Oncogene* 5:1297–1301, 1990.

59. Yang P, Hirose T, Hasegawa T, et al.: Prognostic implication of the p53 protein and Ki-67 antigen immunohistochemistry in malignant fibrous histiocytoma. *Cancer* 76(4):618–25, 1995.

60. Wurl P, Meye A, Schmidt H, et al.: High prognostic significance of Mdm2/p53 co-overexpression in soft tissue sarcoma of the extremities. *Oncogene* 16:1183–5, 1998.

61. Gerdes J: Ki-67 and other proliferation markers useful for immunohistological diagnostic and prognostic evaluations in human malignancies. *Semin Cancer Biol* 1(3):199–206, 1990.

62. Levine EA, Holzmayer T, Bacus S, et al.: Evaluation of newer prognostic markers for adult soft tissue sarcomas. *J Clinl Oncol* 15(10):3249–57, 1997.

63. Rudolph P, Kellner U, Chassevent A, et al.: Prognostic relevance of a novel proliferation marker, ki-s11, for soft-tissue sarcoma. A multivariate study. *Am J Pathol* 150(6):1997–2007, 1997.

64. Sreekantaiah C, Ladanyi M, Rodriguez E, Chaganti RS: Chromosomal aberrations in soft tissue tumors. Relevance to diagnosis, classification, and molecular mechanisms. *Am J Pathol* 144(6):1121–34, 1994.

65. Limon J, Mrozek K, Mandahl N, et al.: Cytogenetics of synovial sarcoma: Presentation of ten new cases and review of the literature. *Genes Chromosom Cancer* 3(5):338–45, 1991.

66. Brizel DM, Rosner GL, Harrelson J, et al.: Pretreatment oxygenation profiles of human soft tissue sarcomas. *Int J Radiat Oncol Biol Phys* 30(3):635–42, 1994.

67. Brizel DM, Rosner GL, Prosnitz LR, Dewhirst MW: Patterns and variability of tumor oxygenation in human soft tissue sarcomas, cervical carcinomas, and lymph node metastases. *Int J Radiat Oncol Biol Phys* 32(4):1121–5, 1995.

68. Brizel DM, Scully SP, Harrelson JM, et al.: Tumor oxygenation predicts for the likelihood of distant metastases in human soft tissue sarcoma. *Cancer Res* 56(5):941–3, 1996.

69. Nordsmark M, Hoyer M, Keller J, et al.: The relationship between tumor oxygenation and cell proliferation in human soft tissue sarcomas. *Int J Radiat Oncol Biol Phys* 35(4):701–8, 1996.

70. Nordsmark M, Keller J, Nielsen OS, et al.: Tumor oxygenation assessed by polarographic needle electrodes and bioenergetic status measured by 31P magnetic resonance spectroscopy in human soft tissue tumours. *Acta Oncol* 36(6):565–71, 1997.

71. Brizel DM, Scully SP, Harrelson JM, et al.: Radiation therapy and hyperthermia improve the oxygenation of human soft tissue sarcomas. *Cancer Res* 56(23):5347–50, 1996.

72. Angelov L, Davis A, O'Sullivan B, et al.: Neurogenic sarcomas: Experience at the University of Toronto. *Neurosurgery* 43(1):56–64 (Discussion 64–5), 1998.

73. Spiro IJ, Suit HD: Radiation-induced bone and soft tissue sarcomas: Clinical aspects and molecular biology. *Cancer Treat Res* 91:143–55, 1997.

74. Patel SG, See AC, Williamson PA, et al.: Radiation induced sarcoma of the head and neck. *Head Neck* 21(4):346–54, 1999.

75. Murray EM, Werner D, Greeff EA, Taylor DA: Postradiation sarcomas: 20 cases and a literature review. *Int J Radiat Oncol Biol Phys* 45(4):951–61, 1999.

76. Catton C, Davis A, Bell R, et al.: Soft tissue sarcoma of the extremity. Limb salvage after failure of combined conservative therapy. *Radiother Oncol* 41(3):209–14, 1996.

77. Pearlstone D, Janjan NA, Feig B, et al.: Re-resection with brachytherapy for locally recurrent soft tissue sarcoma arising in a previously irradiated field. *Cancer J Sci Am* 5(1):26–33, 1999.

78. Catton C, Swallow CJ, O'Sullivan B: Approaches to local salvage of soft tissue sarcoma after primary site failure. *Semin Radiat Oncol* 9(4):378–88, 1999.

79. Begg CB, Cramer LD, Hoskins WJ, Brennan MF: Impact of hospital volume on operative mortality for major cancer surgery. *JAMA* 280(20):1747–51, 1998.

80. Birkmeyer JD, Finlayson SR, Tosteson AN, et al.: Effect of hospital volume on in-hospital mortality with pancreaticoduodenectomy. *Surgery* 125(3):250–6, 1999.

81. Gustafson P, Dreinhover KE, Rydholm A: Soft tissue sarcoma should be treated at a tumor center. A comparison of quality of surgery in 375 patients. *Acta Orthop Scand* 65(1):47–50, 1994.

82. Clasby R, Tilling K, Smith MA, Other AN: Variable management of soft tissue sarcoma. *Br J Surg* 84:1692–6, 1997.

83. Jane MJ, Hughes PJ: Disease incidence and results of extremity lesion treatment: Mersey region soft tissue sarcomas (1975–1985). *Sarcoma* 2:89–96, 1998.

84. Wiklund T, Huuhtanen R, Blomqvist C, et al.: The importance of a multidisciplinary group in the treatment of soft tissue sarcomas. *Eur J Cancer* 32A(2):269–73, 1996.

85. Rydholm A: Centralization of soft tissue sarcoma. The southern Sweden experience. *Acta Orthop Scand Suppl* 273:4–8, 1997.

86. Rydholm A: Improving the management of soft tissue sarcoma. Diagnosis and treatment should be given in specialist centres. *BMJ* 317(7151):93–4, 1998.

87. Giuliano AE, Eilber FR: The rationale for planned reoperation after unplanned total excision of soft tissue sarcoma. *J Clin Oncol* 3:1344–8, 1985.

88. Noria S, Davis A, Kandel R, Levesque J, et al.: Residual disease following unplanned excision of soft-tissue sarcoma of an extremity (see Comments). *J Bone Joint Surg Am* 78(5):650–5, 1996.

89. Davis AM, Kandel RA, Wunder JS, et al.: The impact of residual disease on local recurrence in patients treated by initial unplanned resection for soft tissue sarcoma of the extremity. *J Surg Oncol* 66(2):81–7, 1997.

90. Karakousis CP, Driscoll DL: Treatment and local control of primary extremity soft tissue sarcomas. *J Surg Oncol* 71(3):155–61, 1999.

91. Storm HH: Survival of adult patients with cancer of soft tissue or bone in Europe. *Eur J Cancer* 34(14):2212–17, 1998.

SKIN TUMORS

CHAPTER 28

Skin Cancer

MICHAEL POULSEN

The great majority of skin cancers will be cured and this has resulted in a certain degree of complacency in its management. Despite the overall favorable outlook there remains a subset of patients who remain at higher risk of relapse and indeed may even succumb to the disease. There are many prognostic factors known, but the relationships between these variables are complex and it is difficult to differentiate the independent variables from the dependent ones.

In contrast to the low recurrence rate, the risk of subsequent skin cancer elsewhere is about 50% at 5 years.[1] The factors, which are prognostic for recurrence, are not the same as the factors, that predict for further skin cancer. Fair skin, male gender, high accumulation of solar exposure, and multiple previous basal cell carcinoma (BCC) or squamous cell carcinomas (SCCs) predict for further skin cancers.

The major types of nonmelanomatous skin cancer (NMSC) to be considered in this chapter are BCC, SCC and Merkel cell carcinoma (MCC).

TUMOR-RELATED FACTORS

The histologic type of cancer is one of the most important predictors of outcome, and accordingly histologic confirmation of the diagnosis is highly desirable. Tumors that are most likely to metastasize are those least likely to be diagnosed clinically. Clinical diagnosis is highest for BCCs (85% correct) and is lower for SCCs (53%).[2] MCC is rarely diagnosed clinically, even in special centers.

BCCs can be classified into several morphological types: nodular, ulcerative, superficial, morpheaform, infiltrating, and pigmented. Infiltrating, sclerotic, and multifocal lesions are associated with a higher relapse than nodular lesions (12–30% vs. 1–6%).[1] It has been suggested that the architectural differences between circumscribed and diffuse BCCs may correlate with the pattern and

Prognostic Factors in Cancer, 2nd edition, Edited by Mary K. Gospodarowicz
ISBN 0-471-40633-3   Copyright © 2001 Wiley-Liss, Inc.

expression of certain cellular antigens and biosynthetic products such as $\beta_2 =$ microglobulin and prostaglandins.[3] BCC's that exhibit poor palisading and consist of infiltrating strands and micronodules have a more aggressive pattern of spread and will have a higher recurrence rate.[4]

Three histologic variants of SCC are recognized: spindle-cell SCC, adenoid, and verrucous. Spindle-cell SCC may infiltrate deeply and show biologically aggressive behavior. Verrucous lesions tend to be more locally aggressive and cytologically well differentiated. Deeper invasion and greater cytological atypia are associated with higher recurrence rates.[5] Lesions that penetrate to the reticular dermis have a high recurrence rate. Well-differentiated SCCs have a lower recurrence rate than moderate to poorly differentiated SCCs.[6]

There is a decline in the cure rate for recurrent as opposed to primary skin cancers.[6] This is because the extent of tumor may be underestimated, as the tumor is embedded in a sclerotic matrix and tends to be ill defined.

International Union Against Cancer (UICC) (1997) staging of skin cancer relies predominantly on tumor size (see Appendix 28A). About 90% of skin cancers will be T1, and this will limit the practical application of the staging system. Tumor control is closely related to the size of the tumor. For tumors less than 1 cm, the local control with radiotherapy was 97% for BCC and 91% for SCC. For tumors 1–5 cm, the local control was 87% and 76%, respectively, and for lesions >5 cm, the local control was 87% and 56%, respectively.[7] The critical size, after which the recurrence rate increases, is 2 cm.[6] Rowe et al.[8] looked at all studies on prognosis of SCC published since 1940, and these have been summarized in Table 28.1.

Perineural infiltration occurs in about 5% of patients with carcinoma of the skin and is more common in SCC than BCC.[9] Recurrence rates with surgery are high

TABLE 28.1 Influence of Tumor Variables on Local Recurrence and Metastasis of SCC

Factor	Local Recurrence (%)	Metastasis (%)
Size <2 cm	7.4	9.1
>2 cm	15.2	30.3
Depth <4 mm	5.3	6.7
>4 mm	17.2	45.7
Well differentiated	13.6	9.2
Poorly differentiated	28.6	32.8
Site		
Sun exposed skin	7.9	5.2
Ear	18.7	11
Lip	10.5	13.7
Scar carcinoma	N/A	33.9
Previous treatment	23.3	30.3
Perineural	47.2	47.3
Immunosuppression	N/A	12.9

Source: After Reference 8.

and Goepfert et al.[10] reported a 47% local recurrence rate and a 34.8% metastatic rate. Further studies are necessary to define if radiation therapy to the primary site and the course of the nerve improves the results. Outcome is correlated with the extent of involvement. There is no recognized prognostic staging system for perineural spread. At its earliest extent, the pathologist may see tumor involvement in one or two nerve filaments well within the excision specimen. In its most advanced stage, patients will present with unexplained cranial nerve palsies, pain, and the feeling of ants crawling over the skin (formication). Branches of the fifth and seventh nerves are most commonly involved. The extent of perineural involvement as well as the adequacy of its excision should be evaluated in the histologic report. In a 10-year retrospective review of the Prince of Wales Hospital experience in Sydney, the incidence of perineural involvement was 5%. Following radiation therapy, only 5% recurred. Most of these patients did not have clinical signs of nerve involvement. In 45 patients who presented with advanced perineural disease with established signs, the 5-year local control was 42% and the survival was 54%. For patients with pathological evidence of perineural spread in the excision specimen and no clinical signs or symptoms, the 5-year local control was 92%.[11] In a series of 25 patients with clinical evidence of perineural spread, Mendelhall et al.[12] reported 20% local control with surgery alone and 38% with combined surgery and radiation therapy and 5-year absolute survival rates of 31% and 33%, respectively.

The significance of positive margins was well described by Gooding et al.[13] who found a crude recurrence rate of 35% in 66 incompletely excised BCCs, which were observed. Involved deep margins have a higher relapse rate than involved lateral margins (33% versus 17%),[14] and the risk will be higher if both lateral and deep margins are involved. The risk of recurrence with a positive margin will increase if the lesion has previously failed.[15] Positive margins with SCC are more serious, and these patients require additional therapy.

Advanced skin cancers also exhibit a number of prognostic variables. These lesions are a heterogeneous group. For instance, a T4 tumor could be a 1.5-cm BCC of the pinna, invading cartilage, or 6-cm SCC of the temple, eroding bone and infiltrating into the orbit. Lee et al.[16] investigated the prognostic variables of 68 patients with T4 tumors of the head and neck treated with radiation therapy. The three most important predictors of local control and cause-specific survival were bone involvement, recurrent lesions, and perineural spread. In this study, size was not prognostic. This may be because the absolute size in two dimensions of the tumor did not reflect the true tumor burden, or because the radiation dose was tailored to the tumor size. Likewise the histologic subtype did not appear to be important.

The histologic subtype is important in predicting the risk of nodal and distant recurrence. Metastases in BCCs are rare (<1 per 4000 cases), and for SCCs the incidence is 0.6%,[17] but has been reported higher in some series.[18] Tumors arising in middle-aged men on the temple, ear, forehead, hand or lip that are more than 1 cm in size or greater than 4 mm thick or undifferentiated are at higher risk of nodal secondaries.[1]

Over the past decade, other morphological and biological factors have been studied in order to identify aggressive types of skin cancer. These have included nuclear features, nuclear organizer region status, tumor angiogenesis, overexpression of p53 protein, tumor–extracellular matrix interactions, apoptotic index, bcl–2 protein expression, clonal heterogeneity, and DNA repair capacity.[19] The value of these remains to be determined in routine practice.

Merkel cell carcinoma is an important histologic group to identify because it carries a poor prognosis. Patients are at risk of local recurrence in the dermal lymphatics as well as nodal and distant recurrence.[20–24] The prognosis of MCC shows a sex differentiation, with better survival in women than men.[25] A number of prognostic variables have been defined. Nodal involvement was associated with a median survival of 13 months compared to 40 months for patients with uninvolved nodes.[21] The majority of patients have tumors less than 2 cm in size, so it is difficult to determine if tumor size is prognostic. In the M.D. Anderson series,[21] all patients with tumors >5 cm died of their tumor. Tumor site, sex, and age did not appear to be prognostic. A multivariate analysis on the Queensland Radium Institute data suggested that male sex and nodal disease were independent prognostic variables.[20]

Skin appendage tumors are rare, and may arise from the sweat glands, hair follicles, or sebaceous glands. They are often difficult to diagnose. Most are slow growing or benign, but there are rare cases that are highly malignant and the morphologic criteria may not correlate with the biologic behavior.

HOST-RELATED FACTORS

Tumors of the midface (nose, periocular area, and perioral area), ear, scalp, and forehead have the highest risk of recurrence.[1] Metastatic rates for SCCs of the sun exposed skin, ear, and lip were 5.2%, 8.8%, and 13.7%, respectively.[8] Recurrences are also reported to be higher in younger patients,[26] especially women. This may be due to compromised margins in order to preserve cosmesis.

Tumors associated with chronic inflammation or scars and those occurring on the lower extremities are more likely to recur than tumors associated with keratoses.[27] The risk of nodal metastasis is highest in tumors arising from burns or X-ray scars (10–30%) and lowest for those arising in normal skin (3%).[18] Tumors on the scalp and neck are at higher risk of metastasis than other sites, and may spread to the parotid or cervical nodes. The presence of solar changes in the adjacent skin is not prognostic.[6]

Patients with immunosuppression (e.g., following organ transplantation) need extra care in the management of their skin cancers. The risk of skin cancers (especially SCC) developing increases with the years of suppression (from 7% at 1 year to 70% at 20 years) and is independent of the agent of immunosuppression.[28] The ratio of SCC to BCC is the reverse to the general population. In one study the risk of SCC was 253-fold and the risk of BCC was 10-fold.[29] The overall metastatic rate per patient is 12.9%.[8] The problem is worse for fair-skin population living in sunny climates. Transplant recipients with a human leukocyte antigen (HLA) mismatch donor have a higher risk of SCC than those with an HLA matched donor.[30] This suggests a genetic link in the tumor susceptibility. Skin cancer accounted for 27% of deaths after the fourth year in a group of cardiac transplants.[31] Chronic lymphatic leukemia also results in immunosuppression and the development of skin cancers, which are more aggressive.[32]

Gorlin's syndrome or nevoid BCC syndrome should be thought of when a young patient presents with multiple BCCs. It is transmitted by an autosomal dominant gene and is associated with palmer and plantar pitting and facial changes with well-developed supraorbital ridges and hypertelorism. The syndrome is associated with increased risk of other malignancies such as ameloblastoma, SCC in jaw cysts, medulloblastoma, meningioma, craniopharyngioma, ovarian fibroma, cardiac fibroma, renal fibroma, neurofibroma, rhabdomyosarcoma, and adrenal cortical adenoma.[2] There is some evidence to suggest that radiation therapy may stimulate the development of new lesions and should therefore be avoided.

ENVIRONMENT-RELATED FACTORS

Early diagnosis results in improved outcome for NMSC. This is achieved primarily by community education programs and encouraging the use of general-practitioner screening rather than national screening programs, which are unlikely to be cost-effective.

Treatment modality does not appear to be a strong prognostic variable. Most reported studies have been retrospective and suggest that both surgery and radiation therapy can achieve 5-year local control rates of 85–95%. One randomized trial[33] compared surgery to radiation therapy in selected untreated BCC of less than 4 cm of the face. The study concluded that surgery was superior to radiation therapy both in terms of local control and cosmesis. The relative risk of failure with surgery was 0.7% and with radiation therapy was 7.5% ($p = 0.001$). The failure rate with surgery was lower than that commonly quoted in the literature, and radiation therapy was given by three different techniques, none of which involved megavoltage therapy. Ashby and McEwan[2] summarized the results of 19 publications reporting the use of radiation therapy for NMSC, which included more than 9143 patients. Cure rates varied from 86% to 97%, and the crude recurrence rate was 7.3%. For SCC, the failure rate appears to be lower for Mohs' micrographic surgery, irrespective of site or previous treatment. The recurrence rates for non-Mohs' modalities versus Mohs' micrographic surgery was 7.9% and 3.1%, respectively.[8]

Some authors also have reported that tumor control is related to the modality of radiation used. Lovett et al.[7] found that the control with superficial X rays was superior to that of electrons. In a multivariate analysis, the type of beam and dose per fraction, as well as recurrent presentation and tumor diameter, were highly significant prognostic factors. The authors suggest the poorer results of electrons may be related to the lack of bolus or inattention to the field margins. Other authors have failed to find an adverse recurrence rate with electrons where small lesions had a 2.2 % recurrence rate for both superficial and electron beam.[34]

Access to the full range of treatment modalities is desirable, particularly in the management of advanced cases such as tumors involving bone, cartilage or nerves, or lesions that have recurred. These tumors are better managed with combined surgery and radiation therapy than by surgery or radiation alone.[35] Access to multidisciplinary care is difficult or impossible to achieve in countries such as Australia where there are large areas of the country with very low population densities.

SUMMARY

Most prognostic variables for skin cancer are easily obtainable, relatively inexpensive, and achieved through a thorough history, physical examination, and histologic diagnosis. Recognition of them will allow the appropriate selection of therapy and an improved outcome. Appendix 28B summarizes current prognostic factors in skin cancer.

▬▬▬ **APPENDIX 28A**

TNM Classification: Carcinoma of the Skin (excluding eyelid, vulva, and penis)

T—Primary Tumor

TX Primary tumor cannot be assessed
T0 No evidence of primary tumor
Tis Carcinoma in situ

T1 Tumor 2 cm or less in greatest dimension
T2 Tumor more than 2 cm but not more than 5 cm in greatest dimension
T3 Tumor more than 5 cm in greatest dimension
T4 Tumor invades deep extradermal structures, that is, cartilage, skeletal muscle, or bone

N—Regional Lymph Nodes

NX Regional lymph nodes cannot be assessed
N0 No regional lymph-node metastasis
N1 Regional lymph-node metastasis

M—Distant Metastasis

MX Distant metastasis cannot be assessed
M0 No distant metastasis
M1 Distant metastasis

Stage Grouping

Stage 0	Tis	N0	M0
Stage I	T1	N0	M0
Stage II	T2	N0	M0
	T3	N0	M0
Stage III	T4	N0	M0
	Any T	N1	M0
Stage IV	Any T	Any N	M1

Source: Sobin LH, Wittekind Ch (eds.): *TNM classification of malignant tumors*, 5th ed. New York, Union Internationale Contre le Cancer Wiley-Liss, 1997.

■■■■■■■ **APPENDIX 28B**

Prognostic Factors in Skin Cancer

Prognostic Factors	Tumor Related	Host Related	Environment Related

Essential	Size
	Involvement of
	  cartilage or bone
	Nodes
	Histologic type
	Perineural infiltration
		Site
		Chronic inflammation,
		  burns, radiation scars
			Surgical margins
			Radiation dose

Additional	Differentiation
	Thickness
		Age
		Sex
		Genetic factors
			Radiation
			  modality
			Multidisciplinary
			  care

New and promising	p53 expression Bcl-2 protein expression Clonal heterogeneity Apoptotic index Tumor angiogenesis		

REFERENCES

1. Preston DS, Stern RS: Non melanomatous cancers of the skin. *N Eng J Med* 327:1649–62, 1992.

2. Ashby MA, McEwan L: Treatment of non melanomatous skin cancer: A review of recent trends with special reference to the Australian scene. *Clin Oncol* 2:284–94, 1990.

3. Murphy G, Elder DE: Non-meloncytic tumors of the skin (3rd series). Published by Armed Forces Institute of Pathology, Washington D.C. *Atlas of Tumor Pathology*. 58, 1991.

4. Lang PG, Maize JC: Histologic evolution of recurrent basal cell carcinoma and treatment implications. *J Am Acad Dermatol* 14:186, 1986.

5. Breuninger H, Black B, Rassner G: Microstaging of squamous cell carcinoma. *Am J Clin Pathol* 94:624–7, 1990.

6. Friedman RJ, Rigel DS, Kopf AW, et al.: *Cancer of the skin*. Philadelphia, Saunders, 1991.

7. Lovett R, Perez C, Shapiro S, Garcia D: External irradiation of epithelial skin cancer. *Int J Radiat Oncol Biol Phys* 19:235–42, 1989.

8. Rowe DE, Carroll R, Day C: Prognostic factors for local recurrence, metastasis, and survival in squamous cell carcinoma of the skin, ear and lip. *J Am Acad Dermatol* 26:976–90, 1992.

9. Bourne RG: The Costello Memorial Lecture: The spread of squamous cell carcinoma of the skin via the cranial nerves. *Aust Radiol* 24:106–14, 1980.

10. Goepfert H, Dictyhel W, Medina J, et al.: Perineural invasion in squamous cell carcinoma of the head and neck. *Am J Surg* 148:542–7, 1884.

11. Lehmann M, Hook C, Fisher R, Milross C: A retrospective review of a single institution's experience in the management of cutaneous head and neck malignancy demonstrating perineural infiltration. Published in RACR Book of Abstracts. Paper presented at the RACR Annual Scientific Meeting, 1998.

12. Mendenhall W, Parsons J, Mendenhall N, et al.: Carcinoma of the skin of the head and neck with perineural spread. *Head Neck* 11:301–8, 1989.

13. Gooding CA, White G, Yatsuhashi M: Significance of marginal extension in excised basal cell carcinoma. *N Eng J Med* 273:923–4, 1965.

14. Liu F, Maki E, Warde P, et al.: A management approach to incompletely excised basal cell carcinomas of the skin. *Int J Radiat Oncol Biol Phys* 20(3): 423–9, 1991.

15. Richmond J, Davie R: The significance of incomplete excision in patients with basal cell carcinoma. *Br J Plast Surg* 40:63–7, 1987.

16. Lee R, Mendenhall W, Parsons J, Million R: Radical radiotherapy for T4 carcinoma of the skin of the head and neck: A multivariate analysis. *Head Neck* 15:320–4, 1993.

17. Harris T: Squamous cell carcinoma. In Emmett A, O'Rourke M (eds.): *Malignant skin tumors*. London, Churchill Livingstone, 1991, pp. 143–51.

18. Moller R, Reyman F, Hou Jensen K: Metastases in dermatological patients with squamous cell carcinoma. *Arch Dermatol* 115:703, 1979.

19. Staibona S, Boscaino A, Salvatore G, et al.: The prognostic significance of tumor angiogenesis in non-aggressive and aggressive basal cell carcinoma of human skin. *Hum Pathol* 27:695–9, 1996.

20. Meeuwissen J, Bourne R, Kearsley J: The importance of postoperative radiation therapy in the treatment of Merkel cell carcinoma. *Int. J. Radiat Oncol Biol Phys* 31:325–31, 1995.

21. Morrison W, Peters L, Silva E, et al.: The essential role of radiation therapy is securing locoregional control of Merkel cell carcinoma. *Int J Radiat Oncol Biol Phys* 19:583–9, 1987.

22. Smith DE, Bielamowicz S, Anderson P, Peddada AV: Cutaneous neuroendocrine (Merkel cell) carcinoma. A report of 35 cases. *Am J Clin Oncol* 18(3):199–203, 1995.

23. Boyle F, Pendlebury S, Bell D: Further insights into the natural history and management of primary cutaneous neuroendocrine (Merkel cell) carcinoma. *Int J Radiat Oncol Biol Phys* 31:315–23, 1995.

24. Pacella J, Ashby M, Ainslie J, Minty C: The role of radiation therapy in the management of primary cutaneous neuroendocrine tumors: Experience of the Peter MacCallum Cancer Institute (Melbourne Australia). *Int J Radiation Oncol Biol Phys* 14:1077–84, 1988.

25. Meland NB, Jackson IT: Merkel cell tumor diagnosis, prognosis and management. *Plast Reconstr Surg* 77:632–8, 1996.

26. Leffell D, Headington J, Wong D, Swanson N: Aggressive growth basal cell carcinoma in young adults. *Arch Dermatol* 127:1663–7, 1991.

27. Edwards M, Hirsh R, Broadwater J, et al.: Squamous cell carcinoma arising in previously burned or irradiated skin. *Arch Surg* 124:115–7, 1989.

28. Bouwes-Bavinck JN, Hardie J, Green A, et al.: The risk of skin cancer in renal transplant recipients in Queensland, Australia. A follow-up study. *Transplantation* 15:715–21, 1996.

29. Hartevelt M, Bavinck J, Kootte A, Vermeer J: Incidence of skin cancer after renal transplantation in the Netherlands. *Transplantation* 49:506–9, 1990.

30. Bowes-Bavinck JN, Vermeer BJ, van der Woude FJ, et al.: Relation between skin cancer and HLA antigens in renal transplant recipients. *N Engl J Med* 325:843–9, 1991.

31. Ong CS, Keogh AM, Kossard S, et al.: Skin cancer in Australian heart transplant recipients. *J Am Acad Dermatol* 40:27–34, 1999.

32. Weimar VM, Ceilley RI, Goeken JA: Aggressive biological behavior of basal carcinomas and squamous cell carcinomas in patient with chronic lymphatic leukemia. *J Dermatol Surg Oncol* 5:609–14, 1979.

33. Avril M, Auperin A: Basal cell carcinoma of the face: Surgery or radiation therapy? Results of a randomised study. *Br J Cancer* 76:100–6, 1997.

34. Griep C, Davelaar J, Scholten A, et al.: Electron beam therapy is not inferior to superficial x ray therapy in the treatment of skin carcinoma. *Int J Radiat Oncol Biol Phys* 32:1347–50, 1995.

35. Mendenhall W, Parsons J, Mendenhall N, Million R: T2-T4 carcinoma of the skin of the head and neck treated with radical irradiation. *Int J Radiat Oncol Biol Phys* 13:975–81, 1987.

■■■■■ CHAPTER 29

Cutaneous Malignant Melanoma

PETER J. HEENAN, LAWRENCE L. YU, and DALLAS R. ENGLISH

The most important prognostic factor in patients with cutaneous malignant melanoma (CMM) is the anatomic extent of disease and, specifically, presence of metastasis (See Appendix 29A). In those patients without clinical metastasis at the time of diagnosis, direct measurement of tumor thickness by the method of Breslow[1] remains the most accurate single prognostic factor.[2–7] The improvement in survival rates recorded over time has been associated with a decrease in tumor thickness,[8–11] and geographical differences in prognosis have been related to differences in tumor thickness.[4,11] Furthermore, the prognostic effects of such features as the histologic type and level of invasion are overridden by the effect of tumor thickness.[7] The measurement of tumor thickness by means of an ocular micrometer is also more reproducible among pathologists than the recognition of histologic subtypes and the assessment of level of invasion according to anatomical landmarks, both of which are more prone to subjective interpretation and interobserver variation.[12]

It is also apparent, however, that although tumor thickness remains the best available single prognostic index, it provides only a rough guide to the outcome for an individual patient.[11,13] Increasing efforts have been made, therefore, to discover more accurate means of assessing the risk of metastasis in patients with melanoma by using multifactorial prognostic models[5,14–16] and by searching for molecular markers of metastatic potential. Prognostic models, however, although yielding impressive results in some studies,[5,15,16] may not always be accurate in their application to individual patients,[17] and the search for molecular markers of metastatic potential, although providing initially promising results, has as yet failed to identify prognostic factors that are as accurate or as practically applicable as the measurement of tumor thickness.

Prognostic Factors in Cancer, 2nd edition, Edited by Mary K. Gospodarowicz
ISBN 0-471-40633-3 Copyright © 2001 Wiley-Liss, Inc.

TUMOR-RELATED PROGNOSTIC FACTORS

Anatomic Extent of Disease

Tumor Thickness   Although tumor thickness measured by the method of Breslow[1] is the most accurate and most reproducible single histological index of prognosis, it is an imprecise guide to the behavior of the neoplasm.[13] The prognostic limitations of this method are exposed by the apparently paradoxical lethal behavior of some thin CMM, whereas some thick CMM metastasize late or not at all.[5,11] Thus, the demonstration of an inverse relation between survival rates and thickness, although providing valuable epidemiological information, fails to identify those individual tumors that have already begun the metastatic process, albeit subclinically, at the time of diagnosis of the primary tumor. Claims for improvement in the accuracy of assessment of prognosis according to various breakpoints[18,19] in tumor thickness have been counterbalanced by other reports concluding that the relationship between prognosis and tumor thickness is linear,[20-22] as originally proposed by Breslow et al.[23] Technical problems in applying the Breslow technique of direct measurement of tumor thickness using an ocular micrometer may also lead to inaccuracy and to interobserver variation.[13,24] Measurement of tumor thickness from the top of the granular layer of the epidermis means that almost the full depth of epidermis, which can vary greatly between different neoplasms and between different locations in the same neoplasm, is incorporated as an extraneous measurement beyond that of the invasive tumor itself. For these reasons, Schmoeckel and Braun-Falco[24] excluded the epidermis from their measurement, which was taken from the uppermost to the lowermost melanoma cells. This modification, however, has not been widely accepted, although it would seem to offer a more strictly accurate measurement of the depth of tumor invasion.

Level of Invasion   Univariate analysis of level of invasion[25] demonstrates strong correlation with prognosis,[15,21,22,25-27] but tumor thickness overrides the effect of level of invasion[19,23,26,28] and is more reproducible among pathologists.[12] Because some studies have indicated that level of invasion is important in assessing metastatic potential in thin CMM,[19,22,29] however, level of invasion is still recorded by most pathologists.

Mitotic Rate   Although the prognostic importance of mitotic rate and the method of counting mitoses has varied between different reports,[7] it is generally believed that a high mitotic rate is associated with an increased risk of metastasis.[5-7,30] Mitotic rate is included in most recommended prognostic models, measured as the number of mitoses per square millimeter in the zone of highest mitotic activity in the invasive tumor.[5]

Growth Phase   The introduction of the growth phase concept by Clark et al.[5] offered an explanation for the apparent failure of most so-called "thin" CMM to metastasize. Radial growth phase,[5] according to that concept, implies that some invasive CMM have not developed the potential for metastasis at the time of diagnosis. Complete excision of these cases therefore should be curative, as it is for in situ (Level 1) CMM, which are also deemed to be in radial growth phase. Vertical growth phase,[5] on the other hand, means that the tumors may have developed metastatic potential. Obviously, however, because many tumors fulfilling the histological criteria for vertical growth phase do not develop clinical metastases,[13] the recognition of vertical growth phase must be coordinated with other prognostic factors in the prediction of tumor behavior. The histological criteria for the radial and vertical growth phase are subtle and prone to subjective interpretation,[31,32] which limits the usefulness of this concept in routine reporting.

Histologic Type The widespread acceptance of the classification of Clark et al.[25] is based on its clinicopathological correlations, and on the didactic value of recognizing morphologic variations as an aid to the diagnostic process rather than on its prognostic implications.[33] It was acknowledged by Clark et al.,[25] and further suggested by other observers that nodular CMM may be a variant of the commonest form of melanoma, that is, superficial spreading melanoma, in which expansile growth of the neoplastic cells has produced a nodule that has overgrown the preexisting adjacent epidermal component.[34,35] According to Ackerman,[34] CMM is only one biological entity, a belief that is supported, to some extent, by pathological and epidemiological evidence that anatomic site may be important in determining some of the differences in growth pattern.[35] Lentigo maligna melanoma (CMM arising in Hutchinson's melanotic freckle), according to some reports, has the most favorable prognosis of the histologic types,[21,36] but others have concluded that invasive CMM of all histologic subtypes have similar behavior and that their prognosis is much more closely related to tumor thickness than to their histologic classification.[2,4,37]

Although it has been reported that acral lentiginous melanoma has a worse prognosis than nodular melanoma and superficial spreading melanoma,[21] its apparently more aggressive behavior may be related to the anatomic site rather than its histologic type.[38]

Ulceration The presence of ulceration (i.e., complete loss of the epidermis overlying invasive melanoma), according to many studies,[7,21,26,28] is a strong indicator of poor prognosis, independent of tumor thickness and rated by some as the second most important prognostic factor. According to other studies, however, the effect of ulceration cannot be separated from that of tumor thickness.[6,11] The recommended method of measuring tumor thickness of ulcerated lesions from the base of the ulcer[1] seems to predispose to underestimation of tumor thickness, possibly accounting, at least in part, for the otherwise unexplained and apparently independent correlation between ulceration and poor prognosis.

Tumor-Infiltrating Lymphocytes The presence of tumor-infiltrating lymphocytes (TIL) infiltrating the invasive tumor in vertical growth phase CMM, classified as brisk, nonbrisk, or absent, has correlated strongly with prognosis.[5,39] Other studies, however, have found no significant correlation between this attribute and survival,[6,21] possibly due to variation in the definitions of the categories used for the assessment of TIL.

Regression   The presence of regression in primary CMM has been associated with poorer survival rates in several studies,[5,7] but others have shown either no significant correlation[7,11,30,40] with prognosis or a protective effect.[6] This variation may be due to the use of different definitions of regression and to difficulty in the assessment of the histologic criteria.[41] Nevertheless, the presence of regression in thin CMM has been associated with an increased risk of metastasis.[22,42–44]

Vascular Invasion   Although the presence of melanoma cells in lymphatic and/or blood vessels is a sign that the metastatic process has commenced and, therefore, is generally regarded as an indicator of poor prognosis,[5] vascular invasion is inconsistently recorded and prone to confusion with shrinkage artefact.[45]

Cell Type   CMM composed predominantly of spindle cells has been associated with a better prognosis than those consisting of epithelioid cells,[11,45] but this has not been a consistent finding.[5,46]

Cross-sectional Profile   An exophytic growth pattern (verrucose, polypoid) of CMM portends a poor prognosis,[11] but this effect may depend on tumor thickness.[47]

Prognostic Models

Multifactorial prognostic models have been developed with the aim of improving the accuracy of assessment of survival beyond the use of tumor thickness alone. In 1989, Clark et al.[5] introduced a model based on the recognition of growth phase. In that study, for patients with vertical growth phase CMM, six further factors were found to be independent predictors of survival: mitotic rate, tumor infiltrating lymphocytes, tumor thickness, anatomic site, sex, and regression.

Because the histological criteria for some of these factors are subtle and prone to subjective interpretation, models of this type may not lend themselves to consistent reproduction.[6,17] More recently a prognostic model devised on the basis of tumor thickness, site of the primary melanoma, age of the patient, and sex of the patient, was found to predict more accurately the outcome for patients with primary CMM than did tumor thickness alone.[16]

New and Promising Prognostic Factors   Studies including measurement of tumor volume, nuclear volume and assessment of DNA aneuploidy have produced promising results, but they are not yet in routine use, due largely to the limitations imposed by the techniques involved. The use of the reverse-transcriptase polymerase chain reaction (RT-PCR) to detect circulating melanoma cells and the assessment of serum $S100\beta$-protein levels have also produced varied results in their relation to clinical stage and survival. Other factors, dependent mainly on their demonstration by immunostaining, have yielded conflicting or promising results and have not yet been accepted for routine use. These include the proliferation markers proliferating-cell nuclear antigen (PCNA), MIB1 (Ki-67); the tumor suppressor genes p53 and p16, NM23; adhesion molecules such as intercellular adhesion molecule 1 (ICAM-1) and $\alpha_v\beta_3$; CD44; growth factors; TA-90; tumor angiogenesis assessed by endothelial cell markers; and melastatin, a novel melanocyte-specific metastasis suppressor gene.

Regional Lymph-Node Status   The regional lymph-node status is a powerful prognostic indicator. The number of lymph nodes involved and the presence of extracapsular extension also influence prognosis.[48] Although lymph-node metastasis confers a bad prognosis, the reason for the poor prognosis is that these patients also have visceral metastases. The fact that the regional node group is the most common site of clinically evident metastasis, often preceding clinically evident visceral metastasis, produces the clinical impression that there is an orderly progression of melanoma metastasis which, if correct, would suggest that visceral metastases could be prevented if the regional lymph nodes were to be removed before any microscopic metastases became clinically evident. This is the rationale for elective lymph-node dissection (ELND). All the clinical trials to date, however, have shown no overall survival benefit in patients who have undergone ELND.[49] One trial, on the bases of multiple subgroup comparisons demonstrated a survival benefit;[50] this result has been questioned, however, on its statistical validity.[51]

While there is no doubt that clinically palpable macroscopic metastases confer a poor prognosis, the clinical significance of microscopic melanoma metastases remains uncertain. A recent clinical trial found that survival is not affected by the presence or absence of microscopic metastases.[52] Studies comparing angiogenesis, proliferation, and apoptosis also suggest that macroscopic and microscopic metastases may be different diseases.[53] Therefore, if microscopic melanoma metastases are clinically "inert" and tend to remain dormant for a prolonged period of time, it would be inappropriate to elevate the clinical staging on the finding of microscopic melanoma deposits in sentinel or other regional lymph nodes. Alternatively, if microscopic metastases have the same prognostic significance as macroscopic metastases, then most of the previous pathological studies on regional lymph nodes should be interpreted with caution, because the traditional method of lymph-node examination underestimates the incidence of microscopic melanoma metastases by about 10%.[54] The routine method of pathological examination of lymph nodes is sufficient for the detection of large metastases (involving a large proportion of the lymph node). For cases with tiny metastases (a few cells), however, this method would underestimate the true incidence of lymph-node metastasis.[54] Immunohistochemical melanocytic markers and the examination of multiple levels are required to identify these tiny microscopic metastases.[54] Therefore, all previous studies relating to the prognostic significance of the number of lymph nodes involved should be interpreted with caution. The observed results may merely be a reflection of the advanced stage of their disease (larger lymph-node metastasis is easier to detect than micrometastasis) rather than an effect of the number of lymph nodes involved per se.

Sentinel Lymph-Node Status   The sentinel lymph-node biopsy procedure is a recently developed, minimally invasive, experimental staging procedure currently undergoing clinical trial. It should be emphasized that, before the results of this trial are known, the procedure should only be performed in the context of a clinical trial.

The sentinel lymph node is defined as the first node (or nodes) in a nodal basin draining from the site of a primary cutaneous melanoma. If the sentinel node contains metastatic melanoma, regional lymphadenectomy [selective lymph-node dissection (SLND)] and, sometimes, adjuvant therapy are offered. The rationale of SLND is similar to that for ELND, and is based on the hypothesis that melanoma progression is an orderly process, lodging first at the sentinel node before dissemination to the rest of the regional nodes and to distant sites.[55] Many studies have reported that the sentinel lymph-node status is an accurate indicator of the status of the remainder of the nodal basin and that treatment decisions can be based on the status of the sentinel node alone.[56] Although the final results of the SLND trial are not yet available, preliminary results (more than 50% cases accrual) have shown no survival benefit.[57] This is not unexpected, as no overall survival benefit for ELND has been demonstrated after numerous trials. Proponents of SLND argue that this procedure eliminates unnecessary lymphadenectomy in about 80% of cases compared with ELND. However, the reported data show that in only about 20% of the SLND specimen do the nonsentinel lymph nodes harbor additional metastases.[58] The value of sentinel lymph-node biopsy as a staging tool is also questionable, as yet, in view of the uncertain biological potential of microscopic melanoma metastases and the lack of an effective adjuvant therapy. In summary, sentinel lymph-node biopsy is an experimental staging procedure that, on the present evidence, would only be justified in the hope that an effective adjuvant therapy can be found in the future.

HOST-RELATED PROGNOSTIC FACTORS

Age

In large-population-based series of cases, age is inversely associated with relative survival.[59,60] For example, in Europe, the 5-year relative survival among patients 75 years or older at diagnosis was 64%, whereas in patients less than 55 at diagnosis it was about 80%.[59] Differences in survival by age in US Surveillance, Epidemiology, and End Results (SEER) data are smaller.[60] The main problem with population-based series is that data on other prognostic factors, particularly tumor thickness, are not available. Thus, the poorer relative survival among the elderly may in part be due to increased average tumor thickness. The effect of age on melanoma-specific survival has been examined in several clinical studies. In some, but not all analyses, age has remained a prognostic indicator, even after adjustment for tumor thickness and other prognostic variables.[6,59,61–63]

Gender

Women have higher relative survival rates than men,[59,60] which in some studies at least, is not explained by differences in tumor thickness or other prognostic variables.[16,63] In some series, the difference in survival between men and women appears to be greatest at younger ages;[60,64] the reasons for this are unknown.

Race

Five-year relative survival in black Americans diagnosed in 1989–95 was 67.6%, whereas in white Americans it was substantially higher at 88%.[60] Most of this difference was due to more advanced stage at diagnosis in blacks: only 56% of melanomas in blacks were localized compared with 82% in whites. For localized tumors, the 5-year relative survival was 95% in whites and 91% in blacks.

Socioeconomic Status

Survival is poorer in patients of low socioeconomic status.[65–68] Part of this association is probably due to greater average thickness of melanomas in patients of low socioeconomic status. Survival from melanoma in eastern Europe was substantially lower than in western Europe, and the average thickness of melanoma at diagnosis was greater in eastern Europe than in western Europe.[59] Only one study has examined the effects of tumor thickness and socioeconomic status together, and found that the effect of socioeconomic status was independent of tumor thickness.[68] The authors speculated that factors such as poor nutrition or immunological defects might be responsible for the poor survival among the most disadvantaged patients.

ENVIRONMENT-RELATED PROGNOSTIC FACTORS

Geography, Access to Care

Relative survival rates in Europe and the united states are similar,[59] although within Europe there are substantial variations from east to west. As already discussed, these differences are probably due to differences in tumor thickness and stage at diagnosis.

Anatomic Site

Recent analyses of clinical series from the United States suggest that patients with melanomas on the head, neck, trunk, palms, or soles, or who have subungual melanomas have poorer survival than those with melanomas on the limbs (excluding volar and subungual subsites),[16,63,64] which is in accord with the results of a population-based analysis from western Australia.[11] These findings were independent of tumor thickness. However, in another population-based series, from Scotland, anatomic site was not related to survival after adjustment for tumor thickness.[69]

Pregnancy

There is no evidence that pregnancy affects prognosis for patients with CMM.[70] Although melanomas detected during pregnancy were thicker than those in nonpregnant women in a recent study, these melanomas were not associated with a less favorable prognosis for a given tumor thickness.[71]

TREATMENT

Surgical Treatment of Primary CMM

The effect of various forms of surgical excision of primary CMM has been a controversial topic, mainly in terms of the putative influence of different margins of excision on survival and the risk of local recurrence.[72] Wide excision of the primary tumor beyond complete excision of the tumor itself has no effect on survival; thus, the sole remaining reason for wide excision is to diminish the risk of local recurrence.[72] Evidence supporting a strong correlation between margins of excision and risk of local recurrence, however, is meager. The recent recognition that many so-called local recurrences are, in fact, metastases[28,73,74] suggests that prevention of these lesions is beyond the scope of surgery, as they are part of the same metastatic process that produces more distant cutaneous metastases, lymph-node, and visceral metastases. In other words, the presence of cutaneous metastases after complete excision of the primary tumor is an indication that the metastatic process had already begun at the time of primary treatment. It is likely, therefore, that wider excision of primary CMM beyond complete excision of the tumor itself has no effect on prognosis or the risk of local recurrence.

Surgical Resection of Isolated Metastases

Resection of isolated metastases, according to some reports, may relieve symptoms and, in some cases, prolong survival, especially in patients with solitary metastases in the skin, subcutis, lung or brain.[75]

Adjuvant Therapy

Despite the tremendous expansion in research and clinical trials of adjuvant therapy, there is no conclusive evidence that any of these forms of treatment confer any benefit in survival to patients with metastatic melanoma. Although chemotherapy and immunotherapy may prolong the disease-free interval, this modest effect must be assessed with the prospect of high toxicity.

UICC/AJCC TNM STAGING SYSTEM FOR CUTANEOUS MELANOMA (APPENDIX 29A)

In the 1997 International Union Against Cancer (UICC) Staging System[76] for cutaneous malignant melanoma, tumors with satellites within 2 cm of the primary tumor are classified as pT4 and included in Stage III, as are lesions with in-transit metastases. This staging is supported by the fact that so-called local recurrences of primary CMM that have been completely excised are metastases.[28,73,74] In order to ensure the consistent application of this staging, the correct classification by pathologists of so-called local recurrences as either (1) true persistence of incompletely excised melanoma, or (2) metastasis (as in satellites, in-transit metastases), is essential.[74]

The subdivisions of tumor thickness as equal to or less than 0.75 mm, greater than 0.75 mm to 1.5 mm, greater than 1.5 mm to 4.0 mm, and greater than 4.0 mm, remain arbitrary, as are their correlation with levels 2, 3, 4, and 5. Some Level 3 melanomas, for example, are less than 0.75 mm thick, and many Level 4 melanomas are 1.5 mm thick or less.

The TNM staging system retains level of invasion, stating that in case of discrepancy between tumor thickness and level of invasion, the TT category should be based on the less favorable finding. Buzaid et al.,[28] however, found that level of invasion provided statistically significant information only in patients with tumor thickness equal to or less than 1 mm, and that stratification of tumor thickness with cutoff points of 1 mm, 2 mm, and 4 mm resulted in the best fit for the data. They accordingly recommended that the staging system be modified to incorporate those new tumor thickness groupings and that level of invasion be eliminated,[28] although it would seem appropriate to retain level of invasion for tumors of less than 1.00-mm thickness.

Buzaid et al.,[28] also suggested that the size of lymph nodes involved by metastases should be deleted from the current staging system and replaced by the number of positive nodes, which is a more powerful prognostic factor. Most of these recommended changes[28] have been included in the new proposed AJCC staging system for cutaneous melanoma.[77]

SUMMARY

The rapid expansion of the search for more precise prognostic indicators has produced promising but, as yet, inconclusive results. Beyond tumor thickness, which remains the most accurate guide and the host factors age, anatomic site, and gender, none of the many potential markers has emerged as a proven and practical guide to more accurate assessment of prognosis, especially when applied to individual patients (See Appendix 29B).

■■■■■■■ **APPENDIX 29A**

TNM Classification: Malignant Melanoma of Skin

pT — Primary Tumor

pTX Primary tumor cannot be assessed

pT0 No evidence of primary tumor

pTis Melanoma in situ (Clark Level I) (atypical melanocytic hyperplasia, severe melanocytic dysplasia, not an invasive malignant lesion)

pT1 Tumor 0.75 mm or less in thickness and invades the papillary dermis (Clark Level II)

pT2 Tumor more than 0.75 mm but not more than 1.5 mm in thickness and/or invades to the papillary-reticular dermal interface (Clark Level III)

pT3 Tumor more than 1.5 mm but not more than 4.0 mm in thickness and/or invades the reticular dermis (Clark Level IV)

    pT3a Tumor more than 1.5 mm but not more than 3.0 mm in thickness

    pT3b Tumor more than 3.0 mm but not more than 4.0 mm in thickness

pT4 Tumor more than 4.0 mm in thickness and/or invades subcutaneous tissue (Clark Level V) and/or satellite(s) within 2 cm of the primary tumor

    pT4a Tumor more than 4.0 mm in thickness and/or invades subcutaneous tissue

    pT4b Satellite(s) within 2 cm of the primary tumor

N — Regional Lymph Nodes

NX Regional lymph nodes cannot be assessed

N0 No regional lymph-node metastasis

N1 Metastasis 3 cm or less in greatest dimension in any regional lymph node(s)

N2 Metastasis more than 3 cm in greatest dimension in any regional lymph node(s) and/or in-transit metastasis

N2a Metastasis more than 3 cm in greatest dimension in any regional lymph node(s)

N2b In-transit metastasis

N2c Both

M — Distant Metastasis

MX Distant metastasis cannot be assessed

M0 No distant metastasis

M1 Distant metastasis

M1a Metastasis in skin or subcutaneous tissue or lymph node(s) beyond the regional lymph nodes

M1b Visceral metastasis

Stage Grouping

Stage 0	pTis	N0	M0
Stage I	pT1	N0	M0
	pT2	N0	M0
Stage II	pT3	N0	M0
Stage III	pT4	N0	M0
	Any pT	N1, N2	M0
Stage IV	Any pT	Any N	M1

Source: Sobin LH, Wittekind Ch (eds.): *TNM classification of malignant tumors*, 5th ed. New York. Union Internationale Contre le Cancer Wiley-Liss, 1997.

■■■■■■ **APPENDIX 29A1**

Proposed TNM Classification

Classification

T — Classification

T1	< or = 1.0 mm	a: without ulceration
T1		b: with ulceration or level IV or V
T2	1.01–2.0 mm	a: without ulceration
T2		b: with ulceration
T3	2.01–4.0 mm	a: without ulceration
T3		b: with ulceration
T4	>4.0 mm	a: without ulceration
T4		b: with ulceration

N — Classification

N1	One lymph node	a: micrometastasis[a]
		b: macrometastasis[b]
N2	2–3 lymph nodes	a: micrometastasis[a]
		b: macrometastasis[b]
		c: in-transit met(s)/satellite(s) without metastatic lymph nodes
N3	4 or > metastatic lymph nodes, matted lymph nodes, or combinations of in-transit met(s)/ satellite(s), or ulcerated melanoma and metastatic lymph node(s)	

M — Classification

M1	Distant skin, SQ, or lymph node mets	Normal LDH
M2	Lung mets	Normal LDH
M3	All other visceral or any distant mets	Normal LDH Elevated LDH

mets: metastases

[a]Micrometastases are diagnosed after elective or sentinel lymphadenectomy

[b]Macrometastases are defined as clinically detectable lymph node metastases confirmed by therapeutic lymphadenectomy or when any lymph node metastasis exhibits gross extracapsular extension

■■■■■ **APPENDIX 29B**

Prognostic Factors in Cutaneous Malignant Melanoma

Prognostic Factors	Tumor Related	Host Related	Environment Related
Essential	Primary CMM — Tumor thickness *Metastases* — Cutaneous Lymph nodes Systemic	Age Gender Anatomic site	Completeness of primary excision
Additional	Primary CMM: Mitotic rate Ulceration Regression Level of invasion Tumor infiltrating lymphocytes (TIL) Growth phase Cell type Cross-sectional profile		Lymph-node dissection Excision of isolated metastases Chemotherapy[b] Immunotherapy[b] Radiotherapy[b]
New and promising	Tumor suppressor genes[a] Proliferation markers[a] Angiogenesis[a] Adhesion molecules[a] Growth factors[a] Serum S100β protein[a] RT-PCR for circulating melanoma cells[a]		Polyvalent melanoma cell vaccines[b] Gene therapy[b]

[a]Not in routine use.
[b]No proven survival benefit.

REFERENCES

1. Breslow A: Thickness, cross-sectional area, and depth of invasion in the prognosis of cutaneous melanoma. *Ann Surg* 172:902–8, 1970.
2. Eldh J, Boeryd B, Peterson L-E: Prognostic factors in cutaneous malignant melanoma in Stage I. *Scand J Plast Reconstr Surg* 12:243–55, 1978.
3. McGovern VJ, Shaw HM, Milton GW, et al.: Prognostic significance of the histological features of malignant melanoma. *Histopathology* 3:385–93, 1979.

4. Heenan PJ, Holman CDJ: Survival from invasive cutaneous malignant melanoma in Western Australia and the Oxford region: A comparative histological study of high and low incidence populations. *Pathology* 15:147–52, 1983.

5. Clark WH, Jr., Elder DE, Guerry DG, IV, et al.: Model predicting survival in stage I melanoma based on tumor progression. *J Natl Cancer Inst* 81:1893–904, 1989.

6. Barnhill RL, Fine JA, Roush GC, et al.: Predicting five-year outcome for patients with cutaneous melanoma in a population-based study. *Cancer* 78:427–32, 1996.

7. Vollmer R: Malignant melanoma: A multivariate analysis of prognostic factors. *Pathol Annu* 24:383–407, 1989.

8. English DR, Heenan PJ, Holman CDJ, et al.: Melanoma in Western Australia in 1980–81: Incidence and characteristics of histological types. *Pathology* 19:383–92, 1987.

9. Balch CM, Soong S-J, Milton GW, et al.: Changing trends in cutaneous melanoma over a quarter century in Alabama, USA, and New South Wales, Australia. *Cancer* 52:1748–53, 1983.

10. Schneider JS, Moore DH, Sagebiel RW: Early diagnosis of cutaneous malignant melanoma at Lawrence Livermore National Laboratory. *Arch Dermatol* 126:767–9, 1990.

11. Heenan PJ, English DR, Holman CDJ, et al.: Survival among patients with clinical stage I cutaneous malignant melanoma diagnosed in Western Australia in 1975/1976 and 1980/1981. *Cancer* 68:2079–87, 1991.

12. Heenan PJ, Matz LR, Blackwell JB, et al.: Inter-observer variation between pathologists in the classification of cutaneous malignant melanoma in Western Australia. *Histopathology* 8:717, 1984.

13. Green MS, Ackerman AB: Thickness is not an accurate gauge of prognosis of primary cutaneous melanoma. *Am J Dermatopathol* 15:461–73, 1993.

14. Soong SJ, Shaw HM, Balch CM, et al.: Predicting survival and recurrence in localized melanoma: A multivariate approach. *World J Surg* 16:191–5, 1992.

15. Garbe C, Büttner P, Bertz J, et al.: Primary cutaneous melanoma. Identification of prognostic groups and estimation of individual prognosis for 5093 patients. *Cancer* 75:2484–91, 1995.

16. Schuchter L, Schultz DJ, Synnestvedt M, et al.: A prognostic model for predicting 10-year survival in patients with primary melanoma. *Ann Intern Med* 125:369–75, 1996.

17. Rowley MJ, Cockerell CJ: Reliability of prognostic models in malignant melanoma: A 10-year follow-up study. *Am J Dermatopathol* 13:431–7, 1991.

18. Day CL, Jr. Lew RA, Mihm MC, Jr, et al.: The natural break points for primary tumor thickness in clinical stage I melanoma (Letter). *N Engl J Med* 305:1155, 1981.

19. Büttner P, Garbe C, Bertz J, et al.: Primary cutaneous melanoma. Optimized cutoff points of tumor thickness and importance of Clark's level for prognostic classification. *Cancer* 75:2499–2506, 1995.

20. Keefe M, MacKie RM: The relationship between risk of death from clinical stage I cutaneous melanoma and thickness of primary tumor: No evidence of steps in risk. *Br J Cancer* 64:598–602, 1991.

21. Balch C, Soong SJ, Shaw H, et al.: An analysis of prognostic factors in 8500 patients with cutaneous melanoma, in Balch C, Houghton A, Sober AJ, et al. (eds.): *Cutaneous melanoma*, 2d ed. Philadelphia, Lippincott, 1992, pp.165–87.

22. Mansson-Brahme E, Carstensen J, Erhardt K, et al.: Prognostic factors in thin cutaneous malignant melanoma. *Cancer* 73:2324–32, 1994.

23. Breslow A, Cascinelli N, van der Esch E, et al.: Stage I melanoma of the limbs: Assessment of prognosis by levels of invasion and maximum thickness. *Tumori* 64:273–84, 1978.

24. Schmoeckel C, Braun-Falco O: Prognostic index in malignant melanoma. *Arch Dermatol* 114:871–3, 1978.

25. Clark WH, Jr., From L, Bernardino EA, et al.: The histogenesis and biologic behavior of primary human malignant melanomas of the skin. *Cancer Res* 29:705–27, 1969.

26. Balch CM, Murad T, Soong S-J, et al.: A multifactorial analysis of melanoma: Prognostic histopathological features comparing Clark's and Breslow's staging methods. *Ann Surg* 188:732–42, 1978.

27. Morton DL, Davtyan DG, Wanek LA, et al.: Mulivariate analysis of the relationship between survival and the microstage of primary melanoma by Clark level and Breslow thickness. *Cancer* 71:3737–43, 1993.

28. Buzaid AC, Ross MI, Balch CM, et al.: Critical analysis of the current American Joint Committee on Cancer staging system for cutaneous melanoma and proposal of a new staging system. *J Clin Oncol* 15:1039–51, 1997.

29. Kelly JW, Sagebiel RW, Clyman S, et al.: Thin level IV malignant melanoma: A subset. *Ann Surg* 202:98–103, 1985.

30. Sober AJ, Day CL, Jr, Fitzpatrick TB, et al.: Factors associated with death from melanoma from 2 to 5 years following diagnosis in clinical stage 1 patients. *J Invest Dermatol* 80S:53S–5S, 1983.

31. Solomon AR, Ellis CN, Headington JT: An evaluation of vertical growth in thin superficial spreading melanomas by sequential serial microscopic sections. *Cancer* 52:2338–41, 1983.

32. Sagebiel RW: Problems in microstaging of melanoma vertical growth. *Monogr Pathol* 30:94–109, 1988.

33. Heenan PJ, Elder DE, Sobin LH. *Histological typing of skin tumors. WHO international histologic classification of tumors.* Berlin-New York, Springer-Verlag, 1996.

34. Ackerman AB: Malignant melanoma: A unifying concept. *Hum Pathol* 11:591–5, 1980.

35. Heenan PJ, Armstrong BK, English DR, et al.: Pathological and epidemiological variants of cutaneous malignant melanoma, in Elder DE (ed.): *Pathobiology of malignant melanoma,* Basel, Karger, 1987, pp. 107–46.

36. McGovern VJ, Shaw HM, Milton GW, et al.: Is malignant melanoma arising in a Hutchinson's melanotic freckle a separate disease entity? *Histopathology* 4:235–42, 1980.

37. Koh HK, Michalik E, Sober AJ, et al.: Lentigo malignant melanoma has no better prognosis than other types of melanoma. *J Clin Oncol* 2:994–1001, 1984.

38. Slingluff CL, Vollmer R, Seigler HF: Acral melanoma: A review of 185 patients with identification of prognostic variables. *J Surg Oncol* 45:91–8, 1990.

39. Clemente CG, Mihm MC, Jr., Bufalino R, et al.: Prognostic value of tumor infiltrating lymphocytes in the vertical growth phase of primary cutaneous melanoma. *Cancer* 77:1303–10, 1996.

40. Kelly JW, Sagebiel RW, Blois MS: Regression in malignant melanoma. A histologic feature without independent prognostic significance. *Cancer* 56:2287–91, 1985.

41. Kang S, Barnhill RL, Mihm MC, et al.: Regression in malignant melanoma: An interobserver concordance study. *J Cutan Pathol* 20:126–9, 1993.

42. Sondergaard K, Hou-Jensen K: Partial regression in thin primary cutaneous malignant melanomas clinical stage 1. A study of 486 cases. *Virchows Archiv (A)* 408:241–7, 1985.

43. Ronan SC, Eng AM, Briele HA, et al.: Thin malignant melanomas with regression and metastases. *Arch Dermatol* 123:1326–30, 1987.

44. Blessing K, McLaren KM, McLean A, et al.: Thin malignant melanomas (less than 1.5 mm) with metastasis: A histological study and survival analysis. *Histopathology* 17:389, 1990.

45. Sondergaard K. Schou G: Survival with primary cutaneous malignant melanoma, evaluated from 2012 cases. *Virchows Arch (A)* 406:179–95, 1985.

46. Ronan SG, Han MC, Das Gupta TK: Histologic prognostic indicators in cutaneous malignant melanoma. *Semin Oncol* 15:558–65, 1988.

47. McGovern VJ, Shaw HM, Milton GW: Prognostic significance of a polypoid configuration in malignant melanoma. *Histopathology* 7:663–72, 1983.

48. Balch CM, Soong SJ, Murad TM, et al.: A multifactorial analysis of melanoma: III. Prognostic factors in melanoma patients with lymph node metastases (stage II). *Ann Surg* 193:377–88, 1981.

49. Hochwald SN, Coit DG: Role of elective lymph node dissection in melanoma. *Semin Surg Oncol* 14:276–82, 1998.

50. Balch CM, Soong SJ, Bartolucci AA, et al.: Efficacy of an elective regional lymph node dissection of 1 to 4 mm thick melanomas for patients 60 years of age and younger. *Ann Surg* 224:255–66, 1996.

51. Piepkorn M, Weinstock MA, Barnhill RL: Theoretical and empirical arguments in relation to elective lymph node dissection for melanoma. *Arch Dermatol* 133:995–1002, 1997.

52. Cascinelli N, Morabito A, Santinami M, et al.: Immediate or delayed dissection of regional lymph nodes in patients with melanoma of the trunk: A randomised trial. Lancet 351:793–6, 1998.

53. Barnhill RL, Piepkorn MW, Cochran AJ, et al.: Tumor vascularity, proliferation and apoptosis in human melanoma micrometastases and macrometastases. *Arch Dermatol* 134:991–4, 1998.

54. Yu LL, Flotte TJ, Tanabe KK, et al.: Detection of microscopic melanoma metastases in sentinel lymph nodes. *Cancer* 86:617–27, 1999.

55. Reintgen D, Balch CM, Kirkwood J, et al.: Recent advances in the care of the patient with malignant melanoma. *Ann Surg* 225:1–14, 1997.

56. Reintgen D, Cruse CW, Wells K, et al.: The orderly progression of melanoma nodal metastases. *Ann Surg* 220:759–67, 1994.

57. Morton DL: Management of regional lymph nodes in melanoma patients. *Melanoma Res* 7(Suppl. 1):S22, 1997.

58. Thompson JF, McCarthy WH, Bosch CMJ, et al.: Sentinel lymph node status as an indicator of the presence of metastatic melanoma in regional lymph nodes. *Melanoma Res* 5:255–60, 1995.

59. Smith JA, Whatley PM, Redburn JC: Improving survival of melanoma patients in Europe since 1978. EUROCARE Working Group. *Eur J Cancer* 34:2197–2203, 1998.

60. Ries LAG, Kosary CL, Hankey BF, et al. (eds.): *SEER cancer statistics review, 1973–1996*. Bethesda, MD, National Cancer Institute, 1999.

61. Halpern AC, Schuchter LM: Prognostic models in melanoma. *Semin Oncol* 24(Suppl. 4):S2–7, 1997.

62. Sahin S, Rao B, Kopf AW, et al.: Predicting ten-year survival of patients with primary cutaneous melanoma: Corroboration of a prognostic model. *Cancer* 80:1426–31, 1997.

63. Margolis DJ, Halpern AC, Rebbeck T, et al.: Validation of a melanoma prognostic model. *Arch Dermatol* 134:1597–1601, 1998.

64. Kemeny MM, Busch E, Stewart AK, et al.: Superior survival of young women with malignant melanoma. *Am J Surg* 175:437–44 (Discussion, 44–45), 1998.

65. Vågerö D, Persson G: Risks, survival and trends of malignant melanoma among white and blue collar workers in Sweden. *Soc Sci Med* 19:475–8, 1984.

66. Bonett A, Roder D, Esterman A: Epidemiological features of melanoma in South Australia: Implications for cancer control (see Comments). *Med J Aust* 151:502–4, 6–9, 1989.

67. Geller AC, Miller DR, Lew RA, et al.: Cutaneous melanoma mortality among the socioeconomically disadvantaged in Massachusetts. *Am J Public Health* 86:538–44, 1996.

68. MacKie RM, Hole DJ: Incidence and thickness of primary tumors and survival of patients with cutaneous malignant melanoma in relation to socioeconomic status (see Comments). *Br Med J* 312:1125–8, 1996.

69. MacKie RM, Hole D, Hunter JA, et al.: Cutaneous malignant melanoma in Scotland: Incidence, survival and mortality, 1979–1994. The Scottish Melanoma Group. *Br Med J* 315:1117–21, 1997.

70. Holly EA, Cress RD: Melanoma and pregnancy, in Gallagher RP and Elwood JM (eds.): *Epidemiological aspects of cutaneous malignant melanoma*. Boston, Kluwer, 1994, pp. 209–21.

71. Travers RL, Sober AJ, Berwick M, et al.: Increased thickness of pregnancy-associated melanoma. *Br J Dermatol* 132:876–83, 1995.

72. Heenan PJ, English DR, Holman CDJ, et al.: The effects of surgical treatment on survival and local recurrence of cutaneous malignant melanoma. *Cancer* 69:421–6, 1992.

73. Heenan PJ, Ghaznawie M. The pathogenesis of local recurrence of melanoma at the primary excision site. *Br J Plastic Surg* 52:209–13, 1999.

74. Yu LL, Heenan PJ: The morphological features of locally recurrent melanoma and cutaneous metastases of melanoma. *Hum Pathol* 30:551–5, 1999.

75. Balch CM: Surgical treatment of advanced melanoma, in Balch CM, Houghton AN, Sober AJ, Soong S-J (eds.): *Cutaneous melanoma*, 3d ed. St. Louis, Quality Medial Publishing, 1998, pp. 373–88.

76. Sobin LH, Wittekind C (eds.): *TNM classification of malignant tumors*, 5th ed. New York, International Union Against Cancer Wiley-Liss, 1997.

77. Balch CM, Buzaid AC, Atkius MB, et al.: A new American Joint Committee on Cancer staging system for cutaneous melanoma. *Cancer* 88:1484–91, 2000.

BREAST CANCER

CHAPTER 30

Breast Cancer

PATRICK L. FITZGIBBONS

Breast cancer is a heterogeneous disease that exhibits a wide variety of clinical presentations, histologic types, and growth rates. Because of these variations, determining prognosis for an individual patient at the time of initial diagnosis requires careful assessment of multiple clinical and pathological parameters. This evaluation includes consideration of an expanding list of tumor- and patient-related prognostic factors, which are especially important for decisions related to systemic treatment and predictions for overall survival.

TUMOR-RELATED PROGNOSTIC FACTORS

Essential Factors

The anatomic disease extent, such as tumor size, presence of regional lymph node involvement, or distant metastases, is an important prognostic factor. The TNM system[1,2] is the universally accepted method of classifying the anatomic extent of disease (see Appendix 30A).

Nodal Status The most important disease-related prognostic factor in primary invasive breast cancer is the status of the axillary lymph nodes.[3-7] About 70% of patients with axillary nodal metastases will develop recurrence within 10 years, compared with 20 to 30% of those with negative nodes. The absolute number of involved nodes is also of prognostic importance. Relapse-free survival and overall survival are poorer among patients with four or more involved nodes than those with one to three involved nodes, and the prognosis is substantially worse for those with 10 or more axillary nodal metastases.[7]

The current American Joint Committee on Cancer (AJCC) cancer staging manual states that the prognosis for patients with an isolated axillary micrometas-tasis (pN1a), defined as a single-nodal metastasis ≤2 mm in diameter, is the

Prognostic Factors in Cancer, 2nd edition, Edited by Mary K. Gospodarowicz
ISBN 0-471-40633-3 Copyright © 2001 Wiley-Liss, Inc.

same as that of patients with negative lymph nodes.[6] Recent studies have shown, however, that micrometastases do have an adverse impact on patient survival.[8-10] Axillary micrometastases can be found in about 10% of "node-negative" breast cancer patients by serial step sectioning,[8] and in up to 20% by cytokeratin immunohistochemistry or molecular assays,[9-12] but the impact on patient survival of micrometastases found by these methods is unsettled. Furthermore, while the prognosis for patients with histologically confirmed micrometastases is still somewhat controversial, few data are available on the prognostic significance of isolated cytokeratin-positive cells in the absence of a histologically identified tumor focus. Until these issues are resolved in clinical trials, it is premature to recommend changes in staging and treatment based solely on finding a single, occult micrometastasis, particularly those that are not histologically evident.[13]

Sentinel lymph-node sampling in place of formal axillary dissection has achieved widespread use because of its effectiveness in predicting axillary nodal status and its reduced morbidity. There is high concordance between sentinel lymphadenectomy and axillary dissection, and reported false negative rates are relatively low. The procedure may replace axillary dissection for many patients, but it has not yet been shown to have disease-free and overall survival rates equivalent to axillary dissection.

Tumor Size Tumor size is an important predictor of tumor behavior in breast cancer for both node-negative and node positive patients;[5,14-16] among node-negative patients, tumor size is the most powerful predictor of outcome. For patients with tumors 1.0 cm or smaller (T1a and T1b), the frequency of nodal metastases is 10 to 20%,[5,17] and the 10-year disease free survival is about 90%.[17-19] Fewer than 2% of patients with T1a or T1b cancers and negative axillary nodes will die of disease within 5 years.[5] Precise assessment of tumor size is necessary to properly stratify patients for treatment purposes, particularly for the steadily increasing proportion of pT1 cancers. Underestimating tumor size by gross examination is more frequent in this subset of breast cancers than in those larger than 2.0 cm.

Histologic Grade Histologic grade is an important determinant of prognosis that also allows risk stratification within a given tumor stage.[20-24] For most breast cancers histologic grade is a more meaningful prognostic feature than histologic classification, and helps to explain the favorable prognosis of most special histologic types. About 10% of low-grade (well-differentiated) tumors recur within 5 years, compared with about 30% of high-grade (poorly differentiated) cancers.

A number of histologic grading systems have been proposed, but the Nottingham Combined Histologic Score (Elston-Ellis modification of the Scarff-Bloom-Richardson system) is the most commonly recommended.[22,23] This grading system combines a quantitative assessment of tubule formation, nuclear pleomorphism, and mitotic activity to produce a histologic grade (Table 30.1). Several studies have validated this approach.[23]

TABLE 30.1 Nottingham Combined Histologic Score

Feature	Score[a]
Tubule formation	
>75% of the tumor	1
10% to 75% of the tumor	2
<10% of the tumor	3
Nuclear pleomorphism	
Small regular nuclei	1
Moderate increase in size, variation in shape, etc.	2
Marked variation in size, nucleoli, chromatin clumping, etc.	3
Mitotic count[b]	
<10 mitoses per 10 HPF	1
10–20 mitoses per 10 HPF	2
>20 mitoses per 10 HPF	3

[a]The score for each feature is added to produce a grade as follows: 3–5 points = Grade I; 6–7 points = Grade II; 8–9 points = Grade III.
[b]This tabulation corresponds to the use of 25× objective with a field diameter of 0.59 mm and a field area of 0.274 mm^2.

Histologic Type Invasive breast carcinoma can be roughly divided into two general categories: infiltrating ductal (syn: no special type; ordinary; NOS), and special-type carcinomas. Infiltrating ductal carcinoma comprises about 70% of breast cancers and is usually not further subclassified. For ordinary invasive ductal breast carcinoma, tumor size and histologic grade are the most important pathologic variables.

Invasive lobular carcinoma is usually considered together with ductal carcinoma because of similarities in prognosis, biologic behavior, and treatment. Indeed, many breast cancers exhibit mixtures of ductal and lobular features. There are several histologic subtypes of invasive lobular carcinoma (i.e., classic, pleomorphic, alveolar, and solid). While these subtypes share a single-file or targetoid histologic growth pattern, a propensity for multifocality and multicentricity within the breast, and a distinctive pattern of distant metastasis,[25] only the relatively uncommon "classic" invasive lobular carcinoma has a better prognosis than ordinary infiltrating ductal carcinoma.

The special-type carcinomas, which include tubular, mucinous, medullary, and papillary carcinomas, are associated with a favorable prognosis compared with ordinary invasive ductal carcinoma. In general, these special histologic types have a lower frequency of lymph-node metastasis and improved overall survival when compared by tumor stage, but this good prognosis depends upon the application of strict diagnostic criteria.

When diagnosing special type carcinomas, the characteristic features should comprise at least 90% of the tumor.[26] A tumor that has some of the features of a special type carcinoma (e.g., abundant extracellular mucin; a diffuse single-file growth pattern), but that does not fulfill these diagnostic criteria, should be identified as an ordinary or no-special-type carcinoma and classified primarily by histologic grade.

Mitotic Figure Count An increased rate of cell proliferation strongly correlates with reduced survival in breast cancer. Assessing the number of mitotic figures in histologic sections provides an inexpensive yet relatively accurate assessment of cell proliferation, and is part of the Nottingham combined histologic score recommended for all invasive breast cancers. The mitotic figure count is usually reported as the number of mitotic figures found in 10 consecutive high-power fields (HPF) in the most mitotically active part of the tumor.[27-29] High mitotic rates correlate with poor clinical outcome.[30] Immunohistochemical stains for nuclear proliferation markers such as Ki-67 (MIB-1), and flow cytometric measurement of the fraction of cells in the S phase are also useful methods of measuring cell proliferation but are considered optional (see Additional Factors in this section).

Hormone Receptor Status Estrogen receptor and progesterone receptor determinations are established procedures in the routine management of patients with breast cancer and are considered an essential part of the evaluation of most newly diagnosed primary invasive tumors. However, these determinations are primarily used as predictors of response to therapeutic and adjuvant hormonal therapy; their prognostic power is relatively weak. Most published studies have used ligand-binding assays to determine receptor status, but immunohistochemistry has recently become the preferred method for most cases.[31] Concordance between these methodologies is good, and there is some evidence that immunohistochemistry may be superior to ligand binding assay in predicting clinical outcome.[32]

Effect of Tumor Recurrence or Metastasis Following Primary Therapy
Ipsilateral breast tumor recurrence (IBTR) following breast conservation and radiation is usually limited to the breast, and is effectively treated by salvage mastectomy in most patients. Important factors affecting survival following IBTR include the length of the disease-free interval, estrogen receptor status, and original axillary lymph node status. Patients whose first recurrence is found more than 5 years after initial diagnosis have significantly better survival than those with a disease-free interval shorter than 2 years.[33,34] Chest-wall recurrence following mastectomy is often viewed as an ominous finding, but not all such patients have poor clinical outcome. Stage I and IIa patients who develop a single chest-wall recurrence that can be locally controlled have 10-year survivals comparable to those without chest-wall recurrence.[35]

The site of first relapse following primary therapy is also a powerful predictor of clinical outcome: patients whose first recurrence is a metastasis to liver or brain have much poorer survival than those with recurrence in the breast, chest wall, or axilla. Bone metastasis has an intermediate impact on survival.

Additional Factors

c-erbB-2 (Her2-neu)   The c-erbB-2 (Her2-*neu*) gene carried on chromosome 17 codes for a cell-membrane glycoprotein growth factor receptor. Since normal cells with two copies of the gene express very low levels of the protein, immunohistochemical stains show at most only very faint membrane expression of c-erbB-2. Twenty to 30% of breast cancers have amplification of the c-erbB-2 gene and overexpression of the membrane protein. Such cases can be detected by fluorescence in situ hybridization (FISH), which shows increased gene copy number, or by immunohistochemistry, in which protein overexpression is revealed by strong membrane staining.

c-erbB-2 abnormalities in breast cancer are associated with high histologic grade, reduced overall survival,[36-41] resistance to tamoxifen,[42-44] poorer response to methotrexate-based treatment regimens,[36,37] and better responsiveness to doxorubicin-based treatment regimens.[36,39,40,45] Although useful as a prognostic factor, c-erbB-2 analysis currently enjoys more clinical utility as a predictive marker for treatment response.

Peritumoral Vascular Invasion   Finding nests of tumor within blood vessel or lymphatic spaces in the breast parenchyma outside the tumor is associated with an increased risk of local recurrence and reduced overall survival.[46-48] By contrast, invasion of lymphovascular spaces within the tumor is of little or no prognostic significance. Distinguishing true vascular spaces from retraction artifact may require special stains for endothelial cells or vascular elements (e.g. type IV collagen, laminin, CD31, CD34, Factor VIII-related antigen), but this is not considered necessary for routine prognostic determination.[49,50]

MIB-1 (Ki-67)   Ki-67 is a nuclear protein found in the G_1 through M phases of the cell cycle and is considered a useful marker of cell proliferation. Many studies have found a relationship between the percentage of Ki-67 positive cells (as detected by anti-Ki-67 stains of frozen sections) and clinical outcome.[51-55] These studies suggest that measuring Ki-67 expression can be useful in stratifying patients into good and poor prognostic groups. The monoclonal antibody MIB-1 recognizes Ki-67 but can be used in formalin-fixed paraffin-embedded tissue sections. Besides being of more practical utility, several studies suggest that MIB-1 may have greater predictive value than anti-Ki-67 in breast cancer.[56,57]

S-Phase Fraction by Flow Cytometry   Measuring S-phase fraction (SPF), which is defined as the number of tumor cells that are in the DNA synthesizing, or S phase, of the cell cycle, is another method of assessing the rate of cell proliferation. SPF may be determined by either flow cytometry or image analysis, but most studies that correlate SPF with clinical outcome have used flow cytometry.

A high SPF indicates a rapidly proliferating tumor, and such tumors are associated with an increased risk of recurrence and death from disease. The prognostic significance of SPF applies to both node-negative and node-positive invasive breast cancers,[58,59] but the significance of SPF appears to be less following treatment. One study of node-negative patients found that treatment with cyclophosphamide, methotrexate, and 5-fluorouracil (CMF) was equally effective in patients with either high or low SPF.[60] Similarly, a study of node-positive patients treated with cyclophosphamide, doxorubicin, 5-fluorouracil (CAF) found that SPF did not correlate with response to treatment[61]

p53 The tumor suppressor gene p53 encodes for a nuclear protein involved in the regulation of cell proliferation. This protein is normally undetectable by immunohistochemical assays because of its very short half-life. However, about one-third of breast cancers have mutations of the p53 gene, which usually result in the production of a stable p53 protein that accumulates in the nucleus. Thus, p53 overexpression by routine immunohistochemical stains identifies tumors with p53 gene mutation. Abnormalities of p53 are usually the result of spontaneous somatic mutations, but patients with germline p53 mutations (LiFraumeni syndrome) also have an increased incidence of breast cancer.

Analysis of p53 status by immunohistochemistry has been shown to be a powerful independent prognostic factor in breast cancer.[62] p53 immunopositivity is associated with poor prognostic features such as high histologic grade, increased cell-proliferation rates, and aggressive clinical behavior.[63-66] p53 can also be useful as a predictive marker by identifying patients more likely to respond to chemotherapy.[67-69] p53 overexpression is a significant prognostic factor that can be useful in identifying subsets of node-negative patients for whom aggressive treatment may be needed.[70,71]

New and Promising Factors

DNA Ploidy Analysis Abnormal DNA content (aneuploidy) is associated with high histologic grade, large tumor size, and a slightly less favorable prognosis compared with diploid tumors. The utility of DNA ploidy analysis as a prognostic factor for breast cancer is hampered by lack of standardization among laboratories in cell-preparation methods, differences in software programs used to analyze histograms, the effect of debris on cell cycle analysis of fixed tissues, and lack of consensus about cutoffs to define DNA diploidy and aneuploidy. The DNA Cytometry Consensus Conference[58] concluded that neither DNA index nor DNA ploidy status has independent prognostic significance for breast cancer.

Tumor Angiogenesis Tumor growth and metastasis appear to depend on the growth of new blood vessels in and adjacent to the tumor, and there have been reports of an association between the density of tumor microvessels and risk of metastasis.[72-75] However, significant methodological differences among studies have prevented tumor angiogenesis from becoming a routine measure of prognosis in breast cancer. These differences include the specificity of antibodies used to measure vascular density, the methods used to count new vessels (e.g., vessel density in one hot spot, mean vessel density of three hot spots, highest value in three hot spots), and the types of treatment patients have received. Furthermore, some reports have found that measurement of microvessel density is of no significant prognostic value,[76–78] or too variable to be clinically useful.[76,79,80]

Epidermal Growth-factor Receptor and Transforming Growth Factor-α

The epidermal growth-factor receptor (EGFR) is found in the cell membrane of breast epithelial cells and modulates cell proliferation. The receptor binds both epidermal growth factor and transforming growth factor-α, and is closely related to c-erbB-2. Overexpression of EGFR occurs in some breast cancers and is associated with increased tumor growth, absence of estrogen receptor, and poor response to tamoxifen.[81–83]

Studies of the prognostic significance of EGFR expression have provided mixed results, with only some showing a correlation between EGFR and poorer disease-free survival.[81–86] Transforming growth factor-α competes with EGF for the EGF receptor and also appears to have a promoting effect on the growth of some breast cancers.[87]

bcl-2   bcl-2 has been reported to be a marker of good prognosis and responsiveness to tamoxifen. The presence of bcl-2 correlates with the presence of estrogen receptor, and bcl-2 positive tumors show better response to tamoxifen and longer disease-free survival compared with bcl-2 negative tumors.[88,89] Hellemans et al.[90] found no prognostic significance for bcl-2 expression in node-negative patients, but among node-positive patients, bcl-2 negativity correlated with shorter survival.

pS2   pS2 is a cytoplasmic protein that is expressed only after estrogen stimulation and appears to function as a growth factor. Since pS2 is only produced if there is a functioning estrogen receptor-related pathway, measurement of pS2 might serve as a predictor of tumor behavior and/or responsiveness to hormonal therapy.[91,92] Several studies have shown that pS2-positive tumors have a better prognosis and a better response to tamoxifen than pS2-negative tumors,[91,93,94] and that pS2-negative tumors have a poor prognosis.[92]

PATIENT-RELATED PROGNOSTIC FACTORS

Essential Factors

Age   Determining the effect of patient age on breast cancer prognosis is confounded by many factors, such as screening rates, menopausal status, and differences in treatment. Consequently, significant differences in study designs have resulted in a lack of consensus regarding the prognostic effect of patient age. For example, several studies have shown significantly poorer overall survival among very young patients (e.g., younger than 35 years) and those older than 75 years,[95,96] while others have found that the prognosis for young patients was the same or better than that of older patients.

In a study restricted to premenopausal women, de la Rochefordiere and colleagues found that overall survival and disease-free survival were poorer for those younger than 34 years, and this difference was independent of tumor stage, hormone receptor status, and type of treatment.[97] These findings were confirmed by two subsequent studies, both of which showed significantly worse prognosis for young patients even after other prognostic factors were considered by multivariate analysis.[98,99] While these studies provide strong evidence that very young age is an adverse prognostic feature, the effect of age on prognosis in older women remains unclear, largely because of significant differences in treatment in this age group.

Additional Factors

Pregnancy Many early studies of breast cancer arising during pregnancy or lactation reported extremely poor outcomes, and anecdotal experience of highly aggressive malignancies in such patients would seem to support the conclusion that pregnancy-associated cancers have a poor prognosis. However, while the overall survival of all breast cancer patients diagnosed during pregnancy is worse than for nonpregnant patients, this difference does not appear to be significant when analyzed by tumor stage. Most recent studies have found that the prognosis for breast cancer arising during pregnancy is most closely related to tumor stage, and is similar to carcinoma not arising in pregnancy, at least among node-negative patients.[100–103]

The poorer outcome seen in the overall patient group appears to be related to factors such as patient age and more advanced disease at the time of diagnosis. Delays in diagnosis of breast cancer during pregnancy may be caused by changes in the breast that affect clinical examination, a lower index of suspicion for breast changes that occur during pregnancy or lactation, and to possible reluctance to recommend mammography for this group of women.

Race and Socioeconomic Status Population-based studies performed in the United States have found that black and Hispanic women are significantly more likely to die from breast cancer than white women,[103,104] but analyses of the prognostic effect of ethnicity on breast cancer survival have produced conflicting results. Some studies find little difference in outcome after other prognostic variables are analyzed, but in others, poorer survival rates among black patients are seen even after adjusting for such things as stage of disease.[105,106] One recent study found that socioeconomic status, but not race, was a significant predictor of survival even after adjusting for stage of disease.[107] Besides socioeconomic status and related issues like nutrition, behavior, and life style, many other factors that might affect survival, such as younger age at diagnosis, delays in diagnosis, and access to care and treatment, must be considered before determining the prognostic effect of race.[108,109]

Heredity A woman who has a first-degree relative with breast cancer is at significantly increased risk for developing breast cancer herself. Those who inherit one of the breast cancer susceptibility genes *BRCA1* or *BRCA2* have an estimated lifetime breast cancer risk of 56%.[110] While inheritance of *BRCA1* or *BRCA2* is a significant risk factor for developing breast cancer, it remains unclear whether the overall prognosis of hereditary breast cancer is different than sporadic tumors, or whether *BRCA1* or *BRCA2* can be considered prognostic factors.

Preliminary studies have shown that, compared with sporadic breast cancer, hereditary breast cancers exhibit a variety of poor prognostic features, such as young patient age, high histologic grade, absence of hormone receptors, aneuploidy, and high proliferation markers. Paradoxically, however, studies performed to date have not shown poor clinical outcomes. Multiple studies report survival among breast cancer patients with *BRCA1* and *BRCA2* mutations similar to that of sporadic breast cancers.[111–114] Whether this represents a statistical anomaly, such as lead-time bias in an intensively screened population, or some other effect related to heritable breast cancer is as yet undetermined.

Gender Overall survival for breast cancer was once thought to be worse for men than women,[115] but as in some of the other patient-related prognostic factors, this is probably related to tumor stage at diagnosis rather than a significant biologic difference. A recent study showed that tumor stage at the time of diagnosis is higher for men than women.[116] These authors found that the prognosis for breast cancer was the same for men and women once stage was considered.

ENVIRONMENT-RELATED PROGNOSTIC FACTORS

Essential Factors

Effect of Local and Systemic Treatment Prospective randomized trials have found no significant differences in overall or disease-free survival between modified radical mastectomy and breast conservation (with radiation) in the treatment of stage I and II invasive breast cancer.[117] The overall survival of patients treated by mastectomy ranged from 59% to 82%, compared with 54% to 79% for those treated by conservation.[118]

Some studies have suggested that complete axillary dissection may improve overall survival.[119] This is supported by studies showing the effect of adjuvant radiation therapy to the axillary nodes.[120]

Patients who have a complete response to doxorubicin-containing chemotherapeutic regimens have a significant survival advantage compared with those who show partial or no response to treatment.[121] Both the total chemotherapy dose and dose intensity of adjuvant chemotherapy also appear to be related to clinical outcome. In a study of Stage II breast cancer patients treated within a conventional range of doses, those given moderate and high dose regimens had better disease-free and overall survivals than those treated with a lower dose.[122]

Other studies have assessed the impact of the sequence or timing of treatment on clinical outcome. In a study of node-positive patients, Bonadonna et al.

found that sequential therapy—four courses of doxorubicin followed by eight of CMF—was significantly better than alternate therapy, wherein two courses of CMF alternated with one of doxorubicin.[123] In a study comparing the effect of preoperative (neoadjuvant) chemotherapy with postoperative therapy, no differences were found in disease-free survival or overall survival.[124] In the latter study patients treated preoperatively were more likely to have breast conservation, but the incidence of tumor recurrence and death from disease was not significantly different in the two groups.

Additional Factors

Effect of Screening   Screen-detected cancers are smaller, less likely to have metastasized to axillary lymph nodes, more likely to be in situ, and more likely to be of favorable histologic grade than those that present as palpable masses.[125] Not surprisingly, the long-term survival of such patients is better than those who present symptomatically,[126] but this prognostic difference may be partly related to lead-time bias.

Effect of Delays in Diagnosis   There is some evidence that a delay between the detection of a breast mass and the onset of treatment can affect patient outcome. One study found that an interval longer than 3 months was associated with reduced survival.[127]

SUMMARY

Managing patients with breast cancer involves assessing and clearly reporting multiple prognostic factors. At a minimum these include determining the clinical stage (axillary lymph-node status and the presence or absence of distant metastases), and careful analysis of the primary tumor characteristics (tumor size, histologic type and grade, and hormone receptor status). While these data are necessary to stratify breast cancer patients into broad prognostic categories, there are significant differences in outcome within each category. Measurement of additional prognostic factors often provides significant information that can be useful in clinical decisions related to treatment.

■■■■■■■■ **APPENDIX 30A**

TNM Classification of Breast Tumors

T — Primary Tumor

TX   Primary tumor cannot be assessed

T0   No evidence of primary tumor

Tis   Carcinoma in situ: intraductal carcinoma, or lobular carcinoma in situ, or Paget disease of the nipple with no tumor

T1   Tumor 2 cm or less in greatest dimension

      T1mic Microinvasion 0.1 cm or less in greatest dimension

      T1a More than 0.1 cm but not more than 0.5 cm in greatest dimension

      T1b More than 0.5 cm but not more than 1 cm in greatest dimension

      T1c More than 1 cm but not more than 2 cm in greatest dimension

T2   Tumor more than 2 cm but not more than 5 cm in greatest dimension

T3   Tumor more than 5 cm in greatest dimension

T4   Tumor of any size with direct extension to chest wall or skin only as described in T4a to T4d

T4a Extension to chest wall

T4b Edema (including peau d'orange), or ulceration of the skin of the breast, or satellite skin nodules confined to the same breast

T4c Both 4a and 4b, above

T4d Inflammatory carcinoma

N — Regional Lymph Nodes

NX Regional lymph nodes cannot be assessed (e.g., previously removed)

N0 No regional lymph node metastasis

N1 Metastasis to movable ipsilateral axillary node(s)

N2 Metastasis to ipsilateral axillary node(s) fixed to one another or to other structures

N3 Metastasis to ipsilateral internal mammary lymph node(s)

M — Distant Metastasis

MX Distant metastasis cannot be assessed

M0 No distant metastasis

M1 Distant metastasis

pN — Regional Lymph Nodes

pN1 Metastasis to movable ipsilateral axillary node(s)

    pN1a Only micrometastasis (none larger than 0.2 cm)

    pN1b Metastasis to lymph node(s), any larger than 0.2 cm

    pN1bi Metastasis to 1–3 lymph nodes, any more than 0.2 cm and all less than 2.0 cm in greatest dimension

    pN1bii Metastasis to 4 or more lymph nodes, any more than 0.2 cm and all less than 2.0 cm in greatest dimension

    pN1biii Extension of tumor beyond the capsule of a lymph node metastasis less than 2.0 cm in greatest dimension

    pN1biv Metastasis to a lymph node 2.0 cm or more in greatest dimension

pN2 Metastasis to ipsilateral axillary lymph nodes that are fixed to one another or to other structures

pN3 Metastasis to ipsilateral internal mammary lymph node(s)

Stage Grouping

Stage 0	Tis	N0	M0
Stage I	T1	N0	M0
Stage IIA	T0	N1	M0
	T1	N1[2]	M0
	T2	N0	M0
Stage IIB	T2	N1	M0
	T3	N0	M0
Stage IIIA	T0	N2	M0
	T1	N2	M0
	T2	N2	M0
	T3	N1, N2	M0
Stage IIIB	T4	Any N	M0
	Any T	N3	M0
Stage IV	Any T	Any N	M1

Source: Sobin LH, Wittekind Ch (eds.): *TNM classification of malignant tumors*, 5th ed. New York, Union Internationale Contre le Cancer Wiley-Liss, 1997.

Prognostic Factors in Breast Cancer Related to Overall Survival

Prognostic Factors	Tumor Related	Host Related	Environment Related

Essential	Extent of disease
	  Nodal status
	  Tumor size
	  Presence of metastases
	Histologic grade
	Histologic type
	Mitotic figure count
	Hormone receptor status
	Effect of tumor recurrence
	  or metastasis after
	  primary therapy
		Age	Effect of local and
			  systemic treatment

Additional	c-erbB-2 (Her2-*neu*)
	Peritumoral vascular
	  invasion
	MIB1 (Ki-67)
	S-phase fraction by flow
	  cytometry
	p53
		Pregnancy
		Race
		Socioeconomic
		  status
		Heredity
		Gender
			Effect of screening

New and
  promising
	Cytokeratin staining of
	  histologically negative
	  axillary lymph nodes
	DNA ploidy analysis
	Tumor angiogenesis
	Epidermal growth-factor
	  receptor (EGFR)
	Transforming growth
	  factor-alpha
	bcl-2
	pS2
			Effect of delay in
			  diagnosis

REFERENCES

1. Fleming ID, Cooper JS, Henson DE, et al. (eds.): *AJCC Manual for Staging of Cancer*, 5th ed. Philadelphia, Lippincott-Raven, 1997.
2. Sobin LH, Wittekind Ch (eds.): *TNM classification of malignant tumors*, 5th ed. New York, Union Internationale Centre le Cancer Wiley-Liss, 1997.
3. Rajakariar R, Walker RA: Pathological and biological features of mammographically detected invasive breast cancer. *Br J Cancer* 71:150–4, 1995.

4. Fisher ER, Anderson S, Redmond C, Fisher B: Pathologic findings from the National Surgical Adjuvant Breast Project Protocol B-06: 10-year pathologic and clinical prognostic discriminants. *Cancer* 71:2507–14, 1993.

5. Carter CL, Allen C, Henson DE: Relation of tumor size, lymph node status, and survival in 24,740 breast cancer cases. *Cancer* 63:181–7, 1989.

6. Veronesi U, Galimberti V, Zurrida S, et al.: Prognostic significance of number and level of axillary nodal metastases in breast cancer. *Breast* 2:224–8, 1993.

7. Jatoi I, Hilsenbeck SG, Clark GM, Osborne CK: Significance of axillary lymph node metastasis in primary breast cancer. *J Clin Oncol* 17:2334–40, 1999.

8. International (Ludwig) Breast Cancer Study Group: Prognostic importance of occult axillary lymph node micrometastases from breast cancers. *Lancet* 335:1565–8, 1990.

9. Sedmak DD, Meineke TA, Knechtges DS, Anderson J: Prognostic significance of cytokeratin-positive breast cancer metastases. *Mod Pathol* 2:516–20, 1989.

10. Trojani M, de Mascarel I, Bonichon F, et al.: Micrometastases to axillary lymph nodes from carcinoma of breast: Detection by immunohistochemistry and prognostic significance. *Br J Cancer* 50:303–6, 1987.

11. de Mascarel I, Bonichon F, Coindre JM, Trojani M: Prognostic significance of breast cancer axillary lymph node micrometastases assessed by two special techniques: Reevaluation with longer follow-up. *Br J Cancer* 66:523–7, 1992.

12. Cote RJ, Peterson HF, Chaiwun B, et al.: International Breast Cancer Study Group: Role of immunohistochemical detection of lymph-node metastases in management of breast cancer. *Lancet* 354:896–900, 1999.

13. Hermanek P, Hutter RVP, Sobin LH, Wittekind C: Classification of isolated tumor cells and micrometastasis. *Cancer* 86:2668–73, 1999.

14. Fisher ER, Sass R, Fisher B, et al.: Pathologic findings from the National Surgical Adjuvant Breast Project for breast cancer (protocol no 4). Discrimination for tenth year treatment failure. *Cancer* 53:712–23, 1984.

15. Leitner SP, Swern AS, Weinberger D, et al.: Predictors of recurrence for patients with small (one centimeter or less) localized breast cancer (T1a,b N0 M0). *Cancer* 76:2266–74, 1995.

16. McKinney CD, Frierson HF, Fechner FE, et al.: Pathologic findings in nonpalpable invasive breast cancer. *Am J Surg Pathol* 16:33–6, 1992.

17. Rosen PP, Groshen S, Kinne DW, Norton L: Factors influencing prognosis in node-negative breast carcinoma: Analysis of 767 T1N0M0/T2N0M0 patients with long-term follow up. *J Clin Oncol* 11:2090–2100, 1993.

18. Seidman JD, Schnaper LA, Aisner SC: Relationship of the size of the invasive component of the primary breast carcinoma to axillary lymph node metastasis. *Cancer* 75:65–71, 1995.

19. Kollias J, Elston CE, Ellis IO, et al.: Early-onset breast cancer — histopathological and prognostic considerations. *Br J Cancer* 75:1318–23, 1997.

20. Henson DE, Ries L, Freedman LS, Carriaga M: Relationship among outcome, stage of disease, and histologic grade for 22,616 cases of breast cancer. *Cancer* 68:2142–9, 1991.

21. Bloom HJG, Richardson WW: Histological grading and prognosis in breast carcinoma: A study of 1049 cases of which 359 have been followed for 15 years. *Br J Cancer* 11:359–77, 1957.

22. Elston CW, Ellis JO: Pathological prognostic factors in breast cancer: Experience from a long study with long-term follow-up. *Histopathology* 19:403–10, 1991.

23. Le Doussal V, Tubiana-Hulin M, Friedman S, et al.: Prognostic value of histologic grade nuclear components of Scarff-Bloom-Richardson (SBR). An improved score modification based on multivariate analysis of 1262 invasive ductal breast carcinomas. *Cancer* 64:1914–21, 1989.

24. Neville AM, Bettelheim R, Gelber RD, et al.: Factors predicting treatment responsiveness and prognosis in node-negative breast cancer. *J Clin Oncol* 10:696–705, 1992.

25. Dixon AR, Ellis IO, Elston CW, et al.: A comparison of the clinical metastatic patterns of invasive lobular and ductal carcinomas of the breast. *Br J Cancer* 63:634–5, 1991.

26. Page DL, Jensen RA, Simpson JF: Routinely available indicators of prognosis in breast cancer. *Br Cancer Res Treat* 51:195–208, 1998.

27. Quinn CM, Wright NA: The clinical assessment of proliferation and growth in human tumors: Evaluation of methods and application as prognostic variables. *J Pathol* 160:93–102, 1990.

28. Van Diest PJ, Baak JPA, Matze-Cok P, et al.: Reproducibility of mitosis counting in 2469 breast cancer specimens. *Hum Pathol* 23:603–7, 1992.

29. Baak JPA: Mitosis counting in tumors. *Hum Pathol* 21:683–5, 1990.

30. Clayton F: Pathologic correlates of survival in 378 lymph node negative infiltrating ductal breast carcinomas. Mitotic count as the single best predictor. *Cancer* 68:1309–17, 1991.

31. Allred DC, Harvey JN, Berardo M, Clark GM: Prognostic and predictive factors in breast cancer by immunohistochemical analysis. *Mod Pathol* 11:155–168, 1998.

32. Harvey JN, Clark GM, Osbore CK, Allred DC: Estrogen receptor status by immunohistochemistry is superior to the ligand binding assay for predicting response to adjuvant endocrine therapy in breast cancer. *J Clin Oncol* 17:1474–81, 1999.

33. Hietanen P, Miettinen M, Makinen J: Survival after first recurrence of breast cancer. *Eur J Cancer Clin Oncol* 22:913–9, 1986.

34. Kurtz JM, Spitalier JM, Amalric R, et al.: The prognostic significance of late local recurrence after breast-conserving therapy. *Int J Radiat Oncol Biol Phys* 18:87–93, 1990.

35. Willner J, Kiricuta IC, Kolbl O: Locoregional recurrence of breast cancer following mastectomy: Always a fatal event? Results of univariate and multivariate analysis. *Int J Radiat Oncol Biol Phys* 37:853–63, 1997.

36. Gusterson BA, Gelber RD, Goldhirsch A, et al.: Prognostic importance of c-erbB-2 expression in breast cancer. *J Clin Oncol* 10:1049–56, 1992.

37. Stal O, Sullivan S, Wingren S, et al.: c-erbB-2 expression and benefit from adjuvant chemotherapy and radiotherapy of breast cancer. *Eur J Cancer* 31:2185–90, 1995.

38. Muss HB, Thor AD, Berry DA, et al.: c-erbB-2 expression and response to adjuvant therapy in women with node-positive early breast cancer. *N Engl J Med* 330:1260–6, 1994.

39. Thor AD, Berry DA, Budman DR, et al.: erbB-2, p53 and efficacy of adjuvant therapy in lymph node-positive breast cancer. *J Natl Cancer Inst* 90:1346–60, 1998.

40. Paik S, Bryant J, Park C, et al.: ErbB-2 and response to doxorubicin in patients with axillary lymph-node positive, hormone receptor-negative breast cancer. *J Natl Cancer Inst* 90:1361–70, 1998.

41. Andrulis IL, Bull SB, Blackstein ME, et al.: neu/cerbB-2 amplification identifies a poor-prognosis group of women with node-negative breast cancer. *J Clin Oncol* 16:1340–49, 1998.

42. Carlomagno C, Perrone F, Gallo C, et al.: c-erbB-2 overexpression decreases the benefit of adjuvant tamoxifen in early-stage breast cancer without axillary lymph node metastases. *J Clin Oncol* 14:2702–8, 1996.

43. Wright C, Nicholson S, Angus B, et al.: Relationship between c-erbB-2 protein product expression and response to endocrine therapy in advanced breast cancer. *Br J Cancer* 65:118–21, 1992.

44. Elledge RM, Green S, Ciocca D, et al.: Her-2 expression and response to tamoxifen in estrogen receptor positive breast cancer. *Clin Cancer Res* 4:7–12, 1998.

45. Clark GM: Should selection of adjuvant chemotherapy for patients with breast cancer be based on erbB-2 status? *J Natl Cancer Inst* 90:1320–1, 1998.

46. Pinder S, Ellis IO, O'Rourke S, et al.: Pathological prognostic factors in breast cancer. Vascular invasion: Relationship with recurrence and survival in a large series with long term follow up. *Histopathology* 24:41–7, 1994.

47. Nime FA, Rosen PP, Thaler HT, et al.: Prognostic significance of tumor emboli in intramamammary lymphatics in patients with mammary carcinoma. *Am J Surg Pathol* 1:25–30, 1977.

48. Davis BW, Gelber R, Goldhirsch A, et al.: Prognostic significance of peritumoral lymphatic invasion in clinical trials of adjuvant therapy for breast cancer with axillary lymph node metastasis. *Hum Pathol* 16:1212–8, 1985.

49. Saigo PE, Rosen PP: The application of immunohistochemical stains to identify endothelial-lined channels in mammary carcinoma. *Cancer* 59:51–4, 1987.

50. Lee AK, DeLellis RA, Wolfe HJ: Intramammary lymphatic invasion in breast carcinomas: Evaluation using ABH isoantigens as endothelial markers. *Am J Surg Pathol* 10:589–94, 1986.

51. Sahin AA, Ro J, Ro JY, et al.: Ki-67 immunostaining in node-negative stage I/II breast carcinoma. Significant correlation with prognosis. *Cancer* 68:549–57, 1991.

52. Gaglia P, Bernardi A, Venesio T, et al.: Cell proliferation of breast cancer evaluated by anti-BrdU and anti-Ki-67 antibodies: Its prognostic value on short-term recurrences. *Eur J Cancer* 29A:1509–13, 1993.

53. Veronese SM, Gambacorta M, Gottardi O, et al.: Proliferation index as a prognostic marker in breast cancer. *Cancer* 71:3926–31, 1993.

54. Railo M, Nordling S, Von Boguslawsky K, et al.: Prognostic value of Ki-67 immunolabeling in primary operable breast cancer. *Br J Cancer* 68:579–83, 1993.

55. Molino A, Micciolo R, Turazza M, et al.: Ki-67 imunostaining in 322 primary breast cancers: Association with clinical and pathological variables and prognosis. *Int J Cancer* 74,433–7, 1997.

56. Keshgegian AA, Cnaan A: Proliferation markers in breast carcinoma. Mitotic figure count, S-phase fraction, proliferating cell nuclear antigen, Ki-67 and MIB-1. *Am J Clin Pathol* 104:42–9, 1995.

57. Pinder SE, Wencyk P, Sibbering DM, et al.: Assessment of the new proliferation marker MIB-1 in breast carcinoma using image analysis; Associations with other prognostic factors and survival. *Br J Cancer* 71:146–9, 1995.

58. Hedley DW, Clark GM, Cornelisse CJ, et al.: Consensus review of the clinical utility of DNA cytometry in carcinoma of the breast. *Cytometry* 14:482–5, 1993.

59. Wenger CR, Clark GM: S-phase fraction and breast cancer: A decade of experience. *Breast Cancer Res Treat* 51:255–65, 1998.

60. Dressler LG, Eudey L, Gray R, et al.: Prognostic potential of DNA flow cytometry measurement in node-negative breast cancer patients: Preliminary analysis of an Intergroup study (INT0076). *J Natl Cancer Inst Monogr* 11:167–72, 1992.

61. Muss HB, Thor AD, Berry DA, et al.: c-erbB-2 expression and response to adjuvant therapy in women with node-positive early breast cancer. *N Engl J Med* 330:1260–6, 1994.

62. Elledge RM, Allred DC: Prognostic and predictive value of p53 and p21 in breast cancer. *Br Cancer Res Treat* 52:169–188, 1998.

63. Cattoretti G, Rilke F, Andreola S: p53 expression in breast cancer. *Int J Cancer* 41:178–183, 1988.

64. Thor AD, Moore DM, Edgerton SM, et al.: Accumulation of p53 tumor suppressor gene protein: An independent marker of prognosis in breast cancers. *J Natl Cancer Inst* 84:845–55, 1992.

65. Tsuda H, Hirohashi S: Association among p53 gene mutation, nuclear accumulation of the p53 protein and aggressive phenotypes in breast cancer. *Int J Cancer* 57:498–503, 1994.

66. Barnes DM, Dublin EA, Fisher CJ, et al.: Immunohistochemical detection of p53 protein in mammary carcinoma: An important new independent indicator of prognosis. *Hum Pathol* 24:469–76, 1993.

67. Thor AD, Berry DA, Budman DR, et al.: ErbB-2, p53 and efficacy of adjuvant therapy in lymph node-positive breast cancer. *J Natl Cancer Inst* 90:1346–60, 1998.

68. Hawkins DS, Demers GW, Galloway DA: Inactivation of p53 enhances sensitivity to multiple chemotherapeutic agents. *Cancer Res* 56:892–8, 1996.

69. Bergh J, Norberg T, Sjogren S, et al.: Complete sequencing of the p53 gene provides prognostic information in breast cancer patients, particularly in relation to adjuvant systemic therapy and radiotherapy. *Nat Med* 1:1029–34, 1995.

70. Allred DC, Clark GM, Elledge R, et al.: Accumulation of mutant p53 is associated with increased proliferation and poor clinical outcome in node negative breast cancer. *J Natl Cancer Inst* 85:200–6, 1993.

71. Silvestrini R, Benini E, Daidone MG, et al.: p53 as an independent prognostic marker in lymph node negative breast cancer patients. *J Natl Cancer Inst* 85:965–70, 1993.

72. Weidner N, Semple JP, Welch WR, Folkman J: Tumor angiogenesis and metastasis-correlation in invasive breast carcinoma. *N Engl J Med* 324:1–8, 1991.

73. Toi M, Kashitani J, Tominaga T: Tumor angiogenesis is an independent prognostic indicator in primary breast carcinoma. *Int J Cancer* 55:371–4, 1993.

74. Ogawa Y, Chung YS, Nakata B, et al.: Microvessel quantitation in invasive breast cancer by staining for factor VIII-related antigen. *Br J Cancer* 72:1297–301, 1995.

75. Heimann T, Ferguson D, Powers C, et al.: Angiogenesis as a predictor of long-term survival for patients with node-negative breast cancer. *J Natl Cancer Inst* 88:1764–6, 1996.

76. Axelsson K, Ljung BM, Moore DH, IInd, Thor AD, et al.: Tumor angiogenesis as a prognostic assay for invasive ductal breast carcinoma. *J Natl Cancer Inst* 87:997–1008, 1995.

77. Goulding H, Rashid NFNA, Roberston JFR, et al.: Assessment of angiogenesis in breast cancer. An important factor in prognosis? *Hum Pathol* 26:1196–200, 1995.

78. Khanuja PS, Fregene T, Gimotty P, et al.: Angiogenesis does not predict recurrence in patients with primary breast cancer. *Proc Am Soc Clin Oncol* 12:67, 1993.

79. Hansen S, Grabau DA, Rose C, et al.: Angiogenesis in breast cancer: a comparative study of the observer variability of methods for determining microvessel density. *Lab Invest* 78:1563–73, 1998.

80. Vermeulen PB, Libura M, Libura J, et al.: Influence of investigator experience and microscopic field size on microvessel density in node-negative breast carcinoma. *Br Cancer Res Treat* 42:165–72, 1997.

81. Fox SB, Smith K, Hollyer J, et al.: The epidermal growth factor receptor as a prognostic marker: Results of 370 patients and review of 3009 patients. *Br Cancer Res Treat* 29:41–9, 1994.

82. Toi M, Tominaga T, Osaki A, Toge T: Role of epidermal growth factor receptor expression in primary breast cancer: Results of a biochemical study and an immunocytochemical study. *Br Cancer Res Treat* 29:51–8, 1994.

83. Nicholson S, Wright C, Sainsbury JRC, et al.: Epidermal growth factor receptor (EGFR) as a marker for poor prognosis in node-negative breast cancer patients: neu an tamoxifen failure. *Steroid Biochem Molec Biol* 37:811–4, 1990.

84. Sainsbury JRC, Farndon JR, Needham GK, et al.: Epidermal growth factor receptor status as a predictor of early recurrence and death from breast cancer. *Lancet* i:1398–402, 1987.

85. Lewis S, Locker A, Todd JH: Expression of epidermal growth factor receptor in breast carcinoma. *J Clin Pathol* 43:385–9, 1990.

86. Mansour EG, Ravdin PM, Dressler L: Prognostic factors in early breast cancer. *Cancer* 74:381–400, 1994.

87. Normanno N, Ciardiello F, Brandt R, Salomon DS: Epidermal growth factor related peptides in the pathogenesis of human breast cancer. *Br Cancer Res Treat* 29:11–27, 1994.

88. Elledge RM, Green S, Howes L, et al.: bcl-2, p53, and response to tamoxifen in estrogen receptor-positive metastatic breast cancer: A Southwest Oncology Group study. *J Clin Oncol* 15:1916–22, 1997.

89. Visscher DW, Sarker F, Tabaczka P, Crissman J: Clinicopathologic analysis of bcl-2 immunostaining in breast carcinoma. *Mod Pathol* 9:642–6, 1996.

90. Hellemans P, van Dam PA, Weyler J, et al.: Prognostic value of bcl-2 expression in invasive breast cancer. *Br J Cancer* 72:354–60, 1995.

91. Schwartz LH, Koerner FC, Edgerton SM, et al.: pS2 expression and response to hormonal therapy in patients with advanced breast cancer. *Cancer Res* 51:624–8, 1991.

92. Predine J, Spyratos F, Prud'homme JR, et al.: Enzyme-linked immunosorbent assay of pS2 in breast cancers, benign tumors, and normal breast tissues: Correlation with prognosis and adjuvant hormonal therapy. *Cancer* 69:2116–23, 1992.

93. Henry JA, Piggott NH, Mallick UK, et al.: pNR-2/pS2 immunohistochemical staining in breast cancer: Correlation with prognostic factors and endocrine response. *Br J Cancer* 63:615–22, 1991.

94. Soubeyran I, Quenel N, Coindre JM, et al.: pS2 protein: A marker improving prediction of response to neoadjuvant tamoxifen in post-menopausal breast cancer patients. *Br J Cancer* 74:1120–5, 1996.

95. Host H, Lund E: Age as a prognostic factor in breast cancer. *Cancer* 57:2217–21, 1986.

96. Adami HO, Malker B, Holmberg L, et al.: The relation of survival and age at diagnosis in breast cancer. *N Engl J Med* 315:559–63, 1986.

97. de la Rochefordiere A, Asselain B, Campana F, et al.: Age as a prognostic factor in premenopausal breast carcinoma. *Lancet* 341:1039–43, 1993.

98. Nixon AJ, Neuberg D, Hayes DF, et al.: Relationship of patient age to pathologic features of the tumor and prognosis for patients with stage I or II breast cancer. *J Clin Oncol* 12:888–94, 1994.

99. Albain KS, Allred DC, Clark GM: Breast cancer outcome and predictors of outcome: Are there age differentials? *J Natl Cancer Inst Monogr* 16:35–42, 1994.

100. Gallenberg MM, Loprinzi CL: Breast cancer and pregnancy. *Semin Oncol* 16:369–76, 1989.

101. DiFronzo LA, O'Connell TX: Breast cancer in pregnancy and lactation. *Surg Clin N Am* 76:267–78, 1996.

102. Petrek JA, Dukoff R, Rogatko A: Prognosis of pregnancy-associated breast cancer. *Cancer* 67:869–72, 1991.

103. Ries LAG, Kosary CL, Hankey BF, et al. (eds.): SEER Cancer Statistics Review: 1973–1994. Bethesda, MD, National Cancer Institute; also, NIH Pub. 97–2789. Bethesda, MD, 1997, Table IV-1.

104. Eley JW, Hill HA, Chen VW, et al.: Racial differences in survival from breast cancer. Results of the National Cancer Institute Black/White cancer survival study. *JAMA* 272:222–7, 1994.

105. El-Tamer MB, Homel P, Wait RB: Is race a poor prognostic factor in breast cancer? *J Am Coll Surg* 189:41–5, 1999.

106. Perkins P, Cooksley CD, Cox JD: Breast cancer: Is ethnicity an independent prognostic factor for survival? *Cancer* 78:1241–7, 1996.

107. Franzini L, Williams AF, Franklin J, et al.: Effects of race and socioeconomic status on survival of 1,332 black, Hispanic, and white women with breast cancer. *Ann Surg Oncol* 4:111–8, 1997.

108. Edwards MJ, Gamel JW, Vaughan WP, Wrightson WR: Infiltrating ductal carcinoma of the breast: The survival impact of race. *J Clin Oncol* 16:2693–9, 1998.

109. Richardson JL, Langholz B, Bernstein L, et al.: Stage and delay in breast cancer diagnosis by race, socioeconomic status, age and year. *Br J Cancer* 65:922–6, 1992.

110. Streuwing JP, Hartge P, Wacholder S, et al.: Cancer risk with 185delAG and 5382insC mutations of *BRCA1* and the 6174delT mutation of *BRCA2* among Ashkenazi Jews. *N Engl J Med* 336:1401–8, 1997.

111. Eisinger F, Stoppa-Lyonnet D, Longy M, et al.: Germline mutation at *BRCA1* affects the histoprognostic grade in hereditary breast cancer. *Cancer Res* 56:471–4, 1996.

112. Blackwood MA, Weber BL: *BRCA1* and *BRCA2*: From molecular genetics to clinical medicine. *J Clin Oncol* 16:1969–77, 1998.

113. Lynch BJ, Holder JA, Buys SS, et al.: Pathobiologic characteristics of hereditary breast cancer. *Hum Pathol* 29:1140–4, 1998.

114. Lee JS, Wacholder S, Struewing JP, et al.: Survival after breast cancer in Ashkenazi Jewish *BRCA1* and *BRCA2* mutation carriers. *J Natl Cancer Inst* 91:259–63, 1999.

115. Crichlow R: Carcinoma of the male breast. *Surg Gynecol Obstet* 134:1011, 1972.

116. Guinee VF, Olsson H, Moller T, et al.: The prognosis of breast cancer in males. A report of 335 cases. *Cancer* 71:154–61, 1993.

117. Early Breast Cancer Trialists' Collaborative Group. Effects of radiotherapy and surgery in early breast cancer. An overview of the randomized trials. *N Engl J Med* 333:1444–55, 1995.

118. Winchester DP, Cox J: Standards for diagnosis and management of invasive breast carcinoma. *CA Cancer J Clin* 48:83–107, 1998.

119. Shukla HS, Melhuish J, Mansel RE, Hughes LE: Does local therapy affect survival rates in breast cancer? *Ann Surg Oncol* 6:455–60, 1999.

120. Overgaard M, Hansen PS, Overgaard J, et al.: Postoperative radiotherapy in high-risk premenopausal women with breast cancer who receive adjuvant chemotherapy. *N Engl J Med* 337:949–55, 1997.

121. Rahman ZU, Frye DK, Smith TL, et al.: Results and long term follow up for 1581 patients with metastatic breast carcinoma treated with standard dose doxorubicin-containing chemotherapy. *Cancer* 85:104–11, 1999.

122. Budman DR, Berry DA, Cirrincione CT, et al.: Dose and dose intensity as determinants of outcome in the adjuvant treatment of breast cancer. The Cancer and Leukemia Group B. *J Natl Cancer Inst* 90:1205–11, 1998.

123. Bonadonna G, Zambetti M, Valagussa P: Sequential or alternating doxorubicin and CMF regimens in breast cancer with more than three positive nodes. Ten-year results. *JAMA* 273:542–7, 1995.

124. Fisher B, Bryant J, Wolmark N, et al.: Effect of preoperative chemotherapy on the outcome of women with operable breast cancer. *J Clin Oncol* 16:2672–85, 1998.

125. Olivotto IA, Mates D, Kan L, et al.: Prognosis, treatment, and recurrence of breast cancer for women attending or not attending the Screening Mammography Program of British Columbia. *Breast Cancer Res Treat* 54:73–81, 1999.

126. Barchielli A, Paci E, Balzi D, et al.: Early diagnosis, place of diagnosis and persistent differences at 10 years in breast cancer survival. Hospitals and breast clinic cases prognosis. *Eur J Cancer Prev* 8:281–7, 1999.

127. Richards MA, Westcombe AM, Love SB, et al.: Influence of delay on survival in patients with breast cancer: A systematic review. *Lancet* 353:1119–26, 1999.

GYNECOLOGIC CANCERS

■■■■■■ **CHAPTER 31**

Vulvar Cancer

J. LOU BENEDET and THOMAS G. EHLEN

Vulvar cancer is an uncommon malignancy accounting for approximately 4–5% of all gynecologic cancers. It used to be thought of as predominantly a disease of the elderly, although reports of young, reproductive-age-group women with this disease increasingly appear in the literature. The external location of the vulva should prompt early presentation, but traditionally significant delays in diagnosis have been associated with this cancer.

The past decade has seen a better understanding of the prognostic factors for vulvar cancer, which, in turn, has led to a more individualized approach to therapy. This has led to less aggressive surgery in the earlier stage of the disease with better cosmetic and functional results. It might be expected that, with the increasing life expectancy in many countries and the concomitant aging of the population, an increase in the number of cases being diagnosed would occur in the future.

TUMOR-RELATED FACTORS

Stage

In 1988, the International Federation of Gynaecology and Obstetrics (FIGO), together with the International Union Against Cancer (UICC), revised the staging classification for vulvar cancer.[1,2] Further refinements to the Stage I category were made in 1994.[3,4] Despite the inherent inaccuracies of a clinical staging system for vulvar cancer, particularly as they relate to the ability to accurately assess for the presence or absence of disease in the regional lymph nodes, virtually all studies to date have consistently shown that the extent of disease as measured by the presence or absence of metastasis in the inguinal lymph nodes, as well as tumor size, to be the two most important major predictors for survival and

Prognostic Factors in Cancer, 2nd edition, Edited by Mary K. Gospodarowicz
ISBN 0-471-40633-3 Copyright © 2001 Wiley-Liss, Inc.

recurrence. The UICC-(AJCC TNM) system is an alternative staging system to the FIGO classification (see Appendix 31A).

Involvement of the regional lymph nodes has been shown to be the single most significant prognostic factor for vulvar carcinoma. Homesley et al.[5,6] reported that independent risk factors for positive inguinal-node involvement were the clinical status of the nodes, capillary lymphatic space involvement, tumor differentiation, as well as age and tumor thickness. Podratz et al.[7] noted that bilateral nodal involvement was associated with a 29%, 5-year survival rate as compared to 51% in patients with unilateral involvement. Similarly Rutledge et al.[8] noted that patients with bilaterally positive inguinal nodes were 20.3 times less likely to survive and 7.4 times more likely to have a recurrence than those with bilaterally negative nodes.

As well as bilaterality, the number of positive nodes is a powerful predictor of outcome. Individuals with involvement of one to two unilateral nodes have a significantly different survival rate than individuals with three or more involved nodes.

Origoni et al.[9] reported that the size and location of the metastatic foci within positive nodes appeared to be a significant prognostic predictor in patients with Stage III and IV disease. Similarly, extracapsular spread has generally been regarded as an indicator of increased risk for recurrence and a recent study by van der Velden et al.[10] concluded that extracapsular growth of lymph-node metastasis in the groin was the most important predictor for poor survival in patients with squamous-cell carcinoma of the vulva.

The size of the primary tumor is a significant predictor for survival, recurrence, and for nodal metastasis.[6-8,11-13] Podratz et al.[7] and Andreasson et al.[11] both used multivariate analysis and found that tumor size greater or less than 3–4 cm was an excellent predictor for survival. Fioretti et al.[12] also found the 3 cm size to be statistically significant. Homesley et al.[5] found that lesions up to 8 cm in diameter were at low risk as long as the groin nodes themselves were negative for metastasis. Tumor size correlates with survival, and as such can be used as a prognostic factor. However, tumor size was not found to be an independent predictor of inguinal-node status in the Gynecologic Oncology Group (GOG) studies, as 19% of patients with lesions of 2 cm or more had positive nodes. Smyczek-Gargya et al.[14] in a recent study also confirmed the importance of tumor diameter in a multivariate analysis of prognostic factors in a series of patients with vulvar carcinoma. The importance of tumor size was also emphasized in recently reported studies by Mariani et al.,[15] Rhodes et al.,[16] and Ndubisi et al.[17]

Depth of Invasion

Depth of invasion has been studied extensively as a predictor for lymph-node metastasis and also for survival and recurrence.[6,18-22] Frankman et al.[18] found that the 5-year disease-free survival rate was 98% for those lesions with invasion of 5 mm or less and only 58% for those in which the depth of invasion exceeded this value. Sedlis et al.[21] studied a series of patients with superficial vulvar carcinoma with a measured tumor thickness of 5 mm or less and found a definite correlation between tumor thickness and nodal disease. They noted that the proportion of patients with positive nodes increased steadily with each mm of thickness from 3.1% in tumors ≤ 1 mm to 8.9% in tumors 2 mm thickness, and that in cancers 5 mm thick 33.3% of patients had positive nodes. Hopkins et al.[23] found no deaths in 29 Stage I patients with disease invasive to a depth of 2 mm or less, although one patient with 1 mm of invasion developed a recurrence 2 years later. Berman et al.[22] noted that 11% of patients with depth of invasion of 1 mm or less developed recurrence, as compared to 17% of those with invasion of more than 1 mm. Data from these studies were the major factor underlying the subdivision of the Stage I category of vulvar cancers in 1994.

Histologic Type

Squamous-cell carcinoma accounts for approximately 85% of all vulvar cancers and is by far the most common histologic type. Most of our knowledge concerning prognostic factors in vulvar cancer has been obtained from studying squamous-cell carcinomas, but it would appear that the main prognostic factors identified with squamous-cell carcinomas, namely the presence or absence of lymph-node involvement and tumor size, are also important in other less common forms of vulvar malignancy.

Verrucous carcinoma is a rare malignancy of the genital tract, with metastasis being uncommon, and basal cell carcinoma is another relatively rare vulvar tumor with a tendency to local recurrence and infrequent nodal metastasis. Adenocarcinomas are also extremely uncommon, but may arise in Bartholin's gland, vestibular glands, and rarely sweat gland structures. These lesions appear to have similar prognostic factors to the squamous cell variants.

The importance of histologic grade as a prognostic factor remains unclear. Earlier studies by Rutledge et al.[8] and Podratz et al.[7] reported that histologic grade did not significantly influence survival and recurrence. Hopkins et al.[23] also found that patients with poorly differentiated tumors had significantly worse survival than those with well-differentiated or moderately differentiated tumors, but only in Stage I and II disease. However, grade did not appear to be a factor for patients with Stage III or IV disease. Homesley et al.[5] found that the GOG grading system was important in that the histologic differentiation was not significant for survival when adjusted for the extent of groin-node metastasis and lesion diameter. He did show, however, that tumor differentiation was a highly significant predictor for groin-node metastasis based on the amount of tumor that was undifferentiated in the primary lesion.

Husseinzadeh et al.[24] found cytologic grading to be more significant than histologic grading with regard to nodal metastasis. In more recent studies, Smyczek-Gargya et al.[14] and Pinto[25] both found that grade was an important prognostic factor in multivariate analysis of vulvar cancer. Rhodes et al.[16] also noted the importance of differentiation as an independent prognostic factor in a multivariate analysis of 411 patients with squamous cell carcinoma of the vulva.

Other Important Histologic Features

Several authors[5-7,21,26] have reported that capillary-like space involvement is an adverse prognostic factor and that it is a significant predictor for survival and recurrence. Onnis et al.[26] reported that lymphatic vascular space invasion correlates with lymph-node involvement, and similar findings were also reported in studies by Sedlis et al.[21] and Binder et al.[27] In a series of 272 patients with superficially invasive tumors, Sedlis et al.[21] noted that 21 patients (7.7%) had capillary-like space involvement and positive groin nodes occurred five times as frequently as in patients with negative capillary-like space findings. Although multivariate analysis[21,27] has shown capillary-space involvement to be a significant prognostic factor for superficially invasive tumors, this is only of limited practical use because it appears to be present in only a small proportion of these patients. Homesley et al.,[6] reporting on a larger series of 588 patients, found that 15% had positive capillary-like space involvement and that the frequency of positive groin nodes among patients with this finding was three-times greater than for those without.

Hacker et al.,[20] in a review of Stage I vulvar cancers, noted that the pattern of invasion largely reflected prognosis. They noted that of those with nonconfluent patterns, 28.6% with spray patterns of infiltration had nodal metastasis. Similarly, Magrina et al.[19] also found that, with Stage I tumors, microscopic confluence correlated with patient survival. Kürzl and Messerer[28] found that predictive survival was affected by a dissociated tumor growth pattern. Recent studies by Pinto et al.[25] and Drew et al.[29] also noted the importance of growth patterns as related to prognosis. Ansink et al.[30] in using markers of cell differentiation, such as CK-8, 10, 13 and 14, were able to show that these marker levels were directly related to the growth patterns of the tumor and that these patterns were statistically significant in terms of recurrence and outcome.

Biological and Molecular Markers

Van der Sijde et al.[31] studied a series of 94 women with squamous-cell carcinoma to see the significance of serum squamous-cell carcinoma antigen and found that the levels varied from 10% in patients with Stage I disease to 40% in those with Stage IV disease. No correlation, however, was noted between elevated pretreatment values and the presence of lymph-node metastasis. Forty-two percent of patients with recurrent or progressive disease had elevated levels, but 25% of patients without demonstrable tumor activity were also noted to have elevated serum SCCAg levels. Rose et al.[32] reported that 29% of patients with advanced vulvar cancer had an elevated SCCAg level, supporting the data of van der Sijde, which suggested that the levels appeared to be mainly elevated in individuals with Stage III and IV disease. Also in this study,[32] there appeared to be no association with nodal metastasis.

Several authors[33-35] have studied the prognostic value of CD44 expression in SCC of the vulva. CD44 is a cell adhesion molecule that binds extracellular matrix, and certain isoforms have been implicated in tumor metastasis. These studies[33-35] have essentially shown that the isoforms CD44v4, v5, v6, v7, and v8 do not correlate with survival, but that CD44v3 and v6 appear correlated with poor relapse-free and overall survival of Stage I vulvar cancer patients.

Dolan et al.[36] reported that DNA ploidy in S-phase fraction analyses did not appear to be useful prognostic factors for SCC. Similar results were noted by Siracky et al.[37] who found that 80% had diploid content, and yet many of these had regional-node metastasis. Mariani et al.[15] in a recent study found that ploidy appeared to show a statistically significant relationship with tumor grading, and defined a subset of patients who had pathologic features of high risk. However, when multivariate analysis was used, ploidy status did not have any prognostic role.

Emanuels et al.[38] found that overexpression of p53 is a late event but that neither p53 nor mdm2 expression was a useful marker to predict lymph-node metastasis in vulvar cancer. Several recent studies[38-42] have explored the value of p53 expression and its potential role as a prognostic factor. Kagie et al.[39,40] found that p53 overexpression was common and appeared to play a role in the pathogenesis of vulvar cancer, but did not influence disease-free survival. Similarly McConnell et al.[41] felt that p53 expression was not of prognostic significance, but Scheistroen and the group from the Norwegian Radium Hospital[42] also concluded that p53 overexpression appeared to be involved in the pathogenesis of vulvar cancer and that this was significantly associated with disease-related survival, but that its prognostic impact was observed only in patients with advanced disease.

HOST-RELATED FACTORS

In the literature the prognostic significance of age has been contradictory. Several authors have found that age was a significant predictor for survival and recurrence.[11,18,28,43] Frankman et al.[18] found a 5-year disease-free survival rate of 87% in patients up to 79 years of age and 48% in patients older than 80 years. However, Rutledge et al.,[8] using a univariate Cox proportional hazards model, found that age is a nonsignificant predictor for survival and recurrence. Hopkins[23] also reported that age was not prognostic for survival, either with early- or late-stage diseases. Podratz[7] found that increasing age was directly related to increasing stage and recurrence. Homesley et al.,[5] in a GOG study, found that the odds ratio of increased risk for nodal involvement was related to age, with the risk increasing five-fold between the ages 55 and 65. He also noted that a 75-year-old woman was 13 times more likely to have positive groin nodes than a 55-year-old woman, and that although age was predictive for nodal disease, it had no independent impact on relative survival. In more recent studies, both Pinto et al.[25] and Rhodes et al.[16] found that increasing age was a poor prognostic factor on the basis of multivariate analysis of their clinical material.

One of the problems in assessing the impact of age as a prognostic variable has been that the more elderly patients are often treated less aggressively because of poor general medical conditions, and thus treatment and subsequent pathological assessment is often incomplete.

The importance of immune status has been underlined by recent reports.[44,45] Wright et al.[44] described two patients with HIV who subsequently developed squamous carcinoma of the vulva. In spite of what appeared to be early stage, early disease, these individuals had a rather fulminant course with their illness, and it was felt that the associated HPV with immunosuppression was an important prognostic factor for these women. Similarly, Volgger et al.[45] reported a renal transplantation patient with a microinvasive vulvar cancer who developed aggressive disease and who died 20 months later. The only known factors with respect to prognosis that are host related are patient age and immune state.

ENVIRONMENT-RELATED FACTORS

The importance of the choice of therapy in determining prognosis is best illustrated by data from the 1950s and 1960s, which clearly indicated that radical surgery with inguinal–femoral lymphadenectomy provided the best cure rates and the lowest incidence of recurrence in contrast to patients treated in a less aggressive fashion. Several studies showed that in patients with negative groin nodes, a 5-year disease-free survival rate of approximately 85–90% could be expected. Conversely, in individuals with inguinal-node metastasis the overall 5-year survival rate has been reported as approximately 55%. Currently, postoperative radiotherapy is recommended for patients with positive inguinal lymph nodes where not only the groins but also the pelvic lymph nodes would be irradiated. Pelvic lymphadenectomy is rarely performed today for vulvar cancer.

With a better understanding of the various prognostic factors, a more individualized approach to the management of early vulvar cancer is now possible. This is particularly true for patients with early-stage disease, if after careful histological assessment, the tumor has been shown to be not only small but also superficially invasive. In addition a lateral location of the lesion in these situations has led to conservative tissue-spearing surgery at the primary site, often with clitoral preservation, less disfigurement, and better function.

Several authors[8,20,22,46] have shown that this approach has not compromised survival in carefully selected patients. Iversen et al.[47] showed that the omission of contralateral groin dissection was possible in the presence of a lateral lesion that did not involve midline structures, providing that the ipsilateral nodes themselves were negative for metastasis.

Radiation therapy also plays an important role in the treatment and management of vulvar carcinoma. Most centers[48-52] have used radiation therapy either as an adjunct to primary surgical management in patients with positive resection margins or metastatic disease to the groin lymph nodes. Increasingly combined chemotherapy and radiation has been used, particularly in patients with large lesions where the lesions may involve central structures such as the rectum and/or bladder, in an attempt to permit less radical surgery in those patients. In a GOG study, Sedlis et al.[21] studied patients with positive inguinal lymph nodes, randomized to pelvic-node resection or radiotherapy. Those treated with radiotherapy had an estimated 2-year survival rate of 68%, compared to 54% for those who underwent pelvic lymphadenectomy. Malmström et al.[43] in a series of patients, treated with vulvectomy followed by radiotherapy to the vulvar area and groins, noted survival rates similar to those reported for more aggressive surgery.

The accompanying Appendix 31B relates tumor-, host- and treatment-related prognostic factors in terms that are generally accepted and that show new and promising features.

SUMMARY

A clearer understanding of the important prognostic factors in vulvar cancer has occurred in the past decade, with the presence of disease in regional lymph nodes being the single most important predictor for survival and recurrence (see Appendix 31B). This understanding has led to more individualized and less radical treatment for individuals found to have small, early-stage, superficially invasive tumors. In turn, this less radical treatment has resulted in less morbidity and better cosmetic and functional results for these women without compromising their chances for cure. Further understanding of prognostic factors in the future should allow us to further individualize treatment.

■■■■■■ **APPENDIX 31A**

TNM Classification: Vulva Tumors

T — Primary Tumor

TX   Primary tumor cannot be assessed

T0   No evidence of primary tumor

Tis   Carcinoma in situ (preinvasive carcinoma)

T1   Tumor confined to vulva or vulva and perineum, 2 cm or less in greatest dimension

    T1a Tumor confined to vulva or vulva and perineum, 2 cm or less in greatest dimension and with stromal invasion no greater than 1.0 mm

    T1b Tumor confined to vulva or vulva and perineum, 2 cm or less in greatest dimension and with stromal invasion greater than 1.0 mm

T2   Tumor confined to vulva or vulva and perineum, more than 2 cm in greatest dimension

T3   Tumor invades any of the following: lower urethra, vagina, anus

T4   Tumor invades any of the following: bladder mucosa, rectal mucosa, upper urethral mucosa; or is fixed to pubic bone

N — Regional Lymph Nodes

NX Regional lymph nodes cannot be assessed

N0 No regional lymph-node metastasis

N1 Unilateral regional lymph-node metastasis

N2 Bilateral regional lymph-node metastasis

M — Distant Metastasis

MX Distant metastasis cannot be assessed

M0 No distant metastasis

M1 Distant metastasis (including pelvic lymph node metastasis)

Stage Grouping

Stage 0	Tis	N0	M0
Stage I	T1	N0	M0
Stage IA	T1a	N0	M0
Stage IB	T1b	N0	M0
Stage II	T2	N0	M0
Stage III	T1	N1	M0
	T2	N1	M0
	T3	N0, N1	M0
Stage IVA	T1	N2	M0
	T2	N2	M0
	T3	N2	M0
	T4	Any N	M0
Stage IVB	Any T	Any N	M1

Source: Sobin LH, Wittekind Ch (eds.): *TNM classification of malignant tumors*, 5th ed. New York, Union Internationale Contre le Cancer Wiley-Liss, 1997.

■■■■■■■ **APPENDIX 31B**

Prognostic Factors in Vulvar Cancer

Prognostic Factors	Tumor Related	Host Related	Environmental Related
Essential	T, N, M categories	Age	
Additional	Lymphatic–vascular space involvement Tumor grade Number of involved lymph nodes Extranodal disease Tumor thickness or depth of invasion Extracapsular extension Pattern of invasion	Immune status HIV infection	Surgical margins
New and Promising	CD44, certain isoforms		

REFERENCES

1. FIGO. Changes in gynecologic cancer staging by the International Federation of Gynecology and Obstetrics. *Am J Obstet Gynecol* 162:610–1, 1990.

2. Hermanek P, Sobin LH, (eds.): *UICC International Union Against Cancer: TNM classification of malignant tumors*. 4th ed. New York; Springer-Verlag, 1992.

3. Shepherd J, Sideri M, Benedet J, et al.: Carcinoma of the vulva. *J Epidemiol Biostat* 3(1):111–27, 1998.

4. Vulva, in Sobin LH, Wittekind C, (eds.): *TNM classification of malignant tumours*, 5th ed. New York; Wiley-Liss, 1997, pp. 134–7.

5. Homesley HD, Bundy BN, Sedlis A, et al.: Assessment of current International Federation of Gynecology and Obstetrics staging of vulvar carcinoma relative to prognostic factors for survival (a Gynecologic Oncology Group study). *Am J Obstet Gynecol* 164(4):997–1003, 1991.

6. Homesley HD, Bundy BN, Sedlis A, et al.: Prognostic factors for groin node metastasis in squamous cell carcinoma of the vulva (a Gynecologic Oncology Group study) [see Comments]. *Gynecol Oncol* 49(3):279–83, 1993.

7. Podratz KC, Symmonds RE, Taylor WF, Williams TJ: Carcinoma of the vulva: Analysis of treatment and survival. *Obstet Gynecol* 61(1):63–74, 1983.

8. Rutledge FN, Mitchell MF, Munsell MF, et al.: Prognostic indicators for invasive carcinoma of the vulva. *Gynecol Oncol* 42(3):239–44, 1991.

9. Origoni M, Sideri M, Garsia S, et al.: Prognostic value of pathological patterns of lymph node positivity in squamous cell carcinoma of the vulva stage III and IVA FIGO. *Gynecol Oncol* 45(3):313–6, 1992.

10. Van der Velden J, van Lindert AC, Lammes FB, et al.: Extracapsular growth of lymph node metastases in squamous cell carcinoma of the vulva. The impact on recurrence and survival. *Cancer* 75(12):2885–90, 1995.

11. Andreasson B, Nyboe J: Value of prognostic parameters in squamous cell carcinoma of the vulva. *Gynecol Oncol* 22(3):341–51, 1985.

12. Fioretti P, Gadducci A, Prato B, et al.: The influence of some prognostic factors on the clinical outcome of patients with squamous cell carcinoma of the vulva. *Eur J Gynaecol Oncol* 13(1):97–104, 1992.

13. Grimshaw RN, Murdoch JB, Monaghan JM: Radical vulvectomy and bilateral inguinal-femoral lymphadenopathy through separate incisions: Experience with 100 cases. *Int J Gynecol Cancer* 3:18–23, 1993.

14. Smyczek-Gargya B, Volz B, Geppert M, Dietl J: A multivariate analysis of clinical and morphological prognostic factors in squamous cell carcinoma of the vulva. *Gynecol Obstet Invest* 43(4):261–7, 1997.

15. Mariani L, Conti L, Atlante G, et al.: Vulvar squamous carcinoma: Prognostic role of DNA content. *Gynecol Oncol* 71(2):159–64, 1998.

16. Rhodes CA, Cummins C, Shafi MI: The management of squamous cell vulval cancer: A population based retrospective study of 411 cases [see Comments]. *Br J Obstet Gynaecol* 105(2):200–5, 1998.

17. Ndubisi B, Kaminski PF, Olt G, et al.: Staging and recurrence of disease in squamous cell carcinoma of the vulva. *Gynecol Oncol* 59(1):34–7, 1995.

18. Frankman O, Kabulski Z, Nilsson B, Silfversward C: Prognostic factors in invasive squamous cell carcinoma of the vulva. *Int J Gynaecol Obstet* 36(3):219–28, 1991.

19. Magrina JF, Webb MJ, Gaffey TA, Symmonds RE: Stage I squamous cell cancer of the vulva. *Am J Obstet Gynecol* 134(4):453–9, 1979.

20. Hacker NF, Berek JS, Lagasse LD, et al.: Individualization of treatment for stage I squamous cell vulvar carcinoma. *Obstet Gynecol* 63(2):155–62, 1984.

21. Sedlis A, Homesley H, Bundy BN, et al.: Positive groin lymph nodes in superficial squamous cell vulvar cancer. A Gynecologic Oncology Group Study. *Am J Obstet Gynecol* 156(5):1159–64, 1987.

22. Berman ML, Soper JT, Creasman WT, et al.: Conservative surgical management of superficially invasive stage I vulvar carcinoma. *Gynecol Oncol* 35(3):352–7, 1989.

23. Hopkins MP, Reid GC, Vettrano I, Morley GW: Squamous cell carcinoma of the vulva: Prognostic factors influencing survival. *Gynecol Oncol* 43(2):113–7, 1991.

24. Husseinzadeh N, Wesseler T, et al.: Prognostic factors and the significance of cytologic grading in invasive squamous cell carcinoma of the vulva: A clinicopathologic study. *Gynecol Oncol* 36(2):192–9, 1990.

25. Pinto AP, Signorello LB, Crum CP, et al.: Squamous cell carcinoma of the vulva in Brazil: Prognostic importance of host and viral variables. *Gynecol Oncol* 74(1):61–7, 1999.

26. Onnis A, Marchetti M, Maggino T: Carcinoma of the vulva: Critical analysis of survival and treatment of recurrences. *Eur J Gynaecol Oncol* 13(6):480–5, 1992.

27. Binder SW, Huang I, Fu YS, et al.: Risk factors for the development of lymph node metastasis in vulvar squamous cell carcinoma. *Gynecol Oncol* 37(1):9–16, 1990.

28. Kurzl R, Messerer D: Prognostic factors in squamous cell carcinoma of the vulva: A multivariate analysis. *Gynecol Oncol* 32(2):143–50, 1989.

29. Drew PA, al-Abbadi MA, Orlando CA, et al.: Prognostic factors in carcinoma of the vulva: A clinicopathologic and DNA flow cytometric study. *Int J Gynecol Pathol* 15(3):235–41, 1996.

30. Ansink A, Mooi WJ, van Doornewaard G, et al.: Cytokeratin subtypes and involucrin in squamous cell carcinoma of the vulva. An immunohistochemical study of 41 cases. *Cancer* 76(4):638–43, 1995.

31. Van der Sijde R, de Bruijn HW, Krans M, et al.: Significance of serum SCC antigen as a tumor marker in patients with squamous cell carcinoma of the vulva. *Gynecol Oncol* 35(2):227–32, 1989.

32. Rose PG, Nelson BE, Fournier L, Hunter RE: Serum squamous cell carcinoma antigen levels in invasive squamous vulvar cancer. *J Surg Oncol* 50(3):183–6, 1992.

33. Tempfer C, Sliutz G, Haeusler G, et al.: CV44v3 and v6 variant isoform expression correlates with poor prognosis in early-stage vulvar cancer. *Br J Cancer* 78(8):1091–4, 1998.

34. Tempfer C, Gitsch G, Haeusler G, et al.: Prognostic value of immunohistochemically detected CD44 expression in patients with carcinoma of the vulva. *Cancer* 78(2):273–7, 1996.

35. Tempfer C, Gitsch G, Hanzal E, et al.: Expression of the adhesion molecule CD44v3 is a prognostic factor in vulvar carcinoma. *Anticancer Res* 16(4A):2029–31, 1996.

36. Dolan JR, McCall AR, Gooneratne S, et al.: DNA ploidy, proliferation index, grade, and stage as prognostic factors for vulvar squamous cell carcinomas. *Gynecol Oncol* 48(2):232–5, 1993.

37. Siracky J, Kysela B, Siracka E: Flow cytometric analysis of primary cervical and vulvar carcinomas and their metastases. *Neoplasma* 36(4):437–45, 1989.

38. Emanuels AG, Koudstaal J, Burger MP, Hollema H: In squamous cell carcinoma of the vulva, overexpression of p53 is a late event and neither p53 nor mdm2 expression is a useful marker to predict lymph node metastases. *Br J Cancer* 80(1–2):38–43, 1999.

39. Kagie MJ, Kenter GG, Tollenaar RA, et al.: p53 protein overexpression is common and independent of human papillomavirus infection in squamous cell carcinoma of the vulva. *Cancer* 80(7):1228–33, 1997.

40. Kagie MJ, Kenter GG, Tollenaar RA, et al.: p53 protein overexpression, a frequent observation in squamous cell carcinoma of the vulva and in various synchronous vulvar epithelia, has no value as a prognostic parameter. *Int J Gynecol Pathol* 16(2):124–30, 1997.

41. McConnell DT, Miller ID, Parkin DE, Murray GI: p53 protein expression in a population-based series of primary vulval squamous cell carcinoma and immediate adjacent field change. *Gynecol Oncol* 67(3):248–54, 1997.

42. Scheistroen M, Trope C, Pettersen EO, Nesland JM: p53 protein expression in squamous cell carcinoma of the vulva. *Cancer* 85(5):1133–8, 1999.

43. Malmstrom H, Janson H, Simonsen E, et al.: Prognostic factors in invasive squamous cell carcinoma of the vulva treated with surgery and irradiation. *Acta Oncol* 29(7):915–9, 1990.

44. Wright TC, Koulos JP, Liu P, Sun XW: Invasive vulvar carcinoma in two women infected with human immunodeficiency virus. *Gynecol Oncol* 60(3):500–3, 1996.

45. Volgger B, Marth C, Zeimet A, et al.: Fulminant course of a microinvasive vulvar carcinoma in an immunosuppressed woman. *Gynecol Oncol* 65(1):177–9, 1997.

46. Hoffman MS, Roberts WS, Lapolla JP, Cavanagh D: Recent modifications in the treatment of invasive squamous cell carcinoma of the vulva. *Obstet Gynecol Surv* 44(4):227–33, 1989.

47. Iversen T, Abeler V, Aalders J: Individualized treatment of stage I carcinoma of the vulva. *Obstet Gynecol* 57(1):85–9, 1981.

48. Fairey RN, MacKay PA, Benedet JL, et al.: Radiation treatment of carcinoma of the vulva, 1950–1980. *Am J Obstet Gynecol* 151(5):591–7, 1985.

49. Hacker NF, Berek JS, Juillard GJ, Lagasse LD: Preoperative radiation therapy for locally advanced vulvar cancer. *Cancer* 54(10):2056–61, 1984.

50. Boronow RC, Hickman BT, Reagan MT, et al.: Combined therapy as an alternative to exenteration for locally advanced vulvovaginal cancer. II. Results, complications, and dosimetric and surgical considerations. *Am J Clin Oncol* 10(2):171–81, 1987.

51. Homesley HD, Bundy BN, Sedlis A, Adcock L: Radiation therapy versus pelvic node resection for carcinoma of the vulva with positive groin nodes. *Obstet Gynecol* 68(6):733–40, 1986.

52. Thomas G, Dembo A, DePetrillo A, et al.: Concurrent radiation and chemotherapy in vulvar carcinoma. *Gynecol Oncol* 34(3):263–7, 1989.

CHAPTER 32

Uterine Cervix Cancer

GRAHAM PITSON and ANTHONY FYLES

Carcinoma of the cervix accounts for approximately 20% of all gynecologic cancers and 2% of all malignancies in women. Numerous prognostic factors have been studied in patients with cervical carcinoma, using both univariate and multivariate analysis. Differences in endpoints of analysis, whether survival (disease-free or overall), relapse-free rate, or local control rate, make comparison of such studies difficult. The failure to perform a multivariate analysis, or the use of different covariates in multivariate analyses, can further complicate comparisons between studies. Not all factors are relevant to all patients; for example, depth of tumor invasion and presence of vascular-space invasion can only be reliably determined in patients treated with surgery, whereas hemoglobin level is important in patients treated with radiation. This review concentrates largely on those factors identified using multivariate techniques, such as log rank or Cox regression analysis, in order to account for interactions between various factors. Where available, estimates such as hazard ratios will be included in order to indicate the strengths of the individual variables.

TUMOR-RELATED FACTORS

Tumor stage has long been recognized as the most important determinant of outcome in patients with cervix cancer.[1-7] Although TNM categories now correspond to International Federation of Gynaecology and Obstetrics (FIGO) stages,[8] the majority of the reports in the literature have used the FIGO system (Appendix 32A). The relative risk (RR) of relapse or survival by FIGO stage for representative studies are shown in Table 32.1. Furthermore, several studies have shown a prognostic division by substages. The division of stage IB into IB1 and IB2 based on tumor size stratifies prognosis with respect to survival and pelvic control.[9-11] Within stages II and III, differentiating between unilateral or bilateral

Prognostic Factors in Cancer, 2nd edition, Edited by Mary K. Gospodarowicz
ISBN 0-471-40633-3   Copyright © 2001 Wiley-Liss, Inc.

TABLE 32.1   Effect of FIGO Stage on Relapse and Survival

Stage	5-Year Outcome Johnson[3][a]	(RR) Fyles[1][b]
Stage I	88% (1.00)	78% (1.00)
Stage II	61% (2.66)	61% (1.94)[c]
Stage III	33% (7.08)	41% (3.04)
Stage IV	11% (18.8)	19% (6.59)

[a]Freedom from relapse. [b]Disease-free survival.
[c]Stage IIb only.

TABLE 32.2   Effect of Tumor Size on Relapse in Stage IB [Delgado[9]]

Tumor Size (cm)	Relative Risk
Preclinical	1.00 (95% disease-free at 3 years)
1	1.6
2	1.9
3	2.4
4	2.9
6	4.4
8	6.6

parametrial involvement and unilateral or bilateral sidewall infiltration[1,5,12] also offers prognostic value. Patients with bilateral parametrial infiltration in stage II and bilateral sidewall involvement in stage III have poorer rates of survival and pelvic control compared with unilateral parametrial or sidewall disease.

Tumor size exerts an independent effect on prognosis both in early-stage disease alone[13–15] and in patients with all stages of disease.[10] Most studies have used clinical estimates of tumor size; however, magnetic resonance imaging (MRI) estimates of size have also been shown to correlate with outcome.[16] Relative risk of recurrence as a function of tumor size in Stage I is shown in Table 32.2. The inferior survival reported in patients with barrel-shaped tumors is also probably due to larger tumor volume.[17]

Increasing depth of cervical invasion adversely affects survival. In surgically treated patients both the absolute and proportional depth correlate with outcome.[9,18] Compared to a RR of relapse of 1 for tumors with 3-mm depth of invasion, tumors invading to 10 and 20 mm had a RR of relapse of 3 and 4, respectively. Another study of 827 cases estimated a RR of relapse for outer-third involvement of 2.03 relative to a RR of 1 for inner- and middle-third involvement combined.[14]

Although not included in the FIGO staging scheme, lymph-node metastases have been associated with an increased risk of relapse and poorer survival.

Surgical series have shown pelvic and para-aortic lymph-node metastases to be independent predictors of adverse outcomes.[6,13,15,19] The number of surgically detected pelvic lymph-node metastases was found to be significant in one study[20] and marginally correlated with survival in another,[21] but this finding was not confirmed in other studies.[9,22] Radiotherapy series using imaging to assess nodal disease have shown para-aortic nodal disease to correlate with outcome.[3,10] The import of isolated pelvic-node metastases in patients undergoing radiotherapy is less clear, however, as some series have not found this to be an independent predictor of outcome.[1,10]

Squamous-cell carcinoma and adenocarcinoma are the most commonly occurring histological types of cervical cancers, and account for approximately 80 and 15% of all cases, respectively. Controversy exists as to the prognostic significance of histologic type. Some studies have shown an independent and adverse effect of adenocarcinoma histology in patients treated by surgery or radiation,[1,2,7,11,18,23] and adenosquamous subtypes also have been reported to be independently associated with poor survival.[24] However, a population-based study did not demonstrate an adverse effect for adenocarcinoma or adenosquamous carcinomas[4] nor have several other analyses.[12,14,21] Whether these discrepancies are due to differences in the populations studied, failure to adequately consider all covariates, such as tumor size and referral bias, or an effect of treatment, is unclear. A series of 302 patients specifically examining adenocarcinoma of the cervix found clinical stage, tumor size, grade, lymph-node status and cell subtype to be of independent significance.[25] Small-cell tumors, particularly of the neuroendocrine type, and clear-cell tumors are known for their aggressive behavior although their rarity limits further analysis using multivariate techniques.[1,26]

Histological grade has been shown in some studies to be independently associated with an adverse prognosis;[1,14] however, other studies have not reported such a relationship.[9,10,21] Capillary-lymphatic space invasion has been shown to adversely affect prognosis in surgical patients[21,27] with a RR of 1.7 for disease-free interval in surgical IB patients.[9] Vascular-space invasion when examined separately using immunohistochemical methods has also been reported as an independent prognostic factor.[28]

Biological and Molecular Factors

Recent studies using PCR have consistently found human papilloma virus (HPV) in more than 90% of cases of cervical carcinoma.[29-31] The occurrence of cervical carcinoma without HPV is probably a rare event. Most studies have reported that HPV 16 is more commonly associated with squamous-cell carcinoma, whereas HPV 18 is the most commonly identified serotype in adenocarcinoma. The prognostic importance of HPV serotype is controversial. Examining more recent studies where the rates of HPV detection are higher, HPV 18 has been reported to independently predict poor prognosis.[32] Another series found HPV 18 to be a negative prognostic factor only for patients undergoing surgery.[30] Others, however, have not found HPV serotype to independently predict prognosis.[31]

Levels of squamous-cell carcinoma antigen (SCCAg) have been reported to independently predict a worse outcome in squamous cervical carcinomas.[33,34] However, other series have not found SCCAg to retain independent significance in multivariate analysis when tumor size is taken into account.

Recent studies have examined the role of tumor vascular density on prognosis. Several studies using mean vessel density in "hot spot" areas of maximal tumor vascularity have shown high tumor vascular density to independently predict for a poorer prognosis.[13,27,35-37] However, not all studies have shown this relationship,[38] and the results of vascular density studies may be particularly dependent on the technique used and operator expertise.

Tumor hypoxia measured using polarographic electrodes has been reported to be a negative prognostic factor in both surgical and radiotherapy patients.[38-40] Hypoxia retained significance independent of tumor stage on multivariate analysis performed by Hockel et al.,[40] and confirmatory studies are underway.

Studies examining the role of many molecular markers and oncogenes, such as those discussed below, are often limited by small numbers of patients and either failure to perform a multivariate analysis or failure to include all the major clinical prognostic factors in the multivariate model. Therefore, association reported for many biological markers may be best viewed as preliminary data warranting confirmation in further studies. A study examining the prognostic significance of p53 protein overexpression failed to report any association.[41] Bcl-2 has been reported as correlating with overall survival,[42,43] although this was not confirmed in another small series.[44] Although small studies provided varying results as to the prognostic significance for erb-B2,[41,45] a recent confirmatory multivariate analysis has reported erb-B2 staining to independently adversely affect survival.[46] Promising factors not shown on subsequent multivariate analysis to offer independent prognostic significance include tumor labeling index,[47,48] potential doubling time,[48] epidermal growth factor (EGF) receptor,[49] and S-phase fraction.[48] DNA ploidy was reported to be a significant factor in one series,[14] although a contrary result was found in another series.[50] A low apoptotic index in hypoxic tumors was reported to be a significant adverse pretreatment factor, but was also associated with nodal metastases and lymphovascular-space invasion.[47]

PATIENT-RELATED FACTORS

The significance of patient age on relapse and survival is controversial. A number of retrospective clinical studies have found younger age to be associated with an increased rate of local and/or distant relapse, particularly in patients selected for treatment with radiation therapy.[1,51] Larger retrospective clinical and population-based studies using cancer registry data have reported both an improved prognosis for younger patients (Meanwell, 10,000 patients;[6] Sigurdsson, 400 patients;[4] Chen, 3600 patients[7]) and a nonsignificant reduction in survival (Bjorge, 7000 cases[52]). A study examining the Surveillance, Epidemiology, and End Results (SEER) database included 2000 patients, and found no difference in outcome related to patient age.[53] It appears that the effect of age may be related to the fact that young patients treated by radiation tend to have larger and more advanced stage tumors than those treated surgically.

Low hemoglobin levels have been reported in a number of retrospective series to be associated with a poor prognosis in patients receiving radical radiotherapy. Both a low pretreatment hemoglobin[10,51] and low hemoglobin during treatment[54,55] have been reported to adversely affect outcome. The level of anemia used as a cutoff in these studies varied from 9 g/L to 12 g/L. The relative risk of relapse was reported to be 1.3 for hemoglobin between 10 and 12 g/L, and 2.2 for a hemoglobin less than 10 g/L relative to a hemoglobin of more than 12 g/L.[34] The requirement for transfusions to counteract anemia has also been reported to be associated with a poor outcome.[1] A hematocrit less than 40% was associated with an adverse outcome in patients receiving radiotherapy.[54] No association between hemoglobin level and outcome was reported for patients undergoing radical hysterectomy.[56] Earlier reports associated thrombocytosis with poor survival;[57,58] however, confirmatory studies did not find thrombocytosis to be of significance on multivariate analysis, as it appeared to be associated with overall tumor burden.[59,60]

Other patient-related factors studied in multivariate analysis and found to be significant adverse prognostic influences include low Karnofsky performance status[5] and lack of compliance with screening recommendations.[4]

ENVIRONMENT-RELATED FACTORS

In patients with FIGO stage IB cervical carcinoma treated by radical hysterectomy and postoperative radiation, the presence of positive surgical margins and tumor size were the only independent prognostic factors in predicting survival—a positive surgical margin being associated with a hazard ratio of 14.02. Parametrial extension and involved pelvic lymph nodes also predicted poor outcome in another study.[22]

A Patterns of Care study established that intracavitary radiation therapy in addition to external beam treatment was a significant independent prognostic factor for survival and pelvic control.[5] The same analysis determined that total doses of more than 8500 cGy were associated with improved pelvic control in FIGO stage III cervical carcinoma. Other series also support the idea that the local control of larger tumors is related to the dose given to point A.[61] To some extent these two features may be surrogates for one another, as patients who are not treated with intracavitary brachytherapy generally receive lower total doses due to the limitations of normal tissue toxicity with external beam radiation. Multivariate analysis also showed that a long time interval between surgery and the commencement of radiotherapy predicted for a worse outcome.[62]

The overall treatment time in radiation therapy is inversely correlated with pelvic control and survival[61,63,64] and is consistent with data from other squamous-cell carcinomas such as head and neck tumors.

The addition of concurrent cisplatinum-based chemotherapy to radical radiation has now been shown to improve patient survival in several randomized trials.[65-67] These studies have examined patients with stage II or above, or stage IB tumors greater than 4 cm in diameter without para-aortic lymphadeno-pathy, and have shown an approximate RR for death from disease of 0.5–0.6 with the addition of chemotherapy. Similar proportional benefits with the addition of concurrent chemotherapy to adjuvant radiotherapy in surgical patients with positive pelvic lymph nodes, parametrial extension, or positive surgical margins are suggested in the recently reported Intergroup study.[68]

SUMMARY

In recent years more studies using multivariate analysis techniques have been published on prognostic factors for cervical carcinoma. This approach may allow a clearer determination of the root causes of treatment failure and death by exposing interactions between covariates. Unfortunately not all studies of similar patient groups have examined the same covariates, thereby resulting in discrepancies. Where possible, weight has been given to prognostic factors identified in several multivariate analyses (Appendix 32B).

Essential prognostic factors include tumor stage and size, histologic subtype, lymph-node metastases, and patient performance status. Additional factors necessary in assessing the need for adjuvant radiotherapy include parametrial extension, depth of cervical stromal invasion, capillary–lymphatic-space invasion and surgical margins. There is continuing controversy as to the independent significance of adenocarcinoma subtype and patient age.

Additional prognostic information for radiotherapy patients includes hemo-globin, the extent of pelvic sidewall extension, and treatment-related factors such as radiation treatment duration, use of intracavitary radiation, and concurrent cisplatin-based chemotherapy.

The identification of promising new biologic or molecular prognostic factors is often hampered by the failure to perform an inclusive multivariate analysis and the lack of subsequent confirmatory studies as discussed by Simon (Chapter 4) earlier in this book. However, erb-B2, tumor hypoxia, tumor vascular density, and SCCAg are promising. Future prognostic factor studies in cervical cancer should include the essential prognostic factors at minimum.

■■■■■ **APPENDIX 32A**

TNM Classification: Cervix Uteri

T — Primary Tumor

TNM Categories	FIGO Stages	
TX		Primary tumor cannot be assessed
T0		No evidence of primary tumor
Tis	0	Carcinoma in situ (preinvasive carcinoma)
T1	I	Cervical carcinoma confined to uterus (extension to corpus should be disregarded
T1a	IA	Invasive carcinoma diagnosed only by microscopy. All macroscopically visible lesions — even with superficial invasion — are T1b/Stage IB
T1a1	IA1	Stromal invasion no greater than 3.0 mm in depth and 7.0 mm or less in horizontal spread
T1a2	IA2	Stromal invasion more than 3.0 mm and not more than 5.0 mm with a horizontal spread
		Note: The depth of invasion should not be more than 5 mm taken from the base of the epithelium, either surface or glandular, from which it orginates. The depth of invasion is defined as the measurement of the tumor from the epithelial–stromal junction of the adjacent most superficial epithelial papilla to the deepest point of invasion.
		Vascular space involvement, venous or lymphatic, does not affect classification.
T1b	IB	Clinically visible lesion confined to the cervix or microscopic lesion greater than T1a2/IA2
T1b1	IB1	Clinically visible lesion 4.0 cm or less in greatest dimension
T1b2	IB2	Clinically visible lesion more than 4 cm in greatest dimension
T2	II	Tumor invades beyond uterus but not to pelvic wall or to lower third of the vagina
T2a	IIA	Without parametrial invasion
T2b	IIB	With parametrial invasion
T3	III	Tumor extends to pelvic wall and/or involves lower third of vagina and/or causes hydronephrosis or nonfunctioning kidney
T3a	IIIA	Tumor involves lower third of vagina, no extension to pelvic wall
T3b	IIIB	Tumor extends to pelvic wall and/or causes hydronephrosis or nonfunctioning kidney
T4	IVA	Tumor invades *mucosa* of bladder or rectum and/or extends beyond true pelvis
M1	IVB	Distant metastasis (excludes peritoneal metastasis)

N — Regional Lymph Nodes

NX Regional lymph nodes cannot be assessed

N0 No regional lymph-node metastasis

N1 Regional lymph-node metastasis

M — Distant Metastasis

MX Distant metastasis cannot be assessed

M0 No distant metastasis

M1 Distant metastasis

Stage Grouping

Stage 0	Tis	N0	M0
Stage IA	T1a	N0	M0
Stage IA1	T1a1	N0	M0
Stage IA2	T1a2	N0	M0
Stage IB	T1b	N0	M0
Stage IB1	T1b1	N0	M0
Stage IB2	T1b2	N0	M0
Stage IIA	T2a	N0	M0
Stage IIB	T2b	N0	M0
Stage IIIA	T3a	N0	M0
Stage IIIB	T1	N1	M0
	T2	N1	M0
	T3a	N1	M0
	T3b	Any N	M0
Stage IVA	T4	Any N	M0
Stage IVB	Any T	Any N	M1

Source: Sobin LH, Wittekind Ch (eds.): *TNM classification of malignant tumors*, 5th ed. New York, Union International Centre le cancer Wiley-Liss, 1997.

■■■■■■■ **APPENDIX 32B**

Prognostic Factors in Cancer of the Uterine Cervix

Prognostic Factor	Tumor Related	Host Related	Environment Related
Essential	Stage Tumor size Histological subtype Lymph-node metastases	Performance status	
Additional	Depth of stromal invasion Capillary–lymphatic-space invasion Parametrial extent Pelvic sidewall involvement	Hemoglobin	Radiotherapy duration Radiation dose Use of brachytherapy Concurrent cisplatin
New and promising	Erb-B2 Tumor hypoxia SCC antigen Tumor vascular density		

REFERENCES

1. Fyles AW, Pintilie M, Kirkbride P, et al.: Prognostic factors in patients with cervix cancer treated by radiation therapy: Results of a multiple regression analysis. *Radiother Oncol* 35:107–17, 1995.

2. Jakobsen A, Bichel P, Vaeth M: New prognostic factors in squamous cell carcinoma of cervix uteri. *Am J Clin Oncol* 8:39–43, 1985.

3. Johnson D, Cox R, Billingham G, et al.: Survival, prognostic factors, and relapse patterns in uterine cervical carcinoma. *Am J Clin Oncol* 6:407–15, 1983.

4. Sigurdsson K, Hrafnkelsson J, Geirsson G, et al.: Screening as a prognostic factor in cervical cancer: Analysis of survival and prognostic factors based on Icelandic population data, 1964–1988. *Gynecol Oncol* 43:64–70, 1991.

5. Lanciano R, Won M, Coia L, et al.: Pretreatment and treatment factors associated with improved outcome in squamous cell carcinoma of the uterine cervix: A final report of the 1973 and 1978 Patterns of Care studies. *Int J Radiat Oncol Biol Phys* 20:667–76, 1991.

6. Meanwell C, Kelly K, Wilson S, et al.: Young age as a prognostic factor in cervical cancer: Analysis of population based data from 10,022 cases. *Br Med J (Clin Res Ed)* 296:386–91, 1988.

7. Chen RJ, Lin YH, Chen CA, et al.: Influence of histologic type and age on survival rates for invasive cervical carcinoma in Taiwan. *Gynecol Oncol* 73:184–90, 1999.

8. Sobin L, Wittekind C (eds.): *TNM classification of malignant tumors.* New York, Union Internationale Centre le Cancer Wiley-Liss, 1997.

9. Delgado G, Bundy B, Zaino R, et al.: Prospective surgical-pathological study of disease-free interval in patients with stage IB squamous cell carcinoma of the cervix: A Gynecologic Oncology Group study. *Gynecol Oncol* 38:352–7, 1990.

10. Kapp KS, Stuecklschweiger GF, Kapp DS, et al.: Prognostic factors in patients with carcinoma of the uterine cervix treated with external beam irradiation and IR-192 high-dose-rate brachytherapy. *Int J Radiat Oncol Biol Phys* 42:531–40, 1998.

11. Landoni F, Maneo A, Colombo A, et al.: Randomised study of radical surgery versus radiotherapy for stage Ib-IIa cervical cancer. *Lancet* 350:535–40, 1997.

12. Benstead K, Cowie V, Blair V, et al.: Stage III carcinoma of cervix. The important of increasing age and extent of parametrial infiltration. *Radiother Oncol* 5:271–6, 1986.

13. Obermair A, Wanner C, Bilgi S, et al.: Tumor angiogenesis in stage IB cervical cancer: Correlation of microvessel density with survival. *Am J Obstet Gynecol* 178:314–9, 1998.

14. Lai CH, Hong JH, Hsueh S, et al.: Preoperative prognostic variables and the impact of postoperative adjuvant therapy on the outcomes of Stage IB or II cervical carcinoma patients with or without pelvic lymph node metastases: An analysis of 891 cases. *Cancer* 85:1537–46, 1999.

15. Bolger BS, Dabbas M, Lopes A, et al.: Prognostic value of preoperative squamous cell carcinoma antigen level in patients surgically treated for cervical carcinoma. *Gynecol Oncol* 65:309–13, 1997.

16. Mayr NA, Yuh WT, Zheng J, et al.: Tumor size evaluated by pelvic examination compared with 3-D quantitative analysis in the prediction of outcome for cervical cancer. *Int J Radiat Oncol Biol Phys* 39:395–404, 1997.

17. Perez C, Kao M: Radiation therapy alone or combined with surgery in the treatment of barrel-shaped carcinoma of the uterine cervix. *Int J Radiat Oncol Biol Phys* 11:1903–9, 1985.

18. Samlal RA, van der Velden J, Ten Kate FJ, et al.: Surgical pathologic factors that predict recurrence in stage IB and IIA cervical carcinoma patients with negative pelvic lymph nodes. *Cancer* 80:1234–40, 1997.

19. Kamura T, Tsukamoto N, Tsuruchi N, et al.: Multivariate analysis of the histopathologic prognostic factors of cervical cancer in patients undergoing radical hysterectomy. *Cancer* 69:181–6, 1992.

20. Alvarez R, Soong S, Kinney W, et al.: Identification of prognostic factors and risk groups in patients found to have nodal metastasis at the time of radical hysterectomy for early-stage squamous carcinoma of the cervix. *Gynecol Oncol* 35:130–5, 1989.

21. Sevin BU, Lu Y, Bloch DA, et al.: Surgically defined prognostic parameters in patients with early cervical carcinoma. A multivariate survival tree analysis. *Cancer* 78:1438–46, 1996.

22. Samlal RA, van der Velden J, Schilthuis MS, et al.: Identification of high-risk groups among node-positive patients with stage IB and IIA cervical carcinoma. *Gynecol Oncol* 64:463–7, 1997.

23. Hale R, Buckley C, Fox H, et al.: Prognostic value of c-erbB-2 expression in uterine cervical carcinoma. *J Clin Pathol* 45:594–6, 1992.

24. Look KY, Brunetto VL, Clarke-Pearson DL, et al.: An analysis of cell type in patients with surgically staged stage IB carcinoma of the cervix: A Gynecologic Oncology Group study. *Gynecol Oncol* 63:304–11, 1996.

25. Chen RJ, Chang DY, Yen ML, et al.: Prognostic factors of primary adenocarcinoma of the uterine cervix. *Gynecol Oncol* 69:157–64, 1998.

26. Willen H, Eklund G, Johnsson J, et al.: Invasive squamous cell carcinoma of the uterine cervix. VIII. Survival and malignancy grading in patients treated by irradiation in Lund 1969–1970. *Acta Radiol Oncol* 24:41–50, 1985.

27. Tjalma W, Van Marck E, Weyler J, et al.: Quantification and prognostic relevance of angiogenic parameters in invasive cervical cancer. *Br J Cancer* 78:170–4, 1998.

28. Obermair A, Wanner C, Bilgi S, et al.: The influence of vascular space involvement on the prognosis of patients with stage IB cervical carcinoma: Correlation of results from hematoxylin and eosin staining with results from immunostaining for factor VIII-related antigen. *Cancer* 82:689–96, 1998.

29. Bosch FX, Manos MM, Munoz N, et al.: Prevalence of human papillomavirus in cervical cancer: A worldwide perspective. International biological study on cervical cancer (IBSCC) Study Group. *J Natl Cancer Inst* 87:796–802, 1995.

30. Burger RA, Monk BJ, Kurosaki T, et al.: Human papillomavirus type 18: Association with poor prognosis in early stage cervical cancer. *J Natl Cancer Inst* 88:1361–8, 1996.

31. van Muyden RC, ter Harmsel BW, Smedts FM, et al.: Detection and typing of human papillomavirus in cervical carcinomas in Russian women: A prognostic study. *Cancer* 85:2011–6, 1999.

32. Lombard I, Vincent-Salomon A, Validire P, et al.: Human papillomavirus genotype as a major determinant of the course of cervical cancer. *J Clin Oncol* 16:2613–9, 1998.

33. de Bruijn HW, Duk JM, van der Zee AG, et al.: The clinical value of squamous cell carcinoma antigen in cancer of the uterine cervix. *Tumor Biol* 19:505–16, 1998.

34. Hong JH, Tsai CS, Chang JT, et al.: The prognostic significance of pre- and post-treatment SCC levels in patients with squamous cell carcinoma of the cervix treated by radiotherapy. *Int J Radiat Oncol Biol Phys* 41:823–30, 1998.

35. Cooper R, Wilks D, Logue J, et al.: High tumor angiogenesis is associated with poorer survival in carcinoma of the cervix treated with radiotherapy. *Clin Cancer Res* 4:2795–2800, 1998.

36. Kaku T, Hirakawa T, Kamura T, et al.: Angiogenesis in adenocarcinoma of the uterine cervix. *Cancer* 83:1384–90, 1998.

37. Schlenger K, Hockel M, Mitze M, et al.: Tumor vascularity — A novel prognostic factor in advanced cervical carcinoma. *Gynecol Oncol* 59:57–66, 1995.

38. Sundfor K, Lyng H, Rofstad EK: Tumor hypoxia and vascular density as predictors of metastasis in squamous cell carcinoma of the uterine cervix. *Br J Cancer* 78:822–7, 1998.

39. Fyles AW, Milosevic M, Wong R, et al.: Oxygenation predicts radiation response and survival in patients with cervix cancer [Erratum appears in *Radiother Oncol* 50(3):371, 1999]. *Radiother Oncol* 48:149–56, 1998.

40. Hockel M, Knoop C, Schlenger K, et al.: Intratumoral pO2 predicts survival in advanced cancer of the uterine cervix. *Radiother Oncol* 26:45–50, 1993.

41. Nakano T, Oka K, Ishikawa A, et al.: Immunohistochemical prediction of radiation response and local control in radiation therapy for cervical cancer. *Cancer Detect Prev* 22:120–8, 1998.

42. Tjalma W, De Cuyper E, Weyler J, et al.: Expression of bcl-2 in invasive and in situ carcinoma of the uterine cervix. *Am J Obstet Gynecol* 178:113–7, 1998.

43. Crawford RA, Caldwell C, Iles RK, et al.: Prognostic significance of the bcl-2 apoptotic family of proteins in primary and recurrent cervical cancer. *Br J Cancer* 78:210–4, 1998.

44. Harima Y, Harima K, Shikata N, et al.: Bax and Bcl-2 expressions predict response to radiotherapy in human cervical cancer. *J Cancer Res Clin Oncol* 124:503–510, 1998.

45. Ndubisi B, Sanz S, Lu L, et al.: The prognostic value of HER-2/neu oncogene in cervical cancer. *Ann Clin Lab Sci* 27:396–400, 1997.

46. Nevin J, Laing D, Kaye P, et al.: The significance of Erb-b2 immunostaining in cervical cancer. *Gynecol Oncol* 73:354–8, 1999.

47. Hockel M, Schlenger K, Hockel S, et al.: Hypoxic cervical cancers with low apoptotic index are highly aggressive. *Cancer Res* 59:4525–8, 1999.

48. Tsang RW, Wong CS, Fyles AW, et al.: Tumor proliferation and apoptosis in human uterine cervix carcinoma. *Radiother Oncol* 50:93–101, 1999.

49. Scambia G, Ferrandina G, Distefano M, et al.: Epidermal growth factor receptor (EGFR) is not related to the prognosis of cervical cancer. *Cancer Lett.* 123:135–9, 1998.

50. Konski A, Domenico D, Irving D, et al.: Flow cytometric DNA content analysis of paraffin-embedded tissue derived from cervical carcinoma. *Int J Radiat Oncol Bio Phys* 30:839–43, 1994.

51. Takeshi K, Katsuyuki K, Yoshiaki T, et al.: Definitive radiotherapy combined with high-dose-rate brachytherapy for Stage III carcinoma of the uterine cervix: Retrospective analysis of prognostic factors concerning patient characteristics and treatment parameters. *Int J Radiat Oncol Biol Phys* 41:319–27, 1998.

52. Bjorge T, Thoresen S, Skare G: Incidence, survival and mortality in cervical cancer in Norway, 1956–1990. *Eur J Cancer* 29A:2291–7, 1993.

53. Brewster WR, DiSaia PJ, Monk BJ, et al.: Young age as a prognostic factor in cervical cancer: Results of a population-based study. *Am J Obstet Gynecol* 180:1464–7, 1999.

54. Kapp D, Fischer D, Gutierrez E, et al.: Pretreatment prognostic factors in carcinoma of the uterine cervix: A multivariable analysis of the effect of age, stage, histology and blood counts on survival. *Int J Radiat Oncol Biol Phys* 9:445–55, 1983.

55. Girinski T, Pejovic-Lenfant M, Bourhis J, et al.: Prognostic value of hemoglobin concentrations and blood transfusions in advanced carcinoma of the cervix treated by radiation therapy: Results of a retrospective study of 386 patients. *Int J Radiat Oncol Biol Phys* 16:37–42, 1989.

56. Monk B, Tewari K, Gamboa-Vujicic G, et al.: Does perioperative blood transfusion affect survival in patients with cervical cancer treated with radical hysterectomy? *Obstet Gynecol* 85:343–8, 1995.

57. Hernandez E, Lavine M, Dunton CJ, et al.: Poor prognosis associated with thrombocytosis in patients with cervical cancer. *Cancer* 69:2975–7, 1992.

58. Rodriguez GC, Clarke-Pearson DL, Soper JT, et al.: The negative prognostic implications of thrombocytosis in women with stage IB cervical cancer. *Obstet Gynecol* 83:445–8, 1994.

59. Hernandez E, Heller PB, Whitney C, et al.: Thrombocytosis in surgically treated stage IB squamous cell cervical carcinoma (A Gynecologic Oncology Group study). *Gynecol Oncol* 55:328–32, 1994.

60. Lopes A, Daras V, Cross PA, et al.: Thrombocytosis as a prognostic factor in women with cervical cancer. *Cancer* 74:90–2, 1994.

61. Perez CA, Grigsby PW, Chao KS, et al.: Tumor size, irradiation dose, and long-term outcome of carcinoma of uterine cervix. *Int J Radiat Oncol Biol Phys* 41:307–17, 1998.

62. Yeh S-A, Leung S, Wang C-J, et al.: Postoperative radiotherapy in early stage carcinoma of the uterine cervix: Treatment results and prognostic factors. *Gynecol Oncol* 72:10–15, 1999.

63. Lanciano R, Pajak R, Martz K, et al.: The influence of treatment time on outcome for squamous cell cancer of the uterine cervix treated with radiation: A Patterns-of-Care study. *Int J Radiat Oncol Biol Phys* 25:391–7, 1993.

64. Fyles A, Keane T, Barton M, et al.: The effect of treatment duration in the local control of cervix cancer. *Radiother Oncol* 25:273–9, 1992.

65. Morris M, Eifel PJ, Lu J, et al.: Pelvic radiation with concurrent chemotherapy compared with pelvic and para-aortic radiation for high-risk cervical cancer [see Comments]. *N Engl J Med* 340:1137–43, 1999.

66. Rose P, Bundy B, Watkins E, et al.: Concurrent cisplatin-based radiotherapy and chemotherapy for locally advanced cervical cancer. *New Engl J Med* 340:1144–53, 1999.

67. Keys H, Bundy B, Stehman F, et al.: Cisplatin, radiation and adjuvant hysterectomy compared with radiation and adjuvant hysterectomy for bulky stage IB cervical carcinoma. *New Engl J Med* 340:1154–61, 1999.

68. Peters W, Liu P, Barrett R, et al.: Cisplatin, 5-flourouracil plus radiation therapy are superior to radiation therapy as adjunctive therapy in high-risk, early stage carcinoma of the cervix after radical hysterectomy and pelvic lymphadenectomy: Report of a Phase III inter-group study [Abstract 1]. *Gynecol Oncol* 72:443, 1999.

CHAPTER 33

Endometrial Cancer

J. LOU BENEDET and DIANNE M. MILLER

In many industrialized countries, endometrial cancer has surpassed cervical cancer as the most common form of malignancy affecting the female genital tract. This has occurred due to the effectiveness of screening programs in reducing both the incidence and mortality rates for cervical cancer. Improvement in life expectancy for many women also has led to an increased number of patients being diagnosed with endometrial cancer, which is predominantly a disease of postmenopausal women.

Endometrial cancer most often presents with the symptom of postmenopausal bleeding. Because this manifestation is often found early in the course of the disease and is significantly alarming, women generally present themselves promptly to their physicians for investigation. The majority of endometrial cancers are thus diagnosed as stage I lesions. In certain situations, however, this condition has the potential to behave in an aggressive fashion, resulting in recurrence and ultimately death. The identification of those factors that place patients at high risk for recurrence has been the primary focus of much of the research on this condition in the past 20 years.

Although endometrial cancer is predominantly a disease of postmenopausal women, approximately 20–25% of cases will occur before menopause and a further 5% occur before age 40. Obesity, particularly upper body obesity,[1] nulliparity, and late menopause have all been associated with an increase in risk for endometrial cancer. Use of exogenous unopposed estrogen[2] and tamoxifen[3] have also been associated with an increased risk for the development of endometrial cancer. Use of oral contraceptive tablets[4] and smoking[5], however, have been associated with a decrease in the risk for endometrial cancer and women who develop endometrial cancer while on exogenous estrogen appear to have favorable prognosis.

Prognostic Factors in Cancer, 2nd edition, Edited by Mary K. Gospodarowicz
ISBN 0-471-40633-3 Copyright © 2001 Wiley-Liss, Inc.

TUMOR-RELATED FACTORS

Stage

In 1988, the International Federation of Gynaecology and Obstetrics (FIGO) recommended that the staging for endometrial cancer be based on a surgical–pathological system rather than a purely clinical system. This new system was changed to emphasize both intra- and extrauterine factors, which were felt to be important in the prognosis of this condition. Clinical staging, traditionally, was most important when patients were treated primarily with either preoperative irradiation or exclusively with radiotherapy. Uterine size as related to direct tumor growth and involvement of the myometrium, cervical involvement by tumor extension, and histologic grade of the tumor as well as extrauterine deposits or lesions, were all important prognostic factors that were emphasized by earlier staging systems, but were better characterized with the new surgical staging system. A major advantage of the surgical staging system was that greater precision in assessing extent of disease, which historically has been proven to be the most important single prognostic factor in endometrial cancer, would thus become more accurate. The International Union Against Cancer (UICC) and American Joint Committee on Cancer (AJCC) adapted the FIGO system and both classifications are now identical and compatible with FIGO (see Appendix 33A).

Data from the *FIGO Annual Report*, Volume 23, on over 7000 patients treated for endometrial cancer, from 1990 to 1992, has shown that stage-for-stage survival is much better using a surgical staging system compared with clinical staging. The difference is probably a reflection that surgical staging more accurately details the true extent of the disease, which then in turn can be more optimally treated. The differences are also noted even within a given stage, once again reflecting that clinically staged patients had more disease outside of the uterus than might have been expected and that had not been recognized when the patients were staged clinically. It is also apparent that the histologic grade of the tumor and the degree of myometrial invasion within the subgroups are important factors, which are significant prognostically. The degree of myometrial penetration has been noted to be a consistent indicator of survival and recurrence for endometrial cancer.

When the disease does involve the cervix (stage II), prognosis is poorer and survival drops from approximately 80% to the 50% range. One reason for this appears to be related to a 12% frequency of para-aortic lymph-node metastasis in this group of patients.[6] Several studies have shown that the presence of extrauterine disease affecting adnexal or other intrapelvic or abdominal structures carries with it a poorer prognosis for survival and a high likelihood of recurrence. These patients have also been noted to account for a significant proportion of those with positive peritoneal washings and if the latter prognostic indicator is corrected for, this finding then is greatly diminished in its significance. Creasman[7] showed that clinical diagnosis of stage II disease was often incorrect, with only 45% of patients truly having a surgical–pathological stage II lesion after prior clinical diagnosis.

Histologic Differentiation

The grade of tumor has been universally accepted as one of the more sensitive indicators for prognosis in endometrial cancers. The histologic differentiation has also been correlated with depth of myometrial invasion[6,8] and lymph node metastasis.[9] Creasman et al.[10] noted a higher percentage of pelvic and para-aortic lymph-node involvement with both increasing stage and grade, but the largest percentage increase was noted when Grade 3 lesions were compared to Grade 2. Several studies[9,11–14] have shown that, within the stage I group,[15] tumor differentiation as expressed by Grade 3 versus Grade 1 and 2 is a most significant independent variable for survival and recurrence.

Lurain and coworkers,[12] in studying prognostic factors in Stage I patients who recurred, found that those with Grade 3 tumors were five-times as likely to develop recurrence than patients with Grade 1 or 2 tumors.

Myometrial Invasion

The degree of myometrial penetration has also been noted to be a consistent indicator of survival and recurrence for endometrial cancer.[1–5,8–11,16] Lutz et al.[11,12] noted that the depth of myometrial penetration appeared to be less important than the proximity of the invading tumor to the uterine serosa. Patients whose tumors invaded to within 5 mm of serosa had a 65% 5-year survival as compared to 97% for those whose tumors were greater than 10 mm from the serosal surface. Lurain et al.[12] found that depth of myometrial invasion was significantly associated with disease recurrence in a univariate analysis but not in a multivariate analysis. This more than likely reflects the fact that the histology and grade are more important predictors of both lymph-node metastasis and recurrence and that the myometrial invasion is closely linked to tumor grade. Genest et al.[15] were able to show that tumors invading the outer third of the myometrium in Stage I cases had a significantly poorer prognosis than lesions involving the inner one-third (95% 5-year survival versus 70%). Similarly, DiSaia et al.[17] noted that 8% of patients with endometrial involvement only experienced a recurrence and 5% died of disease, as contrasted to 36% of deaths in patients with deep muscle involvement.

Peritoneal Cytology

The use of cytologic sampling of peritoneal fluid or washing has become routine as an adjunct to staging for patients with endometrial cancer. Creasman et al.[10] noted that 12% of their patients had positive washings, and Morrow et al.[14] noted that, in 32 patients with positive washings as the only positive risk factor, recurrence was observed in 18.8%. Similar findings have also been reported by others,[12,18] but Kadar et al.[13] found that this risk factor was only important when there was extrauterine disease present.

Hysteroscopy, when used for diagnosis, may result in positive peritoneal cytology. The prognostic significance of this is unknown; however, Rose reported a case of probable disease dissemination via this route.[19]

Lymph Node Involvement

In the past, it was thought that early-stage endometrial cancer infrequently spread to lymph nodes and, when it did, the para-aortic lymph nodes were the primary site of metastasis. In 1970, Lewis et al.[9] reported a series of 129 patients with adenocarcinoma of the uterus treated by radical hysterectomy and lymphadenectomy. In this study, 13.2% of patients had lymph-node involvement or 11.2% when the cervix was free of disease. They also noted that the incidence of node involvement was related to the degree of differentiation of the tumor and the depth of myometrial invasion. They found that the survival rate in patients with positive nodes was significantly less than in patients where no evidence of metastasis could be demonstrated. Rutledge,[20] in an excellent review of the role of radical hysterectomy in adenocarcinoma of the endometrium, surveyed the literature for the preceding 20 years and noted that approximately 10% of patients with Stage I disease had metastasis to the pelvic lymph nodes. He also found that the incidence of nodal metastasis increased as the degree of myometrial invasion increased, as well as when the tumors being more undifferentiated. In a more recent study, Creasman et al.[10] reporting on the Gynecologic Group (GOG) results noted an 11% incidence of pelvic node metastasis in stage I carcinomas and 6% with para-aortic metastasis. They also found that the grade of tumor and the depth of myometrial invasion correlated well with nodal disease. In analyzing the site of tumor location with regard to lymph-node metastasis, they noted that, if only the fundus was involved, 8% of the patients had pelvic-node metastasis. This percentage doubled if the lower uterine segment was also involved and 4% of fundal lesions metastasized to para-aortic nodes, while lower segment lesions had over three times the incidence of para-aortic metastasis. Morrow et al.[14] noted that patients with positive para-aortic lymph-node metastasis accounted for nearly 25% of all recurrences. They also found that para-aortic and pelvic-node positivity correlated well with clinical findings.

Currently, considerable debate has occurred over the value of routine lymph-node sampling in what would appear to be low grade, that is, G1 or G2 tumors with minimal or no myometrial invasion. The incidence of nodal involvement in such cases is extremely low and the overall survival with simple hysterectomy for such patients is in the neighborhood of 90+%. Some authorities have argued that lymphadenectomy in these patients constitutes an unnecessary risk for complications, as many are elderly and obese and have coexisting medical conditions. What is perhaps even more controversial is the extent to which para-aortic and pelvic lymph nodes should be removed or sampled. Some would argue that sampling is simply too imprecise and defeats the purpose of surgical staging of endometrial cancer. Nonetheless, resolution of this issue will await further data and studies.

Trimble et al.[21] reviewed the data from the National Cancer Institute database and found that lymph-node sampling did not confer a survival advantage.

Histopathology

The histological type of endometrial cancer is a prognostic factor for survival. The vast majority, however, are adenocarcinoma with an endometrioid pattern with or without benign squamous metaplasia (adenoacanthoma). Zaino et al.[22] in a review found that the relatively common villoglandular subtype of adenocarcinoma had a very good prognosis when compared with other stage I and II endometrial cancers. When compared on a stage-for-stage basis, these lesions have a much better prognosis than patients with clear-cell carcinoma or papillary serous carcinoma of the endometrium.[6,23–25] Data from Volume 23 of the *FIGO Annual Report* showed that the papillary serous and clear-cell types were two to three times more likely to be stage III or IV at the time of diagnosis, compared to the more common endometrioid variety. Lurain et al.[12] noted that, in a study of 227 patients with adenocarcinoma or adenoacanthoma, 8.8% suffered a recurrence, compared to 35.7% of patients with adenosquamous, 25% of 16 papillary adenocarcinomas, and four of seven patients with the clear-cell variety. Symonds[24] also noted that these types of tumors were more likely to metastasize and have an adverse outcome. Christopherson et al.[23] in a detailed review of 1224 cases, noted that 5.5% were clear-cell adenocarcinomas, and the histologic type was found to have a particularly poor outcome. Similarly, Wilson et al.,[25] in a review of patients treated at the Mayo Clinic, noted that 13% of patients in their series had these uncommon histologic subtypes and the overall survival in these patients was only 33%, as contrasted to that of patients with endometrioid lesions, where the survival was 92%.

Hendrickson et al.[26] were the first to call attention to papillary serous endometrial carcinoma and indicated its highly aggressive behavior. Since then, several reports[19,25,27,28] have confirmed the aggressive nature of this particular subtype of endometrial cancer. Abeler and Kjorstad[19] reviewed all endometrial cancers treated at the Norwegian Radium Hospital between 1970 and 1977, and found a frequency of papillary serous carcinoma of the endometrium to be 1.1% of all patients. They found that this tumor occurred more frequently in older women and was extremely aggressive. They were unable, however, to relate this to a higher proportion having lymphatic-space invasion or deep myometrial infiltration as reported by others. Gallion and coworkers,[27] in reporting their experience with papillary serous endometrial cancer, noted that 38% had more extensive disease than had been appreciated clinically. They also noted a 50% frequency of lymphatic space involvement as compared to 14% for non-papillary serous tumors. Furthermore, 75% of these patients developed a recurrence and all eventually died of disease. They also noted that 70% of patients with any degree of myometrial invasion developed recurrence. Aquino-Parsons et al.[29] reported on a small series of patients with papillary serous or clear-cell carcinoma confined to the endometrial curettings and absent in the hysterectomy specimen. In this series there were no recurrences with surgery as the only treatment.

Extrauterine Disease

Several studies[6,12,25,27] have shown that the presence of extrauterine disease affecting adnexal or other intrapelvic or abdominal structures carries with it a poor prognosis for survival and a high likelihood of recurrence. These patients have also been noted, to account for a significant proportion of those patients with positive peritoneal washings and, if the latter prognostic indicator is corrected for this finding, then its significance is greatly diminished.[30] A study by Connell et al.[31] showed that adnexal involvement had little if any independent prognostic value. Instead, adnexal involvement was accompanied by many other adverse pathologic factors.

Hormone Receptor Status

The presence of steroid receptors, particularly progesterone receptors (PgR), may be associated with lesser virulence. Endometrial cancer is known to be a hormone-sensitive and dependent tumor when steroid receptors are present. This would indicate that the tumor has retained some of the biologic properties of the host tissue, which in turn could lead to a better outcome.[32] Kadar et al.[33] studied 137 surgically staged women with clinical Stage I and II endometrial cancers and noted that increasing steroid-receptor concentrations were associated with an increase in survival. They found with a multivariate analysis that only the (PgR) concentration affected survival independently, but that this effect disappeared when the analysis was restricted to women with disease confined to the uterus. They concluded that the receptor status of the primary tumor was of limited prognostic significance unless extrauterine disease was present. Klein et al.[34] noted that receptor status correlated with clinical stage and grade of tumor but not with myometrial invasion. When they subjected their data to a multivariate analysis, PgR emerged as a significant prognostic factor next to clinical stage, whereas estrogen receptor (ER) had no significant prognostic relevance.

Friberg and Norén,[35] in studying the prognostic value of steroid receptors in Stage II patients, concluded that patients who died did not have significantly different ER and PgR concentrations from those who survived.

One of the main values of receptor study and assays at this time is to determine which patients would be suitable for hormone therapy.

Lymphatic-Vascular-Space Involvement

Several studies[13,36,37] in the literature have identified lymphatic-vascular-space involvement (LVS) as an important prognostic factor for endometrial cancer. Gal et al.[37] noted that LVS involvement correlated with other prognostic indicators, such as histological grade, depth of myometrial invasion, peritoneal spread, and lymph-node involvement. LVS is also an independent prognostic indicator for decreased survival in patients with clinical stage I endometrial cancer. In Gal et al.'s[37] study, it proved to be the only prognostic indicator that was positive in all patients who died from endometrial adenocarcinoma. The study by Creasman et al.[10] also identified LVS involvement as an important prognostic factor that was present in 15% of their patients. Pelvic lymph nodes were positive approximately four times as often when LVS was present and there was a sixfold increase in positive para-aortic nodes. In a recent review of the GOG data, Morrow et al.[14] reported that, in those patients where LVS involvement was the single positive risk factor, the recurrence rate was 26.5%. Feltmate et al.[38] showed that LVS involvement was an important independent prognostic factor in Stage II disease as well.

Flow Cytometry

The use of flow cytometry and estimation of tumor ploidy has been consistent in indicating the prognostic value of these factors with regards to survival and recurrence.[24,39–41] Symonds[24] noted that DNA analysis appeared to be most useful when histologic studies were inconclusive in regarding risk assignment, and noted a definite correlation between DNA index and the risk of metastasis.

Iversen et al.[39] studied both the DNA ploidy and steroid receptors as predictors for the disease course in patients with endometrial cancer. Both the death and recurrence rates were significantly lower among patients with diploid and receptor-rich tumors. Single-factor analysis in the first data set of this study showed significant prognostic value for ploidy, surgical stage, grade, and depth of myometrial invasion. In a stepwise analysis, histological grade lost significance and myometrial invasion became of borderline significance. When the receptor data were included, both ER and PgR values were of significance in the single-factor analysis; however, in the stepwise analysis, only ploidy and surgical stage were significant. This would suggest that the prognostic importance of receptor status on survival 13 dependent on and included in the information already obtained by ploidy.

Oncogenes

Amplification of certain oncogenes and increases in their oncoproteins have been shown to be prognostic in a variety of cancers. Berchuck et al.[42] noted that, although only 9% of endometrial cancers had overexpression of HER-2/neu, when present it was associated with an increased incidence of death from persistent or recurrent cancer. Similarly, Hetzel et al.[43] showed that HER-2/neu overexpression was a major prognostic factor in endometrial cancer when subjected to multivariate analysis. Fujimoto et al.[44] studied ras oncogene activation in endometrial cancer and found that there did not appear to be any relationship between point mutation and clinical prognostic factors such as clinical stage, depth of myometrial invasion, grade, histologic type, and ascitic cytology. Ozsaran[45] showed that p53 expression is more common in the aggressive histologic subtypes of endometrial cancer.

Other Cell Markers

A multitude of other markers, such as heat-shock proteins,[46] and cytosolic cathepsin D,[47] have been examined and found to correlate with prognosis. These discoveries await clinical applicability.

Combinations of prognostic factors beyond what is currently incorporated in staging can better predict outcome than individual characteristics. This has led to attempts to develop prognostic indices to predict outcome.[48]

Virtually all of the tumor-related prognostic factors, as grade, depth of myometrial invasion, together with anatomic extent of disease, as well as cytology and lymph-node status, can be viewed as essential, and are the basic elements of the current staging system. Staging has been shown to be the single most important prognostic factor for this disease. These factors are also the current determinants of therapy and the basis of clinical practice guidelines in those jurisdictions where they exist.

Although cell type is not included in the current staging system, it is an essential prognostic factor, as certain histologic subtypes and variants almost invariably would affect the selection of therapy. Appendix 33B summarizes the various prognostic factors in terms of those that are essential, that is, those currently used to select treatment and used in clinical practice guidelines, as well as additional factors and factors that are known to influence prognosis but not necessarily as the basis of treatment; new and promising factors are also listed.

HOST-RELATED FACTORS

Age

Age as a prognostic factor for endometrial cancer has been recognized for many years. Several authors[11–15] have shown that younger patients have improved survival as compared to older patients. Abeler and Kjorstad,[8] in a multivariate analysis, showed that age at the time of diagnosis was the most important prognostic factor. These observations can be related to the fact that the younger women, in general, tend to have earlier, better differentiated lesions with less myometrial invasion. In addition, a relative lack of immunocompetence may be more prevalent in older patients. Approximately 5–10% of endometrial cancers will occur in premenopausal women, often in association with altered gonadal steroid function. These patients may have some delay in diagnosis because the symptom of bleeding or spotting from these lesions not is always appreciated at the outset, permitting the tumors to theoretically invade deeper into the myometrium. Nonetheless, there is no evidence to suggest that these patients have a worse prognosis than the postmenopausal woman.

Medical Conditions

Endometrial cancer has not only been regarded as a disease of postmenopausal women but also as a disorder that is more common in women who are obese, hypertensive, and diabetic. Bokhman[49] postulated that there were two main types of endometrial cancer. The first and most common type was associated with these factors, as well as other manifestations of abnormal function of the hypothalamic hypophyseal complex. The second type occurred in women where these factors were either not prominent or absent. Bokhman noted that the latter type accounted for 35% of patients and that the cancers were more likely to be higher grade with a tendency to deep myometrial invasion and a much poorer prognosis than for patients in the former type (58.8% 5-year survival rate versus 85.6%).

Race

The incidence of endometrial cancer appears to be less in African-American women; however, more of these women appear to have high-grade, high-stage tumors, and the frequency of unfavorable histologies is also higher.[50]

TREATMENT-RELATED FACTORS

Schneider et al., in a series of 100 consecutive women presenting with endometrial cancer,[51] were able to show that preoperative evaluation with tumor markers and magnetic resonance imaging accurately predicted those with high-stage disease. Cheng et al. used ultrasound to identify women at high risk for nodal metastases.[52]

Total abdominal hysterectomy and bilateral salpingo-oophorectomy (TAH/BSO) has been accepted as the mainstay of therapy for early-stage endometrial cancer. Combinations of this surgery with various forms of radiation treatment have also been used extensively in an attempt to further improve survival and lower recurrences. Radiotherapy has often been given as adjuvant therapy, but it has also been used as primary treatment for this disease. What has emerged from the literature on endometrial cancer treatment is that there is no agreement upon the treatment method that is superior with respect to survival for this disease. In his review, Rutledge[20] noted that the recurrence and survival rates were no different for patients treated by radical hysterectomy or TAH/BSO. What he did note was that the site of recurrence was different. His review indicated that there were subsets and groups of patients where disease spreads early beyond the local site and is not detected by the usual clinical means, and that the treatment methods employed can affect local recurrence but not survival in such patients.

Aalders et al.[36] carried out a randomized study in endometrial cancer where patients received TAH/BSO and postoperative intracavitary radium treatments. Patients were then randomized to no further treatment or to treatment with external beam therapy. This study concluded that only patients with poorly differentiated tumors (Grade 3), which infiltrated more than half the myometrial thickness, might benefit from additional external therapy. This study showed that, in spite of similar death and recurrence rates for these two groups of patients, patients who received external beam therapy had a 1.9% vaginal- or pelvic-wall recurrence, as compared to 6.9% for those who did not receive external beam therapy. This study also emphasized the significance of tumor cells in endothelial-lined spaces. These patients had a death and recurrence rate of 26.7%, and no difference was found between the two treatment groups in regards to the death rate.

SUMMARY

Most patients presenting with endometrial cancer will be diagnosed with Stage I lesions. It is this group of patients which have been studied extensively in an attempt to understand the prognostic factors so that therapy can be individually tailored to the patient's risks for recurrence and/or death from this disease. Certain histological subtypes, for example, papillary serous endometrial cancer and clear-cell cancers, carry a poor prognosis, but fortunately, these are found in only a small proportion of endometrial cancer patients. Studies that have been carried out have clearly indicated the intra- and extrauterine factors that are important for prognosis and have led to the current surgical staging system for endometrial cancer. However, much of the information regarding prognosis can be gleaned from careful preoperative assessment of these patients. Such information as uterine size, grade, histologic type, and radiological evidence of disease beyond the uterus can be obtained. Similarly, information regarding ploidy and receptor status is also available on the basis of curettage specimens. With increasing use of hysteroscopy, more precise assessment of the extent of disease in the uterine cavity and also possible extension and involvement of the cervix may be possible.

A major concern regarding surgical staging has been the fact that many of these patients are elderly and obese with significant medical problems, and that the risk from pelvic and para-aortic-node sampling may markedly increase morbidity. Most studies have shown that this has not been a factor. Similarly, concerns have been expressed regarding those patients who, because of adverse factors, may require postoperative extended-field radiation, which can be compromised by postoperative adhesions. Most importantly, it has yet to be clearly demonstrated that, once disease has been discovered outside of the pelvic cavity, the usual treatments can affect survival. Undoubtedly, recurrence patterns will be affected, but a clear demonstration of survival advantage is not available. Intraoperative immediate histologic assessment of the uterine specimen with careful clinical assessment of nodal areas and the abdominal cavity can provide sufficient information regarding the risk of nodal metastasis without resorting to routine lymphadenectomy in all patients with this disease. Appendix 33B provides a summary of the clinically relevant prognostic factors in endometrial cancer.

■■■■■■ **APPENDIX 33A**

TNM Classification: Endometrial cancer

T — Primary Tumor

TNM Categories	FIGO Stages	
TX		Primary tumor cannot be assessed
T0		No evidence of primary tumor
Tis	0	Carcinoma in situ (preinvasive carcinoma)
T1	I	Tumor confined to corpus uteri
T1a	IA	Tumor limited to endometrium
T1b	IB	Tumor invades up to or less than one half of myometrium
T1c	IC	Tumor invades to more than one half of myometrium
T2	II	Tumor invades cervix but does not extend beyond uterus
T2a	IIA	Endocervical glandular involvement only
T2b	IIB	Cervical stromal invasion
T3 and/or N1	III	Local and/or regional spread as specified in T3a, b, N1, and FIGO III A, B, C below
T3a	IIIA	Tumor involves serosa and/or adnexa (direct extension or metastasis) and/or cancer cells in ascites or peritoneal washings
T3b	IIIB	Vaginal involvement (direct extension or metastasis)
N1	IIIC	Metastasis to pelvic and/or para-aortic lymph nodes
T4	IVA	Tumor invades bladder *mucosa* and/or bowel *mucosa*
M1	IVB	Distant metastasis (*excluding* metastasis to vagina, pelvic serosa, or adnexa, *including* metastasis to intra-abdominal lymph nodes other than para-aortic, and/or pelvic nodes)

N — Regional Lymph Nodes

NX Regional lymph nodes cannot be assessed

N0 No regional lymph-node metastasis

N1 Regional lymph-node metastasis

M — Distant Metastasis

MX Distant metastasis cannot be assessed

M0 No distant metastasis

M1 Distant metastasis

Stage Grouping

Stage 0	Tis	N0	M0
Stage IA	T1a	N0	M0
Stage IB	T1b	N0	M0
Stage IC	T1c	N0	M0
Stage IIA	T2a	N0	M0
Stage IIB	T2b	N0	M0
Stage IIIA	T3a	N0	M0
Stage IIIB	T3b	N0	M0
Stage IIIC	T1	N1	M0
	T2	N1	M0
	T3a,b	N1	M0
Stage IVA	T4	Any N	M0
Stage IVB	Any T	Any N	M1

Source: Sobin LH, Wittekind Ch (eds.): *TNM classification of malignant tumors*, 5th ed. New York, Union Internationale Contre le Cancer Wiley-Liss, 1997.

███████ **APPENDIX 33B**

Prognostic Factors in Endometrial Cancer

Prognostic Factors	Tumor Related	Host Related	Environment Related
Essential	Stage Grade Depth of myometrial invasion Positive peritoneal cytology		
Additional	Lymph-node metastasis	Age Race Ancillary medical conditions	
New and promising	Ploidy Flow cytometry Oncogenes		Availability of: MRI Ultrasonography Laparoscopic biopsy Access to care

REFERENCES

1. Swanson CA, Potischman N, Wilbanks GD, et al.: Relationship of endometrial cancer risk to past and contemporary body size and body fat distribution. *Cancer Epidemiol Biomark Prev* 4:321–7, 1993.

2. Woodruff DJ, Pickar JH: Incidence of endometrial hyperplasia in postmenopausal women taking conjugated estrogens (Premarin) with medroxyprogesterone acetate or conjugated estrogens alone. The Menopause Study Group. *Am J Obstet Gynecol* 170:1213–23, 1994.

3. Killackey MA, Hakes TB, Pierce VK: Endometrial adenocarcinoma in breast cancer patients receiving antiestrogens. *Cancer Treat Rep* 69(2):237–8, 1985.

4. The Centers for Disease Control and Steroid Hormone Study. Oral contraceptive use and the risk of endometrial cancer. *JAMA* 249:1600–4, 1983.

5. Lawrence C, Tessaro I, Durgerian S, et al.: Smoking, body weight, and early-stage endometrial cancer. *Cancer* 59(9):1665–9, 1987.

6. Boronow RC, Morrow CP, Creasman WT, et al.: Surgical staging in endometrial cancer: Clinical-pathologic findings of a prospective study. *Obstet Gynecol* 63(6):825–32, 1984.

7. Creasman WT, DeGeest K, DiSaia PJ, Zaino RJ: Significance of true surgical pathologic staging: A Gynecologic Oncology Group Study. *Am J Obstet Gynecol* 181(1):31–4, 1999.

8. Abeler VM, Kjorstad KE: Endometrial adenocarcinoma in Norway. A study of a total population. *Cancer* 67(12):3093–103, 1991.

9. Lewis BV, Stallworthy JA, Cowdell R: Adenocarcinoma of the body of the uterus. *J Obstet Gynaecol Br Commonw* 77(4):343–8, 1970.

10. Creasman WT, Morrow CP, Bundy BN, et al.: Surgical pathologic spread patterns of endometrial cancer. A Gynecologic Oncology Group Study. *Cancer* 60(8, Suppl.):2035–41, 1987.

11. Connelly PJ, Alberhasky RC, Christopherson WM: Carcinoma of the endometrium. III. Analysis of 865 cases of adenocarcinoma and adenoacanthoma. *Obstet Gynecol* 59(5):569–75, 1982.

12. Lurain JR, Rice BL, Rademaker AW, et al.: Prognostic factors associated with recurrence in clinical stage I adenocarcinoma of the endometrium. *Obstet Gynecol* 78(1):63–9, 1991.

13. Kadar N, Malfetano JH, Homesley HD: Determinants of survival of surgically staged patients with endometrial carcinoma histologically confined to the uterus: Implications for therapy. *Obstet Gynecol* 80(4):655–9, 1992.

14. Morrow CP, Bundy BN, Kurman RJ, et al.: Relationship between surgical-pathological risk factors and outcome in clinical stage I and II carcinoma of the endometrium: A Gynecologic Oncology Group study. *Gynecol Oncol* 40(1):55–65, 1991.

15. Genest P, Drouin P, Gerig L, et al.: Prognostic factors in early carcinoma of the endometrium. *Am J Clin Oncol* 10(1):71–7, 1987.

16. De Muelenaere GF: Prognostic factors in endometrial carcinoma. *S Afr Med J* 49(41):1695–8, 1975.

17. DiSaia PJ, Creasman WT, Boronow RC, Blessing JA: Risk factors and recurrent patterns in stage I endometrial cancer. *Am J Obstet Gynecol* 151(8):1009–15, 1985.

18. Turner DA, Gershenson DM, Atkinson N, et al.: The prognostic significance of peritoneal cytology for stage I endometrial cancer. *Obstet Gynecol* 74(5):775–80, 1989.

19. Abeler VM, Kjorstad KE: Serous papillary carcinoma of the endometrium: A histopathological study of 22 cases. *Gynecol Oncol* 39(3):266–71, 1990.

20. Rutledge F: The role of radical hysterectomy in adenocarcinoma of the endometrium. *Gynecol Oncol* 2:331–47, 1974.

21. Trimble EL, Kosary C, Park RC: Lymph node sampling and survival in endometrial cancer. *Gynecol Oncol* 71(3):340–3, 1998.

22. Zaino RJ, Kurman RJ, Brunetto VL, et al.: Villoglandular adenocarcinoma of the endometrium: A clinicopathologic study of 61 cases: A Gynecologic Oncology Group study. *Am J Surg Pathol* 22(11):1379–85, 1998.

23. Christopherson WM, Alberhasky RC, Connelly PJ: Carcinoma of the endometrium: I. A clinicopathologic study of clear-cell carcinoma and secretory carcinoma. *Cancer* 49(8):1511–23, 1982.

24. Symonds DA: Prognostic value of pathologic features and DNA analysis in endometrial carcinoma. *Gynecol Oncol* 39(3):272–6, 1990.

25. Wilson TO, Podratz KC, Gaffey TA, et al.: Evaluation of unfavorable histologic subtypes in endometrial adenocarcinoma. *Am J Obstet Gynecol* 162(2):418–26, 1990.

26. Hendrickson M, Ross J, Eifel P, et al.: Uterine papillary serous carcinoma: A highly malignant form of endometrial adenocarcinoma. *Am J Surg Pathol* 6(2):93–108, 1982.

27. Gallion HH, van Nagell JRJ, Powell DF, et al.: Stage I serous papillary carcinoma of the endometrium. *Cancer* 63(11):2224–8, 1989.

28. Sherman ME, Bitterman P, Rosenshein NB, et al.: Uterine serous carcinoma. A morphologically diverse neoplasm with unifying clinicopathologic features. *Am J Surg Pathol* 16(6):600–10, 1992.

29. Aquino-Parsons C, Lim P, Wong F, Mildenberger M: Papillary serous and clear cell carcinoma limited to endometrial curettings in FIGO stage 1a and 1b endometrial adenocarcinoma: Treatment implications. *Gynecol Oncol* 71(1):83–6, 1998.

30. Kadar N, Homesley HD, Malfetano JH: Positive peritoneal cytology is an adverse factor in endometrial carcinoma only if there is other evidence of extrauterine disease. *Gynecol Oncol* 46(2):145–9, 1992.

31. Connell PP, Rotmensch J, Waggoner S, Mundt AJ: The significance of adnexal involvement in endometrial carcinoma. *Gynecol Oncol* 74(1):74–9, 1999.

32. Creasman WT: Prognostic significance of hormone receptors in endometrial cancer. *Cancer* 71:1467–70, 1993.

33. Kadar N, Malfetano JH, Homesley HD: Steroid receptor concentrations in endometrial carcinoma: Effect on survival in surgically staged patients. *Gynecol Oncol* 50(3):281–6, 1993.

34. Kleine W, Maier T, Geyer H, Pfleiderer A: Estrogen and progesterone receptors in endometrial cancer and their prognostic relevance. *Gynecol Oncol* 38(1):59–65, 1990.

35. Friberg LG, Norén H: Prognostic value of steroid hormone receptors for 5-year survival in stage II endometrial cancer. *Cancer* 71(11):3570–4, 1993.

36. Aalders J, Abeler V, Kolstad P, Onsrud M: Postoperative external irradiation and prognostic parameters in stage I endometrial carcinoma: Clinical and histopathologic study of 540 patients. *Obstet Gynecol* 56(4):419–27, 1980.

37. Gal D, Recio FO, Zamurovic D, Tancer ML: Lymphovascular space involvement—A prognostic indicator in endometrial adenocarcinoma. *Gynecol Oncol* 42(2):142–5, 1991.

38. Feltmate CM, Duska LR, Chang Y, et al.: Predictors of recurrence in surgical stage II endometrial adenocarcinoma. *Gynecol Oncol* 73(3):407–11, 1999.

39. Iversen OE, Utaaker E, Skaarland E: DNA ploidy and steroid receptors as predictors of disease course in patients with endometrial carcinoma. *Acta Obstet Gynecol Scand* 67(6):531–7, 1988.

40. Britton LC, Wilson TO, Gaffey TA, et al.: Flow cytometric DNA analysis of stage I endometrial carcinoma. *Gynecol Oncol* 34(3):317–22, 1989.

41. Ambros RA, Kurman RJ: Identification of patients with stage I uterine endometrioid adenocarcinoma at high risk of recurrence by DNA ploidy, myometrial invasion, and vascular invasion. *Gynecol Oncol* 45(3):235–9, 1992.

42. Berchuck A, Rodriguez G, Kinney RB, et al.: Overexpression of HER-2/neu in endometrial cancer is associated with advanced stage disease. *Am J Obstet Gynecol* 164:15–21, 1991.

43. Hetzel DJ, Wilson TO, Keeney GL, et al. HER-2/neu expression: A major prognostic factor in endometrial cancer. *Gynecol Oncol* 47(2):179–85, 1992.

44. Fujimoto I, Shimizu Y, Hirai Y, et al.: Studies on ras oncogene activation in endometrial carcinoma. *Gynecol Oncol* 48(2):196–202, 1993.

45. Ozsaran AA, Turker S, Dikmen Y, et al.: p53 staining as a prognostic indicator in endometrial carcinoma. *Eur J Gynaecol Oncol* 20(2):156–9, 1999.

46. Nanbu K, Konishi I, Mandai M, et al.: Prognostic significance of heat shock proteins HSP70 and HSP90 in endometrial carcinomas. *Cancer Detect Prev* 22(6):549–55, 1998.

47. Falcon O, Chirino R, Leon L, et al.: Low levels of cathepsin D are associated with a poor prognosis in endometrial cancer. *Br J Cancer* 79(3-4):570–6, 1999.

48. Nordstrom B, Bergstrom R, Strang P: Prognostic index models in stage I and II endometrial carcinoma. *Anticancer Res* 18(5B):3717–24, 1998.

49. Bokhman JV: Two pathogenetic types of endometrial carcinoma. *Gynecol Oncol* 15(1):10–7, 1983.

50. Hicks ML, Phillips JL, Parham G, et al.: The National Cancer Data Base report on endometrial cancer in African-American women. *Cancer* 83(12):2629–37, 1998.

51. Schneider J, Centeno M, Saez F, et al.: Preoperative CA-125, CA 19-9 and nuclear magnetic resonance in endometrial carcinoma: Correlation with surgical stage. *Tumor Biol* 20(1):25–9, 1999.

52. Cheng WF, Chen CA, Lee CN, et al.: Preoperative ultrasound study in predicting lymph node metastasis for endometrial cancer patients. *Gynecol Oncol* 71(3):424–7, 1998.

CHAPTER 34

Cancer of the Ovary and Fallopian Tube

SERGIO PECORELLI, LUCIA ZIGLIANI, and FRANCO E. ODICINO

OVARIAN CANCER

In both treatment and management of carcinoma of the ovary, a series of endpoints has been identified. Such endpoints are widely mentioned in the literature and will be analyzed in this chapter by following the guidelines suggested in the first part of this book, "Principles of Prognostic Factors." Overall, the probability of cure of ovarian cancer is low, 41.6% 5-year survival (Volume 23 of the *FIGO Annual Report on the Results of Treatment in Gynecological Cancer*), even though in the last 20 years it has increased at least by one third.[1] The improvement of overall survival thus represents the main objective of prospective clinical research, with study designs derived from the results obtained in other fields of clinical and basic research.

The different prognostic factors are discussed according to their subdivision into *essential, additional*, and *new and promising*. Each of these factors will be cross-referenced to *tumor-, host-* and *environment-related* characteristics, although some of them cannot be strictly classified under these specific categories. Prognostic factors will be dealt with in four different *scenarios*, chosen according to the importance they have in the management of this cancer.

SCENARIO I: OVERALL SURVIVAL (APPENDIX 34B.1)

Essential

Tumor-related Prognostic Factors It is fundamental to differentiate between frankly malignant epithelial ovarian tumors and those of borderline

---

* This section on ovarian cancer was written by S. Pecorelli, L. Zigliani, and F. Odicino.

Prognostic Factors in Cancer, 2nd edition, Edited by Mary K. Gospodarowicz
ISBN 0-471-40633-3   Copyright © 2001 Wiley-Liss, Inc.

malignancy (otherwise classified as "of *low malignant potential*").[2] The diagnosis of borderline tumors depends on the absence of stromal invasion in the primary ovarian tumor, but it does not consider the extraovarian spread of the disease.[3,4] Borderline tumors represent 5–10% of ovarian neoplasms and are mainly diagnosed in early stages. They have an overall 5-year survival ranging from 85% to 95%.[1] The only subgroup of borderline tumors with a poor prognosis are advanced-stage mucinous tumors (5% of the whole group of borderline tumors, 15% of those with mucinous histology), which have the histological appearances of borderline malignancy but are associated with pseudomyxoma peritonei: it has recently been established that most, if not all, ovarian mucinous tumors associated with pseudomyxoma peritonei are metastatic tumors of gastrointestinal origin (mostly appendiceal neoplasms, and rarely pancreas and colon cancers). Among true mucinous ovarian borderline tumors, those defined as endocervical mucinous borderline tumor (EMBT) have a better prognosis compared with those defined as intestinal mucinous borderline tumor (IMBT) and rare mixed epithelial borderline tumor (MEBT).[5] The biology of borderline tumors is not clear. They share some histological characteristics with the frankly malignant tumors, although their clinical behavior is much less aggressive, even when diagnosed with extraovarian spread (peritoneal implants). Those implants can be subdivided into three different categories: (a) benign implants (endosalpingosis); (b) "noninvasive" implants; (c) "invasive" implants, the latter often suggesting the adoption of an adjuvant postsurgical treatment.[6] Apart from the obvious necessity to differentiate borderline malignancies from frankly malignant (invasive) ovarian epithelial tumors, the assessment of the extent of the disease (staging) is of paramount importance.

Ovarian cancers are staged following the definitions set by the International Federation of Gynecology and Obstetrics (FIGO) in its nomenclature updated in 1988 by its Committee on Gynecologic Oncology. The International Union Against Cancer (UICC) and American Joint Committee on Cancer (AJCC) adapted the FIGO system and published the TNM classification for ovarian cancer (see Appendix 34A.1). Staging ovarian cancer requires a surgical procedure with final aims of removing as much disease as possible (tumor debulking), and defining the true extent of the cancer. The *stage* of the disease is the most important prognostic factor in invasive ovarian cancer, more than in borderline tumors. Staging enables the clinician to plan appropriate treatment. Most scientific papers are unanimous in recognizing the stage's independent prognostic significance.[7]

In early-stage cancers, the prognostic value of the *histological grade* has been widely assessed,[8] even if methods for grade assessment are not uniform and subjective, hence loaded with a high inter- and intraobserver variability. In early-stage ovarian cancer, the risk of dying of the disease is almost doubled when tumors are moderately or poorly differentiated, compared with those that are well differentiated.

In patients diagnosed with advanced-stage disease, overall survival is not only related to the *initial tumor burden*, but tends to decrease with the increase of *postsurgical residual tumor mass*, thus representing one of the most predictive factors of survival. It should be kept in mind, however, that this prognostic factor is not only tumor related but also host and environment related, since the biological characteristics of the tumor itself are challenged by the patient's response to the tumor's presence. Moreover, the intrinsic biologic tumor's aggressiveness and the patient's reactivity to the disease determine the modality and the sites of the tumor spread, which are subsequently challenged by the ability of the surgeon to debulk as much tumor as possible. Although in the scientific literature different cutoffs to define the "optimal" residual disease have been proposed (<2 cm, <1 cm, <0.5 cm) and from time to time accepted, cytoreduction should now be considered truly "optimal" when the surgeon leaves no gross residual disease.[9,10] In patients with small-volume residual disease, prognosis is directly related to the number of implants.

Host-related Prognostic Factors   *Age* and *performance status* have been thoroughly evaluated. Both demonstrated their impact on prognosis, even if not always as independent variables.[9,11] Their impact on clinical management is clear: an older patient is more likely to be affected by physical impairment thus lowering the possibility of undergoing an extensive surgical debulking, and of submitting to a more aggressive (and often more toxic) chemotherapy. The same applies to patients with low performance status. Patients with low performance status are less likely to be recruited to randomized clinical trials.

Environment-related Prognostic Factors   Several articles in the literature have addressed the influence of quality of care in patients affected by ovarian cancer treated in different settings. It has been noted that patients treated by the *gynecologic oncologist* live better and longer than those treated by the general obstetrician/gynecologist or by the general surgeon. The gynecologic oncologist more thoroughly assesses the extent of disease (intensive surgical staging), particularly in early clinical stage tumors. Moreover, the gynecologic oncologist is more frequently able to optimally debulk ovarian cancer (small-size residual tumor), which independently impacts on survival.[12]

Finally, the gynecologic oncologist can more appropriately plan the treatment and is more often involved in clinical research trials, thus offering the patient the best and most updated therapy. The *type of chemotherapy* is of prognostic importance for all categories of ovarian cancer patients. Meta-analyses published in the scientific literature have shown that platinum-based chemotherapy is superior to non-platinum-based chemotherapy (in early and advanced stages), and that combination platinum-based chemotherapy has been proven to be superior to single-drug chemotherapy (advanced-stage patients).[9]

Additional

Tumor-related Prognostic Factors   Among pathological factors that better define prognosis of ovarian cancer patients, but do not alter the therapeutic plan, the *histological grade* in advanced-stage disease is important. Cases that are clearly at one extreme of the grading system (from well to poorly differentiated) can be allotted to good or bad prognostic categories. In spite of all the efforts made by gynecologic pathologists worldwide, a universal grading system has not been agreed upon. All techniques to define the histological grading are subjective and therefore have a high degree of inter- and intraobserver variability. In view of this, in advanced ovarian cancer patients, the impact of the histological grading on prognosis is not so strong as in patients with early-stage disease, although it provides the clinician with fundamental information.[13,14] Any statement about the prognostic significance of *histological type* in frankly malignant epithelial ovarian cancer must be tempered by the fact that there is a high degree of subjectivity in assigning the histological type. The histological type has not been proven to be a prognostic factor in ovarian carcinoma: stage for stage and grade for grade, the serous and endometrioid types have the same prognosis. Although Stage III–IV mucinous carcinoma have an unusually poor prognosis, no conclusion can be drawn as for the impact of histological type on overall survival. The same applies to clear-cell carcinoma, which is usually thought to be the histological type with the worst prognosis among malignant epithelial ovarian tumors.[10,15]

DNA ploidy of frankly malignant ovarian carcinomas, as determined in either flow or image cytometry, has emerged as an important independent prognostic factor in most studies. Patients with aneuploid tumors have a worse prognosis compared with those with diploid tumors. This applies to both advanced- and early-stage disease.[16,17]

In borderline tumors, the impact of DNA ploidy on prognosis is more controversial, although a high prognostic significance has been observed in many studies.

Lymph-node involvement is supposed to have a lower impact on prognosis compared to intra-abdominal spread, and often does not alter the therapeutic strategy. Nevertheless, it has been observed in selected studies that an inverse correlation exists between *lymph-node status* and overall survival with a lower 5-year survival in patients with positive lymph nodes. The assessment of the impact of lymph-node status on prognosis is, however, limited by the inconsistency in the collected information, especially in those affected by advanced-stage disease.[18]

Both absolute levels and half-life of *CA125* have been demonstrated to be good prognostic indicators. An absolute CA125 value >70 U/mL after the second cycle of chemotherapy has been shown to be the best of all prognostic factors, although it is not reliable enough to be used alone to indicate a change in therapy. The serum CA125 half-life of less than 20 days correlates significantly with survival and with tumor regression (response to chemotherapy).[19]

Host-related Prognostic Factors It is well established that the genetic loss of *BRCA1* is important in the pathogenesis of hereditary breast and ovarian cancer. However, the role of BRCA1 in nonfamilial cancers, which represent the vast majority of these diseases, is not yet clear. BRCA1 is important for monitoring genome integrity. Women who carry germline mutations in BRCA1 develop ovarian cancer at a younger median age compared with noncarriers.

A series of studies has implicated BRCA1 mutations as both a favorable and an unfavorable prognostic factor. It was reported recently that women with ovarian cancer who carry the Ashkenazi mutations in BRCA1 had more favorable survival compared to controls. Studies from other groups have not confirmed the favorable survival of BRCA1 carriers. A Swedish population-based study on women with BRCA1-associated ovarian cancer evidenced a transient survival advantage — lasting for 2 to 3 years — in patients with this 17q mutation that did not persist over time. On the contrary, a U.S. case control study showed a highly significant survival advantage in BRCA1-carrier patients affected by advanced ovarian cancer.[20]

Surgical assessment of a clinically complete remission after primary surgery and first-line chemotherapy (second look) provides prognostic information of great importance, since there are no clinical methods with sufficiently high sensitivity able to define a patient as free of disease: 30 to 40% of patients with clinically complete remission and normal CA125 present subclinical persistence of disease at second look. Nevertheless, patients with pathologically complete remission develop a relapse within an unpredictable period and only half of them survive 5 years. The prognostic significance of a complete surgically assessed remission is therefore of utmost importance, since these patients survive longer compared to those who do not achieve it, even though not all of them can be considered "cured."[13]

At present, the achievement of a pathologically complete remission should be considered an additional prognostic factor, up to when ongoing controlled clinical trials show the best management of these patients.

Environment-related Prognostic Factors Several investigators have studied the role of ultraradical surgery to optimally debulk the tumor. The most commonly used procedure was partial bowel resection. The role of splenectomy or peritoneal stripping of the diaphragm also has been evaluated. It appears that these operative procedures are prognostically of benefit only if the patient has been rendered grossly free of any residual disease. The role of pelvic and paraortic lymphadenectomy is still a topic for discussion among researchers. Whether lymphadenectomy is only diagnostic or is also therapeutic has not yet been established. It does appear, however, that there is a role for lymphadenectomy, particularly in early-stage disease in order to identify those patients with more advanced disease. Without lymphadenectomy a significant number of patients with apparent early disease but with nodal metastases would be unknown and therefore would not have optimal treatment. According to some studies, there seems to be a correlation between lymph-node status and overall survival with decreased 5-year survival in patients with positive pelvic/paraortic nodes. On the contrary, survival seems to be better in patients with FIGO Stage IIIC based on lymph-node status compared only with those patients with Stage IIIC based on intra-abdominal spread of the disease.

These data should not be considered as conclusive, but suggestive of the true prognostic impact of lymph-node status on overall survival.[18] Based upon evidence from two large prospective randomized trials, which showed that pacli-taxel plus cisplatin was superior to cyclophosphamide plus cisplatin in terms of response rate, progression-free survival, and overall survival, the combination of taxane plus platinoid represents the new standard regimen. This combination has demonstrated survival benefits for patients with suboptimally as well as optimally debulked disease. Toxicities with the paclitaxel/cisplatin regimen are accept-able even if higher than those observed with the cyclophosphamide/cisplatin regimen.[21,22] For this reason, carboplatin has replaced cisplatin in the association with paclitaxel, since, up to now, it has shown a more favorable toxicity profile with equivalent efficacy. Randomized clinical trials are under way in Europe and North America to evaluate the impact of this combination regimen.

New and Promising

Tumor-related Prognostic Factors   Many studies and published data refer to this category. Only prognostic factors, which have been considered relevant both by clinicians and researchers, are mentioned here. Among pathological and histological prognostic factors, the *quantitative morphometric analyses* of ovarian carcinoma are thought to provide objective and reproducible data. Measurements of nuclear variables, such as nuclear area, nuclear volume, or shortest nuclear axis, provide important independent prognostic information.[23] However, there is currently no consensus on a particular nuclear variable that would offer the most powerful prognostic information, since different studies have yielded conflicting results. The study of *cellular proliferative activity*, which can be measured with different methods (i.e., mitotic counts), flow cytometric determination of the S-phase fraction, proliferation antigens such as proliferating-cell nuclear antigen (PCNA), and MIB-1 (for detection of Ki-67 antigen), could not identify a single independent prognostic factor. Studies on the prognostic value of these different variables showed conflicting results.[24] To solve the questions raised, further studies are needed. Studies evaluating the measurement of cellular expression of silver-stained nucleolar organizer region (AgNOR) proteins as a prognostic factor have produced conflicting results and have failed to establish such counts as an independent prognostic factor. This is also due to the fact that it is not clear whether *AgNOR counts* reflect the proliferative activity or the ploidy of the tumor. Many ovarian carcinomas contain *steroid receptors*, and although there have been both claims and denials that receptor-positive neoplasms have better prognosis than receptor-negative tumors, no clear agreement has been reached.[25] Studies on tumor *angiogenesis* as assessed by microvessel counts have failed to establish that this is an independent prognostic factor.

Since the relations between the tumor and the *immune system (cellular or humoral)* are far from being understood, no specific immune reaction is likely to become — in the short run — a significant prognostic factor. Although many specific aspects of this area of research (oncologic immunology) have been thoroughly examined, some of the most important of these raised more questions, which are still open. It is difficult to strictly classify most of these aspects as being tumor or host related. *Macrophage colony stimulating factor* (CSF-1) and *interleukin-6* (IL-6) have been shown to have some promise in small studies. Markedly elevated levels of CSF-1 in the serum and ascites in epithelial ovarian cancer patients have been associated with a poor prognosis. Many other cytokines, chemokines, and growth factors seem to play important roles in the natural history of ovarian carcinoma, and may prove to be of prognostic significance in wider trials. Recently, the *heat-shock protein* (HSP) family was proposed as a class of antiapoptotic genes, in addition to Bcl-2 an inhibitor of apoptosis protein families of genes. HSP27, HSP60, HSP70, HSP90 showed some correlation with prognosis (and response to chemotherapy HSP27)[26,27] in ovarian epithelial cancer, although in multivariate analyses most of them failed to demonstrate an independent value.

An increasingly high number of molecular biology studies on cancer of the ovary have been published in the last few years. Many of these examined the role of *p53* in the development, progression, and response to treatment of ovarian carcinoma. Mutation of p53 and overexpression of mutant p53 products are more common in advanced-stage (40–60%) than in early-stage disease (15%). Some studies have suggested that p53 overexpression in Stage III–IV disease is associated with a 10–20% decrease in 5-year survival.[28,29] Among other tumor suppressor genes, *loss of heterozygosity* (LOH) at the retinoblastoma (RB) gene locus has been frequently observed. However, reduced RB expression deserves further evaluation, especially as an adverse prognostic factor in Stage I disease. LOH analysis is a new tool allowing a deeper and more specific evaluation of DNA, hence highlighting genetic anomalies, which might turn into clinically useful prognostic factors. Although this phenomenon is more often present in advanced-stage disease, only a few loci have been identified as prognostic indicators of a survival disadvantage. None of these has been shown to be an independent prognostic factor in multivariate analysis.[30] *Comparative genomic hybridization* (CGH), a new technique that can thoroughly and simultaneously analyze thousands of genes, is now being applied to the study of ovarian cancer. CGH could play a key role thanks to its more precise and wide range of genetic analysis, enabling the identification of different patterns of increased/decreased gene expression possibly relevant to different histological types of ovarian cancer, although up to the present results have yet to be achieved.[31]

Overexpression of *c-erbB-2, ras,* and *myc* oncogenes are observed in a high number of ovarian cancer cases. Attempts to correlate these observations with prognosis have failed mainly due to methodological bias and untargeted study designs.

A series of new methods for investigating carcinogenesis, and thus prognosis of ovarian cancer, require further evaluation, although some of these proved to be scientifically valid, but not clinically useful at this time. Among them are measurements of genomic alterations, patterns of gene expression, mismatch repair enzymes, regulators of apoptosis (*bcl-2, bax*), adhesion molecules (*integrins, cadherins*), proteases (*uPA*), and suppressors of metastasis (*nm23*).[32]

Host-related Prognostic Factors The area of research of *oncologic immunology* has been studied in depth. However, no significant immunologic aspect has been identified as a significant prognostic factor. The significance of the lymphocyte infiltration in tumor tissues now seems to be better understood, since both interconnections and properties of complex cellular elements are being clarified. The *macrophage, T-lymphocytes, NK cells*, and recently *dendritic cells* are under evaluation. One of these or a combination of cellular elements or cytokincs may be possible prognostic markers.

Possible connections of the immune system and the function of different oncosuppressor genes (*BRCA1, BRCA2, OVCA1, OVCA2*) represent an important area of research, thus becoming a useful tool for prognosis and also, it is hoped, for therapy.[20]

Environment-related Prognostic Factors   The primary purpose of surgery in ovarian cancer is to debulk the disease to there being "no gross residual disease." Unfortunately, not all patients with advanced stage are optimally debulked despite maximum surgical effort. *Interval debulking surgery* (IDS), defined as a surgical procedure performed midway through a chemotherapy regimen in patients who did not achieve an optimal debulking at initial surgery, has been demonstrated to significantly lengthen progression-free and overall survival in a multi-institutional randomized trial. IDS was demonstrated to be an independent prognostic factor in reducing the risk of death by one-third. Data from this European study, although promising, will need further confirmation by other clinical control trials (the North American study GOG-152 is underway). Significance of interval debulking surgery may become an important improvement in prognosis in advanced ovarian cancer patients.[33]

Platinum-based *intraperitoneal chemotherapy* in patients with small residual disease after primary debulking surgery showed superior outcomes in two large randomized trials. However, long-term follow-up data are lacking; this promising approach therefore cannot be considered a standard treatment yet.

SCENARIO II: RESPONSE TO TREATMENT (APPENDIX 34B.2)

Essential

Tumor-related Prognostic Factors   In advanced-stage ovarian cancer patients, both the *substage* (FIGO IIIA and IIIB versus IIIC and IV) and the amount of *residual disease* (FIGO IIIC and IV) have been identified to be of prognostic importance in terms of response to first-line chemotherapy. However, these factors have a major importance for disease outcome on prognosis rather than chemotherapy response.

Additional

Host-related Prognostic Factors   Both *age* and *performance status* of the patient influence the choice and intensity of the administered chemotherapy regimen.

Environment-related Prognostic Factors   In two large prospective randomized trials, the combination of *paclitaxel and cisplatin* compared to cisplatin + cyclophosphamide showed a survival benefit not only for the optimally debulked patients, but also for those affected by suboptimal debulked disease. In the meta-analysis performed by the Advanced Ovarian Cancer Trialist Group (AOCTG), however, the preceding observation (survival advantage in suboptimally debulked patients) was noticed for the cyclophosphamide + adriamycin + cisplatin (CAP) regimen, too.[9]

New and Promising

Tumor-related Prognostic Factors   Numerous genes and/or proteins have been implicated in some series as important in platinum or taxane drug resistance. Among them are mutated *p53*, elevated *glutathione* (GSH), *lung resistance related protein* (LRP), *P-glycoprotein* (P-gp), *multidrug resistance protein* (MRP1) and *bcl-2/bax*. However, results have not always been consistent among studies. Definitive conclusions about the relevance of these molecular markers for drug resistance await further studies.[34]

SCENARIO III: RESPONSE TO SALVAGE THERAPY (APPENDIX 34B.3)

Essential

Tumor-related Prognostic Factors   The efficacy of a second-line/salvage chemotherapy is strictly related to the initial characteristics of the patient. Since these characteristics are relevant to both tumor and host, they will be dealt with only in this paragraph. According to the response to the previous chemotherapeutic treatment, three different prognostic groups are usually considered: (1) patients with no response to first-line chemotherapy, (2) patients with partial response and subsequent progression of disease, (3) patients who achieved a complete response but relapsed after a variable period of time. Second-line chemotherapy will have little or no efficacy at all on the first two groups, while in the third one it will be more effective according to the length of the chemotherapy-free interval. Moreover, it has been shown that, at the time of relapse, serous histological type, number of disease sites (≤ 2), and maximum size of the largest lesions (≤ 5 cm) are independently related to the response to second-or-more line chemotherapy.[35,36]

Additional

Tumor-related Prognostic Factors   Time from the last treatment (platinum-free interval <6 vs. ≥ 6 months) has been observed not to be an independent prognostic factor, since it correlated with tumor size.

New and Promising

Tumor-related Prognostic Factors Small studies were undertaken to evaluate whether immunophenotyping of advanced epithelial ovarian cancer could predict response to initial and second-line chemotherapy. Among several factors [c-erb-B-2, epidermal growth-factor receptor (EGFR), p53, tumor necrosis factor alpha (TNFα), estrogen receptor (ER), progesterone receptor (PgR), P-glycoprotein 170 (P170)], only the expression of the Ki67-defined antigen showed a significant correlation with the response to second-line chemotherapy.

SCENARIO IV: FERTILITY PRESERVATION (APPENDIX 34B.4)

Essential

Tumor-related Prognostic Factors In the past few years, the issue of conservative surgery in ovarian cancer patients has become important. The onset of an ovarian neoplasm in a fertile woman wishing to preserve the possibility of childbearing has raised many questions. In these cases, different prognostic factors should be taken into consideration in order to provide the patient with the best and most adequate conservative treatment. Histology represents the major aspect to be considered: in most cases, tumors of borderline malignancy do not contraindicate conservative treatment. Among frankly malignant tumors, conservative treatment is only performed in early-stage patients. In these patients, the histological degree of differentiation represents the major prognostic factor. Those with well-differentiated tumors (G1) are generally considered at low risk, while it is less certain how to tackle these with moderate differentiation (G2). It seems that the worsening prognosis from G1 to G2 is greater than that from G2 to G3.

Environment-related Prognostic Factors Quality of care is of paramount importance when dealing with the conservative treatment of ovarian cancer. These patients should be managed pre- and postoperatively by a gynecologic oncologist with the fundamental collaboration of an expert gynecologic pathologist.

FALLOPIAN TUBE CANCER

Carcinoma of the Fallopian tube is a very rare neoplasm representing 0.2–0.5% of gynecologic malignancies. Its prevalence is 2.9–3.6 cases/1,000,000 women/year. Only 83 cases observed in the years 1990 to 1992 were reported to the Editorial Office of the *FIGO Annual Report on the Results of Treatment in Gynecological Cancer*, thus limiting the possibility of a thorough analysis of the prognostic factors in this malignancy.[37] In 1991, the FIGO Committee on Gynecologic Oncology designed a specific staging classification for carcinoma

This section on Fallopian tube cancer was written by S. Pecorelli, L. Zigliani, and F. Odicino.

of the Fallopian tube, which up to that time was staged according to the ovarian cancer staging system (Table 34.1). Staging for Fallopian tube cancer is by the surgical pathological system. Operative findings prior to tumor debulking can be modified by histopathologic as well as clinical or radiological evaluation. The UICC and AJCC adapted the FIGO system and published the TNM classification for ovarian cancer (see Appendix 34A.2).

FIGO stage represents the most important prognostic factor. Stage I patients comprise more than one-third of all patients and show an 80% 5-year survival, while in Stage II, III, and IV patients 5-year survival is 50%, 35%, and 0%, respectively.[38,39] Most of the Fallopian tube carcinoma cases are histologically classified as serous adenocarcinoma, while other histological types are rare. The histological type has never been shown to be of prognostic significance for the outcome of the disease. The degree of differentiation and the degree of nuclear atypia both seem to be of limited prognostic impact, even though it is not clear whether the lack of prognostic importance is due to methodological limitations in defining the degree of differentiation or to the low impact on prognosis of the degree of differentiation itself.[40] The prognostic significance of the lymphatic spread of the disease is not yet clear. Pelvic, paraortic and groin lymph-node involvement are considered regional metastases and are reported in 30–50% of cases undergoing primary surgery. Fallopian tube carcinoma frequently causes distant relapses, especially in the lymph nodes.

Together with the stage, the amount of residual disease is considered the most important prognostic factor, thus highlighting the role of cytoreductive surgery (Appendix 34B.5). Although the importance of adjuvant treatment in early-stage disease is not clear, the improved prognosis observed in patients with advanced disease who were administered chemotherapy underlines a key role for adjuvant chemotherapy. Among biological factors, ploidy and overexpression of *p53* have shown some relevance regarding prognosis. In particular, p53 alterations seem to have a prognostic impact in stage 0 (carcinoma in situ).[41]

■■■■■ **APPENDIX 34A.1**

TNM Classification: Ovarian Cancer

T — Primary Tumor

TNM Categories	FIGO Stages	
TX		Primary tumor cannot be assessed
T0		No evidence of primary tumor
T1	I	Tumor limited to the ovaries
T1a	IA	Tumor limited to one ovary; capsule intact, no tumor on ovarian surface; no malignant cells in ascites or peritoneal washings
T1b	IB	Tumor limited to both ovaries; capsule intact, no tumor on ovarian surface; no malignant cells in ascites or peritoneal washings
T1c	IC	Tumor limited to one or both ovaries with any of the following: capsule ruptured, tumor on ovarian surface, malignant cells in ascites or peritoneal washings
T2	II	Tumor involves one or both ovaries with pelvic extension
T2a	IIA	Extension and/or implants on uterus and/or tube(s); no malignant cells in ascites or peritoneal washings
T2b	IIB	Extension to other pelvic tissues; no malignant cells in ascites or peritoneal washings
T2c	IIC	Pelvic extension (2a or 2b) with malignant cells in ascites or peritoneal washings
T3 and/or N1	III	Tumor involves one or both ovaries with microscopically confirmed peritoneal metastasis outside the pelvis and/or regional lymph-node metastasis
T3a	IIIA	Microscopic peritoneal metastasis beyond pelvis
T3b	IIIB	Macroscopic peritoneal metastasis beyond pelvis 2 cm or less in greatest dimension
T3c and/or N1	IIIC	Peritoneal metastasis beyond pelvis more than 2 cm in greatest dimension and/or regional lymph-node metastasis
M1	IV	Distant metastasis (excludes peritoneal metastasis)

N — Regional Lymph Nodes

NX Regional lymph nodes cannot be assessed

N0 No regional lymph-node metastasis

N1 Regional lymph-node metastasis

M — Distant Metastasis

MX Distant metastasis cannot be assessed

M0 No distant metastasis

M1 Distant metastasis

Stage Grouping			
Stage IA	T1a	N0	M0
Stage IB	T1b	N0	M0
Stage IC	T1c	N0	M0
Stage IIA	T2a	N0	M0
Stage IIB	T2b	N0	M0
Stage IIC	T2c	N0	M0
Stage IIIA	T3a	N0	M0
Stage IIIB	T3b	N0	M0
Stage IIIC	T3c	N0	M0
	Any T	N1	M0
Stage IV	Any T	Any N	M1

Source: Sobin LH, Wittekind Ch (eds.): *TNM classification of malignant tumors*, 5th ed. New York, Union Internationale Contre le Cancer Wiley-Liss, 1997.

■■■■■■■■ **APPENDIX 34A.2**

TNM Classification: Fallopian Tube

T — Primary Tumor

TNM Categories	FIGO Stages	
TX		Primary tumor cannot be assessed
T0		No evidence of primary tumor
Tis	0	Carcinoma in situ (preinvasive carcinoma)
T1	I	Tumor confined to Fallopian tube(s)
T1a	IA	Tumor limited to one tube, without penetrating the serosal surface; no ascites
T1b	IB	Tumor limited to both tubes, without penetrating the serosal surface; no ascites
T1c	IC	Tumor limited to one or both tube(s) with extension onto or through the tubal serosa, or with malignant cells in ascites or peritoneal washings
T2	II	Tumor involves one or both Fallopian tube(s) with pelvic extension
T2a	IIA	Extension and/or metastasis to uterus and/or ovaries
T2b	IIB	Extension to other pelvic structures
T2c	IIC	Pelvic extension (2a or 2b) with malignant cells in ascites or peritoneal washings
T3 and/or N1	III	Tumor involves one or both Fallopian tube(s) with peritoneal implants outside the pelvis and/or positive regional lymph nodes
T3a	IIIA	Microscopic peritoneal metastasis outside the pelvis
T3b	IIIB	Macroscopic peritoneal metastasis outside the pelvis 2 cm or less in greatest dimension
T3c and/or N1	IIIC	Peritoneal metastasis more than 2 cm in greatest dimension and/or positive regional lymph nodes
M1	IV	Distant metastasis (excludes peritoneal metastasis)

N — Regional Lymph Nodes

NX Regional lymph nodes cannot be assessed

N0 No regional lymph-node metastasis

N1 Regional lymph-node metastasis

M — Distant Metastasis

MX Distant metastasis cannot be assessed

M0 No distant metastasis

M1 Distant metastasis

Stage Grouping

Stage 0	Tis	N0	M0
Stage IA	T1a	N0	M0
Stage IB	T1b	N0	M0
Stage IC	T1c	N0	M0
Stage IIA	T2a	N0	M0
Stage IIB	T2b	N0	M0
Stage IIC	T2c	N0	M0
Stage IIIA	T3a	N0	M0
Stage IIIB	T3b	N0	M0
Stage IIIC	T3c	N0	M0
	Any T	N1	M0
Stage IV	Any T	Any N	M1

Source: Sobin LH, Wittekind Ch (eds.): *TNM classification of malignant tumors*, 5th ed. New York, Union Internationale Contre le Cancer Wiley-Liss, 1997.

APPENDIX 34B.1

Prognostic Factors for Overall Survival

Prognostic Factors	Tumor Related	Host Related	Environment Related
Essential	• Stage (tumor burden) • Histology — borderline — mucin ous — EMBT / IMBT/MEBT, others; borderline — benign/noninvasive implants, invasive implants; frankly malignant — frankly malignant • Grade (early stage — frankly malignant) • Initial tumor mass • Residual disease	• Age • Performance status • Residual disease	• Initial tumor mass vs. post-surgical residual disease • Quality of care — gynecologic oncologist, obstetrician/gynecologist, general surgeon • DDP based CT (early and advanced stages) • Combination of DDP-based first-line CT (advanced stages)
Additional	• Grade (advanced stage - frankly malignant) • Histology frankly malignant Stage III–IV — mucinous, others • DNA ploidy (frankly malignant) • Lymph-node status • CA125	• BRCA1 • pCR at second look	• Ultraradical surgery • Lymphadenectomy (early stages) • Combination of DDP + TAX-based first-line CT (suboptimally + optimally debulked pts)
New and Promising	• Quantitative morphometric analyses • Cellular proliferative activity • AgNOR counts • Tumor angiogenesis • Cytokines, chemokines, growth factors • Apoptosis • LOH • Other oncogenes	• Oncologic immunology • Oncogenes	• Interval debulking surgery (IDS) • Intraperitoneal CT (in small residual volumes)

■■■■■■■ **APPENDIX 34B.2**

Prognostic Factors for Response to First-line Treatment

Prognostic Factors	Tumor Related	Host Related	Environment Related
Essential	• FIGO substage • Residual disease		
Additional		• Age • Performance status	• CP vs. CAP CT (suboptimally debulked) • CP vs. TP CT (optimally debulked)
New and Promising	• p53 • Oncogenes • Molecular markers/proteins		

■■■■■■■ **APPENDIX 34B.3**

Prognostic Factors for Response to Salvage Therapy

Prognostic Factors	Tumor Related	Host Related	Environment Related
Essential	• Platinum CT sensitivity • Serous histological type • Number of disease sites (≤ 2) • Size of lesions (≤ 5 cm)		
Additional	• Platinum-free interval		
New and Promising	• Oncogenes		

■■■■■ **APPENDIX 34B.4**

Prognostic Factors for Fertility Preservation

Prognostic Factors	Tumor Related	Host Related	Environment Related

Essential	• Histology ⸺ frankly malignant
	• Stage ＼borderline
	• Grade malignant
			• Quality
			  of care ⸺ gynecologic
			           oncologist
			          ＼gynecologic
			           pathologist

Additional			
New and Promising			

■■■■■ **APPENDIX 34B.5**

Prognostic Factors in Fallopian Tube Cancer

Prognostic Factors	Tumor Related	Host Related	Environment Related

Essential	• Stage
	• Residual disease
			• Quality
			  of care ⸺ gynecologic
			           oncologist/
			           pathologist
			          ＼obstetrician/
			           gynecologist
			          ＼general surgeon
			• Adjuvant CT (advanced stages)

Additional	• Grade + degree of nuclear atypia • Histological type • Lymph-node status • Ploidy • p53		
New and Promising		• p53 alterations	

REFERENCES

1. Pecorelli S, Odicino F, Maisonneuve P, et al.: Carcinoma of the ovary. *J Epidemiol Biostat* 3(1):75, 1998.

2. Link CJ, Kohn E, Reed E: The relationship between borderline ovarian tumors and epithelial ovarian carcinoma: epidemiologic, pathologic and molecular aspects. *Gynecol Oncol* 60:347, 1996.

3. Bell DA, Scully RE: Serous borderline tumors of the peritoneum. *Am J Surg Pathol* 14:230, 1990.

4. Michael H, Roth LM: Invasive and non-invasive implants in ovarian serous tumors of low malignant potential. *Cancer* 57:1240, 1986.

5. Prat J: Ovarian tumors of borderline malignancy (tumors of low malignant potential): A critical appraisal. *Adv Anat Pathol* 6:247, 1999.

6. Gersherson DM: Contemporary treatment of borderline ovarian tumors. *Cancer Invest* 17:206, 1999.

7. Villa A, Parazzini F, Acerboni S, et al.: Survival and prognostic factors of early ovarian cancer. *Br J Cancer* 77:123, 1998.

8. Scully RE: *Histological typing of ovarian tumors (WHO International Histological Classification of Tumors)* 2nd ed. Berlin-New York, Springer- Verlag, 1999.

9. Advanced Ovarian Cancer Trialist Group: Chemotherapy in advanced ovarian cancer: An overview of randomised clinical trials. *BMJ* 303:884, 1991.

10. Makar AP, Baekelandt M, Tropé C, et al.: The prognostic significance of residual disease, FIGO substage, tumor histology, and grade in patients with FIGO III ovarian cancer. *Gynecol Oncol* 56:175, 1995.

11. DiSilvestro P, Peipert JF, Hogan JW, et al.: Prognostic value of clinical variables in ovarian cancer. *J Clin Epidemiol* 50:501, 1997.

12. Bristow RE, Montz FJ, Lagasse LD, et al.: Survival impact of surgical cytoreduction in stage IV epithelial ovarian cancer. *Gynecol Oncol* 72:278, 1999.

13. Tropé C: Prognostic factors in ovarian cancer. *Cancer Treat Res* 95:287, 1998.

14. Friedlander ML: Prognostic factors in ovarian cancer. *Semin Oncol* 25:305, 1998.

15. Tammela J, Geisler JP, Eskew PN, et al.: Clear cell carcinoma of the ovary: Poor: prognosis compared to serous carcinoma. *Eur J Gynecol Oncol* 19:438, 1998.

16. Reles AE, Gee C, Schellschmidt I, et al.: Prognostic significance of DNA content and S-phase fraction in epithelial ovarian carcinomas analyzed by image cytometry. *Gynecol Oncol* 71:3, 1998.

17. Rice LW, Mark SD, Berkowitz RS, et al.: Clinicopathologic variables, operative characteristics, and DNA ploidy in predicting outcome in ovarian epithelial carcinoma. *Obstet Gynecol* 86:379, 1995.

18. Di Re F, Baiocchi G, Fontanelli R, et al.: Systematic pelvic and paraortic lymphadenectomy for advanced ovarian cancer: Prognostic significance of node metastases. *Gynecol Oncol* 62:360, 1996.

19. Meier W, Stieber P, Hascholzner U, et al.: Prognostic significance of CA125 in patients with ovarian cancer and secondary debulking surgery. *Anticancer Res* 17:2945, 1997.

20. Lynch HT, Watson P: BRCA1, pathology, and survival. *J Clin Oncol* 16:395, 1998.

21. McGuire WP, Hoskins WJ, Brady MF, et al.: Cyclophosphamide and cisplatin compared with paclitaxel and cisplatin in patients with stage III and IV ovarian cancer. *N Engl J Med* 334:1, 1996.

22. Tropé C, Picard MJ, Stuart G, et al.: Improved survival with paclitaxel-cisplatin compared with cyclophosphamide-cisplatin in advanced ovarian cancer after a median follow-up of 39 months: Update of the EORTC, NOVOCA, NCIC, Scottish Intergroup Study. *Int J Gynecol Cancer* 9:57, 1999.

23. Liu CQ, Sasaki H, Fahey MT, et al.: Prognostic value of nuclear morphometry in patients with TNM stage T1 ovarian clear adenocarcinoma. *Br J Cancer* 79:1736, 1999.

24. Altavilla G, Marchetti M, Padovan P, et al.: Predictive value of proliferative cellular nuclear antigen (PCNA) and Ki67 antigen in advanced stage serous papilliferous ovarian cancer. *Eur J Gynaecol Oncol* 17:524, 1996.

25. Hemplin RE, Piver MS, Eltabbakh GH, et al.: Progesterone receptor status is a significant prognostic variable of progression free survival in advanced epithelial ovarian cancer. *Am J Clin Oncol* 21:447, 1998.

26. Arts HJ, Hollema H, Lemstra W, et al.: Heat shock protein 27 (HSP27) expression in ovarian carcinoma: relation in response to chemotherapy and prognosis. *Int J Cancer* 84:234, 1999.

27. Schneider J, Jimenez E, Marembach K, et al.: Co-expression of the MDR1 gene and HSP27 in human ovarian cancer. *Anticancer Res* 18:2967, 1998.

28. Anttila MA, Ji H, Juhola MT, et al.: The prognostic significance of p53 expression quantitated by computerized image analysis in epithelial ovarian cancer. *Int J Gynecol Pathol* 18:42, 1999.

29. Eltabbakh GH, Belinson JL, Kennedy AW, et al.: p53 is not an independent prognostic factor for patients with primary ovarian epithelial cancer. *Cancer* 80:892, 1997.

30. Saretzki G, Hoffmann U, Rohlke P, et al.: Identification of allelic losses in benign, borderline, and invasive epithelial tumors and correlation with clinical outcome. *Cancer* 80:1241, 1997.

31. Wolf NG, Abdul-Karim FW, Farver C, et al.: Analysis of ovarian borderline tumors using comparative genomic hybridization and fluorescence in situ hybridization. *Genes Chromosomes Cancer* 25:307, 1999.

32. Tai YT, Lee S, Niloff E, et al.: Bax Protein Expression and Clinical Outcome in Epithelial Ovarian Cancer. *J Clin Oncol* 16:2583, 1998.

33. van der Burgh MEL, Van Lent M, Buyse M, et al.: The effect of debulking surgery after induction chemotherapy on the prognosis in advanced epithelial ovarian cancer. *N Eng J Med* 332:629, 1995.

34. Izquierdo MA, van der Zee AG, Vermorken JB, et al.: Drug resistance associated marker LRP for prediction of response to chemotherapy and prognosis in advanced ovarian carcinoma. *J Natl Cancer Inst* 87:1230, 1995.

35. Eisenhauer EA, Vermorken JB, van Glabbecke M: Predictors of response to subsequent chemotherapy in platinum pre-treated ovarian cancer: A multivariate analysis of 704 patients. *Ann Oncol* 8:963, 1997.

36. Markman M: Prognostic factors in salvage therapy of ovarian cancer. *Ann Oncol* 8:937, 1997.

37. Pecorelli S, Odicino F, Maisonneuve P, et al.: Carcinoma of the Fallopian tube. *J Epidemiol Biostat* 3(1):63, 1998.

38. Baekelandt M, Kockx M, Wesling S, et al.: Primary adenocarcinoma of the Fallopian tube. Review of the literature. *Int J Gynecol Cancer* 3:65, 1993.

39. Nordin AJ: Primary carcinoma of the Fallopian tube: A 20 year literature review. *Obstet Gynecol Surv* 48:349,1994.

40. Wheeler JE: Diseases of the Fallopian tube in Kurman RJ (ed.): *Blaustein's pathology of the female genital.* New York, Springer Verlag, 1994.

41. Zheng W, Sung CJ, Cao P, et al.: Early occurrence and prognostic significance of p53 alteration in primary carcinoma of the Fallopian tube. *Gynecol Oncol* 64:38, 1997.

CHAPTER 35

Gestational Trophoblastic Disease

HEXTAN Y.S. NGAN and LING-CHUI WONG

Gestational trophoblastic disease (GTD) is a disease of the proliferative trophoblastic allografts and includes partial mole (PM), complete hydatidiform mole (CM), invasive mole, metastatic mole, choriocarcinoma (CC), and placental site trophoblastic tumor (PSTT). While CC and PSTT are definitely neoplastic, the various types of molar pregnancies are basically benign, but with a potential to behave like a malignant disease that requires chemotherapy. This potential malignant behavior is identified by the failure of regression of the human chorionic gonadotrophin (hCG) in the absence of a normal pregnancy and is termed gestational trophoblastic tumor (GTT) or gestational persistent trophoblastic disease (GPTD). The criteria for the diagnosis of postmolar GTT varies among different centers in the world.[1] Basically, if the hCG level fails to fall satisfactory over 3–4 weeks, or when there is a rise in the hCG level over 2–3 weeks, GTT is diagnosed and further investigations should be done to assess the extent of the disease. The risk or predictive factors of PTD following mole will be discussed in the first major section below.

In GTT, unlike other solid malignancies, metastasis does not always mean poor prognosis. If the metastatic lesion is a mole rather than CC, the prognosis is much better. However, histological confirmation is uncommon because most cases of GTT are treated with chemotherapy. Thus, other prognostic factors in addition to metastasis have to be taken into consideration in assessing the prognosis of a GTT. The prognostic factors of GTT are be discussed in the second major section below. PSTT arises from the intermediate trophoblasts and behaves quite differently from that of GTT and will be discussed separately in the final major section below.

Prognostic Factors in Cancer, 2nd edition, Edited by Mary K. Gospodarowicz.
ISBN 0-471-40633-3 Copyright © 2001 Wiley-Liss, Inc.

RISK FACTORS FOR PERSISTENT TROPHOBLASTIC DISEASE FOLLOWING MOLES

Tumor-related Factors

Histological Features   Histologically, there are two types of hydatidiform moles. PM has varying-sized chorionic villi with focal hydropic changes and trophoblastic hyperplasia. Embryonic or fetal tissues are often identified. Most of them are triploid in karyotype. The chance of PM progressing to GTT is lower (0.5–7.7%) than CM.[2,3] CM has generalized hydropic swelling of the chorionic villi and diffuse trophoblastic hyperplasia. Embryonic or fetal tissues are usually absent. Most of them are 46 XX in karyotype, and both sets of the haploid chromosomes are paternal in origin. The percentage of CM progressing to GTT varies from 5.6–36%,[4–7] depending on the criteria used for diagnosis.

Apart from the histological type of the hydatidiform mole, histopathological gradings assessing the degree of trophoblastic hyperplasia and atypia, placental-bed reaction had been considered as having inconclusive prognostic significance. Using multivariate analysis, Ayhan et al.[8] showed that trophoblastic hyperplasia was a powerful predictor of GTT in 82 cases of GTD. In the same study, marked nuclear atypia and necrosis, hemorrhage, though significant on univariate analysis, were not significant on multivariate analysis. These findings need further validation from a larger study.

Anatomic Extent of Disease   Hydatidiform mole may be locally invasive or metastatic. Invasive mole is usually diagnosed on hysterectomy, which is rarely performed nowadays. In the old days, metastatic moles were found in the vagina or lung on postmortem or rarely in a surgical pulmonary lobectomy specimen. They have the same potential to progress to GTT and the same HCG criteria are used for diagnosis. Vaginal or lung metastasis do not increase the risk of GTT.[9]

Molecular/Genetic Factors and Tumor Marker   DNA ploidy study by flow cytometry showed that CM is mainly diploid and PM is mainly triploid. Aneuploidy CM seems to have a higher risk for progressing to GTT,[10] but the evidence is inconclusive. Similarly, proliferative index assessed by flow cytometry seems to be predictive, as shown in some studies,[11] but not in others.[12] Proliferative activity as assessed by immunohistochemistry for PCNA and Ki67 also showed that they have no prognostic significance.[13,14] Telomerase activity also has been recently found to be a potential prognostic indicator in predicting GPTD.[15,16]

Chromosomal analysis of CM showed mainly 46 XX of androgenic origin. About 10–20% of CM are heterozygous, with 4–15% of 46 XY. Some studies have shown that heterozygous CM such as 46 XY has a higher risk of progressing to GTT,[17] which was not confirmed by others.[18,19]

Since activation of proto-oncogene may turn a benign lesion to a malignant one, expression of epidermal growth factor receptor and c-erbB-2 expression in

CM were studied. However, no significant difference was observed between those that regressed and those that progressed to GTT.[20,21]

HCG is the diagnostic marker for GTT. However, HCG molecules in GTD are heterogeneous or degraded in serum and urine. Free β-subunits, free α-subunits, core-hCG, or nicked HCG may interfere with the assay of the hCG.[22] It is thus important to choose an appropriate assay kit. In the management of GTT, a kit that measures the total β-hCG is appropriate. Some studies showed that CM with high free β-subunits to total β-hCG ratio or high preevacuation serum hCG have higher risk of progressing to GTT, but confirmation is required.[23]

Clinical Parameters   Large uterine size, bilateral luteal cysts, and complications of the cysts, symptoms of preeclampsia or hyperthyroidism and history of previous molar pregnancy are associated with higher risk of GTT. However, nowadays, with the early diagnosis of molar pregnancy by ultrasound, some of these symptoms and signs, which occur mainly in second trimester molar pregnancy, are rarely seen. On the other hand, the introduction of Doppler study showed that a low resistant and pulsality index of the uterine arteries in CM predicts a higher risk of progressing to GTT.[24] This finding needs further confirmation.

In one study,[25] twin conception with CM and coexisting fetus is associated with a 55% risk for developing GTT.

Host-related Factors

Demographic   GTD is more common in Asia and Latin America than in the West. However, there is no evidence to show that different geographic or ethnic areas predict a difference in the risk of developing GTT from CM. Extremes of maternal age is one of the risk factor of GTT. A recent multivariate analysis[8] showed that maternal age over 35 was an important risk factor.

Immune Status   CM is an allograft of androgenic origin, and immunological response may play a role in the eradication of trophoblastic cells. Higher levels of serum interleukin-1-β, interleukin-6, and tumor necrosis factor α were observed in CM, which progressed to GTT.[26]

Environment-related Factors

Treatment Related   Treatment of mole is by uterine evacuation. The risk of GTT increases with the use of oxytocics. Thus, termination of molar pregnancy using oxytocics and the like, such as mifepristone, should be avoided.[27]

Quality of Care and Geography   Mole is a benign condition. However, 6–36% progress to GTT, which it diagnosed early, has a good prognosis with almost 100% cure. It is thus important to follow up all patients with molar pregnancy by serial serum hCG assay. A central registry helps to keep track of these patients. A centralized laboratory for the serum hCG assay is not only cost effective but is essential to ensure good quality control.

PROGNOSTIC FACTORS OF GESTATIONAL TROPHOBLASTIC DISEASE

Tumor-related Factors

Histological Factors   CC is an aggressive tumor, and unless treated early has a poor prognosis. Since most cases of GTT have no histological confirmation, a high hCG status in the absence of pregnancy or nongestational hCG secreting tumor after normal pregnancy is assumed to be CC. On the other hand, a high hCG status after molar pregnancy could be due to invasive or metastatic mole, which has a more favorable prognosis. The assessment of this risk factor was reflected in the type of antecedent pregnancy, where more weight was given to antecedent normal pregnancy or abortion than to molar pregnancy in various risk-scoring systems, such as the World Health Organization (WHO)[28] (Table 35.1) or the Charing Cross scoring system.[29]

Anatomic Extent of Disease   GTTs spread locally and systematically. Hematogenous spread is early because of the vascular invasive nature of trophoblastic tissues. Hence, anatomical staging has some limitations when considering the prognosis with advancing stage. Indeed, the International Federation of Gynaecology and Obsetrics (FIGO) staging system before 1992 was based purely on anatomical classification and Stage III disease may do as well as a Stage I disease. Therefore, other risk factors (serum hCG and interval

TABLE 35.1   WHO Prognostic Score

Prognostic Factors	Score[a]			
	0	1	2	4
Age (years)	<39	>39	—	—
Antecedent pregnancy	Mole	Abortion	Term	—
Interval (months)	<4	4–6	7–12	>12
HCG (IU/L)	$<10^3$	$10^3 - 10^4$	$10^4 - 10^5$	$>10^5$
ABO groups	—	O × A	B	—
(female × male		A × O	AB	
Largest tumor, including uterine tumor	—	3–5 cm	>5 cm	—
Site of metastasis	—	Spleen Kidney	GI tract Liver	Brain
Number of metastasis	—	1–4	4–8	>8
Prior chemotherapy	—	—	Single drug	2 or more drugs

[a]*Total score*: <4 = low risk; 5–8 = medium risk; >8 = high risk.

TABLE 35.2 FIGO Staging of Gestational Trophoblastic Disease (1992)

Stage		Substage
I	Disease confined to the uterus	A = no risk factor[a]
II	Disease extends outside uterus, but is limited to the genital structures (adnexa, vagina, broad ligament)	B = one risk factor
III	Disease extends to the lungs with or without known genital tract involvement	C = two risk factors
IV	All other metastatic sites	

[a]*Risk factors*: (1) HCG >100 000 IU/L; (2) interval of disease >6 months from termination of the antecedent pregnancy.

between treatment and precedent pregnancy) were added in the FIGO staging after 1992 (Table 35.2) to improve the prediction of prognosis.[30] The International Union Against Cancer (UICC) and American Joint Committee on Cancer (AJCC) have adopted the 1992 FIGO proposal and published a TNM classification (see Appendix 35A).

The site of metastasis is of prognostic significance. Metastasis to brain and liver has poor outcome, whereas metastasis to vagina or lung is of little significance.[31] Metastasis to other organs, such as the gastrointestinal (GI) tract, spleen, or kidneys are probably of intermediate significance.

In GTT, the extent of the disease is also reflected in the size of the largest tumor, the number of metastases, and the number of metastatic sites. Indeed, these factors are incorporated in various risk-scoring systems.[28,29,32] Recent studies using multivariate analysis showed that the number of sites of metastasis is probably one of the more important prognostic factors.[33]

Molecular/Genetic Factors and Tumor Marker Serum HCG is not only the diagnostic marker for GTT but is also of prognostic significance. The higher the level of serum hCG at the time of diagnosis of GTT (not molar pregnancy), the worse the prognosis. A level greater than 100,000 IU/L predict poor prognostic outcome.[34,35] In fact, serum hCG probably reflects the total body burden of viable tumor, and in multivariate analysis, other factors, such as size of tumor or number of metastatic sites become insignificant.[36]

Several proto-oncogenes were studied, and epidermal growth factor receptor, c-erbB-2, mdm2, p53, and p21, though expressed to various degrees in mole or CC, did not show themselves as having prognostic importance.[37–39]

Clinical Parameters The duration of GTT as measured by the time from the termination of the previous pregnancy to the diagnosis of GTT is of prognostic significance. Various studies showed that duration ranging from 4 to 12 months had prognostic significance.[29,40,41] This probably reflects late diagnosis with possible extensive spread of the tumor leading to poorer prognosis.

Host-related Factors

Demographic   Old age is an important prognostic factor. One study showed that age greater than 39 years has poorer outcome.[29] In a multivariate analysis, age was not an independent prognostic factor.[33] However, good performance status would affect the result of treatment, since chemotherapy of high risk GTT tends to be quite toxic.

Immune Status   The human leukocyte antigen (HLA) typing and blood group of the patient and her partner have been shown to be of prognostic significance.[42] The mortality rate for incompatible blood group mating such as A × O or O × A was greater than A × A or O × O. Patients with group B or AB had a poorer prognosis irrespective of her partner's blood group. However, recent studies failed to confirm the significance of blood group in GTT.

Environment-related Factors

Treatment Related   GTT is treated by chemotherapy. Appropriate treatment includes early prompt treatment as well as the use of effective regimens. Early diagnosis and treatment are most difficult in GTT following normal pregnancy. A high index of suspicion is important and pregnancy tests should be performed for unexplained irregular bleeding and a solitary lung nodule or unusual cerebral signs in a young woman. High-risk GTT should be treated by multiple-agent chemotherapy. Various studies showed poor outcome if a single agent was used to treat high-risk disease.[40,43] Inadequate chemotherapy allows for the emergence of drug-resistant tumor refractory to subsequent treatment. Prophylactic chemotherapy following mole with high-risk factors in developing GTT decreases the percentage of patients progressing to GTT.[44] However, patients developing GTT after prophylactic chemotherapy following evacuation of molar pregnancy may also have poorer outcome due to theoretical emergence of drug-resistant tumor.

Socioeconomic   GTT occurs in women of reproductive age. Psychosocial studies showed some effect on self-esteem. However, there was no evidence of any adverse effect on prognosis.[45,46]

Quality of Care   Since GTT is not a common gynecological disease, it is important that treatment be performed in a center with expertise in its management. Thus, centralization of GTT is essential to have a good treatment outcome.

PROGNOSTIC FACTORS FOR PLACENTAL-SITE TROPHOBLASTIC TUMOR

PSTT is a rare disease and little is known about its prognostic factors. PSTT also has a spectrum of biologic behavior, but the aggressive form tends to be lethal. The treatment is by hysterectomy, if localized in the uterus. Chemotherapy, however is not as effective as it is in GTT. The main prognostic factors are presence of metastasis and last known pregnancy more than 2 years prior to presentation with PSTT.

SUMMARY

Gestational trophoblastic disease is a highly curable disease. The anatomic extent of disease, although important, does not accurately predict the course of the illness. Nonanatomic prognostic factors, including hCG level, site of metastasis, and the temporal progress of the disease in relation to pregnancy, are essential pieces of information in the management of this disease (see Appendix 35B).

■■■■■■ **APPENDIX 35A**

TM Classification: Gestational Trophoblastic Tumors

T — Primary Tumor

TM Categories	FIGO Stages[a]	
TX		Primary tumor cannot be assessed
T0		No evidence of primary tumor
T1	I	Tumor confined to uterus
T2	II	Tumor extends to other genital structures: vagina, ovary, broad ligament, Fallopian tube by metastasis or direct extension
M1a	III	Metastasis to the lung(s)
M1b	IV	Other distant metastasis with or without lung involvement

[a]Stages I to IV are subdivided into A to C according to the number of risk factors: A without risk factors; B with one risk factor; C with two risk factors.

M — Metastasis

MX Metastasis cannot be assessed

M0 No distant metastasis

M1 Distant metastasis

    M1a Metastasis to lung(s)

    M1b Other distant metastasis with or without lung involvement

Stage Grouping

Stage	T	M	Risk Factors
IA	T1	M0	Without
IB	T1	M0	One
IC	T1	M0	Two
IIA	T2	M0	Without
IIB	T2	M0	One
IIC	T2	M0	Two
IIIA	Any T	M1a	Without
IIIB	Any T	M1a	One
IIIC	Any T	M1a	Two
IVA	Any T	M1b	Without
IVB	Any T	M1b	One
IVC	Any T	M1b	Two

Source: Sobin LH, Wittekind Ch (eds.): *TNM classification of malignant tumors*, 5th ed. New York, Union Internationale Contre le Cancer Wiley-Liss, 1997.

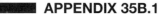 **APPENDIX 35B.1**

Risk or Predictive Factors for GTT Following Mole

Prognostic Factors	Tumor Related	Host Related	Environment Related
Essential	Hydatidiform mole	Age	Central registry follow-up
Additional	Trophoblastic hyperplasia Aneuploidy Proliferative index Serum HCG Clinical parameters Coexisting fetus Doppler index	Immune markers	Oxytocics
New and promising			

■■■■■ **APPENDIX 35B.2**

Prognostic Factors for GTT

Prognostic Factors	Tumor Related	Host Related	Environment Related

Essential	Choriocarcinoma
	Type of antecedent
	  pregnancy
	Site of metastasis
	  (liver/brain)
	Number of sites of
	  metastasis
	Serum HCG level
	Interval from previous
	  pregnancy and treatment
			Expertise in
			  treatment (early
			  and appropriate)
			Failure of previous
			  chemotherapy

Additional	Number of metastases Size of tumor	Age Blood group HLA	
New and promising			

REFERENCE

1. Kohorn EI: Evaluation of the criteria used to make the diagnosis of nonmetastatic gestational trophoblastic neoplasia. *Gynecol Oncol* 48:139–47, 1993.

2. Bagshawe KD, Lawler SD, Paradinas FJ, et al.: Gestational trophoblastic tumors following initial diagnosis of partial hydatidiform mole. *Lancet* 335:1074–6, 1990.

3. Szulman AE, Ma HK, Wong LC, Hsu C: Residual trophoblastic disease in association with partial hydatidiform mole. *Obstet Gynecol* 57:392–4, 1981.

4. Bagshawe KD, Wilson H, Dublon P, et al.: Follow-up after hydatidiform mole: Studies using radioimmunoassay for urinary human chorionic gonadotrophin (HCG). *J Obstet Gynaecol Br Commonw* 80:461–8, 1973.

5. Curry SL, Hammond CB, Tyrey L, et al.: Hydatidiform mole: diagnosis, management, and long-term follow-up of 347 patients. *Obstet Gyneco* 45:1–8, 1975.

6. Nakano R, Sasaki K, Yamoto, M, Hata, H: Trophoblastic disease: Analysis of 342 patients. *Gynecol Obstet Invest* 11:237–42, 1980.

7. Lurain JR, Brewer JI, Torok, EE, Halpern B: Natural history of hydatidiform mole after primary evacuation. *Am J Obstet Gynecol* 145:591–5, 1983.

8. Ayhan A, Tuncer ZS, Halilzade H, Kucukali T.: Predictors of persistent disease in women with complete hydatidiform mole. *J Reprod Med* 41:591–4, 1996.

9. Wong LC, Ngan HY, Collins RJ, Ma HK: Vaginal metastases in gestational trophoblastic disease. *Asia Oceania J Obstet Gynaecol* 16:123–6, 1990.

10. Martin DA, Sutton GP, Ulbright TM, et al.: DNA content as a prognostic index in gestational trophoblastic neoplasia. *Gynecol Oncol* 34:383–8, 1989.

11. Lage JM.: Flow cytometric analysis of nuclear DNA content in gestational trophoblastic disease. *J Reprod Med* 36:31–5, 1991.

12. Hemming JD, Quirke P, Womack C, et al.: Flow cytometry in persistent trophoblastic disease. *Placenta* 9:615–21, 1988.

13. Cheung AN, Ngan HY, Chen WZ, et al.: The significance of proliferating cell nuclear antigen in human trophoblastic disease: an immunohistochemical study. *Histopathology* 22:565–8, 1993.

14. Cheung AN, Ngan HY, Collins RJ, Wong YL: Assessment of cell proliferation in hydatidiform mole using monoclonal antibody MIB1 to Ki-67 antigen. *J Clin Pathol* 47:601–4, 1994.

15. Cheung AN, Zhang DK, Ngan HY, et al.: Telomerase activity in gestational trophoblastic disease. *J Clin Pathol* 52:588–92, 1999.

16. Bae SN, Kim SJ: Telomerase activity in complete hydatidiform mole. *Am J Obstet Gynecol* 180:328–33, 1999.

17. Wake N, Seki T, Fujita H, et al.: Malignant potential of homozygous and heterozygous complete moles. *Cancer Res* 44:1226–30, 1984.

18. Mutter GL, Pomponio RJ, Berkowitz RS, Genest DR: Sex chromosome composition of complete hydatidiform moles: relationship to metastasis. *Am J Obstet Gynecol* 168:1547–51, 1993.

19. Cheung AN, Sit AS, Chung LP, et al.: Detection of heterozygous XY complete hydatidiform mole by chromosome in situ hybridization. *Gynecol Oncol* 55:386–92, 1994.

20. Cameron B, Gown AM, Tamimi HK: Expression of c-erb B-2 oncogene product in persistent gestational trophoblastic disease. *Am J Obstet Gynecol* 170:1616–21, 1994.

21. Balaram P, John M, Rajalekshmy TN, et al.: Expression of epidermal growth factor receptor in gestational trophoblastic diseases. *J Cancer Res Clin Oncol* 123:161–6, 1997.

22. Cole LA, Kohorn EI, Kim GS: Detecting and monitoring trophoblastic disease. New perspectives on measuring human chorionic gonadotropin levels. *J Reprod Med* 39:193–200, 1994.

23. Mungan T, Kuscu E, Ugur M, et al.: Screening of persistent trophoblastic disease with various serum markers. *Eur J Gynaecol Oncol* 19:495–7, 1998.

24. Gungor T, Ekin M, Dumanli H, Gokmen O: Color Doppler ultrasonography in the earlier differentiation of benign molehydatidiforms from malignant gestational trophoblastic disease. *Acta Obstet Gynecol Scand* 77:860–2, 1998.

25. Fishman DA, Padilla LA, Keh P, et al.: Management of twin pregnancies consisting of a complete hydatidiform mole and normal fetus. *Obstet Gynecol* 91:546–50, 1998.

26. Shaarawy M, Darwish NA: Serum cytokines in gestational trophoblastic diseases. *Acta Oncol* 34:177–82, 1995.

27. Stone M, Bagshawe KD: An analysis of the influences of maternal age, gestational age, contraceptive method, and the mode of primary treatment of patients with hydatidiform moles on the incidence of subsequent chemotherapy. *Br J Obstet Gynaecol* 86:782–92, 1979.

28. WHO scientific group: Gestational trophoblastic disease. *Tech Rep Ser* 692:7–81, 1983.

29. Bagshawe KD: Risk and prognostic factors in trophoblastic neoplasia. *Cancer* 38:1373–85, 1976.

30. FIGO Oncology Committee: FIGO Oncology Committee Rep. *Int J Gynaecol Obstet* 39:149–50, 1992.

31. Miller DS, Lurain JR: Classification and staging of gestational trophoblastic tumors. *Obstet Gynecol Clin North Am* 15:477–90, 1988.

32. Dijkema HE, Aalders JG, de Bruijn HW, et al.: Risk factors in gestational trophoblastic disease, and consequences for primary treatment. *Eur J Obstet Gynecol Reprod Biol* 22:145–52, 1986.

33. Soper JT, Evans AC, Conaway MR, et al.: Evaluation of prognostic factors and staging in gestational trophoblastic tumor. *Obstet Gynecol* 84:969–73, 1994.

34. Ngan H, Lopes ADB, Lauder IJ, et al.: An evaluation of the prognostic factors in metastatic gestational trophoblastic disease. *Int J Gynecol Cancer* 4:36–42, 1994.

35. Lurain JR, Brewer JI, Mazur MT, Torok EE: Fatal gestational trophoblastic disease: an analysis of treatment failures. *Am J Obstet Gynecol* 144:391–5, 1982.

36. Rodabaugh KJ, Bernstein MR, Goldstein DP, Berkowitz RS: Natural history of postterm choriocarcinoma. *J Reprod Med* 43:75–80, 1998.

37. Cheung AN, Shen DH, Khoo US, et al.: p21WAF1/CIP1 expression in gestational trophoblastic disease: Correlation with clinicopathological parameters, and Ki67 and p53 gene expression. *J Clin Pathol* 51:159–62, 1998.

38. Cheung AN, Srivastava G, Chung LP, et al.: Expression of the p53 gene in trophoblastic cells in hydatidiform moles and normal human placentas. *J Reprod Med* 39:223–7, 1994.

39. Fulop V, Mok SC, Genest DR, et al.: p53, p21, Rb and mdm2 oncoproteins. Expression in normal placenta, partial and complete mole, and choriocarcinoma. *J Reprod Med* 43:119–27, 1998.

40. Kim SJ, Bae SN, Kim JH, et al.: Risk factors for the prediction of treatment failure in gestational trophoblastic tumors treated with EMA/CO regimen. *Gynecol Oncol* 71:247–53, 1998.

41. Lurain JR, Brewer JI, Torok EE, Halpern B: Gestational trophoblastic disease: treatment results at the Brewer Trophoblastic Disease Center. *Obstet Gynecol* 60:354–60, 1982.

42. Bagshawe KD: Immunological aspects of trophoblastic neoplasia. *Br J Cancer* 28 (Suppl 1):1982, 1973.

43. Lurain JR, Brewer JI: Treatment of high-risk gestational trophoblastic disease with methotrexate, actinomycin D, and cyclophosphamide chemotherapy. *Obstet Gynecol* 65:830–6, 1985.

44. Park TK, Kim SN, Lee SK: Analysis of risk factors for postmolar trophoblastic disease: Categorization of risk factors and effect of prophylactic chemotherapy. *Yonsei Med J* 37:412–9, 1996.

45. Ngan HY, Tang GW: Psychosocial aspects of gestational trophoblastic disease in Chinese residents of Hong Kong. *J Reprod Med* 31:173–8, 1986.

46. Berkowitz RS, Marean AR, Hamilton N, et al.: Psychological and social impact of gestational trophoblastic neoplasia. *J Reprod Med* 25:14–16, 1980.

47. Newlands ES, Bower M, Fisher RA, Paradinas FJ: Management of placental site trophoblastic tumors. *J Reprod Med* 43:53–9, 1998.

UROLOGICAL TUMORS

CHAPTER 36

Squamous-Cell Carcinoma of the Penis

SIMON HORENBLAS

Squamous-cell carcinoma (SCC) of the penis is a rare malignancy, accounting for less than 1% of urological cancers in males in Western countries. From all cancers affecting the penis more than 95% consists of SCC. Rare disorders like melanoma and soft tissue disease will not be considered in this summary. Most information regarding clinical course and prognostic factors has been based on relatively few series and case histories; there are no known prospective clinical trials in the field of penile cancer. Therefore bias, on the basis of referral pattern and institutional treatment preferences, cannot be ruled out. Moreover, there are only a few publications analyzing clinical data with multivariate prognostic factor analysis. For classification purposes, at least six classification systems of SCC of the penis have been proposed. Because the TNM system of the International Union Against Cancer (UICC) is considered the most universal used classification, the others will not be considered here[1] (see Appendix 36A).

TUMOR-RELATED PROGNOSTIC FACTORS

Histology

Growth Pattern Even though various publications have suggested that classification according to growth pattern is of prognostic importance, it is hardly used in daily management or decision making. Traditionally a solid pattern and a cord pattern were defined. The cord pattern was considered a tumor with poor prognostic characteristics and with a tendency to metastasize early.[2–4] Cubilla et al. defined the following patterns of growth: superficial spreading, vertical, multicentric, and verrucous.[5] This retrospective study found a relation between growth pattern and regional metastatic involvement. The metastatic rate was 82% in vertical-growth carcinoma in contrast to no evidence of metastasis in verrucous carcinoma. The majority of patients (42%) had cancer of the superficial spreading type, followed by the vertical-growth type (32%). Whether these growth patterns

---

Prognostic Factors in Cancer, 2nd edition, Edited by Mary K. Gospodarowicz
ISBN 0-471-40633-3 Copyright © 2001 Wiley-Liss, Inc.

form a continuum is not clear. However the association of vertical-growth type, high grade of differentiation, and the very frequent presence of DNA of oncogenic human papilloma virus (HPV) types in vertical-growth carcinoma only, might suggest different pathways. While this approach has been successfully employed in melanoma, it is an unusual way to characterize squamous-cell tumors, and has not been widely accepted among pathologists.[6] Given the lack of multivariate analysis, it is unclear how growth pattern relates to other prognostic indicators.

Vascular Invasion While vascular invasion is a poor prognostic factor in almost all tumors, the prognostic significance in SCC of the penis has not been assessed properly.[7] Despite easy access to the bloodstream through invasion into the spongious/cavernous tissue, hematogenous dissemination is uncommon, and is always preceded by lymphatic spread. Therefore, the current clinical wisdom would have it that vascular invasion in not an important factor.

Histologic Grade Most agree that grade has predictive value for the presence of regional metastasis. Grade is considered to be an essential part of clinical decision making about treatment of the primary tumor and the management of regional lymph nodes. Elective lymph-node dissection has been justified on the basis of high probability of occult metastasis in poorly differentiated tumors.[8-14] In one extensive study, lymph-node involvement was found in 82% of poorly differentiated tumors in contrast to 29% of well-differentiated tumors.[8] However, there is no real consensus on the prognostic value of the grade of differentiation of the primary tumor.[3,10,11,15-18] Grade and lymphatic involvement were independent prognostic factors for survival.[19] The 5-year survival for poorly differentiated tumors was 47%, in contrast to 79% and 68% 5-year survival in well- and moderately differentiated tumors, respectively.[2,7,9,20] Solsona et al.[21] assessed the predictive value of grade for lymph-node involvement. While grade by itself was not predictive, the combination of corpus cavernosum invasion and grade was highly predictive.[21] Of patients with infiltrating poorly differentiated tumors, 80% had lymphatic invasion.

Depth of Penetration The exact depth of penetration has been proposed as a classification criterion, thus obviating interobserver variations by measurement with a microruler. In cancer of the vulva, the probability of lymphatic invasion is related to infiltration of the tumor.[22] However, the usefulness of this measurement in penile cancer has not been properly assessed. Instead of an exact measurement, infiltration into the various structures of the penis has been assessed. Infiltration into the cavernous tissue was found to be an indicator of poor prognosis.[7,21] In the absence of multivariate analysis the exact value of this finding is unclear. Clinical evidence of infiltration into the various structures of the penis is considered to be a classification criterion.

Extent of Local Disease

The extent of disease is of prognostic significance with respect to local recurrence and to disease, related survival. Until 1978, the size of the tumor was considered

TABLE 36.1

	TNM 1978	TNM 1987
Ta		Noninvasive verrucous carcinoma
T1	Tumor <2 cm, strictly superficial or exophytic	Tumor invades subepithelial connective tissue
T2	Tumor >2 cm but less than 5 cm in its largest dimension, or tumor with minimal extension	Tumor invades corpus spongiosum or cavernosum
T3	Tumor >5 cm in its largest dimension or tumor with deep extension, including urethra	Tumor invades urethra or prostate
T4	Tumor infiltrating neighboring structures	Tumor invades other adjacent structures
N0	No evidence of lymph-node involvement	No regional lymph-node metastasis
N1	Evidence of involvement of movable unilateral regional lymph nodes	metastasis in a single superficial inguinal lymph node
N2	Evidence of involvement of movable bilateral regional lymph nodes	Metastasis in multiple or bilateral superficial inguinal lymph nodes
N3	Evidence of involvement of fixed regional lymph nodes	Metastasis in deep inguinal or pelvic lymph node(s), unilateral or bilateral
M0	No evidence of distant metastasis	No evidence of distant metastasis
M1	Evidence of distant metastasis	Evidence of distant metastasis

to be a classification criterion of the primary tumor (Table 36.1). A univariate analysis showed the prognostic significance of the size of the tumor.[23] Disease-related survival in node-negative patients for lesions smaller than was 2 cm and lesions larger than 5 cm was 94% and 52%, respectively. However, lesion size alone can be misleading. Some tumors present as very large, with minimal infiltration, while others show a significant amount of infiltration despite their small size. A comparison of clinical and pathological data showed a difference of 26%.[23] In the majority of cases, the clinical T category underestimated the infiltration in the subepithelial or cavernous tissue. This was especially seen in the smaller tumors. In the larger tumors, infection and edema masked the real size of the tumor, which gave a false impression of infiltration. Realizing the importance of infiltration, the TNM classification system was replaced in 1987 with a new classification (Table 36.1). The size of the primary tumor was replaced by depth of infiltration. This, however, is considered a histopathological criterion, which means there is no reliable clinical method for defining the precise depth of infiltration of the penis. This modification, which results in the removal of a useful clinical parameter, is awaiting a formal prognostic factor analysis.

In conclusion, the size of tumor and the depth of infiltration have been shown to be of prognostic importance. Simple measurement of the size of the tumor remains clinically important.

Extent of Regional Disease

Regional lymph-node involvement is the most important prognostic factor for disease-related survival. Five-year survivals for patients with no lymph-node involvement and those with positive regional lymph-node involvement are 93% and 50%, respectively.[8] These data also show that a cure can be achieved even in patients with lymph-node metastases. In daily clinical practice, the accurate evaluation of the lymph nodes has been hindered by the presence of inflammatory enlargement of the inguinal nodes, while small metastatic deposits are not detected with physical examination or imaging. Size and the number of involved nodes further determine prognosis. The N classification of the latest TNM system has been altered to reflect differences between a single and multiple lymph nodes. While previous reports have shown the number of involved lymph nodes to be of importance, the exact number of involved lymph nodes is only available after histopathological examination.[19,24] A distinction between superficial and deep inguinal lymph nodes was introduced. This again is not viewed as a clinical parameter, as there is no reliable way of distinguishing the superficial inguinal lymph nodes from the deep ones. Besides, there is no evidence that these lymph nodes should be considered separately, as two distinct regions. The prognosis of disease with fixed regional lymph nodes was poor, with an average 5-year survival of 17%.[19,25–29]

Distant Metastasis

Hematogenous spread is a late event in the natural history of SCC of the penis and is always preceded by lymphatic spread. This stage of the disease leads invariably to the death of the patient.

DNA Content

In a study of 26 patients, Gustaffson et al. found that high-grade tumors tended to be nondiploid, and that ploidy did not add significant prognostic information.[30] A study of verrucous carcinoma found only diploid tumors.[31] The largest study of all again found no prognostic information additional to that obtained by traditional pathologic assessment.[32]

HOST-RELATED PROGNOSTIC FACTORS

Patient Demographics

Based on data collected by the International Agency for Research on Cancer, the incidence rates in developed countries vary from 0.4 to 0.9/100.000 (age-adjusted to "the world standard population").[33] This is in contrast to other parts of the world where incidence rates as high as 7.9/100.000 have been

TABLE 36.2   Incidence Rates of Penile Carcinoma/100,000[a]

Brazil, Recife	7.9
Puerto Rico	3.6
Brazil, Sao Paulo	2.5
Columbia	2.4
India, Bombay	2.1
Costa Rica	1.9
Singapore: Indian population	1.0
United States, Connecticut: black population	0.9
Philippines, Rizal	0.9
Denmark	0.9
The Netherlands	0.9
United States, Los Angeles: black population	0.8
German Democratic Republic	0.8
Canada	0.7
United States, Connecticut: white population	0.7
Singapore: Chinese population	0.5
Norway	0.4
Sweden	0.0[b]
Kuwait	0.0[b]
Israel	0.0[b]

[a]Age adjusted to "world standard population," based on cancer incidence in five continents, also see following footnote.
[b]Less than 10 cases/100,000, not further specified.

found.[34,35] A summary of incidence rates is given in Table 36.2. The following reasons for these different figures are suggested: access to health care, difference in hygiene related to water supply, difference in sexual attitude (number of sexual partners, use of condoms, legal status of prostitution, and public health control of prostitutes), and difference in smoking habits. These reasons are based on the following observations.

Phimosis/Presence or Absence of Foreskin

The extreme rarity of penile cancer after neonatal circumcision is well documented.[36–38] Less than 30 cases have been reported in the last 50 years, of which less than ten occurred among northern American Jewish males.[39–48] It is difficult to understand in what way "a piece of skin the size of a quarter" is instrumental in cancer promotion.[49] A complete circumcision prevents the most prominent finding associated with penile cancer: an unretractable foreskin. Reported incidence of phimosis in patients with penile cancer range from 42% to 92%. Chronic irritations with or without bacterial inflammation are the most common resulting conditions. A Swedish case-control study of 244 patients with penile cancer estimated that 45% of cancer patients suffered at least one episode of balanitis in contrast to 8% in the control group.[50] In this study, phimosis and balanitis represented significant independent risk factors. Studies in China and India, using multivariate analyses, corroborate these findings.[51,52]

Much speculation has been given to the presumed carcinogenic effect of the chronic presence of smegma. Analysis has shown that smegma consists of flakes of epidermis, necrotic epithelial debris, and the products of bacterial action on these desquamated cells.[53-55] Evidence that smegma is a carcinogen is at best ambiguous.[56-58] Phimosis after the age of 6 years is considered a pathologic condition and should be treated. This could lead to a decrease of the incidence of penile cancer.

Human Papilloma Virus

Recent findings on the oncogenic potential of the sexually transmittable human papilloma viruses (HPV) have renewed interest and research in its role in penile carcinoma. The association of HPV with cancer of the cervix is well established. In almost all of the cases the presence of HPV-DNA is found in the tumor. The ubiquitous presence of HPV-DNA has not been confirmed in penile carcinoma. On average, 50% of the tumors are found to be HPV positive, with a predominance of HPV-16. Similar to the hypothesis for vulva cancer,[59,60] penile cancer may develop in two distinct settings:

1. HPV-linked penile cancer, developing in a younger population and associated with sexually related risk factors.
2. HPV-negative penile cancer, occurring in an older population and unrelated to sexual practice.

These two settings also could easily explain the epidemiological differences as shown earlier. While knowledge on HPV is essential for the etiology of cancer of the penis, it does not play a role of prognostic importance, the same as with the findings in cervical cancer.

Smoking

There is extensive epidemiological evidence to support an association between smoking and anogenital SCC.[50-52,61] It has been suggested that smoking could predispose to anogenital cancer by an effect on the immune system. The majority of studies indicate that smoking relatively close to the time of diagnosis is associated with a particularly great increase in risk, which supports the hypothesis that smoking has a late-stage or promotional role.

New Prognostic Factors

Clinically useful determinants for early lymphatic invasion are eagerly awaited. A recent publication showed renewed interest in sentinel-node involvement.[62] Assuming the sequential metastatic spread presence, absence of lymphatic involvement of a sentinel node could determine the likehood of further prognosis. The individual drainage pattern of the tumor was visualized using lymphoscintigraphy and a gamma detector. However promising, though, this first report on more than 50 patients needs further proof of reliability.

■ **APPENDIX 36A**

TNM Classification: Penis Cancer

T — Primary Tumor

TX   Primary tumor cannot be assessed

T0   No evidence of primary tumor

Tis   Carcinoma in situ

Ta   Noninvasive verrucous carcinoma

T1   Tumor invades subepithelial connective tissue

T2   Tumor invades corpus spongiosum or cavernosum

T3   Tumor invades urethra or prostate

T4   Tumor invades other adjacent structures

N — Regional Lymph Nodes

NX   Regional lymph nodes cannot be assessed

N0   No regional lymph-node metastasis

N1   Metastasis in a single superficial inguinal lymph node

N2   Metastasis in multiple or bilateral superficial inguinal lymph nodes

N3   Metastasis in deep inguinal or pelvic lymph node(s), unilateral or bilateral

M — Distant Metastasis

MX   Distant metastasis cannot be assessed

M0   No distant metastasis

M1   Distant metastasis

Stage Grouping			
Stage 0	Tis	N0	M0
	Ta	N0	M0
Stage I	T1	N0	M0
Stage II	T1	N1	M0
	T2	N0, N1	M0
Stage III	T1	N2	M0
	T2	N2	M0
	T3	N0, N1, N2	M0
Stage IV	T4	Any N	M0
	Any T	N3	M0
	Any T	Any N	M1

Source: Sobin LH, Wiitekind Ch (eds.): *TNM classification of malignant tumors*, 5th ed. New York, Union Internationale Contre le Cancer Wiley-Liss, 1997.

■■■■■■ **APPENDIX 36B**

Prognostic Factors for SCC of the Penis

Prognostic Factors	Tumor Related	Host Related	Environment Related
Essential	Grade Lymph-node invasion Stage	Phimosis	Incidence of oncogenic- HPV
Additional	Size primary tumor and infiltration		
New and promising	Sentinel-node involvement		

REFERENCES

1. Sobin LH, Wittekind Ch (eds.): TNM classification of malignant tumours, 5th ed. New York, Union Internationale Contre le Cancer Wiley-Liss, 1997.

2. Salaverria JC, Hope-Stone HF, Paris AMI, et al.: Conservative treatment of carcinoma of the penis. *Br J Urol* 51:32–37 1979.

3. El-Demiry MIM, Oliver RTD, Hope-Stone HF, Blandy JP: Reappraisal of the role of radiotherapy and surgery in the management of carcinoma of the penis. *Br J Urol* 56:724–8 1984.

4. Frew IDO, Jefferies JD, Swinney J: Carcinoma of penis. *Br J Urol* 39:398–404 1967.

5. Cubilla AL, Barreto J, Caballero C, et al.: Pathologic features of epidermoid carcinoma of the penis, a prospective study of 66 cases. *Am J Surg Pathol* 17:753–63 1993.

6. Murphy WM: Diseases of the penis and scrotum in Murphy WM (ed.): *Urologic pathology*, 2d ed. Philadelphia, Saunders, 1997.

7. Fraley EE, Gang Z., Manivel C, Niehaus GA: The role of ilio-inguinal lymphadenectomy and significance of histological differentiation in treatment of carcinoma of the penis. *J Urol* 142:1478–82 1989.

8. Horenblas S., von Tinteren H: Squamous cell carcinoma of the penis. IV. Prognostic factors od survival: Analysis of tumor, nodes and metastatic classification system. *J Urol* 151:1239–43 1994.

9. Fraley EE, Gang Z., Sazama R, Lange PH: Cancer of the Penis. Prognosis and Treatment Plans. *Cancer* 55:1618–24 1985.

10. Darai E, Karaitianos I, Durand JC: Traitement des Aires Ganglionnaires Inguinales dans le Cancer de la Verge A Propos de 85 Cas Traités á l'Institut *Curie Ann Chir*, 42:748–52 1988.

11. Jensen MS: Cancer of the penis in Denmark 1942 to 1962 (511 cases). *Danish Med Bull* 24:66–72 1977.

12. Hardner GJ, Bhanalaph T, Murphy GP, et al.: Carcinoma of the penis. Analysis of therapy in 100 consecutive cases. *J Urol* 108:428–430 1972.

13. Maiche AG, Pyrhönen S: Clinical staging of cancer of the penis: By size?, By localization?, Or by depth of infiltration. *Eur J Urol*,18:16–22 1990.

14. Fraley EE, Gang Z., Manivel C, Niehaus GA: The role of ilio-inguinal lymphadenectomy and significance of histological differentiation in treatment of carcinoma of the penis. *J Urol* 142:1478–82 1989.

15. Baker BH, Spratt JS, Perez-Mesa C, et al.: Carcinoma of the penis. *J Urol* 116:458–61 1976.

16. Ekström T, Edsmyr F: Cancer of the penis: A clinical study of 229 cases. *Acta Chir Scand* 115:25 1958.

17. Wajsman Z, Moore RH, Merrin CE, Murphy GP: Surgical treatment of penile cancer. *Cancer* 40:1697–701 1977.

18. Hanash KA, Furlow WL, Utz DC, Harrison EG: Carcinoma of the penis. A clinicopathologic study. *J Urol*, 104(2):291–7 1970.

19. Horenblas S, von Tinteren H, Delemarre JFM, et al.: Treatment of the regional lymph nodes. *J Urol* 149:492–7 1993.

20. Maiche AG, Pyrhönen S, Karkinen M: Histological grading of squamous cell carcinoma of the penis. A new scoring system. *Br J Urol* 67:522–6 1991.

21. Solsona E, Iborra I, Ricos JV, et al.: Corpus cavernosum invasion and tumor grade in the prediction of lymph node condition in penile carcinoma. *Eur Urol*, 22:115–8 1992.

22. Hacker NF, Berek JS, Lagasse LD, et al.: Individualization of treatment for stage I squamous cell vulvar carcinoma. *Obstet Gynecol* 63:155–62, 1984.

23. Horenblas S, van Tinteren H, Delemarre JFM, et al.: Squamous cell carcinoma of the penis. Accuracy of TNM-classification system, role of lymphangiography, CT-scan and fine needle aspiration cytology. *J Urol* 146:1279–83 1991.

24. Srinivas V, Morse MJ, Herr HW, et al.: Penile cancer: Relation of extent of nodal metastasis to survival. *J Urol* 137:880–2 1987.

25. Jackson SM: The treatment of carcinoma of the penis. *Br J Surg* 53:33–5 1966.

26. Murrel DS, Williams JL: Radiotherapy in the treatment of carcinoma of the penis. *Br J Urol*, 37:211–22 1965.

27. Whitmore WF, Vagaiwala MR: A technique of ilioinguinal lymph node dissection for carcinoma of the penis. *Surg Gynecol Obstet* 159:573 1984.

28. Koch MO, McDougal S: Penile carcinoma: The case for primary lymphadenectomy. *Cancer Treat Res* 46:55–64 1989.

29. Lichtenauer P, Ott G, Dröge KH: Zur klassifizierung, verlauf und behandlung des penis-carcinoms (statistische auswertung von 317 bioptisch nachgewiesen penis-carcinomen). *Urologe A*, 12:66–70 1973.

30. Gustafsson O, Tribukait B, Nyman CR, Borgstrom E: DNA pattern and histopathology in carcinoma of the penis. A prospective study. *Scan J Urol Nephrol Suppl* 110:219–22 1988.

31. Masih AS, Stoler MH, Farrow GM, et al.: Penile verrucous carcinoma: A clinicopathologic, human papillomavirus typing and flow cytometric analysis. *Mod Pathol*, 5:48–55 1992.

32. Hall TC: Basal cell carcinoma of the penis. *J Urol* 99:314–15 1968.

33. Muir C, et al. (eds.): *Cancer incidence in five continents*. Lyon, International Agency for Research on Cancer, 1987.

34. Waterhouse J, et al. (eds.): *Cancer incidence in five continents*. Lyon, International Agency for Research on Cancer, 1982.

35. Reddy CRRM, Gopal Rao T, Venkatarathnam G, et al.: A study of 80 patients with penile carcinoma combined with cervical biopsy study of their wives. *Int Surg* 62:549–53 1977.

36. Wolbarst AL: Circumcision and penile cancer. *Lancet* I:150 1932

37. Bleich AR: Prophylaxis of penile carcinoma. *JAMA* 143:1054 1950.

38. Licklider S: Jewish penile carcinoma. *J Urol* 86:98 1961.

39. Sufrin G, Huben R: Benign and malignant lesions of the penis, in Gillenwater JY, et al. (eds.): *Adult and pediatric urology*, 2d ed. Chicago, Year Book Med. Pub., 1991, pp. 1643–81.

40. Dean AL: Epithelioma of the penis. *J Urol* 33:252 1935.

41. Marshall VF: Typical carcinoma of the penis in a male circumcised in infancy. *Cancer* 6:1044 1953.

42. Reitman PH: An unusual case of penile carcinoma. *J Urol* 69:547 1953.

43. Paquin AJ, Pearce JM: Carcinoma of the penis in a man circumcised in infancy. *J Urol* 74:626 1955.

44. Amelar RD: Carcinoma of the penis due to trauma occurring in a male patient circumcised at birth. *J Urol* 75:728 1956.

45. Ledlie RCB, Smithers DW: Carcinoma of the penis in a man circumcised in infancy. *J Urol* 76:756 1956.

46. Kaufman JJ, Sternberg TH: Carcinoma of the penis in a circumcised man. *J Urol* 90:449 1963.

47. Melmed EP, Pyne JR: Carcinoma of the penis in a Jew circumcised in infancy. *Br J Surg* 54:729–31 1967.

48. Rogus BJ: Squamous cell carcinoma in young circumcised man. *J Urol* 138:861–2 1987.

49. Wiswell ThE: Prepuce presence portends prevalence of potentially perilous periurethral pathogens. *J Urol* 148:739–42 1992.

50. Hellberg D, Nilsson S: Genital cancer among wives of men with penile cancer. A study between 1958 and 1982. *Br J Obstet Gynecol* 96:221–5 1989.

51. Brinton LA: Epidemiology of cervical cancer—overview, in Munoz N,: Bosch FX, Shah KV, Meheus A (eds.): *The epidemiology of cervical cancer and human papillomavirus*. Lyon, International Agency for Research on Cancer, 1992, pp. 3–23.

52. Harish K, Ravi R: The role of tabacco in penile carcinoma. *Br J Urol* 75:375–7 1995.

53. Shabad AL: Some aspects of etiology and prevention of penile cancer. *J Urol* 92:696 1964.

54. Schellhammer PF, Jordan GH, Schlossberg SM: Tumors of the penis, in Walsh PC, Retik AB, Stamey ThA, Vaughan ED (eds.): *Campbell's urology*, Vol. 2, 16th ed., Philadelphia, Saunders, 1992, pp. 1264–98.

55. Parkash S, Subramanyan K, Chaudhuri S: Human subpreputial collection: Its nature and formation. *J Urol* 110:211–2 1973.

56. Pratt-Thomas HR, Heins HC, Latham, et al.: The carcinogenic effect of human smegma: An experimental study. *Cancer*, 9:671 1956.

57. Fishman M, Shear MJ, Friedman H, Stewart H: Studies in carcinogenesis. XVII. Local effect of repeated application of 3,4-Benzpyrene and of human smegma to the vagina and cervix of mice. *J Natl Cancer Inst* 2:361–1942.

58. Heins HC, Dennis EJ, Pratt-Thomas HR, Charleston SC: The possible role of smegma in carcinoma of the cervix. *Am J Obstet Gynecol* 76:726 1958.

59. Crum CP, Nuovo GJ: *Genital papillomaviruses and related neoplasms.* New York, Raven Press, 1991.

60. Higgins GD, Davy M, Roder D, et al.: Increased age and mortality associated with cervical carcinomas negative for human papillomavirus RNA. *Lancet*, 338:910–3 1991.

61. Daling JR, Sherman KJ, Hislop TG, et al.: Cigarette smoking and the risk of anogenital cancer. *Am J Epidemiol* 135:180–9 1992.

62. Horenblas S, Jansen L, Meinhardt W, et al.: Detection of occult metastasis in squamous cell carcinoma of the penis using a dynamicsentinel node procedure. *J Urol* 163:100–4 2000.

CHAPTER 37

Prostate Cancer

LOUIS DENIS and GERALD P. MURPHY

Prostate cancer became an endemic disease in the Western world mainly because of the aging of the population. The peak age incidence hovers around 70. The introduction of prostatic-specific antigen (PSA) assay for the diagnosis of prostate cancer resulted in a considerable shift in the detection of disease toward earlier stages that are potentially curable. In countries where PSA is widely used for the detection of prostate cancer,[1] up to 75% of patients present with localized disease. This has given great expectations to patients and their physicians. However, conclusive proof that mortality is decreasing due to population screening is still lacking.[2] The problem is enhanced by the heterogeneous behavior of the prostate.

The International Union Against Cancer (UICC) TNM (tumor, nodules, metastasis) classification of malignant tumors is the means by which the prognosis of most solid cancers can be staged and defined at diagnosis.[3] However, the TNM system does not include all relevant prognostic parameters in prostate cancer, especially the PSA.[4] There is a need to evaluate prognostic factors not only at diagnosis but also after treatment.[5] The need to fine-tune the staging process in early prostate cancer drives the search for better prognostic markers. Needed measures to predict the outcome and support treatment decisions at diagnosis include biologic, pathologic, genetic, molecular, and other nonanatomic prognostic factors. Prognosis could be enhanced further using a neural network methodology, especially for an analysis of risk for each patient.[6,7] However, despite efforts and hopes, no superior marker to the anatomic disease, extent, histologic grade, on PSA is available today.[8]

Within the scope of this chapter, we will present prognostic factors relevant for the treatment and outcomes in localized and advanced prostate cancer according to relationship to the tumor, the host, and the environment. A relevance-based subdivision into essential, additional, and promising prognostic factors is also presented.

Prognostic Factors in Cancer, 2nd edition, Edited by Mary K. Gospodarowicz.
ISBN 0-471-40633-3 Copyright © 2001 Wiley-Liss, Inc.

TUMOR-RELATED FACTORS

Anatomic Extent of Disease

The UICC/American Joint Committee on Cancer (AJCC) TNM classification is now universally accepted and widely utilized by the urologist to categorize patients with prostate cancer before treatment[3] (see Appendix 37A). The classification's practical application in the routine clinic has been established.[9] The procedures to assess T, N, and M categories include physical examination, imaging, biochemical tests (primarily PSA), and skeletal imaging. With the exception of the digital rectal examination (DRE) that indicates the T category, physical examination contributes little to the assessment of the anatomic disease extent. Imaging by transrectal ultrasound (TRUS) or by transrectal magnetic resonance imaging (MRI) failed to improve the accuracy of clinical staging of prostate cancer. The search for improved methodology of these tests is being pursued.[7] At this point, however, TRUS is used mainly to direct the needle in transrectal biopsy. Frequently no tumor is palpable or visible by imaging, and consequently an elevated serum PSA is the only indication for prostate biopsy. In the absence of a precise anatomic zone to be biopsied, the six-core biopsy has become the routine in patients being classified as having T1c (nonpalpable) disease.[10] The margin of error in the diagnosis of organ-confined tumor (T1–T2) is considerable.[7]

Tumor size in localized disease correlates clearly with patterns of progression. A tumor volume of 1 cc has 20% probability of capsular invasion, 1% of seminal vesicle invasion, and 1% of metastatic disease.[11] The data from retrospective study of 1000 patients with pT3 disease after radical prostatectomy showed that tumor grade and volume correlate with cause-specific survival and progression ($p = 0.002$ and less than 0.0001).[12] It is evident that tumor extent has a higher risk of progression and death. The prognostic significance of seminal vesicle invasion decreases the progression-free survival considerably.[13] The prognosis of stage T3bNo also depends on the extent of the seminal vesicle invasion.[14]

The presence of pelvic lymph-node involvement carries a poor prognosis. This was demonstrated in a study on 475 patients treated with radiotherapy after pelvic lymphadenectomy where, with a mean follow-up of 67 months, the cancer mortality was 7% for patients with lymph-node-negative disease versus 30% for patients with lymph-node involvement.[15] Tumor extent and size are predictive for the overall outcome and local control in patients treated with curative intent. Even a simple measurement like the maximum diameter of the prostate tumor can serve as an independent predictor of PSA failure after radical prostatectomy. In a cohort of 434 patients, only 15% of men with tumor of diameter <1 cm had biochemical failure, compared with 73% of men with tumor with a maximum diameter >2 cm.[16]

The independent prognostic value of tumor extent and volume has been confirmed in patients with *advanced disease* (T3–T4, N1, or M1) in the trials of the National Prostatic Cancer Project and the European Organization for Research and Treatment of Cancer (EORTC). More specifically, a number of studies[17] have confirmed that in asymptomatic patients, the number of lesions on the bone scan is an independent prognostic factor. A number and amount of tumor on positive biopsies are useful to predict tumor volume.[18]

Finally, there is the possible prognostic significance of tumor location in the prostate. We know that approximately 70% of prostate cancer arises from the peripheral zone, 20% from the transition zone, and less than 10% from the central zone of the prostate.[19] It has been reported that patients with transition-zone tumors tend to have better prognosis than patients with peripheral-zone tumors.[20] On the contrary, it is reported that anterior tumors have a worse prognosis.[21] This observation was made in a study of 785 patients where it was also noted that African-American men have a greater percentage of anterior tumors than do Caucasian men. The lesson from these observations is that when there are elevated serum PSA levels and a negative set of biopsies, it is recommended that both the transition and the anterior zones of the prostate be biopsied.

Histopathologic Features

Grade The histologic grade plays a key role in determining progression and overall survival.[22] Broder designed the first grading system about 75 years ago, and it was followed by many other grading systems. Over the last two decades, the Gleason system became the preferred grading system for categorizing prostatic cancer. The system recognizes five grades that, depending on their relative presence in the tissue, are combined to form the Gleason score that is a strong predictor for progression in survival at any stage of the disease.[23] In a selected series of 652 patients treated with radical prostatectomy, the patients with Gleason score 6, 7, and 8 or more had no evidence of the disease (NED) survival of 91.2%, 75%, and 34.5%, respectively.[24]

In a landmark analysis of the prognostic factors for prostate cancer by the Veterans Administration Cooperative Urological Research Group (VACURG), it was shown that grade according to the Gleason sum and the presence or absence of metastatic disease were the most powerful prognostic factors both in localized and advanced disease.[25] Here, combined grading and staging identified groups of patients in categories scoring from 3 to 15, followed up by mortality data on 1032 patients. There were no cancer deaths in the lowest prognostic factor categories, while 50% of the patients with the highest category died of prostatic cancer. The histologic grade, the tumor size, and the serum levels of acid phosphatase in patients with localized disease allowed the formation of three risk groups that showed progression in 5 years in 7%, 9%, and 31% of cases. In contrast, in patients with metastatic disease and a Gleason sum above 8, the mortality was 75%. The relative amount of the highest grade in the specimen is important, and organ-confined prostate cancer that is considered for radical prostatectomy may contain small foci of Gleason score 7.[26] The importance of the grading is highlighted by the results of a population-based study of long-term survival in patients with clinically localized prostate cancer.[27] The adapted 10-year survival results are presented in Table 37.1 where the impact of higher grades is substantial.

TABLE 37.1 Ten-year Survival in Localized PCA by Histological Grade

	Radical Prostatectomy	Radiation Treatment	Conservative Treatment
G1	94	90	93
G2	87	76	77
G3	67	53	45

Ploidy   It has been suggested that correlation of the content of DNA in the tumor cells, assessed by cytology or histology, can be used as a possible additional prognostic parameter to grade. Low-grade tumors are mostly diploid and high-grade tumors mostly aneuploid. Ploidy has been reported as inferior to the prediction provided by Gleason grading. If an accurate Gleason sum is a concern, ploidy can be helpful and should be a consideration in second-opinion pathological consults.[28]

Markers   The extensive search for tumor products that can could be used as diagnostic and/or prognostic factors has produced a long list of potential markers that are currently under investigation for possible clinical use.[29,30] Out of a long list of potential prognostic factors, presented in Table 37.2, *mitotic figures, cell adhesion markers, neuroendocrine markers, microvessel density, epidermal growth factors*, and *mutations of the androgen receptor* are candidates for clinical applications. The clinical application will certainly require more study, especially since they have to exhibit prognostic independence from PSA. PSA replaced prostatic acid phosphatase (PAP) as the marker of prostate cancer after a decade of intensive laboratory and clinical investigation. It is somewhat paradoxical that a tissue rather than a tumor-specific marker proved to be useful as a diagnostic and prognostic marker for prostate cancer. In fact, PSA emerged as a potent and independent prognostic marker at diagnosis and at relapse for localized and metastatic disease.[43,44] The prognostic significance is extremely valuable in patients with T1c disease and in patients offered surgical or radiation treatment.[31,32] Its addition to the clinical stage and Gleason sum, PSA helps to predict risk of occult extraprostatic extension.[33] Undetectable levels of PSA are expected after complete eradication of the cancer by radical prostatectomy, but the lowest level of PSA is a strong surrogate marker for response after radiation therapy.[34] It is obvious that a decreasing PSA profile curve and the lowest level of PSA values that were close to 0.2 ng/mL had the best progression-free survival.[35,36] Identical conclusions were reached in locally advanced or metastatic disease treated with hormones. Here pretreatment PSA was not predictive of outcome, but all patients with N1-3M0 disease who failed to achieve undetectable PSA levels had a relapse by 8 years.[37] Again, the PSA decline is an independent prognostic marker in this cohort of patients.[38] Intense research focused on the aspects of PSA in its different forms, such as, free PSA, complex PSA (C-PSA), and the hK2 and hK1 kallikreins, as well as the prostate-specific membrane antigen (PSMA), with the latter emerging as a potential additional prognostic factor in clinical use.[39] A clearer understanding is emerging but more factors for

TABLE 37.2   List of Potential Prognostic Factors Under Investigation for Clinical Use

Potential Prognostic Markers

Proliferation and apoptotic markers
   Ki 67 antigen, nuclear nonhistone protein
   Mitotic figures
   Apoptotic bodies
   bcl 2, apoptosis suppressing oncoprotein
   High-mobility protein I (Y)

Enzymes and secretory proteins
   5 alpha reductase
   Telomerase
   Antioxidant enzymes
   Activin and inhibin
   Relaxin
   Androgen receptor gene
   12-lipoxygenase
   Metalloproteinases and inhibitors

Cytoskeletal proteins
   Cytokeratin peptides
   Cell adhesion markers
   Cadherines E
   Oligosaccharide Sialyl-Lewis

Stromal Proteins, Growth Factors, Receptors
   Epidermal growth factors: HER2/neu, HER3, HER4
   Transforming growth factors
   Fibroblast growth factors
   Insulin-like growth factors: IGFI receptor tyrosinase kinase activity
   Nerve growth factors
   Vascular endothelial growth factors
   Platelet-derived growth factors

Genetic Factors
   Chromosomes gain/loss 7, 8p, 8q
   p 53 tumor suppressor
   WAF 1/CIP 1 (p 21 cyclin dependent kinase inhibitor)
   CDKN 2/MTS 1 (p 16—CDK 4)
   c-myc expression
   Rb protein
   Androgen receptor gene mutations
   Metastasis suppressor gene nm 23
   KAT 1 suppressor gene
   Oncoprotein PTI-1
   MMAC 1/PTEN (10 q 23-3)
   p 73 (1 p 36, 2-3)

Source: Provided by D. Bostwick.

evaluating prognosis in the individual patient may require the use of artificial neural networks for analysis.[40]

Other biochemical factors, such as alkaline phosphatase (ALP) and hemoglobin, relate to advanced stages of metastatic disease.

HOST-RELATED FACTORS

Age as well as *comorbidity* are reliable prognostic factors for survival in patients with localized or advanced disease. Another clinical prognostic parameter is the *performance status* used alone or in combination with the pain score in patients with advanced disease. A poor performance status is usually associated with shorter survival.[41] Clinical parameters, including hemoglobin levels, albumin, creatinine, rapid weight loss, and low serum testosterone, represent the vital status of the individual. A high pretreatment serum testosterone level was reported as an independent prognosticator for metastatic relapse after irradiation for localized prostate cancer.[42] Symptoms due to cancer are indicators of a worse prognosis, be it lower urinary tract symptoms (LUTS) or pain from metastatic sites.

The importance of prognostic factors has been highlighted in a number of randomized trials on patients with metastatic disease for evaluation and interpretation of these trials. In the first Intergroup Study (INT 0036) on metastatic prostate cancer patients, prognostic factors associated with the extent of disease included anemia, anorexia, elevated alkaline phosphatase, and number of bone lesions.[45] In a number of trials of the EORTC, multivariate analysis could be used to divide patients with good (3.5 years median survival) and poor (1.75 years median survival) prognosis, respectively, based on performance status, hemoglobin, pain score, alkaline phosphatase and, of course, T category and grade status at entry in the study.[46] It is evident that wider differences can be expected between survival based on prognostic factors than on differences in treatment efficacy. There are no randomized trials comparing curative treatments in most of these cases, but host characteristics usually play a secondary role to tumor characteristics. As expected, stage and grade determine the survival prediction.[47]

The incidence of prostate cancer is higher in African-American men than in age-matched Caucasian men, but contrary to earlier reports, race may not be related to poorer prognosis.[48] Hereditary prostate cancer is a recognized problem and accounts for 9% of all cancers and more than 40% of early onset disease.[49]

ENVIRONMENT-RELATED FACTORS

There are no clear guidelines on the ultimate choice between a number of treatment options ranging from radical perineal prostatectomy to laparoscopic radical prostatectomy for the surgical choices, and conformal radiotherapy to brachytherapy. Without forgetting the choice of watchful waiting, there are also no clear differences in the efficacy, the complications, and the learning curve of each choice.

It has been reported that transurethral resection of the prostate (TURP) influences prognosis adversely. However, the procedure is indicated because of the obstructing mass, which is already a negative prognostic factor.

Almost no data are available on the influence of socioeconomic conditions, quality control of care, and access to care, which certainly will influence treatment outcome and survival. Focused studies on these factors are urgently needed.

SUMMARY

Advances in statistical analyses have been able to single out significant and independent prognostic factors affecting endpoints and outcome of treatment. Unfortunately, the clinical correlation, especially concerning specific time to death, progression-free survival, and quality of life, is not always clear for the individual patient. The organization of several prognostic factors into model predictive systems that use a set of parameters known to have prognostic relevance is an attempt to increase the correlation.

Conventional parameters were used to calculate the risk of second treatment from the CAPSURE database following attempts at local curative treatment. Here low risk rates are PSA <5 ng/mL, stage T1–2N0m0, and Gleason sum<6; high-risk rates are PSA >15 ng/mL, T3–4N+M1, and Gleason sum $\geq$7; and intermediate risk is in between.[50]

The Partin nomogram, extensively validated and constantly reevaluated, uses only three parameters to predict the clinical stage.[33] Correct prediction occurs in 72.4% of cases, and these systems should be improved to serve the individual guideline. We focused attention on the influence of the initial prognostic factors, which should be taken into account when treatment is chosen. It is common sense to let stage and grade as well as age be primary considerations in choosing the treatment of localized disease.

The lack of prospective randomized trials in patients with localized disease and the notorious difficulties in correct staging and grading of early prostate cancer makes it difficult to evaluate the value of the variable. Still, the number of prospective trials where the known prognostic factors could be balanced in the different areas suggesting different risk groups as to outcome of disease should be pursued in clinical research and practice. In clinical research we need to make sure that our trials allow for the separation of patient cohorts into subsets with a wide variety of outcomes, even survival. This will ultimately allow us to establish more stringent entry criteria for certain types of treatment plus predictions of which patient cohorts will do better with one or another treatment or even no treatment at all.

To conclude, the anatomic extent of disease, the total tumor burden, the histologic grade, and serum PSA form the base for prognosis in patients with localized and advanced prostate cancer. These factors are essential in clinical practice. New factors are needed to determine the certainty of dealing with localized disease, the possibility of cure, and the biological aggressiveness of the tumor. Here the preoperative factors define the scenario as presented in

Appendix 37B.1. It is evident that factors defining biological aggression are related to the tumor. In advanced prostate cancer, prognostic factors related to survival and quality of life dominate the clinical picture. These factors are presented in Appendix 37B.2. More research and clinical trials are needed to improve the shortcomings of the actual therapeutic decision making in prostate cancer.

■■■■■■■ **APPENDIX 37A**

TNM Classification: Prostate Cancer

T—Primary Tumor

TX   Primary tumor cannot be assessed

T0   No evidence of primary tumor

T1   Clinically inapparent tumor not palpable or visible by imaging

T1a   Tumor incidental histological finding in 5% or less of tissue resected

     T1b Tumor incidental histological finding in more than 5% of tissue resected

     T1c Tumor identified by needle biopsy (e.g., because of elevated PSA)

T2   Tumor confined within the prostate

     T2a Tumor involves one lobe

     T2b Tumor involves both lobes

T3   Tumor extends through the prostatic capsule

     T3a Extracapsular extension (unilateral or bilateral)

     T3b Tumor invades seminal vesicle(s)

T4   Tumor is fixed or invades adjacent structures other than seminal vesicles: bladder neck, external sphincter, rectum, levator muscles, and/or pelvic wall

N—Regional Lymph Nodes

NX   Regional lymph nodes cannot be assessed

N0   No regional lymph-node metastasis

N1   Regional lymph-node metastasis

M—Distant Metastasis

MX   Distant metastasis cannot be assessed

M0   No distant metastasis

M1   Distant metastasis

     M1a Nonregional lymph node(s)

     M1b Bone(s)

     M1c Other site(s)

G — Histopathological Grading

GX   Grade cannot be assessed

G1   Well differentiated (slight anaplasia)

G2   Moderately differentiated (moderate anaplasia)

G3–4 Poorly differentiated/undifferentiated (marked anaplasia)

Stage Grouping

Stage I	T1a	N0	M0	G1
Stage II	T1a	N0	M0	G2, 3–4
	T1b	N0	M0	Any G
	T1c	N0	M0	Any G
	T1	N0	M0	Any G
	T2	N0	M0	Any G
Stage III	T3	N0	M0	Any G
Stage IV	T4	N0	M0	Any G
	Any T	N1	M0	Any G
	Any T	Any N	M1	Any G

Source: Sobin LH, Wittekind Ch (eds.): *TNM classification of malignant Tumors*, 5th ed. New York, Union Internationale Contre le Cancer, Wiley-Liss, 1997.

■■■■■ **APPENDIX 37B.1**

Prognostic Factors in Localized Prostate Cancer

Prognostic Factors	Tumor Related	Host Related	Environment Related
Essential	Stage Grade PSA level	Age Comorbidity Performance status	Socioeconomic factors
Additional	Ploidy	Prior TURP Race	Access to care Expertise
New and promising	PSMA Kallikreins Microvessel density Mitotic figures Cell adhesion Neuroendocrine differentiation EGFR Androgen receptor		

■■■■■ **APPENDIX 37B.2**

Prognostic Factors in Advanced Prostate Cancer

Prognostic Factors	Tumor Related	Host Related	Environment Related
Essential	T, N, M categories Grade PSA level Pain	Age Comorbidity Performance status	Socioeconomic factors
Additional	Hemoglobin Alkaline phosphatase Creatinine		Access to care Expertise
New and promising	PSMA EGFR Androgen receptor		

REFERENCES

1. Mettlin C, Murphy GP, Rosenthal DS, Menck HR: The National Cancer Database report on prostate carcinoma after the peak in incidence rates in the US. *Cancer* 83:1679–84, 1998.

2. Denis L, Mettlin C, Carter HB, et al.: Early detection and screening, in Murphy G, Partin A, Khoury S, Denis L (eds.): *Prostate cancer*. Paris, SCI, 2000.

3. Sobin LH, Wittekind Ch (eds.): *TNM classification of malignant tumors*, 5th ed. New York, Union Internationale Centre le Cancer Wiley Liss, 1997, pp. 1–225.

4. Hermanek P, Sobin LH, Wittekind Ch: How to improve the present TNM staging system. *Cancer* 86:2189–91, 1999.

5. Blute ML, Bostwick DG, Seay TM, et al.: Pathologic classification of prostate carcinoma: The impact of margin status. *Cancer* 82:902–8, 1998.

6. Yarbro JW, Page DL, Fielding LP, et al.: American Joint Committee on Cancer Prognostic Factors Consensus Conference. *Cancer* 86:2436–46, 1999.

7. Murphy GP, Snow PB, Brandt J, et al.: Evaluation of prostate cancer patients receiving multiple staging tests, including ProstaScint scintiscans. *The Prostate* 42:145–9, 2000.

8. Reiter RE: Prostate cancer diagnostics — obstacles and opportunities [Editorial]. *J Urol* 162:2046–7, 1999.

9. Ohori M, Wheeler TM, Scardino PT: The New American Joint Committee on Cancer and International Union against Cancer TNM classification of prostate cancer. Clinicopathologic correlations. *Cancer* 74:104–14, 1994.

10. Stamey TA: Making the most out of six systematic sextant biopsies. *Urology* 45:1–12, 1995.

11. Bostwick DG, Lee F, Graham SD, et al.: Staging of early prostate cancer: A proposed tumor volume-based prognostic index. *Urology* 41:403–11, 1993.

12. Cheng WS, Frydenberg M, Bergstralh EJ, et al.: Radical prostatectomy for pathologic stage C prostate cancer: Influence of pathologic variables and adjuvant treatment on disease outcome. *Urology* 42:283–91, 1993.

13. Guillonneau B, Vallancien G: Editorial: What is the prognostic significance of seminal vesicle invasion by prostate cancer? [Editorial]. *The Prostate* 36:207–8, 1998.

14. Debras B, Guillonneau B, Bougaran J, et al.: Prognostic significance of seminal vesicle invasion on the radical prostatectomy specimen. *Eur Urol* 33:271–7, 1998.

15. Gervasi LA, Mata JA, Scardino JA, et al.: Prognostic significance of lymph node metastases in prostatic cancer. *J Urol* 142:332–6, 1989.

16. Renshaw AA, Richie JP, Loughlin KR, et al.: Maximum diameter of prostatic carcinoma is a simple, inexpensive, and independent predictor of prostate-specific antigen failure in radical prostatectomy specimens: Validation in a cohort of 434 patients. *Am J Clin Pathol* 111:641–4, 1999.

17. Denis L: Staging and prognosis in prostate cancer. *Eur Urol* 24:13–9, 1993.

18. Sebo TJ, Bock BJ, Cheville JC, et al.: The percent of cores positive for cancer in prostate needle biopsy specimens is strongly predictive of tumor stage and volume at radical prostatectomy. *J Urol* 163:174–8, 2000.

19. McNeal JE, Redwine EA, Freiha FS, Stamey TA: Zonal distribution of prostatic adenocarcinoma: Correlation with histologic pattern and direction. *Am J Surg Pathol* 12:897–906, 1988.

20. Stamey TA, Dietrick DD, Issa MM: Large organ confined impalpable transition zone prostate cancer: Association with metastatic levels of prostate specific antigen. *J Urol* 149:510–5, 1993.

21. Tiguert R, Gheiler EL, Tefilli MV, et al.: Racial differences and prognostic significance of tumor location in radical prostatectomy specimens. *The Prostate* 37:230–5, 1998.

22. Epstein JI, Carmichael M, Partin AW, et al.: Is tumor volume an independent predictor of progression following radical prostatectomy? A multivariate analysis of 185 clinical stage B adenocarcinomas of the prostate with 5 years of follow-up. *J Urol* 149:1478–81, 1993.

23. Gleason DF, Mellinger GT: The Veterans Administration Cooperative Urological Research Group: Prediction of prognosis for prostatic carcinoma by combined histological grading and clinical staging. *J Urol* 111:58–64, 1974.

24. Tefilli MV, Gheiler EL, Tiguert R, et al.: Should Gleason score 7 prostate cancer be considered a unique grade category? *Urology* 53:372–7, 1999.

25. Byar D, Corle D: Analysis of prognostic factors for prostatic cancer in the VACURG studies, in Denis L, Prout G, Schröder F (eds.): *Controlled clinical trials in urologic oncology.* New York, Raven Press, 1984, pp. 147–68.

26. Yang XJ, Lecksell K, Potter SR, Epstein JI: Significance of small foci of Gleason score 7 or greater prostate cancer on needle biopsy. *Urology* 54:528–32, 1999.

27. Lu-Yao GL, Long-Yao S: Population-based study of long-term survival in patients with clinically localized prostate cancer. *Lancet* 349:906–10, 1997.

28. Brinker DA, Ross JS, Trans TA, et al.: Can ploidy of prostate carcinoma diagnosed on needle biopsy predict radical prostatectomy stage and grade? *J Urol* 162:2036–9, 1999.

29. Gao X, Porter AT, Grignon DJ, et al.: Diagnostic and prognostic markers for human prostate cancer. *The Prostate* 31:264–81, 1997.

30. Burton JL, Oakley N, Anderson JB: Recent advances in the histopathology and molecular biology of prostate cancer. *Br J Urol Int* 85:87–94, 2000.

31. Cookson MS, Fleshner NE, Soloway SM, Fair WR: Prognostic significance of prostate-specific antigen in stage T1c prostate cancer treated by radical prostatectomy. *Urology* 49:887–97, 1997.

32. D'Amico AV, Whittington R, Malkowicz SB, et al.: Prostate-specific antigen failure despite pathologically organ-confined and margin-negative prostate cancer: The basis for an adjuvant therapy trial. *J Clin Oncol* 15(4):1465–9, 1997.

33. Partin AW, Nathan MW, Subong ENP: Combination of prostate specific antigen, clinical stage and Gleason score to predict pathological stage of localized prostate cancer. *JAMA* 277:1445–51, 1997.

34. American Society for Therapeutic Radiology and Oncology Consensus Panel: Consensus statement: Guidelines for PSA following radiation therapy. *Int J Radiat Oncol Biol Phys* 37:1035–41, 1997.

35. Jani AB, Chen MH, Vaida F, et al.: PSA-based outcome analysis after radiation therapy for prostate cancer: A new definition of biochemical failure after intervention. *Urology* 54:700–5, 1999.

36. Critz FA, Williams WH, Holladay CT, et al.: Post-treatment PSA ≤0.2 ng/mL defines disease freedom after radiotherapy for prostate cancer using modern techniques. *Urology* 54:968–71, 1999.

37. Zagars GK, Sands ME, Pollack A, von Eschenbach AC: Early androgen ablation for stage D1 (N1T0N3,MO) prostate cancer: Prognostic variables and outcome. *J Urol* 151:1330–3, 1999.

38. Palmberg C, Koivisto P, Visakorpi T, Tammela TLJ: PSA decline is an independent prognostic marker in hormonally treated prostate cancer. *Eur Urol* 36:191–6, 1999.

39. Murphy GP, Partin A: Workshop on prostate markers. *Cancer* 83:2233–8, 1998.

40. Partin AW, Murphy GP, Brawer MK: Report on prostate cancer tumor workshop 1999. *Cancer* 88:955–63, 2000.

41. De Voogt HJ, Suciu S, Sylvester R, et al.: Members of the European Organization for Research and Treatment of Cancer Cooperative Group: Multivariate analysis of prognostic factors in patients with advanced prostatic cancer: Results from 2 European Organization for Research and Treatment of Cancer Trials. *J Urol* 141:883–8, 1989.

42. Zagars GK, Pollack A, von Eschenbach AC: Serum testosterone — a significant determinant of metastatic relapse for irradiated localized prostate cancer. *Urology* 49:327–34, 1997.

43. Cooper EH, Armitage TG, Robinson MRH, et al.: Prostate specific antigen and the prediction of prognosis in metastatic prostate cancer. *Cancer* 66:1025–9, 1990.

44. Fossa SD, Paus E, Lindegaard M, Newling DWW: Prostate-specific antigen and other prognostic factors in patients with hormone-resistant prostatic cancer undergoing experimental treatment. *Brit J Urol* 69:175–9, 1992.

45. Eisenberger MA, Crawford ED, Wolf M, et al.: Investigators of the National Cancer Institute Intergroup Study # 0036: Prognostic factors in stage D2 prostate cancer: Important implications for future trials: Results of a Cooperative Intergroup Study (INT. 0036). *Semin Oncol* 21:613–9, 1994.

46. Sylvester RJ, Denis L, de Voogt H, for the European Organization for Research and Treatment of Cancer (EORTC) Genito-Urinary Tract Cancer Cooperative Group: The importance of prognostic factors in the interpretation of two EORTC metastatic prostate cancer trials. *Eur Urol* 33:134–43, 1998.

47. Zagars GK, von Eschenbach AC, Ayala AG: Prognostic factors in prostate cancer. *Cancer* 72:1709–25, 1993.

48. Witte MN, Kattan MW, Albani J, et al.: Race is not an independent predictor of positive surgical margins after radical prostatectomy. *Urology* 54:869–74, 1999.

49. Smith JR, Freye D, Carpten JD, et al.: Major susceptibility locus for prostate cancer on chromosome 1 suggested by a genome wide search. *Science* 274:1371–4, 1996.

50. Grossfeld GD, Stier DM, Flanders SG, et al.: Use of second treatment following definitive therapy for prostate cancer. Data from CAPSURE database. *J Urol* 160:1398–404, 1998.

CHAPTER 38

Germ-cell Testis Tumors

HANS-JOACHIM SCHMOLL and CHRISTOPH RIE

Prognostic factors are of major importance for the treatment and cure of patients with testicular cancer. The histologic type, seminoma versus nonseminomatous germ-cell tumors (NSGCT) and the (TNM) stage constitute the fundamental prognostic factors that govern clinical practice.[1] (see Appendix 38A) For early stages, prognostic factors are the critical determinants for the decisions about treatment. They don't necessarily predict the survival, which is greater than 98% independent of treatment strategy, but for the risk of relapse with different treatment options. In advanced stages, prognostic factors indicate the chance of survival following chemotherapy, either first-line or salvage. In this chapter, the different prognostic factors, relevant for decision making in early and late stage germ-cell testis tumors, are discussed.

STAGE I SEMINOMA

Prognostic factors in stage I and II seminomas estimate the risk of relapse after orchiectomy followed by either adjuvant radiation therapy or surveillance. Prognostic factors for relapse have been studied in three large surveillance studies. In the Danish Testicular Carcinoma Study Group (DATECA) study, tumor size, histological subtype, necrosis, and invasion of the rete testis predicted for relapse on univariate analysis, but on multivariate analysis, tumor size was the only significant prognostic factor.[2] Univariate analysis of the Princess Margaret Hospital series showed tumor size, age, and the absence or presence of small vessel invasion as being predictive for relapse. On multivariate analysis, age older than 34 years and tumor size greater 6 cm were shown as being predictive for relapse.[3] The prognostic impact of age was not confirmed in the large DATECA surveillance study, and

Special thanks to Mrs. N. Roever (secretary to Professor Schmoll) for making this paper a reality.

Prognostic Factors in Cancer, 2nd edition, Edited by Mary K. Gospodarowicz
ISBN 0-471-40633-3 Copyright © 2001 Wiley-Liss, Inc.

was not analyzed in the Royal Marsden Study, where only vascular invasion was a significant factor predicting for relapse.[4] A number of other candidate histopathological findings have been studied, including ploidy, mitotic rate, S-phase fraction, the presence of syncytiotrophoblasts, the degree of lymphocytic infiltration of the primary tumor, expression of beta human chorionic gonadotrophia (β-hCG), and low molecular-weight keratin on immunohistochemistry, but no significance was observed.[3] However, the choice of treatment (surveillance vs. radiotherapy vs. chemotherapy) has no influence on survival, but results in different adverse effects and the total amount of treatment.[5] The pooled of the three clinical studies revealed tumor diameter and rete testis invasion as significant factors for relapse after orchiectomy without further adjuvant therapy.

STAGE I NONSEMINOMATOUS GERM-CELL CANCER

In clinical stage I NSGCT, the major role of prognostic factors is to identify risk groups for pathological stage II disease (II a,b) or progression on surveillance programs. The most relevant prognostic factor is vascular invasion (both lymphatic or blood vessels).[6] Further important prognostic factors define the risk of lymph-node metastases or the lung metastases. Independently, a high proportion of embryonal carcinoma in the specimen is a prognostic factor that predicts a more advanced disease. Multiple cutoff levels were tested and a 50% cutoff level yielded highest score for sensitivity and specificity in an analysis of the Bonn University Medical Center.[7] A recent prognostic factor is the MIB1 (Ki67) in the tumor, with strong staining being predictive for a more advanced disease. A multivariate analysis compared vascular invasion, percentage of embryonal carcinoma and MIB-1 (Ki67) staining, and identified the Ki67 staining as best parameter to predict pathological stage I disease.[8,9] In a Norwegian study of 68 patients, DNA ploidy was examined, but had no prognostic value.[10] In a large study of 149 patients Heidenreich et al. examined the presence of vascular invasion, percentage of histological subtypes, MIB-1, p53, bcl-2, cathepsin D, and E-cadherin.[11] All patients had stage I disease and underwent retroperitoneal lymph node dissection (RPLND). Of the 149 clinical stage I patients, 63 patients had retroperitoneal lymph-node involvement (pathological stage II). The predictive factors for occult lymph-node metastases in clinical stage I include high percentage of embryonal carcinoma, vascular invasion, high-p53 expression, and E-cadherin; however, on multivariate analysis only vascular invasion and percentage of embryonal carcinoma were significant.[11] In a study performed by Fukuda et al. on 80 patients, vascular endothelial growth factor (VEGF) overexpression was a significant prognostic factor associated with distant metastases in NSGCT.[12] Several other groups compared vascular invasion preorchiectomy alpha-feloprotien (AFP), embryonal carcinoma, yolk sack tumor, or other tumor elements as shown in Table 38.1. For clinically staged patients, only vascular invasion is a significant prognostic factor (Table 38.1). Using a 3-mm threshold to define nonmetastatic lymph nodes, the sensitivity and negative predictive value of CT-based staging was 90%.[13] In a later study, Leibovitch

TABLE 38.1 Multivariate Analyses of Factors Predictive for Occult Metastatic Disease in Clinical Stage I NSGCT

Investigators	Study Endpoint	Number of Points	Significant Factors [increased (I) or decreased (D) risk]
Swedish-Norwegian Testicular Cancer Group[77]	p stage II at RPLD	187	Vascular invasion (I) Elevated preorchiectomy AFP (D) Embryonal carcinoma(I) Yolk sac tumor (D)
	Relapse in p stage I	190	Vascular invasion (I) Orchiectomy–RPLND interval (D) Teratoma elements (D)
	All relapses	258	Vascular invasion (I) Teratoma present (D) Orchiectomy–RPLND interval (D) Elevated preorchiectomy AFP (D)
Medical Research Council[15]	Relapse after orchiectomy and surveillance strategy	259	Vascular invasion (I) Yolk sac tumor (D) Presence of MTU (I)
Royal Marsden Hospital[78]	Relapse after orchiectomy and surveillance strategy	126	Lymphatic invasion (I) Histology (I)
AFIP[18]	p stage II at RPLD	459	Vascular invasion (I) Embryonal carcinoma (I) Yolk sac tumor (D)

combined the proliferation index and radiologic findings and identified two groups, one with MIB-1 staining $<90\%$ and a lymph-node diameter <10 mm, and a second with MIB-1 staining $<80\%$ and a lymph-node diameter <3 mm, with a low risk of occult lymph-node metastasis.[14]

Another question is whether treatment influences the prognosis in stage I NSGCT. Several studies showed that the overall survival for patients initially treated with RPLND is the same as for surveillance at $\geq98\%$. Patients on surveillance have a higher relapse rate (25–30%),[15] but the survival rate is the same as after RPLND because of the excellent salvage therapy.

STAGE II SEMINOMA

In stage II seminoma, prognostic factors are important for identifying the patients who are best treated with radiotherapy or chemotherapy. In 72 patients with clinical stage II seminoma treated with radiotherapy at the Princess Margaret Hospital, the size of retroperitoneal lymph nodes was the most important predictor for relapse and survival. The relapse rate was less than 20% for stage IIA–B, and 30–70% for stage IIC,[16,17] indicating that chemotherapy is the optimal treatment for patients with a stage IIC seminoma.[17]

STAGE II NONSEMINOMATOUS GERM-CELL CANCER

In contrast to stage I, in stage II disease histopathologic findings do not have a major prognostic impact. The presence of vascular invasion is a predictive factor for relapse in stage II NSGCT after RPLND (63.5% relapse rate vs. 24.0%).[18] Several studies demonstrated that the most important factors are the number of infiltrated lymph nodes and the maximum size of involved lymph nodes (Table 38.2). It appears that tumor size less than 2–3 cm and/or less than 6 lymph nodes might reveal a low risk of relapse (20–50%) in comparison to more advanced lymph-node involvement (40–70% relapse rate).[19]

STAGE III SEMINOMA

Seminoma is generally regarded as highly chemotherapy sensitive, even more so than NSCGT. With cisplatin-based chemotherapy, a complete remission (CR) rate of 63% and a disease-free survival at 5 years of 70% in patients with prior irradiation, and a CR rate of 71% and disease-free survival (DFS) at 5 years of 85% in untreated patients have been reported.[20–23] Unfortunately, nearly all of these data derive from small and often retrospective series with a large heterogeneity in the respective patient populations, which partially explains the wide range of CR rates from 38% to 100%, progression-free survival rates from 50% to 100%, and overall survival rates from 71% to 100%.

The large differences between individual centers and study groups have led (in contrast to NSGCT) to somewhat different treatment strategies for advanced seminoma.[24–27] A recent analysis of combined data from four consecutive Memorial Sloan Kettering Cancer Center studies on good-prognosis testicular

TABLE 38.2   Prognostic Factors in Stage II NSGCT

Investigators	Criteria for Low Risk of Relapse
Vogelzang et al. 1983[79]	<2 cm, <6 nodes
Vugrin et al. 1981[80]	<6 nodes, 2cm, no extranodal extension
Pizzocaro and Monfardini, 1984[81]	<3cm, no extranodal extension
Richie and Kantoff, 1991[82]	<6 nodes, <2 cm, no extranodal extension

cancer (according to the MSKCC criteria) evaluated predicting factors for clinical outcome in seminoma patients.[20] Increased levels of hCG or lactate dehydrogenase (LDH) were associated with a significantly inferior survival. Prior irradiation, the presence of visceral metastases, and advanced disease according to the "Indiana classification" also related to an inferior survival, which was not statistically significant. In contrast to NSCGT, an extragonadal location of a primary tumor either in the retroperitoneum or in the mediastinum was not associated with an inferior prognosis as compared to a testicular origin.

The International Germ Cell Cancer Collaborative Group (IGCCCG) has reported a retrospective analysis of prognostic factors in 660 patients with advanced seminoma treated within prospective trials between 1975 and 1990.[28] In this large meta-analysis, a primary extragonadal seminoma again was not associated with a worse prognosis as compared to a testicular origin. The presence of lung metastases and increase in level of hCG were of only borderline statistical significance, whereas the increase in the level of LDH and the presence of a supraclavicular mass were independent prognostic factors for treatment outcome. The most important adverse prognostic factor, however, was the presence of nonpulmonary visceral metastasis (NPVM). The final prognostic model identified two distinct subgroups among seminoma that had significant differences in the response rates and survival:

1. *Good Prognosis Patients Without NPVM, Independent of hCG or LDH*: By definition, the AFP has to be normal for all seminoma. For patients with these characteristics a progression-free survival of 82% and a 5-year overall survival of 86% were estimated. This group represented 90% of patients with advanced seminoma.

2. *Poor Prognosis Patients; Presence of NPVM, Independent of hCG or LDH Levels*: Again, the AFP levels had to be normal. Patients with advanced seminoma and NPVM had an estimated progression-free survival at 5 years of 67% and an overall survival at 5 years of 72%. These represented 10% of all patients with advanced seminoma.

A separate and more detailed analysis of 286 patients with metastatic seminoma from the IGCCCG series has been reported by Fossa et al.[29] The data identified the same prognostic factors as reported in the studies from the MSKCC and the IGCCCG (Table 38.2): stage, LDH level, presence or absence of NPVM, mediastinal or supraclavicular lymph-node involvement, presence or absence and number of lung metastasis, and prior irradiation.[20,28,29] Increased level of hCG was not a significant predictive factor, in contrast to the MSKCC analysis. Similar to the IGCCCG classification, these variables allow an easy definition of prognostic categories within metastatic seminoma, but may be more relevant with respect to patients with a lower tumor burden.

METASTATIC NONSEMINOMATOUS GERM-CELL TUMORS

In contrast to seminoma, the term NSGCT applies to a variety of histologic subtypes, including embryonal carcinomas, choriocarcinomas, yolk sac tumors, and immature teratomas, to differentiated and mature teratomas with a relatively benign biological behavior. Although the metastatic potential of an individual histologic subtype varies and has been used for the prediction of occult metastases in clinical stage I disease, in NSGCT most of the prognostic classifications did not identify histologic subtype as an independent prognostic factor.[26,28,30,31] The more aggressive nature of NSGCT in comparison to seminoma might be reflected in the fact that about half of the patients present with metastatic disease. At the time of initial diagnosis, 20 to 30% of NSGCT patients have large-volume abdominal metastases, supradiaphragmatic lymph-node involvement, pulmonary or nonpulmonary visceral metastases, and require chemotherapy.[32] In these patients, the cure rates vary from 90% or greater to 50% or less, depending on the presence or absence of adverse disease characteristics. With such large differences, the availability of reliable prognostic models gained paramount importance; in particular as risk-adapted treatment strategies emerged.

Historical Models

A large number of possible prognostic factors evolved from clinical trials in metastatic NSGCT (Table 38.3).[26,27,30,31]. Categorical variables reflect tumor volume and extent of metastatic spread. In some analyses hCG, AFP, or LDH either completely replaced clinical findings or at least added to an improved prognostic modeling. However, the proportion of patients in good or poor risk categories varied substantially.[25] When the classifications from the MSKCC, Indiana University, and the European Organization for Research and Treatment of Cancer (EORTC) were compared in an independent cohort of 118 patients, 31% were considered poor risk by the MSKCC criteria, 34% by the Indiana classification, and 61% by the EORTC criteria. The risk assignments were discordant in 52 of 118 (44%) patients.[25] Metastatic disease is diagnosed more frequently with computed tomography (CT), as compared to conventional X-ray imaging, and the use of CT resulted in "stage migration."[33] In patients with large-volume metastatic disease, the addition of etoposide to cisplatin-based combination chemotherapy has resulted in higher response rates and improved long-term survival.[32,34–36] Many analyses of prognostic factors represented single-center experiences, and some have simply been too small and lacked the power to detect all of the relevant prognostic factors.[28,37,38] Differences in remission or survival rates serve as outcome measures in prognostic factor analyses. However, long-term progression-free survival is the superior endpoint in such analyses and more relevant to a patient's ultimate prognosis.[39]

The prognostic model generated from the IGCCCG study was based on the analysis of 5202 patients treated in prospective studies in North America, Europe, New Zealand, and Australia[28] (Table 38.3). The database was sufficiently large to

ERRATUM

Prognostic Factors in Cancer, Second Edition

Editors, M. K. Gospodarowicz, D. E. Henson, R. V. P. Hutter, B. O'Sullivan,
L. H. Sobin, and Ch. Wittekind
Copyright ©2001 Wiley-Liss, Inc.
ISBN 0-471-40633-3

TABLE 38.5 Definitions of Risk Categories in Germ-cell Tumors According to the IGCCCG

Prognosis	% of patients	Tumor	Primary/metastases	Marker	Marker values	Survival
Good prognosis	*56% of patients*	Nonseminomas	Testicular or retroperitoneal primary tumor and only "good" markers; No nonpulmonary visceral metastases		AFP < 1000 ng/m, HCG < 5000 U/L, LDH < 1.5 × upper limit of normal	*Progression-free survival 89%*, *Overall survival 92%*
		Seminoma	Any primary site; No nonpulmonary visceral metastases		Normal AFP, Any hCG, any LDH	
Intermediate prognosis	*28% of patients*	Nonseminoma	Testicular or retroperitoneal primary tumor; No nonpulmonary visceral metastases	Any "intermediate" marker	AFP 1000–10,000 ng/mL, HCG 5000–50,000 U/L, LDH 1.5–10 × upper limit of normal	*Progression-free survival 75%*, *Overall survival 80%*
		Seminoma	Any primary site; Any nonpulmonary visceral metastases		Normal AFP, Any hCG, any LDH	
Poor prognosis	*16% of patients*	Nonseminoma	Mediastinal primary tumor	Any "poor" marker	AFP > 10,000 ng/mL, HCG > 50,000 U/L, LDH > 10 × upper limit of normal	*Progression-free survival 41%*, *Overall survival 48%*
		Seminoma	None			

TABLE 38.3   Definitions of Risk Categories in Germ-cell Tumors According to the IGCCCG

Good prognosis	*56% of patients*	*Progression-free survival 89%* *Overall survival 92%*
Nonseminomas	Testicular or retroperitoneal primary tumor and only "good" markers	AFP < 1000 ng/m HCG < 5000 U/L LDH < 15 × upper limit of normal
	No nonpulmonary visceral metastases	
Seminoma	Any primary site No nonpulmonary visceral metastases	Normal AFP Any hCG, any LDH
Intermediate prognosis	*28% of patients*	*Progression-free survival 75%* *Overall survival 80%*
Nonseminoma	Testicular or retroperitoneal primary tumor Any "intermediate" marker No nonpulmonary visceral metastases	AFP 1000–10,000 ng/mL HCG 5000–50,000 U/L LDH 1.5–10 × upper limit of normal
Seminoma	Any primary site Any nonpulmonary visceral metastases	Normal AFP Any hCG, any LDH
Poor prognosis	*16% of patients*	*Progression-free survival 41%* *Overall survival 48%*
Nonseminoma	Mediastinal primary tumor Any "poor" marker Any nonpulmonary metastases	AFP < 10, 000 ng/mL HCG < 50, 000 U/L LDH < 10 × upper limit of normal
Seminoma	None	

allow a random division of patients into a test set comprising 70% of patients and a validation set with the remaining 30% to evaluate the prognostic model. The model was further validated with the results of two recent prospective clinical trials. Multivariate analysis identified mediastinal primary, hCG, AFP, LDH, and the extent of disease defined by NVPM or the number of tumor sites, as the most important independent prognostic factors. Age and the extent of pulmonary disease were also significant, but to a lesser degree, and were not considered in the final model. In NSGCT, three prognostic groups were identified with progression-free survival rates at 5 years of 89%, 75%, and 41%, respectively (Table 38.4). Its validation with data from a prospective trial in poor-risk patients selected according to the Indiana classification showed the discriminative power of the IGCCCC prognostic model. The three distinct prognostic groups had progression-free survival rates of greater than 80%, 74%, and 50% among these patients.[27,29]

The IGCCCG work has led to the development of a new TNM staging classification that incorporates all the significant prognostic factors defined by the IGCCCG model. (see Appendix 38A)

SALVAGE TREATMENT

The majority of patients who require salvage treatment have NSGCT, as seminoma patients are usually cured with first-line treatment, although few patients with seminoma do relapse with AFP elevations or NSGCT histology. A favorable response rate of 88% and a DFS of 54% were found in 24 seminoma patients, treated with cisplatin-based salvage chemotherapy between 1984 and 1994 at the Indiana University.[23] In all other salvage trials, however, the number of seminoma patients is too small to draw any conclusions.

"Conventional-Dose" Salvage Treatment

The study by Droz et al. reported a series of 203 patients treated with conventional-dose salvage chemotherapy.[40] In multivariate analysis, presence of extragonadal NSGCT, incomplete response to first-line treatment, presence of lung metastases and levels of hCG that were greater than or equal to 10,000 UIL or levels of AFP greater than or equal to 1000 ng/mL were identified as independent adverse prognostic factors. Three prognostic groups were identified with a progression-free survival at 2 years of 43%, 22%, and 0%, respectively. Gerl et al. retrospectively analyzed a series of 67 patients who required salvage treatment for relapsed or refractory germ-cell tumors.[41] Only age younger than 35 years, achievement of a CR after first-line treatment, and remission duration of more than 3 months had prognostic significance. These three variables were used to identify a subgroup of patients with a projected 72% overall survival at 5 years. More recently, Fossa et al. reported a multivariate analysis of 165 patients treated in MRC trials between 1982 and 1986.[42] Among a large number of variables studied, an incomplete response to first-line chemotherapy, a remission duration of less than 2 years, and high levels of AFP of more than 50 kU/L and hCG greater than 100 IU/L at the time of relapse were identified as independent adverse prognostic factors that served to define three prognostic groups with survival rates ranging from 9% to 75%, respectively (Table 38.5). An incomplete response to first-line chemotherapy or a short response duration of less than 6 months after first-line treatment were identified as poor prognostic factors in separate studies from the MSKCC and Norway.[43,44] In a retrospective series of 73 patients with extragonadal NSGCT, only 7% became long-term disease-free survivors, despite incorporation of high-dose chemotherapy in the treatments of about one-third.[37]

"High-Dose" Salvage Treatment

In the past, high-dose chemotherapy was primarily indicated for patients with disease refractory to cisplatin and in patients with multiple relapses who were considered incurable with conventional-dose treatment. Its role as intensification of first salvage treatment has been investigated recently.[45,46] Sensitivity to cisplatin was identified as the most important prognostic factor.[47,48] Patients with primary mediastinal NSGCT had inferior results with high-dose treatment as compared to patients with other primaries.[37,45] Two groups reported on multivariate analyses. Motzer et al. identified hCG levels of more than 100 times the upper normal limit and the absence of retroperitoneal metastases as independent adverse prognostic factors for long-term survival.[49] In 283 patients from four institutions four independent prognostic variables were identified: remission status prior to high-dose treatment, primary mediastinal NSGCT, sensitivity to cisplatin, and hCG levels greater than 1000 U/L prior to high-dose treatment.[50] Patients with absolute refractory disease and hCG levels of more than 1000 U/L did not profit from high-dose treatment and were classified as poor prognosis (Table 38.5).

Posttreatment Marker Decline   In the majority of NSGCT and in some seminoma patients, the hCG or AFP levels are available to measure early treatment response.[51–56] In the majority of these studies, the natural logarithm of a marker was plotted versus linear time and the slope of the regression. Those patients with a slope that exceeded 3 days for hCG and 7 days for AFP were considered to have a delayed marker response. Numerous problems precluded serial measurements of LDH from evaluation as a prognostic factor.[57] Despite the obvious rationale of measuring treatment response early, methodologic limitations have led to conflicting results. In some studies, prolonged marker half-life was a strong indicator for treatment failure. Consequently, the rate of marker decline was used to select patients for early treatment intensification.[58] However, two recent studies failed to show such a relation.[54,56] In one study of 183 patients with NSGCT, the accuracy of correctly predicting long-term progression-free survival was only 57% for a prolonged marker decline of either hCG or AFP.[54] The early analyses have been limited by small numbers of patients and inferior chemotherapy regimens.[37] Apart from the problems in defining inappropriate marker decline, the distribution of other known risk factors for treatment failure, such as pretreatment risk category, pretreatment marker levels, and primary tumor site, differed widely between studies, and competing risks have not been fully appreciated.

Molecular Markers   The discovery of molecular alterations promoted increasing attempts to understand the development and biology of germ-cell tumors. Cytogenetic alterations have been most frequently found on chromosomes 1 and 12, and particularly the isochromosome of the short arm of chromosome 12{i(12p)} has been extensively studied.[59,60] Based on a very small analysis of only 24 patients, the copy number of i(12p) has been found to be a clinically useful prognostic marker, but no further studies have yet confirmed this observation.[61] The tumor suppressor genes p53 and the retinoblastoma gene (RB-1) play important roles in the regulation of the normal cell cycle and trigger apoptosis. Loss of these genes by deletion or mutation have been linked to clinical resistance in many solid tumors. In germ-cell tumors, however, alterations in p53 are rare, which might explain the exquisite sensitivity of germ-cell tumors to chemotherapy.[62,63] Alterations of RB-1 have not been studied in respect to their clinical implications.[64,65] Other prognostic markers investigated included the proliferative capacity in primary tumor specimens, the role of growth factors and their ligands, the degree of cisplatin adduct formation as measure of DNA damage, as well as repair mechanisms of cisplatin-damaged DNA.[66–72] In germ-cell tumors, however, it may still be a long time before even the exciting molecular alterations or mechanisms that are being studied in cell lines or resected tumor specimens will ultimately translate into clinical practice.

ENVIRONMENT-RELATED PROGNOSTIC FACTORS

The expertise of the treating physician is a prognostic factor, as it affects the outcome in cancer patients. There is increasing evidence that for many cancers, centers that do not treat a certain "critical mass" of patients may not achieve the optimal treatment outcome. This finding has been observed in several studies of advanced testicular germ-cell cancer in the United Kingdom and Europe.[73,74] The differences have also been observed when the outcomes of patients with testis cancer in Surveillance, Epidemiology, and End Results (SEER) data have been compared to the outcomes achieved by the expert group at the Memorial Sloan Kettering Cancer Center in New York.[75]

The delay in diagnosis is still a problem in some areas of the world, and there is evidence that delay leads to presentation with higher stage, requiring more complex treatment, and may indeed compromise the survival.[76]

SUMMARY

There are numerous prognostic factors in germ-cell testis tumors that assist in selecting the optimal therapy for an individual patient and in defining the prognosis with respect to the risk of relapse and the overall survival (see Appendix 38B). The work of the International Germ Cell Cancer Collaborative Group has clarified the use of these factors in defining the distinct risk groups, and the consensus achieved has unified the approach to prognosis in this disease. Because germ-cell tumors are one of most curable cancers today, the environment-related factors need to be studied further to ascertain the uniform access to the excellent outcomes.

TNM Classification: Testis

pT — Primary Tumor

pTX Primary tumor cannot be assessed (if no radical orchiectomy has been performed, TX is used)

pT0 No evidence of primary tumor (e.g., histologic scar in testis)

pTis Intratubular germ cell neoplasia (carcinoma in situ)

pT1 Tumor limited to testis and epididymis without vascular/lymphatic invasion; tumor may invade tunica albuginea but not tunica vaginalis.

pT2 Tumor limited to testis and epididymis with vascular/lymphatic invasion, or tumor extending through tunica albuginea with involvement of tunica vaginalis.

pT3 Tumor invades spermatic cord with or without vascular/lymphatic invasion.

pT4 Tumor invades scrotum with or without vascular/lymphatic invasion.

N — Regional Lymph Nodes

NX Regional lymph nodes cannot be assessed

N0 No regional lymph-node metastasis

N1 Metastasis with a lymph-node mass 2 cm or less in greatest dimension or multiple lymph nodes, none more than 2 cm in greatest dimension

N2 Metastasis with a lymph-node mass more than 2 cm but not more than 5 cm in greatest dimension, or multiple lymph nodes, any one mass more than 2 cm but not more than 5 cm in greatest dimension

N3 Metastasis with a lymph-node mass more than 5 cm in greatest dimension

M — Distant Metastasis

MX Distant metastasis cannot be assessed

M0 No distant metastasis

M1 Distant metastasis
   M1a Nonregional lymph node or pulmonary metastasis
   M1b Distant metastasis other than to nonregional lymph nodes and lungs

S — Serum Tumor Markers

SX Serum marker studies not available or not performed

S0 Serum marker study levels within normal limits

	LDH	hCG (mIU/mL)	AFP (ng/mL)
S1	$<1.5 \times N$	and <5000	and <1000
S2	$1.5–10 \times N$	or $5000–50{,}000$	or $1000–10{,}000$
S3	$>10 \times N$	or $>50{,}000$	or $>10{,}000$

N indicates the upper limit of normal for the LDH assay

Stage Grouping

Stage 0	pTis	N0	M0	S0,SX
Stage I	pT1–4	N0	M0	SX
Stage IA	pT1	N0	M0	S0
Stage IB	pT2–4	N0	M0	S0
Stage IS	Any pT/TX	N0	M0	S1–3
Stage II	Any pT/TX	N1–3	M0	SX
Stage IIA	Any pT/TX	N1	M0	S0–1
Stage IIB	Any pT/TX	N2	M0	S0–1
Stage IIC	Any pT/TX	N3	M0	S0–1
Stage III	Any pT/TX	Any N	M1, M1a	SX
Stage IIIA	Any pT/TX	Any N	M1, M1a	S0–1
Stage IIIB	Any pT/TX	N1–3	M0	S2
	Any pT/TX	Any N	M1, M1a	S2
Stage IIIC	Any pT/TX	N1–3	M0	S3
	Any pT/TX	Any N	M1, M1a	S3
	Any pT/TX	Any N	M1b	Any S

Source: Sobin LH, Wittekind Ch (eds.): *TNM classification of malignant tumors*, 5th ed. New York, Union Internationale Contre le Cancer Wiley-Liss, 1997.

▬▬▬▬ **APPENDIX 38B**

Prognostic Factors in Germ-cell Testis Tumors

Prognostic factors	Tumor Related	Host Related	Environment Related
Essential	Seminoma vs. NSGCT T, N, M categories HCG, AFP, LDH Site of metastasis		Expertise of physician
Additional	Number of metastases Size of metastases Histologic type	Delay in diagnosis	
New and promising	Copy number of i(12p)		

REFERENCES

1. Sobin LH, Fleming ID: *TNM classification of malignant tumors, fifth edition (1997). Union Internationale Contre le Cancer and the American Joint Committee on Cancer. Cancer* 80:1803–4, 1997.

2. Von der Maase H, Specht L, Jacobsen GK, et al.: Surveillance following orchidectomy for Stage I seminoma of the testis. *Eur J Cancer* 14:1931–4, 1993.

3. Warde P, Gospodarowicz M, Banerjee D, et al.: Prognostic factors for relapse in Stage I testicular seminoma treated with surveillance. *J Uro* 157:1705–9, 1997.

4. Horwich A, Alsanjari N, A'Hern R, et al.: Surveillance following orchidectomy for Stage I testicular seminoma. *B J Cancer* 65:775–8, 1992.

5. Gospodarowicz M, Warde P, Catton C: Optimum management of early stage seminoma, in Jones W, Appleyard I, Harnden P., et al. (eds).: *Germ cell tumours IV.* London, Libbey, 1998, pp. 153–162.

6. Hoeltl W, Kosak D, Pont J, et al.: Testicular cancer: Prognostic implications of vascular invasion. *J Urol* 137:683–5, 1987.

7. Albers P, Siener R, Hartmann M, et al.: Risk factors for relapse in Stage I non-seminomatous germ-cell tumors: Preliminary results of the German Multicenter Trial. German Testicular Cancer Study Group. *Int J Cancer* 83:828–30, 1999.

8. Albers P, Bierhoff E, Mueller S: Prognostic parameters to identify a low risk group in low stage NSGCT, in Jones W, Appleyard I, Harnden P, et al. (eds.): *Germ cell tumours IV.* London, Libbey, 1998, pp. 89–97.

9. Albers P, Miller GA, Orazi A, et al.: Immunohistochemical assessment of tumor proliferation and volume of embryonal carcinoma identify patients with clinical stage A nonseminomatous testicular germ cell tumor at low risk for occult metastasis. *Cancer* 75:844–50, 1995.

10. Fossa SD, Nesland JM, Waehre H, et al.: DNA ploidy in the primary tumor from patients with nonseminomatous testicular germ cell tumors clinical Stage I. *Cancer* 67:1874–7, 1991.

11. Heidenreich A, Sesterhenn IA, Mostofi FK, et al.: Prognostic risk factors that identify patients with clinical Stage I nonseminomatous germ cell tumors at low risk and high risk for metastasis. *Cancer* 83:1002–11, 1998.

12. Fukuda S, Shirahama T, Imazono Y, et al.: Expression of vascular endothelial growth factor in patients with testicular germ cell tumors as an indicator of metastatic disease. *Cancer* 85:1323–30, 1999.

13. Leibovitch L, Foster RS, Kopecky KK, et al.: Improved accuracy of computerized tomography based clinical staging in low stage nonseminomatous germ cell cancer using size criteria of retroperitoneal lymph nodes. *J Urol* 154:1759–63, 1995.

14. Leibovitch I, Foster RS, Kopecky KK, et al.: Identification of clinical stage A nonseminomatous testis cancer patients at extremely low risk for metastatic disease: A combined approach using quantitive immunohistochemical, histopathologic, and radiologic assessment. *J Clin Oncol* 16:261–8, 1998.

15. Freedman LS, Parkinson MC, Jones WG, et al.: Histopathology in the prediction of relapse of patients with Stage I testicular teratoma treated by orchidectomy alone. *Lancet* 2:294–8, 1987.

16. Gospodarowicz MK, Warde PR, Panzarella T, et al.: The Princess Margaret Hospital Experience in the management of Stage I and II seminoma — 1981 to 1991. *Adv Biosci* 91:177–185, 1994.

17. Warde P, Gospodarowicz M, Panzarella T, et al.: Management of Stage II seminoma [see Comments]. *J Clin Oncol* 16:290–4, 1998.

18. Sesterhenn IA, Weiss RB, Mostofi FK, et al.: Prognosis and other clinical correlates of pathologic review in Stage I and II testicular carcinoma: A report from the Testicular Cancer Intergroup Study. *J Clin Oncol* 10:69–78, 1992.

19. Schmoll HJ: Treatment of testicular tumours based on risk factors. *Curr Opin Urol* 9:431–8, 1999.

20. Mencel PJ, Motzer RJ, Mazumdar M, et al.: Advanced seminoma: treatment results, survival, and prognostic factors in 142 patients. *J Clin Oncol* 12:120–6, 1994.

21. Dirix L, Oosterom A: Chemotherapy for metastatic seminoma, in Horwich A (ed.): *Testicular cancer: Investigation and treatment*. London, Chapman & Hall Medical, 1996, pp. 147–153.

22. Dreicer R, Ritter M: Management of Stage III-IV(c) seminoma, in Raghavan D, Scher H, Leibel S (eds.): *Principles and practice of genitourinary oncology*. New York, Lippincott-Raven, 1997, pp. 697–702.

23. Miller K, Loehrer P, Gonin R, et al.: Salvage chemotherapy with vinblastine, ifosfamide and cisplatin in recurrent seminoma. *J Clin Oncol* 15:1427–31, 1997.

24. Mead GM, Stenning SP, Parkinson MC, et al.: The Second Medical Research Council study of prognostic factors in nonseminomatous germ cell tumors. Medical Research Council Testicular Tumour Working Party [Erratum appears in *J Clin Oncol* 10(5):867, 1992]. *J Clin Oncol* 10:85–94, 1992.

25. Bajorin D, Katz A, Chan E, et al.: Comparison of criteria for assigning germ cell tumor patients to "good risk" and "poor risk" studies. *J Clin Oncol* 6:786–92, 1988.

26. Bosl GJ, Geller NL, Cirrincione C, et al.: Multivariate analysis of prognostic variables in patients with metastatic testicular cancer. *Cancer Res* 43:3403–7, 1983.

27. Birch R, Williams S, Cone A, et al.: Prognostic factors for favorable outcome in disseminated germ cell tumors. *J Clin Oncol* 4:400–7, 1986.

28. International Germ Cell Cancer Collaborative Group: International Germ Cell Consensus Classification: A prognostic factor-based staging system for metastatic germ cell cancers [see Comments]. *J Clin Oncol* 15:594–603, 1997.

29. Fossa SD, Oliver RT, Stenning SP, et al.: Prognostic factors for patients with advanced seminoma treated with platinum-based chemotherapy [see Comments]. *Eur J Cancer* 33:1380–7, 1997.

30. Droz JP, Kramar A, Ghosn M, et al.: Prognostic factors in advanced nonseminomatous testicular cancer. A multivariate logistic regression analysis. *Cancer* 62:564–8, 1988.

31. Stoter G, Sylvester R, Sleijfer DT, et al.: Multivariate analysis of prognostic factors in patients with disseminated nonseminomatous testicular cancer: Results from a European Organization for Research on Treatment of Cancer Multiinstitutional Phase III Study. *Cancer Res* 47:2714–8, 1987.

32. Bosl GJ, Motzer RJ: Testicular germ-cell cancer [Erratum appears in *N Engl J Med* 337(19):1403, 1997]. *N Engl J Med* 337:242–53, 1997.

33. Bosl GJ, Geller NL, Chan EY: Stage migration and the increasing proportion of complete responders in patients with advanced germ cell tumors. *Cancer Res* 48:3524–7, 1988.

34. Beyer J, Bokemeyer C, Schmoll HJ, et al.: Treatment intensification in disseminated germ-cell tumors. *World J Urol* 12:207–13, 1994.

35. Williams SD, Birch R, Einhorn LH, et al.: Treatment of disseminated germ-cell tumors with cisplatin, bleomycin, and either vinblastine or etoposide. *N Engl J Med* 316:1435–40, 1987.

36. Gerl A, Clemm C, Schmeller N, et al.: Advances in the management of metastatic non-seminomatous germ cell tumours during the cisplatin era: A single-institution experience. *Br J Cancer* 74:1280–5, 1996.

37. Saxman SB, Nichols CR, Einhorn LH: Salvage chemotherapy in patients with extragonadal nonseminomatous germ cell tumors: The Indiana University experience. *J Clin Oncol* 12:1390–3, 1994.

38. Nichols CR, Saxman S, Williams SD, et al.: Primary mediastinal nonseminomatous germ cell tumors. A modern single institution experience. *Cancer* 65:1641–6, 1990.

39. Debono DJ, Heilman DK, Einhorn LH, et al.: Decision analysis for avoiding postchemotherapy surgery in patients with disseminated nonseminomatous germ cell tumors [see Comments]. *J Clin Oncol* 15:1455–64, 1997.

40. Droz J, Kramar A, Nichols C: Second line chemotherapy with ifosfamide, cisplatin and either etoposide or vinblastine in recurrent germ cell cancer: Assignment of prognostic groups. American Society of Clinical Oncology, Abstr 704, 1993.

41. Gerl A, Clemm C, Schmeller N, et al.: Prognosis after salvage treatment for unselected male patients with germ cell tumours. *Br J Cancer* 72:1026–32, 1995.

42. Fossa SD, Stenning SP, Gerl A, et al.: Prognostic factors in patients progressing after cisplatin-based chemotherapy for malignant non-seminomatous germ cell tumours. *Br J Cancer* 80:1392–9, 1999.

43. Josefsen D, Ous S, Hoie J, et al.: Salvage treatment in male patients with germ cell tumours. *Br J Cancer* 67:568–72, 1993.

44. Motzer RJ, Geller NL, Tan CC, et al.: Salvage chemotherapy for patients with germ cell tumors. The Memorial Sloan-Kettering Cancer Center experience (1979–1989). *Cancer* 67:1305–10, 1991.

45. Nichols CR, Roth BJ, Loehrer PJ, et al.: Salvage chemotherapy for recurrent germ cell cancer. *Semin Oncol* 21:102–8, 1994.

46. Broun ER, Nichols CR, Gize G, et al.: Tandem high dose chemotherapy with autologous bone marrow transplantation for initial relapse of testicular germ cell cancer. *Cancer* 79:1605–10, 1997.

47. Linkesch W, Greinix H, Hocker P: Long term follow up of phase I/II trial of ultra high carboplatin, VP12, cyclosphosphamide with ABMT in refractory or relapsed NSGC. American Society of Clinical Oncology, Abstr 717, 1993.

48. Siegert W, Beyer J, Strohscheer I, et al.: High-dose treatment with carboplatin, etoposide, and ifosfamide followed by autologous stem-cell transplantation in relapsed or refractory germ cell cancer: A phase I/II study. The German Testicular Cancer Cooperative Study Group. *J Clin Oncol* 12:1223–31, 1994.

49. Motzer RJ, Mazumdar M, Bosl GJ, et al.: High-dose carboplatin, etoposide, and cyclophosphamide for patients with refractory germ cell tumors: Treatment results and prognostic factors for survival and toxicity. *J Clin Oncol* 14:1098–105, 1996.

50. Beyer J, Kramar A, Mandanas R, et al.: High-dose chemotherapy as salvage treatment in germ cell tumors: A multivariate analysis of prognostic variables [see Comments]. *J Clin Oncol* 14:2638–45, 1996.

51. Toner GC, Geller NL, Tan C, et al.: Serum tumor marker half-life during chemotherapy allows early prediction of complete response and survival in nonseminomatous germ cell tumors. *Cancer Res* 50:5904–10, 1990.

52. Murphy BA, Motzer RJ, Mazumdar M, et al.: Serum tumor marker decline is an early predictor of treatment outcome in germ cell tumor patients treated with cisplatin and ifosfamide salvage chemotherapy. *Cancer* 73:2520–6, 1994.

53. Vogelzang NJ, Lange PH, Goldman A, et al.: Acute changes of alpha-fetoprotein and human chorionic gonadotropin during induction chemotherapy of germ cell tumors. *Cancer Res* 42:4855–61, 1982.

54. Stevens MJ, Norman AR, Dearnaley DP, et al.: Prognostic significance of early serum tumor marker half-life in metastatic testicular teratoma. *J Clin Oncol* 13:87–92, 1995.

55. Picozzi VJ, Jr., Freiha FS, Hannigan JF, Jr., et al.: Prognostic significance of a decline in serum human chorionic gonadotropin levels after initial chemotherapy for advanced germ-cell carcinoma. *Ann Intern Med* 100:183–6, 1984.

56. Gerl A, Clemm C, Lamerz R, et al.: Prognostic implications of tumour marker analysis in non-seminomatous germ cell tumours with poor prognosis metastatic disease. *Eur J Cancer* 29A:961–5, 1993.

57. Fossa SD, Poulsen JP, Aaserud A: Alkaline phosphatase and lactate dehydrogenase changes during leucocytosis induced by G-CSF in testicular cancer [Letter; Comment]. *Lancet* 340:1544, 1992.

58. Motzer RJ, Mazumdar M, Bajorin DF, et al.: High-dose carboplatin, etoposide, and cyclophosphamide with autologous bone marrow transplantation in first-line therapy for patients with poor-risk germ cell tumors. *J Clin Oncol* 15:2546–52, 1997.

59. Malek NP, Casper J, Looijenga LH, et al.: Quantification of additional short arms of chromosome 12 in germ cell tumours using the polymerase chain reaction. *Eur J Cancer* 33:1488–94, 1997.

60. Chaganti RS, Rodriguez E, Bosl GJ: Cytogenetics of male germ-cell tumors. *Urol Clin North Am* 20:55–66, 1993.

61. Bosl GJ, Dmitrovsky E, Reuter VE, et al.: Isochromosome of the short arm of chromosome 12: Clinically useful markers for male germ cell tumors [Erratum appears in *J Natl Cancer Inst* 82(7):627, 1990] [see Comments]. *J Natl Cancer Inst* 81:1874–8, 1989.

62. Huddart RA, Titley J, Robertson D, et al.: Programmed cell death in response to chemotherapeutic agents in human germ cell tumour lines. *Eur J Cancer* 31A:739–46, 1995.

63. Schmidt B, Ackermann R, Strohmeyer T: Molecular biology of testicular germ cell tumors: Current status. *J Mol Med* 73:355–67, 1995.

64. Strohmeyer T, Reissmann P, Cordon-Cardo C, et al.: Correlation between retinoblastoma gene expression and differentiation in human testicular tumors. *Proc Natl Acad Sci USA* 88:6662–6, 1991.

65. Chaganti R, Bosl G: Molecular biology of male germ cell tumors, in Horwich A (ed.): *Testicular cancer: Investigation and treatment.* London, Chapman & Hall Medical, 1996, pp. 53–60.

66. Sledge GW, Jr., Eble JN, Roth BJ, et al.: Relation of proliferative activity to survival in patients with advanced germ cell cancer. *Cancer Res* 48:3864–8, 1988.

67. Strohmeyer T: Molecular biologic investigations of proto-oncogenes and growth factors in human testicular tumors. *World J Urol* 12:74–8, 1994.

68. Reed E, Ozols RF, Tarone R, et al.: The measurement of cisplatin-DNA adduct levels in testicular cancer patients. *Carcinogenesis* 9:1909–11, 1988.

69. Motzer RJ, Reed E, Perera F, et al.: Platinum-DNA adducts assayed in leukocytes of patients with germ cell tumors measured by atomic absorbance spectrometry and enzyme-linked immunosorbent assay. *Cancer* 73:2843–52, 1994.

70. Kelland LR: The molecular basis of cisplatin sensitivity/resistance [Comment]. *Eur J Cancer* 30A:725–7, 1994.

71. Schmoll HJ: Prognostic factors for advanced seminoma—A solid basis for clinical trials [Editorial; Comment]. *Eur J Cancer* 33:1347–50, 1997.

72. Hill BT, Shellard SA, Fichtinger-Schepman AM, et al.: Differential formation and enhanced removal of specific cisplatin-DNA adducts in two cisplatin-selected resistant human testicular teratoma sublines. *Anticancer Drugs* 5:321–8, 1994.

73. Collette L, Sylvester RJ, Stenning SP, et al.: Impact of the treating institution on survival of patients with "poor-prognosis" metastatic nonseminoma. European Organization for Research and Treatment of Cancer Genito-Urinary Tract Cancer Collaborative Group and the Medical Research Council Testicular Cancer Working Party [see Comments]. *J Natl Cancer Inst* 91:839–46, 1999.

74. Harding MJ, Paul J, Gillis CR, et al.: Management of malignant teratoma: Does referral to a specialist unit matter? [see Comments]. *Lancet* 341:999–1002, 1993.

75. Feuer EJ, Sheinfeld J, Bosl GJ: Does size matter? Association between number of patients treated and patient outcome in metastatic testicular Cancer [Editorial; Comment]. *J Natl Cancer Inst* 91:816–8, 1999.

76. Moul JW, Paulson DF, Dodge RK, et al.: Delay in diagnosis and survival in testicular cancer: Impact of effective therapy and changes during 18 years. *J Urol* 143:520–3, 1990.

77. Klepp O, Olsson A, Henrikson H: Predicting metastases in clinical Stage I testicular teratoma: Multivariate analysis of a large multicentric study (SWENOTECA), *5th European Conference on Clinical Oncology (ECCO)*, Abstr O787, 1989.

78. Hoskin P, Dilly S, Easton D, et al.: Prognostic factors in Stage I non-seminomatous germ-cell testicular tumors managed by orchiectomy and surveillance: Implications for adjuvant chemotherapy. *J Clin Oncol* 4:1031–6, 1986.

79. Vogelzang NJ, Fraley EE, Lange PH, et al.: Stage II nonseminomatous testicular cancer: A 10-year experience. *J Clin Oncol* 1:171–8, 1983.

80. Vugrin D, Whitmore W, Cvitkovic E, et al.: Adjuvant chemotherapy with VAB-3 of Stage II-B testicular cancer. *Cancer* 48:233–7, 1981.

81. Pizzocaro G, Monfardini S: No adjuvant chemotherapy in selected patients with pathologic Stage II nonseminomatous germ cell tumors of the testis. *J Urol* 131:677–80, 1984.

82. Richie JP, Kantoff PW: Is adjuvant chemotherapy necessary for patients with stage B1 testicular cancer? *J Clin Oncol* 9:1393–6, 1991.

CHAPTER 39

Renal-cell Carcinoma

HEIN VAN POPPEL, GOEDELE BECKERS, and LUC BAERT

A significant problem for clinicians who treat cancer is the application of the known determinants of disease outcome to the individual patient. The clinical course can be affected by the inherent properties of the tumor, the host-related factors, and the treatment applied. Renal-cell carcinoma (RCC) has the reputation of an individual unpredictable outcome with rare cases of spontaneous tumor regression and extended survival despite the presence of metastases. This unpredictable outcome is determined by the genotypic biological behavior and the tumor-host interaction. Refinement of our ability to predict the outcome should facilitate the rational choice of treatment alternatives and provide more reliability in the interaction with the patient. In case of RCC the absence of other effective treatment modalities besides surgery, renders these considerations even more important.

TUMOR-RELATED FACTORS

The anatomic extent of disease, the local extent, the venous or lymphatic invasion, and systemic dissemination remain the most important prognostic factors for RCC. Microscopic features such as nuclear grade, nuclear morphometry, histologic tumor type or subtype, and mitotic activity are widely recognized as relevant prognosticators, but microvascular invasion and microvessel density are gaining more interest. The absence or presence of symptoms and serologic alterations has an obvious impact on prognosis. Recently molecular biology and genetics have been investigated more and more as to their prognostic value, but further research in this promising but expensive field is warranted.

Tumor Extent

The most important prognostic factor in RCC is the anatomical extent of the tumor at the time of diagnosis.[1-9] Through the years different staging systems

Prognostic Factors in Cancer, 2nd edition, Edited by Mary K. Gospodarowicz
ISBN 0-471-40633-3   Copyright © 2001 Wiley-Liss, Inc.

have been developed, the first proposed in 1958.[5] Since then many systems have been based on three main prognostic categories: organ confined, locally advanced, and metastatic disease.

The first staging systems to be used was the Robson staging, proposed over 30 years ago.[1] Currently, the TNM classification is standard.[6] (see Appendix 39A). The TNM system was adapted in 1997, with the main change being the cutpoint diameter of the tumor between stage T1 and T2, which was increased moved from 2.5 cm to 7 cm in an attempt to avoid the overlap in the survival curves between these two stages.[10] Tumor size is not considered to be a relevant independent prognostic factor: RCCs with the same grade, ploidy pattern, nuclear morphometry, and vimentin expression have no significantly better prognosis when the tumors are smaller than 5 cm.[10,11]

Also, in multifocal and bilateral RCC the stage of the individual tumor foci are important. Moreover, the 5-year survival of patients with bilateral RCC was shown to be significantly better (77.8%) than for patients with metachronously occurring lesions (37.5%).[10]

Patients with RCC that is limited to the kidney have the best prognosis. Invasion through the renal capsule decreases survival rates by 15 to 20%.[12] In 4 to 20% of the cases, the tumor can invade the renal vein or the vena cava, with simultaneous lymph-node invasion in 55 to 60% of the cases.[2] The 5-year survival with a tumor thrombus in the vena cava is comparable to that of patients with distant metastases.[10] The locoregional extent rather than the level of the tumor thrombus in the vena cava determines the prognosis.[13]

The incidence of lymph-node invasion varies in different series. Invasion of the lymph nodes occurs in 20 to 30% of cases and is more frequent than invasion into the perirenal fat. Approximately 10% of the patients have positive lymph nodes without distant metastases. This improves the prognosis, with 5-year survival rates of about 52%. The 5-year survival of lymph-node-positive patients with metastases varies between 0 and 11%.[4,14,15]

There is a statistically significant difference between a better prognosis for solitary metastases and one for lung or bony metastases only. It is estimated that solitary metastases occur in only 1.6 to 3.6% of cases, and 5-year survival rates were found to vary between 35 and 50%.[16] Patients with lung metastases fare better than those with bone metastases.[14] Metastases that occur metachronously have a better prognosis with a better outcome that is related to the time interval between the detection of the primary tumor and the appearance of the metastases.[17] When the time between a nephrectomy and the first metastatic localization is longer than 24 months, the prognosis is also significantly better.[18]

Microscopic Features

Histologic Grade   The microscopic finding that significantly correlates most with prognosis in every tumor stage, is the histologic grade.[9] Obviously, patients with high-grade tumors mostly present with more advanced stages at the time of diagnosis and are at a substantially greater risk of local recurrence or distant metastases. Nevertheless, histologic grading is less important as an independent prognostic factor than the nodal (N0 vs. N1–3) or metastatic stage (M0 vs. M1).[19] Grade has probably more prognostic relevance in tumors with intermediate tumor stages.[3,9,20]

The most commonly used grading system is that of Fuhrman et al.[21] The mean 5-year survival rate was reported to be approximately 60% for Grade I, 30% for Grade II and III, and only 10% for Grade IV. This grading system, however, has important limitations. First, there is the interobserver correlation, which is poorer for the Fuhrman grading system than for any other grading system for RCC.[22] A second drawback is the quality of the fixation of the specimens, which can influence the size of the nuclei and nucleoli. Third, most kidney tumors are composed of cells with different grades, and it has not been determined how many cells of a higher grade have to be present to define a higher tumor grade. Finally, the Fuhrman grading system was conceived without taking the different histological tumor types into account. Patients with papillary (chromophilic) RCC are doing better, while those with collecting-duct carcinoma have a much worse prognosis.[23] Sarcomatoid tumors are classified as Fuhrman Grade IV, and have an extremely poor prognosis.[23,24] The presence of sarcomatoid foci in the tumor correlates significantly with the probability of cancer death in all patients, but also with that of disease progression in those with localized RCC.[25]

Because of the problems with the Fuhrman grading, other systems have been proposed. The Erlangen classification is based on pattern and cellular type. Grade I corresponds to all tumors with a solid pattern and clear cells. Grade III encompasses the sarcomatoid and anaplastic tumors, and the tumors with granular cells with field. Grade II are those tumors that have other patterns and cytologic characteristics (tubular, papillary, glandular, cystic, mixed, granular cells without field, and oncocytic cells).[26] However, in this system there is no significant prognostic difference between Grade I and Grade II tumors, although there is a significant difference in survival between Grade I–II and Grade III tumors.

The International Union Against Cancer (UICC) grading system is also still in use.[6] The tumors are categorized between Grade I, well-differentiated, and Grade IV, undifferentiated, and GX when the tumor grade cannot be assessed. Additionally, this system is considered as useful in the intermediate tumor stages.[12]

Nuclear Morphometry   The problems with the different grading systems have prompted the development of quantitative morphometric parameters such as nuclear area, nuclear perimeter and diameter, nuclear roundness, irregularity, ellipticity, and elongation. The mean nuclear volume was significantly correlated with disease-specific survival,[25,27] although this was not always confirmed.[28] Five-year survival rates as high as 97 to 100% were reported for tumors with small nuclear areas (between 32 and 39 μm).[12,29] Therefore, some consider nuclear morphometry to be clearly superior to conventional histological grading in predicting prognosis.[30]

Histologic Tumor Type The renal adenoma, renal oncocytoma, and metanephric adenoma are considered to be benign tumors of the kidney. The distinction between adenoma and carcinoma by morphologic criteria is difficult and the adenoma–carcinoma sequence is still controversial. The tumor size has been commonly used to distinguish between these two entities, but it is well known that some tumors of less than 3 cm can exhibit metastases. It therefore was attempted to further differentiate the two subtypes. Type 1 is the papillary pattern, with small basophilic cells and often multifocal tumors of reduced size, which is probably not a cancer precursor. Type 2 has a solid or tubulopapillary pattern with clear cells, larger size, and is frequently solitary. Morphologically Type 2 might be either a precursor of RCC or could be considered a small carcinoma.[31]

RCC formerly was categorized on the basis of the microscopic aspect of the cytoplasm as either the clear-cell or granular-cell type. However the prognostic significance of these categories was not established. In general the prognosis of a clear-cell RCC is somewhat better than that of the eosinophilic or granular subtype,[32] and papillary tumors have a better prognosis than solid ones. The so-called cystic clear-cell carcinoma is mostly low grade, low stage, and diploid, and has an excellent prognosis.[33] In 1985 Thoenes et al.[34] reported on a new classification that distinguished between the clear-cell, the chromophil (with its eosinophil and basophil variant), the chromophobe (the typical one and the eosinophil variant), and the collecting-duct carcinoma. This Mainz classification was based on morphological criteria, but subsequent genetic studies have confirmed its validity by showing characteristic genetic abnormalities.

The conventional RCC (clear-cell type) is known to have a loss of genetic material on chromosome 3p, and nearly half of them have somatic mutations in the von Hippel-Lindau gene (20% have inactivation of the gene). About 5% have sarcomatoid changes.[24]

The papillary (chromophilic) RCC occurs in about 15% of kidney neoplasms and has a better prognosis than the conventional type.[4,35] Papillary RCC presents trisomy of different chromosomes 3q, 7, 12, 16, 17, and 20 and loss of the Y chromosome.[12,35] Studies have shown a 5-year survival of 80 to 90% for papillary renal cell carcinoma.[36] Chromophobe RCC can exhibit monosomy of chromosomes 1, 2, 6, 10, 13, 17, and 21, as well as hypodiploidy; its prognosis is variable.[35]

Prognosis is much worse in case of a collecting duct carcinoma accounting for about 1% of renal malignancies. The Bellini duct carcinoma and the medullary carcinoma of the kidney arise from the collecting ducts of the renal cortex or medulla. Most of the patients will present metastases at the time of diagnosis and survival is between weeks and months despite surgery or any other treatment.[12,24]

Mitotic Rate The appearance of mitotic figures is more pronounced in more aggressive tumors. The number of mitoses counted was correlated with survival, and tumors with fewer than 1 mitosis per 10 high-power fields have the best prognosis. Indeed, 1 mitosis per 10 high-power fields can decrease the 5-year survival from 67% to 16%.[3] Although it appears very tempting to correlate the evaluation of the mitotic rate with outcome, its application has remained very limited.

Microvascular Invasion   RCC has the particular propensity of invading small vessels (lymphatics or veins), initiating a process of lymph-node and distant metastases. Microscopic invasion of small vessels, defined as tumor growth through its wall, was shown to be important.[37–39] In an unspecified group of patients that underwent nephrectomy, where there was no clinical lymph-node invasion or metastases, tumor progression occurred in 6% of patients without and in 40% of patients with microvascular invasion. The 89% 5-year survival of patients without microvascular invasion was reduced to less than 50% in those with microvascular invasion.[39] Microscopic invasion of small vessels within the tumor is easy to recognize, and the pathological report should mention the presence or absence of this important prognosticator.

Microvessel Density   In most other tumors a higher microvessel density is associated with a higher degree of malignancy. In RCC, however, high-grade tumors showed a lower microvessel density than low-grade cancers. For a mean microvessel density of ≤ 40 per high power field, an inverse relation with patient survival was found[40] for only stage III tumors. Further studies are needed to demonstrate a prognostic relevance of this parameter.

Symptoms   The classic triad of pain, hematuria, and flank mass has become quite uncommon and now occurs in less than 10% of patients. When the classic symptoms are present, the disease is advanced. These symptoms can also occur separately with pain in 41% of the cases, hematuria in 38%, and a palpable mass in 24% of patients. Weight loss and hypertension can occur in about 30% of the patients. Fever and night sweats can also occur. In about 8%, hypercalcemia occurs. None of these symptoms has an independent prognostic value in multivariate analysis.[7,14,15,18,32] Obviously, patients with an asymptomatic tumor have a better 5-year survival rate than those who present with complaints (79% vs. 57%), but they have lower stage disease (77% vs. 54% with Stages I or II).[8,41]

The Stauffer syndrome,[42] is a remarkable syndrome that occasionally accompanies RCC. Patients present with liver-function disorders, a decrease in white blood cell count, fever, and the presence of necrotic nonmetastatic foci in the liver. The presence of this syndrome has no prognostic importance in itself, but its disappearance after nephrectomy correlates with good survival rates, while its reappearance means tumor recurrence and poor prognosis.[43]

Serological Alterations   An accelerated erythrocyte sedimentation rate (ESR) above 30 mm/h, a hemoglobin level below 10 in women and below 12 in men, hypercalcemia or hypoalbuminemia, an elevated alkaline phosphatase, gamma-glutamyl transpeptidase, lactate dehydrogenase (LDH), α-globulin, and serum ferritine all correlate with a higher tumor stage. In a multivariate analysis, however, only the accelerated ESR was shown to have a prognostic impact.[32,44]

Molecular Markers

Genetic Alterations and DNA Ploidy   Most RCCs show loss of genetic material in chromosomes 3p, 4q, 6q, 8p, and 9p and a gain in genetic material in chromosomes 17q and Xq.[36] Because tumor suppressor genes are located on these chromosomes, they are thought to play a role in the tumorigenesis and tumor progression. It is difficult to estimate the clinical relevance of these changes, since genetic instability is a well-known phenomenon in RCC.[45,46] Mutations of the von Hippel-Lindau (VHL) tumor suppressor gene were found in 57% of nonhereditary clear-cell RCC. The presence of those mutations, however, had no prognostic impact.[47]

The changes in ploidy are an expression of genetic instability and can be prognostically relevant. In RCC, a number of studies showed a positive correlation between DNA ploidy and grade, stage, and survival,[48,49] but this finding was not observed in all studies. The intratumoral heterogeneity of DNA[26,50] could be responsible for the lack of correlation between DNA content in a primary tumor and the survival time.[51] Although patients with five or less cytogenetic changes have a better prognosis, the tumor grade remains a better independent prognostic factor to predict disease recurrence.[52]

Proliferation Markers and Oncogenes   In recent years many studies have focused on proliferation markers, mostly on small numbers of patients and with diverging results. Although interesting results have been obtained, at this time there is no clinical relevance for diagnosis or prognosis.

Nucleolar Organizing Regions   Nucleolar organizing regions (NORs) are chromosomal DNA loops encoding ribosomal RNA, detectable by silver staining (AgNOR). The number and the distribution of AgNOR areas is correlated with growth fractions.[19] In a multivariate analysis the AgNOR count correlates with grade and survival. Low values in Stage I and II predict a 100% 5-year survival, while in Grade III tumors they correlate with a long disease-free survival.[53]

Angiogenic Factors   The most studied angiogenic factors are basic fibroblast growth factor (bFGF) and vascular endothelial growth factor (VEGF). Some studies have shown an increase in both factors in patients with N+ or M+ disease.[54] No correlation was found, however, with tumor grade, tumor stage, and tumor volume.[54,55] One study showed that a bFGF above 14 pg/mL is associated with a higher frequency of pulmonary metastases.[56] Patients with lymphocytic infiltration of the tumor were shown to have a better prognosis than those with just a few or no lymphocytes infiltrating the tumor.[57] Tumor infiltrating lymphocytes express angiogenesis factor VEGF, and this could mean that tumor infiltrating lymphocytes could enhance tumor progression.[58] The importance of angiogenetic factors needs further elaboration.

Adhesion Molecules and Proteases   Tissue degradation and remodeling in normal and tumor tissue are controlled by limited proteolysis of the extracellular matrix. This proteolysis results from different proteases for example, urokinase, collagenase and cathepsin. Urokinase-type plasminogen activator and tissue-type plasminogen activator transform plasminogen into plasmin. Urokinase mainly mediates pericellular proteolysis and tissue degradation. Urokinase is elevated in tumor tissue, and urokinase specific inhibitors can block invasion of several metastatic human tumor cell lines in vitro. With values above 0.84 ng/mL, urokinase could correlate with infiltration in the perirenal fat and the development of distant metastases.

Plasminogen activator inhibitor-1 seems to protect the tissues and the tumoral blood vessels against degradation and can inhibit tumor infiltration. A cutoff level of 12 ng/mg protein was shown to correlate with the development of metastases after surgery.[59] CD44 is a transmembrane glycoprotein involved in cell–cell and cell–matrix interactions. Multivariate analysis indicated CD44 expression as independent prognostic factor for overall and disease-free survival.[60] Sialyl Lewis carbohydrate antigen is thought to mediate the interaction of leucocytes or tumor cells with endothelial cells, followed by integrin-mediated adhesion. Cells expressing this antigen may show a higher metastatic potential because of its increased chance of adhering to endothelial cells in blood vessels.[61] Expression of progelatinase A messenger RNA (a Type IV collagenase) seems to have an inverse relationship with patient survival.[62]

Proliferation Markers   Proliferating-cell nuclear antigen (PCNA), Ki-S5 and Ki-67/MIB-1, are markers of active cell proliferation.[12,38,54,63] Several studies have shown that both markers correlate positively with tumor stage.[38,54,63] One study has shown that survival was significantly poorer in patients with a PCNA index greater than 5%.[63] Other studies showed the importance of Ki-67 as a powerful predictor of survival and disease-free survival in M0 tumors, while in T1-2N0M0 tumors and Grade II tumors different prognostic groups could be distinguished according to Ki-67 labeling ($p = 0.0098$).[64] These markers could identify patients that will show tumor recurrence despite diagnosis and treatment in a localized stage. Ki-S5 correlates significantly with stage and tumor grade: patients with low Ki-S5 labeling exhibit more than an 80% disease-free survival.[65] Tissue polypeptide antigen (TPA) is thought to indicate proliferative activity of cancer cells, but is a non-organ-specific prognostic marker that can be useful for monitoring the course of the disease. High levels of this marker might indicate metastatic tumor activity.[66]

Markers of Apoptosis   Metallothionein (MT) is a major cysteine-rich protein, which has a role in the absorption, transport, and metabolism of the important trace metals zinc, copper, and cadmium. MT has a role in the detoxification of these heavy metals. There were significant relationships of MT expression with both higher grade ($p < 0.05$) and invasive growth pattern ($p < 0.01$) of RCC. In the same study the apoptosis index was significantly higher in Grade II

($p < 0.0001$) and Grade III ($p < 0.005$) of RCC than in Grade I.[67] The frequency of apoptosis and the expression of MT may be related to carcinogenesis, but also to progression of RCC.[68]

p53 Suppressor Gene, Bcl-2 Oncogene, c-myc Expression, nm23 Protein Expression, CD95 (Fas/APO-1)   Except in the sarcomatoid variant, mutations in the p53 suppressor gene are rare in RCC. p53 controls a cell cycle checkpoint responsible for maintaining the integrity of the genome by interrupting the cell cycle in the G1 phase for DNA repair or by cell apoptosis when there is severe DNA damage.[69] Bcl-2 oncogene is expressed in about 60% of RCC, but there was no correlation with prognosis or pathological features found.[70] High values of c-myc correlate with T-category and with nuclear grade, but not with nodal involvement, tumor cell type, or the presence of metastases.[71] Also, the expression of this oncogene has no clinical relevance. Decreased expression of nm23-H1 protein could be a strong predictor for poor prognosis in carcinomas of less than 5 cm and can be found in about 50% of the tumors. It cannot, however, predict the presence of metastases. nm23-H2 has no clinical relevance for prognosis.[72] CD95 (Fas/APO-1) values can be increased in some patients with RCC. One study has shown that the disease-specific survival rate was significantly lower in the group that expressed this protein. This protein also could play a role in treatment strategies.[73] All the studies related to oncogenes are based on small numbers of patients, and the results remain irrelevant to actual daily practice.

Glycoprotein Tumor Markers   Increased values of CA-50, CA-19.9, CA-125, and CA-15.3 have been described in RCC. CA-125 and CA-15.3 could be correlated with the clinical stage and tumor grade. Patients with an increased CA-125 have a significantly shorter survival rate.[74]

TuM2-PK   The pyruvate *kinase* isoenzyme *tumor M2*, one of the isoforms of the glycolytic enzyme pyruvate kinase, is strongly overexpressed by tumor cells and released into body fluids. TuM2-PK can be measured in the plasma and was shown to strongly correlate with the Robson tumor stage, and thus have prognostic implications.[75]

Parathyroid Hormone-related Protein   Hypercalcemia is a bad prognostic factor in patients with RCC.[12] The parathyroid hormone-related protein is responsible for this hypercalcemia. Recent studies showed that the amino-terminal region of the parathyroid hormone-related protein displays growth-factor-like activity and can play a role in the growth of RCC. A study of 40 radical nephrectomy specimens showed that in 75% of cases there was a strong expression of this gene, mostly in clear-cell-type tumors. Granular-cell-type tumors express this protein significantly less often. Tumor recurrence was significantly greater in the weakly staining tumors. Therefore, parathyroid hormone-related protein could be an independent prognostic factor for RCC.[76]

Vimentin expression by tumor cells provides important prognostic information for patients with localized RCC; the combination of vimentin expression and histological grade is a better predictor for survival than grade or vimentin expression alone.[77]

HOST-RELATED FACTORS

The unpredictable outcome of RCC is partly due to the interaction of the tumor with its host. Several studies have shown that race, age, gender and tumor side have no influence on the prognosis of an RCC.[7,14,15,18] Performance status is an important issue, but hereditary predisposition, hemodialysis, and exposure to carcinogens also can be relevant in assessing the prognosis of RCC.

Performance Status

Patients' performance status has been shown to be an important prognostic factor. A less-than-normal performance status has a significantly worse prognosis in nonmetastatic as well as in the metastatic tumors.[13–15,78]

Von Hippel-Lindau Disease

The von Hippel-Lindau disease is a rare autosomal-dominant disorder (incidence 1:36,000) that displays the development of bilateral and multifocal renal cysts and tumors, but also hemangioblastoma of the spine and the cerebellum, hemangiomas of the retina, pheochromocytoma, island-cell tumors of the pancreas, and epididymal cystadenomas. Kidney cancers are always of the clear-cell type and have a chromosomal alteration at the level of the short arm of chromosome 3 (3p25). These alterations are mutations of the von Hippel-Lindau tumor suppressor gene, whose product, the von Hippel-Lindau tumor suppressor protein (pVHL), plays a role in angiogenesis in normal cells, as well as in the formation of extracellular matrix and the cell cycle. Despite intense follow-up, 30 to 50% of these patients die from metastatic RCC.[12,79,80]

Tuberous Sclerosis Complex

Tuberous sclerosis complex is also an autosomal-dominant disease, occurring in 1:14,000 humans, mostly women. The mutations are located at the level of chromosomes 9q34 and 16p13. The patients develop hamartomas of the skin, the central nervous system, the lungs, and the heart. Forty to 80% of the patients develop cysts, angiomyolipomas, and malignant tumors at the level of the kidneys. The development of malignancies in the kidneys is, however, less frequent than in von Hippel-Lindau disease.[12,81]

Autosomal-dominant Adult Polycystic Kidney Disease

Autosomal-dominant adult polycystic kidney disease is the most common renal cystic disease, with an incidence of 1:1000 persons. Fifty percent of those patients develop terminal renal failure. The chromosomal alterations are located on chromosomes 16 and 4. Although there is no consensus, most researchers believe that there is an increased incidence of renal tumors. When tumors develop, it is mostly in younger patients with the aggressive histological type.[82]

Familial Renal-Cell Carcinoma

Worldwide about 20 families are described with a familial renal carcinoma. Mostly the tumors are of the papillary type. The incidence is much higher in men than in women and the tumors are mostly detected at younger ages. The mean survival is 52 years.[12,83]

ENVIRONMENT-RELATED FACTORS

The surgical and other treatment modalities that are applied for RCC can have an important impact on the prognosis, although it remains difficult to prove whether the natural history of the disease or the treatment used has more prognostic relevance. Radical nephrectomy is still considered to be standard treatment of the nonmetastatic RCC. Resection of the adrenal is a matter of controversy. Since the incidence of adrenal metastases, diagnosed on histological examination and unrecognized on preoperative ultrasound or CT scan, is low, many authors try to find arguments for dropping the adrenal from consideration as a prognosticator. The probability of an adrenal metastasis is correlated with tumor stage, but not with the localization of the tumor in the upper or lower pole.[84] While some authors advocate an adrenalectomy only in patients with an abnormal adrenal on CT scan or in larger tumors of the upper pole,[85,86] it was shown that 7% of the patients with tumors larger than 5 cm in diameter have micrometastatic adrenal involvement.[87] Therefore not performing an adrenalectomy can have prognostic implications.

The role of lymphadenectomy also remains controversial. Patients with obvious lymph nodes that are pathologically proven to be malignant have a bad prognosis despite nephrectomy and an extensive lymphadenectomy. Survival rates vary between 5% and 30% at 5 years.[79] Probably those patients that could benefit from a lymphadenectomy are those with microscopic invasion that was not recognized before surgery. Although lymph-node dissection in RCC has always been considered a staging procedure rather than as a cure, there can be a subset of patients with microscopic invasion that are cured by the lymphadenectomy.

This has been suggested in nonrandomized single-center studies, but will need confirmation in larger randomized studies.[4,10,15,88]

Smaller tumors can be removed by partial nephrectomy, even in the presence of a normal contralateral kidney. The incidence of local recurrence is low in an elective situation, where an easily resectable small tumor is usually removed in the presence of a normal contralateral kidney.[89] Nevertheless local recurrence can occur when enucleations of the tumor are performed. The major problem with nephron-sparing surgery is the multifocal behavior of RCC that is responsible for recurrence elsewhere in the kidney. This has prognostic importance and implies that patients undergoing partial nephrectomy should continue to have ultrasonographic follow-up of the remnant and contralateral kidney.[90]

Extension of a tumor thrombus in the renal vein or in the vena cava necessitates complete excision. This can result in prolonged survival in patients that have no lymph-node or distant metastases at the time of surgery.[13] Prolonged survival was obtained even with thrombus in the right atrium. Here surgical expertise also becomes an important prognostic factor.[91]

The value of nephrectomy is much debated in case of metastatic RCC. While radical nephrectomy can be proposed because of bleeding and pain, its prognostic value remains uncertain.[14,16,78] Radical nephrectomy can be followed by spontaneous regression of pulmonary metastases in less than 1% of cases.[14,18]

Debulking surgery for tumors invading the colon, the duodenum, and the pancreas results in survival rates of less than 12% after 1 year. Resection of solitary metastases can exhibit prolonged survival, while metastasectomies of lesions that occur more than 2 years after the treatment of the primary tumor have a better prognosis.[16]

Immunotherapy has been shown to induce tumor response in about 20% of patients, and long-standing remissions have been described. The positive prognostic factors for treatment with interferon-alpha, interleukin-2, or combinations are a good performance status, a long disease-free interval, and disease predominantly in the lung.[18,78,79] The administration of interferon in itself has been described as a factor that improves prognosis.[93]

SUMMARY

Renal cell carcinoma (RCC) is reputed to have an unpredictable outcome in the individual patient, although progress has been made in the application of prognostic factors. Essential factors in predicting outcome are the anatomical extent of the tumor at the time of diagnosis, the tumor grade, and the histological type of the tumor. A bad performance status and elevated erythrocyte sedimentation rate imply a worse prognosis. The patients undergoing a radical or a partial nephrectomy have a good prognosis when there is no lymph-node or distant metastatic disease. For an individual patient, the performance of routine adrenalectomy and lymph-node dissection can be of value. The rare patient with solitary metastasis can have a favorable survival prognosis.

■■■■■ **APPENDIX 39A**

TNM Classification: Kidney Cancer

T — Primary Tumour

TX Primary tumor cannot be assessed

T0 No evidence of primary tumor

T1 Tumor 7.0 cm or less in greatest dimension, limited to the kidney

T2 Tumor more than 7.0 cm in greatest dimension, limited to the kidney

T3 Tumor extends into major veins or invades adrenal gland or perinephric tissues but not beyond Gerota fascia

T3a Tumor invades adrenal gland or perinephric tissues but not beyond Gerota fascia

T3b Tumor grossly extends into renal vein(s) or vena cava below diaphragm

T3c Tumor grossly extends into vena cava above diaphragm

T4 Tumor invades beyond Gerota fascia

N — Regional Lymph Nodes

NX Regional lymph nodes cannot be assessed

N0 No regional lymph node metastasis

N1 Metastasis in a single regional lymph node

N2 Metastasis in more than one regional lymph node

M — Distant Metastasis

MX Distant metastasis cannot be assessed

M0 No distant metastasis

M1 Distant metastasis

	Stage Grouping		
Stage I	T1	N0	M0
Stage II	T2	N0	M0
Stage III	T1	N1	M0
	T2	N1	M0
	T3	N0, N1	M0
Stage IV	T4	N0, N1	M0
	Any T	N2	M0
	Any T	Any N	M1

Source: Sobin LH, Fleming ID: TNM classification of malignant tumors, fifth edition (1997). Union Internationale Contre le Cancer and the American Joint Committee on Cancer. *Cancer* 80:1803–4, 1997.

■■■■■■ **APPENDIX 39B**

Prognostic Factors in Renal-cell Carcinoma

Prognostic Factors	Tumor Related	Host Related	Environment Related
Essential	Stage Histologic grade	Hereditary diseases	Radical or partial nephrectomy
Additional	Histologic tumor type Vena cava invasion Nuclear morphometry Mitotic rate Sedimentation rate Symptoms	Performance status	Adrenalectomy Lymph-node dissection
New and promising	Microvascular involvement Genetic alterations DNA ploidy Proliferation markers		Immunotherapy Metastasectomy

REFERENCES

1. Robson CJ, Churchill BM, Anderson W: The results of radical nephrectomy for renal cell carcinoma. *J Urol* 101:297–301, 1969.

2. Golimbu M, Joshi P, Sperber A, et al.: Renal cell carcinoma: Survival and prognostic factors. *Urology* 27:291–301, 1986.

3. Grignon DJ, Ayala AG, El-Naggar A, et al.: Renal cell carcinoma: A clinicopathologic and DNA flow cytometric analysis of 103 cases. *Cancer* 64:2133–40, 1989.

4. Giberti C, Oneto F, Martorana G, et al.: Radical nephrectomy for renal cell carcinoma: Long-term results and prognostic factors on a series of 328 cases. *Eur Urol* 31:40–8, 1997.

5. Flocks RH, Kadesky MC: Malignant neoplasms of the kidney: An analysis of 353 patients followed 5 years or more. *Eur Urol* 79:196, 1958.

6. Sobin LH, Wittekind Ch (eds.): *UICC TNM classification of malignant tumours*, 5th ed. New York, Wiley-Liss, 1997, pp. 180–182.

7. Montie JE: Prognostic factors for renal cell carcinoma. [Editorial]. *J Urol* 152:1397–8, 1994.

8. Trasher JB, Paulson DF: Prognostic factors in renal cancer. *Urol Clin North Am* 20:247–62, 1993.

9. Medeiros LJ, Gelb AB, Weiss LM: Renal cell carcinoma: Prognostic significance of morphologic parameters in 121 cases. *Cancer* 61:1639–51, 1988.

10. Giuliani L, Giberti C, Martorana G, et al.: Radical extensive surgery for renal cell carcinoma: Long term results and prognostic factors. *J Urol* 143:468–73, 1990.

11. Nativ O, Sabo E, Raviv G, et al.: The impact of tumor size on clinical outcome in patients with localized renal cell carcinoma treated by radical nephrectomy. *J Urol* 158:729–32, 1997.

12. Bonsib SM: Risk and prognosis in renal neoplasms. A pathologist's prospective. *Urol Clin North Am* 26:643–60, 1999.

13. Tongaonkar HB, Dandekar NP, Dalal AV, et al.: Renal cell carcinoma extending to the renal vein and inferior vena cava: Results of surgical treatment and prognostic factors. *J Surg Oncol* 59:94–100, 1995.

14. Frank W, Stuhldreher D, Saffrin R, et al.: Stage IV renal cell carcinoma. *J Urol* 152:1998–9, 1994.

15. Lanigan D: Prognostic factors in renal cell carcinoma. *Br J Urol* 75:565–71, 1995.

16. Van Poppel HP, Baert L: Palliative surgical therapy, in Petrovich Z, Baert L, Brady LW (eds.): *Carcinoma of the kidney and testis, and rare urologic malignancies.* Berlin, Springer-Verlag, 1999, pp. 96–109.

17. Landonio G, Baiocchi C, Cattaneo D, et al.: Retrospective analysis of 156 cases of metastatic renal cell carcinoma: Evaluation of prognostic factors and response to different treatments. *Tumori* 80:468–72, 1994.

18. Mani S, Todd MB, Katz K, et al.: Prognostic factors for survival in patients with metastatic renal cancer treated with biological response modifiers. *J Urol* 154:35–40, 1995.

19. Fujii Y, Owada F, Higashi Y, et al.: Prognostic factors of renal cell carcinoma: A multivariate analysis. *Hinyokika Kiyo* 42:85–9, 1996.

20. Bretheau D, Lechevallier E, de Fromont M, et al.: Prognostic value of nuclear grade of renal cell carcinoma. *Cancer* 76:2543–9, 1995.

21. Fuhrman SA, Lasky LC, Limas C: Prognostic significance of morphologic parameters in renal cell carcinoma. *Am J Surg Pathol* 6:655–63, 1982.

22. Lanigan D, Conroy R, Barry-Walsh C, et al.: A comparative analysis of grading systems in renal adenocarcinoma. *Histopathology* 24:473–6, 1994.

23. Goldstein NS: Grading of renal cell carcinoma. *Urol Clin North Am* 26:637–42, 1999.

24. Bostwick DG, Eble JN: Diagnosis and classification of renal cell carcinoma. *Urol Clin North Am* 26:627–35, 1999.

25. Kanamaru H, Sasaki M, Miwa Y, et al.: Prognostic value of sarcomatoid histology and volume-weighted mean nuclear volume in renal cell carcinoma. *Br J Urol* 83:222–6, 1999.

26. Riuz-cerda JL, Hernandez M, Sempere A, et al.: Intratumoral heterogeneity of DNA content in renal cell carcinoma and its prognostic significance. *Cancer* 86:664–71, 1999.

27. Soda T, Fujikawa K, Ito T, et al.: Volume-weighted mean nuclear volume as a prognostic factor in renal cell carcinoma. *Lab Invest* 79:859–67, 1999.

28. Yörukoglu K, Aktas S, Güller C, et al.: Volume-weighted mean nuclear volume in renal cell carcinoma. *Urology* 52:44–7, 1998.

29. Nativ O, Sabo E, Raviv G, et al.: The role of nuclear morphometry for predicting disease outcome in patients with localized renal cell carcinoma. *Cancer* 76:1440–4, 1995.

30. Nativ O, Sabo E, Bejar J, et al.: A comparison between histological grade and nuclear morphometry for predicting the clinical outcome of localized renal cell carcinoma. *Br J Urol* 78:33–8, 1996.

31. Faria V, Reis M, Trigueiros D: Renal adenoma: Identification of two histologic types. *Eur Urol* 26:170–5, 1994.

32. Sene AP, Hunt L, McMahon R, et al.: Renal carcinoma in patients undergoing nephrectomy: Analysis of survival and prognostic factors. *Br J Urol* 70:125–34, 1992.

33. Corica FA, Iczkowski KA, Cheng L, et al.: Cystic renal cell carcinoma is cured by resection: A study of 24 cases with long-term follow-up. *J Urol* 161:408–11, 1999.

34. Thoenes W, Störkel S, Rumpelt HJ: Histopathology and classification of renal cell tumors (adenomas, oncocytomas and carcinomas). *Path Res Pract* 181:125–43, 1986.

35. Dal Cin P, Van Den Berghe H: Genetics of renal cell carcinoma, in Petrovich Z, Baert L, Brady LW (eds.): *Carcinoma of the kidney and testis, and rare urologic malignancies*. Berlin, Springer-Verlag, 1999, pp. 15–31.

36. Onda H, Yasuda M, Serizawa A, et al.: Clinical outcome in localized renal cell carcinomas related to immunoexpression of proliferating cell nuclear antigen, Ki-67 antigen, and tumor size. *Oncol Rep* 6:1039–43, 1999.

37. Samma S, Yoshida K, Ozono S, et al.: Tumor thrombus and microvascular invasion as prognostic factors in renal cell carcinoma. *Jpn J Clin Oncol* 21:340–5, 1991.

38. Mrstik C, Salamon J, Weber R, et al.: Microscopic venous infiltration as predictor of relapse in renal cell carcinoma. *J Urol* 148:271–5, 1992.

39. Van Poppel H, Vandendriessche H, Boel K, et al.: Microscopic vascular invasion is the most relevant prognosticator after radical nephrectomy for clinically nonmetastatic renal cell carcinoma. *J Urol* 158:45–9, 1997.

40. Delahunt B, Bethwaete PB, Thornton A: Prognostic significance of microscopic vascularity for clear cell renal cell carcinoma. *Br J Urol* 80:401–4, 1997.

41. Dinney CP, Awad SA, Gajewski JB, et al.: Analysis of imaging modalities, staging systems, and prognostic indicators for renal cell carcinoma. *Urology* 39:122–9, 1992.

42. Jacobi GH, Philipp T: Stauffer's syndrome — Diagnostic help in hypernephroma. *Clin Nephrol* 4:113–5, 1975.

43. Boxer RJ, Waisman J, Lieber MM, et al.: Non-metastatic hepatic dysfunction associated with renal carcinoma. *J Urol* 119:468–71, 1978.

44. Hannisdal E, Bostad L, Grottum KA, et al.: Erythrocyte sedimentation rate as a prognostic factor in renal cell carcinoma. *Eur J Surg Oncol* 15:333–6, 1989.

45. Diacoumis E, Sourvinos G, Kiaris H, et al.: Genetic instability in renal cell carcinoma. *Eur Urol* 33:227–32, 1998.

46. Bissig H, Richter J, Desper R, et al.: Evaluation of the clonal relationship between primary and metastatic renal cell carcinoma by comparative genomic hybridization. *Am J Pathol* 155:267–74, 1999.

47. Belldegrun A, Franklin JR, Figlin R: Commentary on prognostic factors in renal cell carcinoma. *J Urol* 154:1274, 1995.

48. deKernion JB, Mukamel E, Ritchie AW, et al.: Prognostic significance of the DNA content of renal carcinoma. *Cancer* 64:1669–73, 1989.

49. Jochum W, Schroder S, al-Taha R, et al.: Prognostic significance of nuclear DNA content and proliferative activity in renal cell carcinomas. *Cancer* 77:514–21, 1996.

50. Franklin JR, Figlin R, Belldegrun A: Renal cell carcinoma: Basic biology and clinical behavior. *Semin Urol Oncol* 14:208–15, 1996.

51. Ljungberg G, Stenling R, Roos G: DNA content and prognosis in renal cell carcinoma. A comparison between primary tumors and metastases. *Cancer* 57:2346–50, 1986.

52. Elfving P, Mandahl N, Lundgren R, et al.: Prognostic implications of cytogenetic findings in kidney cancer. *Br J Urol* 80:698–706, 1997.

53. Tannapfel A, Hahn HA, Katalinic A, et al.: Prognostic value of ploidy and proliferation markers in renal cell carcinoma. *Cancer* 77:164–71, 1996.

54. Dosquet C, Coudert MC, Lepage E, et al.: Are angiogenetic factors, cytokines, and soluble adhesion molecules prognostic factors in patients with renal cell carcinoma? *Clin Cancer Res* 3:2451–8, 1997.

55. Wechsel HW, Bichler KH, Feil G, et al.: Renal cell carcinoma: Relevance of angiogenetic factors. *Anticancer Res* 19:1537–40, 1999.

56. Duensing S, Grosse J, Atzpodien J: Increased serum levels of basic fibroblast growth factor are associated with progressive lung metastases in advanced renal cell carcinoma patients. *Anticancer Res* 15:2331–3, 1995.

57. Tomita K, Okui N, Kinura A, et al.: Prognostic significance of histopathological findings (including lymphocyte infiltration) in renal cell carcinoma. *Hinyokika Kiyo* 42:925–30, 1996.

58. Otto T, Blass-Kampmann S, Rübben H: Tumor-infiltrating lymphocytes (TIL) promote angiogenesis in renal cell cancer. *Aktuel Urol* 30:187–190, 1999.

59. Hofmann R, Lehmer A, Hartung R, et al.: Prognostic value of urokinase plasminogen activator and plasminogen activator inhibitor-l in renal cell cancer. *J Urol* 155:858–62, 1996.

60. Paradis V, Ferlicot S, Ghannam E, et al.: CD44 is an independent prognostic factor in conventional renal cell carcinomas. *J Urol* 161:1984–7, 1999.

61. Koga H, Nakashima M, Hasegawa S, et al.: A flow cytometric analysis of the expression of adhesion molecules on human renal cells with different metastatic potentials. *Eur Urol* 31:86–91, 1997.

62. Walther MM, Kleiner DE, Lubensky IA, et al.: Progelatinase A mRNA expression in cell lines derived from tumors in patients with metastatic renal cell carcinoma correlates inversely with survival. *Urology* 50:295–301, 1997.

63. Morel-Quadreny L, Clar-Blanch F, Fenollosa-Enterna B, et al.: Proliferating cell nuclear antigen as a prognostic factor in renal cell carcinoma. *Anticancer Res* 18:677–82, 1998.

64. Aaltomaa S, Lipponen P, Ala-Opas M, et al.: Prognostic value of Ki-67 expression in renal cell carcinomas. *Eur Urol* 31:350–5, 1997.

65. Papadopoulos I, Rudolph P, Weichert-Jacobsen K: Value of p53 expression, cellular proliferation, and DNA content as prognostic indicators in renal cell carcinoma. *Eur Urol* 32:110–7, 1997.

66. Höbarth K, Hallas A, Kramer G, et al.: Tissue polypeptide-specific antigen in renal cell carcinoma. *Eur Urol* 30:89–95, 1996.

67. Zhang XH, Takenaka I: Incidence of apoptosis and metallothionein expression in renal cell carcinoma. *Br J Urol* 81:9–13, 1998.

68. Hellemans G, Soumillion A, Proost P, et al.: Metallothioneins in human kidneys and associated tumors. *Nephron*, 83:331–40, 1999.

69. Fair WR, Heston WD, Cordon-Cardo C: An overview of cancer biology, in Walsh PC, Retik AB, Vaughan ED, Wein AJ (eds.): *Campbell's urology*, 7th ed. Philadelphia, Saunders, 1997, pp. 2259–82.

70. Sejima T, Miyagawa I: Expression of Bcl-2, p53 oncoprotein, and proliferating cell nuclear antigen in renal cell carcinoma. *Eur Urol* 35:242–8, 1999.

71. Lanigan D, McLean PA, Murphy DM: c-myc expression in renal carcinoma: Correlation with clinical parameters. *Br J Urol* 72:143–7, 1993.

72. Nakagawa Y, Tsumatani K, Kurumatani N, et al.: Prognostic value of nm23 protein expression in renal cell carcinomas. *Oncology* 55:370–6, 1998.

73. Kimura M, Tomita Y, Imai T, et al.: Significance of serum-soluble CD95 (Fas/APO-1) on prognosis in renal cell cancer patients. *Br J Cancer* 80:1648–51, 1999.

74. Grankvist K, Ljungberg B, Rasmuson T: Evaluation of five glycoprotein tumour markers (CEA, CA-50, CA-19.9, CA-125, CA-15.3) for the prognosis of renal-cell carcinoma. *Int J Cancer* 74:233–6, 1997.

75. Oremek GM, Teigelkamp S, Kramer W et al.: The pyruvate kinase isoenzyme tumor M2 (TuM2-pK) as a tumor marker for renal carcinoma. *Anticancer Res* 19:2599–2602, 1999.

76. Iwamura M, Wu W, Ohori M, et al.: Parathyroid hormone-related protein is an independent prognostic factor for renal cell carcinoma. *Cancer* 86:1028–34, 1999.

77. Sabo E, Miselevich I, Bejar J, et al.: The role of vimentin expression in predicting the long-term outcome of patients with localized renal cell carcinoma. *Br J Urol* 80:864–8, 1997.

78. Bennett RT, Lerner SE, Taub HC, et al.: Cytoreductive surgery for stage IV renal cell carcinoma. *J Urol* 154:32–4, 1995.

79. Belldegrun A, deKernion JB: Renal tumors, in Walsh PC, Retik AB, Vaughan ED, Wein AJ (eds.): *Campbell's urology*, 7th ed. Philadelphia, Saunders, 1997, pp. 2283–2326.

80. Ohh M, Kaelin WG: The von Hippel-Lindau tumour suppressor protein: New perspectives. *Mol Med Today* 5:257–63, 1999.

81. Pea M, Bonetti F, Martignoni G, et al.: Apparent renal cell carcinomas in tuberous sclerosis are heterogeneous. *Am J Surg Pathol* 22:180–2, 1998.

82. Fick GM, Gabow PA: Hereditary and acquired cystic disease of the kidney. *Kidney Int* 46:951–64, 1994.

83. Zbar B, Glenn G, Lubensky I, et al.: Hereditary papillary renal cell carcinoma: Clinical studies in 10 families. *J Urol* 153:907–12, 1995.

84. Von Knobloch R, Seseke F, Riedmiller H, et al.: Radical nephrectomy for renal cell carinoma: Is adrenalectomy necessary? *Eur Urol* 36:303–8, 1999.

85. Wunderlich H, Schlichter A, Reichelt O, et al.: Real indications for adrenalectomy in renal cell carcinoma. *Eur Urol* 35:272–6, 1999.

86. Motzer RJ, Bander NH, Nanus DM: Renal cell carcinoma. *N Engl J Med* 335:865–75, 1996.

87. Li GR, Soulie M, Escourrou G, et al.: Micrometastatic adrenal invasion by renal carcinoma in patients undergoing nephrectomy. *Br J Urol* 78:826–8, 1996.

88. Herrlinger A, Schrott KM, Schott G, et al.: What are the benefits of extended dissection of the regional renal lymph nodes in the therapy of renal cell carcinoma? *J Urol* 146:1224–7, 1991.

89. Van Poppel H, Bamelis B, Oyen R, et al.: Partial nephrectomy for renal cell carcinoma can achieve long-term tumor control. *J Urol* 160:674–8, 1998.

90. Van Poppel HP, Baert L: Nephron-sparing surgery, in Petrovich Z, Baert L, Brady LW (eds.): *Carcinoma of the kidney and testis, and rare urologic malignancies.* Berlin, Springer-Verlag, 1999, pp. 79–93.

91. Stein JP, Skinner DG: Radical nephrectomy, in Petrovich Z, Baert L, Brady LW (eds.): *Carcinoma of the kidney and testis, and rare urologic malignancies.* Berlin, Springer-Verlag, 1999, pp. 57–78.

92. Fossa S, Jones M, Johnson P, et al.: Interferon-alpha and survival in renal cell cancer. *Br J Urol* 77:286–90, 1995.

CHAPTER 40

Bladder Cancer

PIERFRANCESCO BASSI and FRANCESCO PAGANO

Transitional cell carcinoma of the bladder is the second most common malignancy of the genitourinary tract, and the second most common cause of death among all genitourinary tumors, the 11th most common cancer on a worldwide basis, accounting for 3–4% of all malignancies.[1] Annually, about 220,000 new cases are being diagnosed; three-fourths of these patients are men and a disproportional (two-thirds) number of cases occur in developed countries.[2,3]

It's important to underline that a distinction between superficial bladder cancer (stages Ta, T1, Tis) and invasive bladder cancer (stages T2–T4) must be taken into account due to the different prognosis and treatment approaches.[4] (see Appendix 40A) As a matter of fact, bladder cancer is a heterogeneous disease with considerable variations of its natural history with 5-year survival rates ranging from 97% to 98% of a single, well-differentiated, and small papillary tumor to less than 10% of an invasive bladder cancer extending throughout the bladder wall with distant metastases. Among superficial bladder cancer, tumor recurrence after initial therapy varies from 30% in patients with a solitary papillary tumor to more than 90% in patients with multiple tumors. Intense research efforts are being made to identify and characterize the different types of bladder cancer and their variable biological potential. The desire to predict which superficial bladder cancer will recur or progress to invasive cancer, and which invasive bladder cancer will metastatize has spurred the development of a variety of potential prognostic factors.

In this chapter we provide a contemporary review of such prognostic factors with a particular emphasis to the reliable or potential use in the clinical practice.

Prognostic Factors in Cancer, 2nd edition, Edited by Mary K. Gospodarowicz
ISBN 0-471-40633-3   Copyright © 2001 Wiley-Liss, Inc.

TUMOR-RELATED PROGNOSTIC FACTORS

Essential and Additional Prognostic Factors in Superficial Bladder Cancer

The most relevant behavioral features of superficial bladder cancer are tumor recurrence and progression to muscle invasive tumor. Because of the fundamental differences in the natural history of superficial and muscle-invasive bladder cancer, they will be considered separately. It is likely that recurrence and progression may be biologically disassociated phenomena. Findings from three different studies support this assertion. Torti and colleagues[5] in a series of 241 patients with superficial cancer and a median follow-up of 62 months showed that the risk of progression to muscle invasion did not increase from the first to fifth recurrences, respectively. A recent series by Thompson and colleagues[6] of 124 patients documented 7 late, muscle-invasive tumors as the first recurrence of their disease. Herr and Wartinger,[7] in 61 patients followed for more than 10 years, observed tumor progression in 25 (41%), only 8 of whom had prior superficial recurrences. A recurrence does not necessarily herald progression, and freedom from recurrence is no guarantee against developing muscle invasion. Several variables have been considered as factors affecting tumor recurrence or progression: tumor category (Ta vs. T1), tumor grade, prior recurrence rate, number and size of the tumors, tumor configuration, tumor site, positive urine cytology or presence of associated carcinoma in situ (Tis), and prior response to local therapy.[4]

In newly diagnosed bladder cancer, Parmar et al.[8] found the most important independent risk prognostic factors for progression to be the status at cystoscopy 3 months after the initial transurethral resection (TUR) and the number of tumors at presentation. Slightly different results have been reported in a recent Quebec study of 382 newly diagnosed Ta, T1 tumors.[9] A number of tumors, tumor size, and tumor grade were the most important factors predicting tumor recurrence. Koch et al.[10] followed 642 patients free of disease after TUR, fulguration, or laser surgery. Of 502 patients with Ta/T1 tumors, approximately two-thirds of first recurrences occured within 18 months of diagnosis and more of these patients have died of unrelated causes than of bladder cancer. Recurrences occurred sooner in patients with multifocal, rather than unifocal, disease and sooner in women than in men.

To identify the prognostic variables in superficial bladder cancer, European Organization for Research and Treatment of Cancer-Genitourinary (EORTC-GU) group pooled trials of 576 patients who received one intravesical chemotherapy.[11] The endpoints selected included time to first recurrence, recurrence rate per year, time to invasion, and cancer-specific survival. In the multivariate analysis of prior recurrence rate, tumor size, grade, wall involvement, posterior, and dome involvement were significant factors for time to first recurrence. When recurrence was considered at the first follow-up cystoscopy at 3 months, number of tumors, prior recurrence rate, and tumor size were shown to be independent prognostic factors. The prior recurrence rate, grade, and number of tumors were the most important prognostic factors for recurrence. When the time to invasion endpoint was considered, the prior recurrence rate, grade, tumor size, gender, age, and recurrence at the first cystoscopy were highly correlated with invasion. More interestingly, gender, prior recurrence rate, grade, tumor size, and number of tumors were found to be independent predictors of survival. The use of recurrence rate or time to first recurrence is preferable and recommended as an endpoint of interest in patients with superficial bladder cancer, because a relatively small number of patients experience progression to invasive bladder cancer.

Limited data are available on the outcome of superficial bladder cancer patients undergoing repeated intravesical therapies. Bassi and coworkers[12] evaluated 148 patients with multifocal, recurrent, or persistent superficial bladder tumors who underwent multiple TURs and received two or more intravesical treatments (stages TAm, T1m, Tis, G1–3). The primary endpoint was progression-free survival. The multivariate analysis identified three independent prognostic factors for tumor progression, dynamic stage (considered to have been initially diagnosed as stage T1, to have developed a stage T1 in the follow-up, to have never been diagnosed a stage T1 in the follow-up), dynamic grade (considered to have initially been diagnosed as a Grade 3 tumor, to have developed a Grade 3 tumor, or to have never been diagnosed as Grade 3 tumor), and number (<3 or 3 or more) of positive cystoscopies at 3-year follow-up.

Essential and Additional Prognostic Factors in Invasive Bladder Cancer

Limited good-quality data are available regarding the factors predictive for long-term survival of patients with invasive bladder cancer. The major published series evaluate small patient cohorts, undergoing different therapeutical modalities, in a noncontemporary setting and with unsatisfactory statistical methods. Recently, the problem has been clarified by two large studies. A large series of patients encompassing 21 years was retrospectively evaluated to establish a hierarchy of predictive variables of cancer-specific survival.[13] For multivariate analysis tumor category and grade, the presence of nodal involvement, positive surgical margins, and patient age at surgery were independent predictors for cancer-specific survival in the Frazier series.[13] Different results have been reported by Bassi and coworkers[14] in a homogeneous cohort of patients undergoing radical surgery, such as monotherapy for bladder cancer at a single institution: only tumor category and grade were independent predictors of survival, while variables such as age; gender; tumor grade; perineural, lymphatic, and vascular invasion; ureteral obstruction; and previous superficial bladder cancer history were not shown to be predictive. The anatomic extent of the tumor, namely, the depth of wall invasion, is universally accepted as the most important prognostic factor. Five-year survival ranges from 70% for T2 tumors to 10% for T4 tumors. The prognosis is substantially related to the presence of organ-confined or extravesical disease, respectively.[13–17]

The presence of pelvic lymph-node involvement has been universally associated with poor outcome.[13–22] More recently the role of pelvic lymph-node involvement, an independent predictor of survival in patients with invasive bladder cancer,[14,18,21,22] has been clarified in retrospective studies on large patient series. Furthermore, the prognosis of invasive bladder cancer is directly related to the extent of the lymph-node involvement, namely, number and size of the positive nodes. Patients with N1 disease seem to benefit from pelvic node dissection and radical cystectomy as evidenced by similar outcome in those with node-negative disease and similar pT category of the primary tumor. However, the observed benefit quickly disappears when more than one node is involved . Additional therapy other than surgery seems appropriate in the latter group.

Other variables associated with the extent of the tumor have also been considered in the literature. The presence of obstructive uropathy has been reported by some authors as a prognostic factor,[23] but in a more recent series the independent predictive value of this variable hasn't been confirmed.[14] Positive surgical resection margins have been shown in the Frazier series to be associated with a poor outcome and to be an independent predictor of survival.[13] Transitional-cell carcinoma (TCC) encompasses more than 90% of the all bladder cancers. The remaining proportion of patients have pure squamous-cell carcinomas or adenocarcinoma, rarely mixed histotypes.[4] Even though a direct relationship between tumor extent and survival also has been demonstrated also for these histotypes, no reliable information is available regarding the comparative impact of histological type on outcome.[25,26]

Tumor differentiation, namely grade, has been considered an important prognostic factor for invasive bladder cancer for several decades. Several reports claimed grade to be also an independent predictor of survival.[27-29] Bassi et al.'s recent series on a homogeneous cohort of patients undergoing radical cystectomy as a definitive and single treatment for invasive bladder cancer clearly showed[14] that grade is a significant prognostic factor in univariate analysis, but not multivariate analysis. This observation is simply explained by the fact that the major part of the invasive bladder tumors are of Grade 3.[14,24,29]

New and Promising Prognostic Factors for Superficial and Invasive Bladder Cancer

Next to tumor characteristics and the more sophisticated evaluation of the likelihood of recurrence or progression come DNA-ploidy measurement, immunohistochemical staining of the basement-membrane components, evaluation of cell adherence molecules, growth factors, proteases, cell surface antigens, and blood group antigens, as well as the determination of cell-cycle-related proteins in bladder carcinoma. They are all experimental, and none of them has reached clinical significance or becomes part of clinical routine.

Aneuploidy, as determined by flow cytometry (FCM), has been associated with decreased survival in both low- and high-stage TCC, although the correlations are better and more consistent for low stage tumors.[30] Aneuploidy correlates well with histologic grade and with lymph node metastasis.[30] Nuclear morphometry, an image-analysis technique for evaluation of nuclear shape correlates with metastasis.[31] The estimate of the proliferative activity of tumor cells may be an indicator of prognosis by cell-cycle-related proteins such as Ki-67 and proliferating-cell nuclear antigen (PCNA). These proteins are detected in higher stage tumors[32,33] and are associated with reduced survival, although this association is stronger with lower stage (Ta/T1) than invasive bladder cancers.[32] These techniques have added little prognostic information to that obtained from classic prognosticators.[34]

Cell division is regulated by cell-cycle-associated proteins, including cyclins and their associated kinases. Loss of regulation of proliferation is an early and essential step in cancer development.

Several genes and gene products associated with the regulation of the cell cycle have been the subject of recent intensive investigation, and the p53 and Rb tumor suppressor genes have been shown to be important prognostic factors for patients with bladder cancer. The retinoblastoma tumor suppressor gene was the first tumor suppressor gene identified through the study of patients with retinoblastoma: inactivation of the Rb gene is thought to be an important step in bladder cancer progression. The results of two small studies have suggested that loss of expression of the Rb protein may be of prognostic significance in transitional-cell carcinoma of the bladder. Logothetis et al.[35] studied 43 patients with locally advanced bladder cancer (T2–T4a) and found that tumor with loss of Rb expression had a 3-year survival ($p = 0.01$), suggesting that loss of Rb expression is a prognostic factor in patients with advanced cancer. Cordon Cardo et al.[36] reported that patients with muscle invasive bladder cancer with a loss of Rb expression had a shorter 5-year survival ($p = 0.001$) than those with normal Rb protein expression.

p53 tumor suppressor gene mutations are thought to be the most common genetic defect in human tumors;[37] this protein has an important role in preventing cell-cycle progression by delaying cell division, allowing time for DNA repair. Molecular analysis has shown that abnormal nuclear accumulation of p53 protein in bladder tumors, as detected by immunohistochemical staining, correlates closely with gene mutations detected by DNA sequencing.[38] Large series have shown that abnormal p53 expression is found more frequently in higher grade and higher stage bladder tumors and is a predictor of poor outcome.[39,40] Mutations in p53 have been associated with the progression of superficial bladder cancer.[41–43] Sarkis et al.[41] showed that progression of patients with Ta, T1, and CIS correlated with p53 mutation. Nuclear overexpression of p53 was an independent predictor of death from bladder cancer for patients with CIS and T1 tumors.[41,43] p53 status has been evaluated as a predictor of response to bacillus Calmette-Guérin (BCG) in patients with superficial bladder cancer.[44] Although pretreatment p53 overexpression was an independent predictor for progression, it did not predict response to BCG. However, in patients with residual disease after BCG treatment, post-therapy p53 overexpression was predictive of disease progression. Esrig et al.[39] investigated the role of p53 overexpression in 243 patients treated by radical cystectomy for TCC of the bladder and found that p53 overexpression was the sole independent predictor of relapse (75 vs. 40%, $p < 0.001$). When patients were stratified by stage, nuclear p53 accumulation was associated with an increased risk of disease in patients with stage pTl, pT2, and pT3a, but not pTa or extravesical disease (pT3b, pT4, or lymph-node metastasis). Lipponen[40] investigated the role of p53 overexpression by immunohistochemistry in 212 patients treated by a variety of different modalities and found a 29% incidence of p53 mutations in the entire cohort. Overexpression of p53 protein was an adverse prognostic factor in patients with muscle-invasive disease. However, p53 overexpression was not an independent prognostic factor and provided no more predictive information than could be obtained from tumor stage and mitotic index.

Both p53 and Rb have been evaluated as predictors of response to therapy for muscle-invasive bladder cancer. Pollack et al.[45] recently reevaluated the role of preoperative radiation therapy in patients with stage T3b TCC and found that p53 mutations predicted a poor response to preoperative radiation, while Rb status was the only independent predictor of response to radiation. Logothetis et al.[35] looked at the prognostic significance of Rb status in patients with advanced TCC treated with methotrexate, vinblastine, aoxorubicin, cisplatin (MVAC) chemotherapy and cystectomy: in this study altered Rb expression predicted a poor response to therapy. Sarkis et al. conducted a similar analysis and evaluated the significance of altered p53 expression in patients with muscle invasive TCC treated with neoadjuvant MVAC:[46] they reported that patients with p53 mutations had a significantly higher proportion of cancer deaths, so that p53 mutations predicted a poor response to MVAC chemotherapy. However, Cote et al.[47] presented conflicting results related to p53 expression and response to chemotherapy. In their study, p53 mutations predicted a positive response to chemotherapy.[47]

An alternative pathway to disrupt p53 function without mutation of p53 is through amplification of MDM2. MDM2 inhibits the function of p53 and may contribute to progression in tumors that are immunohistochemically negative for p53. Amplification of the MDM2 gene or overexpression of its product has been reported in some bladder cancer tissues.[48,49] Although Lianes et al.[48] suggest that this pathway may be more important in low-stage tumors, Habuchi et al.[49] hypothesize that this pathway is involved in genetic instability and oncogene expression in higher-stage tumors. Further work is necessary to clearly identify the role of MDM2 in bladder cancer progression.

p21 is a negative cell-cycle regulator transcriptionally regulated by p53 that also prevents the inactivation of Rb. Abnormal immunohistochemical staining of p21 is reported to be a risk factor for progression of TCC in patients with wild-type p53 expression.[50]

Interestingly, two preliminary reports examining the prognostic importance of the combination of altered p53 and Rb expression suggest that patients whose tumors exhibit both p63 and Rb dysfunction have the poorest prognosis, and patients whose tumors exhibit dysfunction of one gene have an intermediate prognosis.[51,52] Although it is impossible to predict which tumors with mutations in both genes will progress, no tumors expressing wild-type p53 and Rb progressed. These results suggest that mutation of the p53 and Rb genes have independent and synergistic roles in the development of bladder cancer. Recently, two other genes, p15 and p16, which encode proteins that also regulate the activity of cyclins, have been studied in bladder cancer:[53] these two genes localized to chromosome 9, at 9p21 are putative tumor suppressors that may be lost early in the pathogenesis of TCC.

Neoangiogenesis may facilitate the transition of cells into the circulation resulting in metastasis.[54] High tumor vascularity in invasive bladder cancers was reported[55] to be a strong predictor of lymph-node metastasis and an independent prognostic indicator for survival, for example, a 2.5-fold greater risk of dying of bladder cancer for patients with high microvessel counts.[56,57] However, there are conflicting reports in the literature regarding the prognostic value of vascular density in bladder cancer. Babkowski et al.[58] evaluated the prognostic significance of microvessel density in 54 patients with stage T1 bladder, but found that vascular density did not correlate with prognosis using any of the three antibodies. The risk of progression to metastatic disease was relatively low in this study compared to those in which microvessel density was found to be prognostic, so this study does not eliminate the possibility that microvessel density could be a marker for metastasis in bladder cancer.

Specific antibodies for cell-surface antigens from human bladder cancer have been produced. Two of these antibodies, M344 and l9A211, are expressed preferentially in low-grade transitional cell carcinoma.[59] The expression of both of these markers has been associated with an increased recurrence rate. Two other antibodies, T138 and T43,[60] preferentially react with higher-stage tumors, and in several studies of locally invasive bladder cancer have shown some prognostic value.

Loss of expression of blood group A, B, and H antigens in bladder cancer have been proposed as prognostic indicators.[59,61] The loss of ABO antigens, however, was found to be relatively common and provides no prognostic information.[59,61] More recently, a group of antibodies reactive with the Lewis X blood group determinant have been studied, including 486 P3/12 and E7.[62] These antibodies were useful for detecting recurrence in low-stage bladder cancers with a reported sensitivity of 81% and a specificity of 86%. The Thomsen-Friedenreich (T) antigen is another blood-group antigen that is expressed in bladder cancers but not in normal urothelial cells.[63] The T antigen is associated with recurrence in low-stage bladder cancers,[63] but offers no prognostic information for invasive bladder cancers.[64]

E-cadherin, an epithelial-cell adhesion molecule[65] appears to act as a tumor suppressor.[66,67] Several recent reports have shown an association between a decrease in E-cadherin expression at the cell border and increased bladder cancer stage.[68] In two of these studies, decreased E-cadherin expression was also associated with a poorer survival.[69,70]

Integrins function as receptors for extracellular matrix proteins.[71] Liebert and her co-workers[72] noted a progressive loss of $\alpha2\beta1$ expression with increasing bladder cancer stage. This finding could result in a loss of cell–cell adhesion similar to E-cadherin loss. The loss of $\alpha2\beta1$ expression was observed in low-stage bladder cancers, suggesting that the loss of this expression occurs early in bladder cancer progression. The expression of another member of the integrin family, the $\alpha6\beta4$ heterodimer is associated with a basal anchoring structure in normal epithelial tissues, including the urinary bladder;[73] however, in invasive bladder cancer, the association between $\alpha6\beta4$ and the anchoring structure is lost. In many cases the $\alpha6\beta4$ integrin is overexpressed, suggesting that the cancer cells utilize this receptor to move through the basement membrane.

The epidermal growth-factor receptor (EGFR) is found on most epithelial cells. Clinically, overexpression of EGFR correlates with tumor stage[74–76] and is associated with a poor prognosis, especially for lower-stage bladder cancers.[76] In a subset analysis, Neal and his coworkers found that EGFR did not predict survival for patients with higher-stage tumor.[76]

The c-erb-B2 oncogene encodes a cellular surface protein. Several studies report that high expression of c-erb-B2 protein is associated with higher stage[77–79] increased metastasis[79] and poorer outcome.[78]

Fibroblast growth factors (FGFs) are a large family of polypeptide growth factors. FGFs contribute significantly to the induction of angiogenesis by their effects on endothelial-cell migration and growth.[73] Since angiogenesis correlates with poor prognosis in bladder cancer, it is expected that expression of FGFs in the urine would be valuable predictors of disease state. Furthermore, FGFs affect many cell types, and treatment with FGFs induces a highly motile, fibroblastoid cell type in a rat bladder cancer epithelial-cell line.[80] Two members of the FGF family, FGF-1 (acidic FGF) and FGF-2 (basic FGF) have been identified in the urine of patients with bladder cancer.[81–83] Levels of expression of FGF-2 correlated with higher-stage and metastasis. Patients with higher-stage tumors were more likely to have a positive urinary test for FGF-1.[81] Bladder cancer cells in tissues were also shown to express FGF-1: a greater numbers of high-stage tumors expressed FGF-1, and expression was related to metastasis.[81–83]

Since penetration of the basement membrane is thought to be an essential step in the progression of bladder cancer, expression by cancer cells of enzymes capable of destroying the basement membrane should correlate with metastasis. Several families of proteases have been evaluated in bladder cancers.[84,85] One group of proteases is the metalloproteinases that degrade collagen IV (also called Type IV collagenase or MMP-2 and MMP-9). Slightly contradictory results were obtained in two reported studies. In the first,[84] the urinary levels MMP-2 were found to be higher in patients with invasive cancers, and immunohistochemical staining revealed that the tumor cells were producing collagenase. In contrast, in the other study,[85] both Type IV collagenases were studied and increased levels were observed in invasive bladder cancers.

A second type of protease, the urokinase plasminogen activator (uPA), is a serine protease that is associated with fibrinolysis. The presence of active uPA can activate other cellular components, including metalloproteinases, and can directly contribute to matrix degradation. Low-stage bladder cancers with low expression of uPA had significantly better survival than high expressors, although these differences were not independent of grade.[86]

A final group of proteases, the cathepsin family of cysteine proteases, has been the subject of preliminary analysis in bladder cancer. The T24 invasive human bladder cancer cell line showed high level of expression of cathepsin B, while the noninvasive human bladder cancer cell line RT4 had low expression.[87] However, in a clinical study of cathepsin D expression in bladder cancers, Dickinson et al. observed the opposite association: a decreasing expression of cathepsin D with increasing bladder cancer stage; invasive bladder tumors expressing cathepsin D had a better outcome than those not expressing it.[88] Cathepsin D expression was not an independent predictor in multivariate analysis. The authors noted that normal urothelium expressed high levels of cathepsin D, and that loss of expression might be related to loss of differentiation in higher-stage tumors.[88]

The intact basement membrane, composed of collagen IV, proteoglycans, laminin, and other extracellular matrix components, presents a physical barrier to tumor-cell invasion and metastasis. A number of investigators have evaluated immunohistochemical staining for extracellular matrix components of the basement membrane, including collagen IV[89–91] and laminin.[66] In general, increasing defects in basement-membrane integrity are noted with increasing stage of tumor. Daher et al.[91] noted the development of gaps in the collagen IV in the basement membrane, and divided their patient cohort into two groups based on intact or defective collagen IV. Of the invasive bladder cancer patients in this study, 29 were observed for a 3-year follow-up period. Of the 16 evaluable patients with intact collagen IV, 11 were still alive at 3 years; of the 13 patients with defective collagen IV, none were alive at 3 years.[91] These data suggest that even within high-stage tumors, evaluation of basement-membrane integrity may be of prognostic significance. Laminin immunohistochemical staining has also been used to evaluate basement-membrane integrity.[66] Disrupted basement-membrane laminin was associated with metastasis. This same group detected the presence of laminin P1, a laminin degradation product, in the blood and urine of patients with invasive cancer.[67] The blood tests were neither highly sensitive nor discriminatory:[66,67] 31% of noncancer patients showed a positive result, and of bladder cancer patients, 57% with intact basement membrane were positive, and only 82% with interrupted basement membrane were positive. The urine tests showed promise for following patients with invasive bladder cancers demonstrating 58% sensitivity, 96% specificity, and 87% positive-predictive value.[67] Unfortunately, no follow-up of these patients was provided.

HOST-RELATED PROGNOSTIC FACTORS

In nearly all populations, men are 2.5–5.0 times more likely to develop bladder cancer than women. Incidence of bladder cancer rises monotonically with age: the disease is rare prior to age 35, and two-thirds of the cases occur in people aged 65 or older.[2,97]

There is a marked racial–ethnic variation in bladder cancer incidence: in the United States, non-Latino white men show the highest incidence of bladder cancer among all races. Their rate is twice those in Latino and African-American men, and 2.5 times higher than those in the chinese and Japanese-American male communities. A similar pattern is observed in women, even though within race, the male rate is about 3–4 times higher than the female rate.[93,94]

In contrast to Europe and the United States, in some regions of Africa, where schistostomiasis is endemic, bladder cancer is the most frequent tumor, with the majority of the patients being diagnosed with squamous-cell carcinoma and one-third having a history of bilharziasis.[26,93–95]

As far as bladder cancer being hereditary, numerous case reports document the clustering of TCC in families, several of which demonstrate an extremely early age of onset of disease, which argues in favor of a genetic component to familial TCC.[96] The results of large epidemiological studies also suggest the existence of familial bladder cancer and first-degree relatives appear to have an increased risk for disease by a factor of 2: familial clustering of smoking does not appear to be a cause of this increased risk.[97] However, further studies are required to identify candidates' genes that might be responsible for this form of bladder cancer.[3]

Age has been reported to be a prognostic factor of outcome in superficial and invasive bladder cancer,[27] but contradictory results have been observed in two large patient series treated with radical surgery.[13,14] Also performance status has been shown to be an ominous variable of survival in patients undergoing systemic chemotherapy for advanced bladder cancer.[98] No reliable information on this variable is reported for patients undergoing definitive surgical therapy for invasive disease: as a matter of fact, in such cases the anesthesiological risk has been taken more frequently into account. Finally, anemia has been found to be an adverse prognostic factor in patients treated with radiation therapy for muscle-invasive bladder cancer,[99–101] but opposite results have been reported in surgically treated bladder cancer.[14]

Since the publication of the classic paper late in the last century postulating the higher incidence of bladder cancer among aniline dye workers, multiple occupational, environmental, and genetic factors have been identified:[94,95] chemical dye exposure, 2-naphthylamine, 4-aminobiphenyl, benzidine, arylamines, cigarette smoking, schistosomiasis, and so on. Cigarette smoking has been shown to be the single most important cause of bladder cancer, there being a good correlation between duration and severity of exposure to smoking and incidence of this tumor; furthermore, smokers who continue experience worse disease-associated outcomes than those who stop or ex-smokers.[97]

TNM Classification: Bladder Cancer

T — Primary Tumor

TX Primary tumor cannot be assessed

T0 No evidence of primary tumor

Ta Noninvasive papillary carcinoma

Tis Carcinoma in situ: "flat tumor"

T1 Tumor invades subepithelial connective tissue

T2 Tumor invades muscle
   T2a Tumor invades superficial muscle (inner half)
   T2b Tumor invades deep muscle (outer half)

T3 Tumor invades perivesical tissue:
   T3a Microscopically
   T3b Macroscopically (extravesical mass)

T4 Tumor invades any of the following: prostate, uterus, vagina, pelvic wall, abdominal wall
   T4a Tumor invades prostate, uterus, or vagina
   T4b Tumor invades pelvic wall or abdominal wall

N — Regional Lymph Nodes

NX Regional lymph nodes cannot be assessed

N0 No regional lymph node metastasis

N1 Metastasis in a single lymph node 2 cm or less in greatest dimension

N2 Metastasis in a single lymph node more than 2 cm but not more than 5 cm in greatest dimension, or multiple lymph nodes, none more than 5 cm in greatest dimension

N3 Metastasis in a lymph node more than 5 cm in greatest dimension

M — Distant Metastasis

MX Distant metastasis cannot be assessed

M0 No distant metastasis

M1 Distant metastasis

Stage Grouping

Stage 0a	Ta	N0	M0
Stage 0is	Tis	N0	M0
Stage I	T1	N0	M0
Stage II	T2a	N0	M0
	T2b	N0	M0
Stage III	T3a	N0	M0
	T3b	N0	M0
	T4a	N0	M0
Stage IV	T4b	N0	M0
	Any T	N1, 2, 3	M0
	Any T	Any N	M1

Source: Sobin LH, Wiitekind Ch (eds.): *TNM classification of malignant tumors*, 5th ed. New York, Union Internationale Contre le Cancer Wiley-Liss, 1997.

■■■■■■ **APPENDIX 40B.1**

Prognostic Factors in Superficial (Ta, T1, Tis) Bladder Cancer

Prognostic Factor	Tumor Related	Host Related	Environment Related
Essential	Number of tumors Grade Recurrence rate		Schistomiasis Cigarette smoking
Additional	T category	Age Race	Socioeconomic status
New and promising	p53 c-erb-B2		

■■■■■ **APPENDIX 40B.2**

Prognostic Factors in Invasive (T2-T4; any T, N+, M+) Bladder Cancer

Prognostic Factors	Tumor Related	Host Related	Environment Related

Essential	T category
	Lymph-node
	  involvement
	Metastases
		Performance
		Status
			Schistomiasis
			Cigarette
			  smoking

Additional	Histologic grade Ureteric obstruction	Age Race	Socioeconomic status
New and promising	p53 Rb gene Neangiogenesis c-erb-B2		

REFERENCES

1. American Cancer Society: *Facts and figures, 1998*. Baltimore, Williams of Wilkins, 1998, pp. 1–18.

2. Parkin DM, Muir CS, Whelan SL: Estimates of the worldwide frequency of sixteen major cancers in 1980. *Int J Cancer*, 41:184–97, 1998.

3. Parker SL, Tong T, Bolden S: Cancer Statistics, 1997. *CA—Cancer J Clin*, 47:5, 1997.

4. Sobin LH, Wiitekind Ch (eds.): *TNM classification of malignant tumors*, 5th ed. New York, Union Internationale Contre le Cancer Wiley-Liss, 1997.

5. Torti FM, Lum BL, Aston D: Superficial bladder cancer: The primacy of grade in the development of invasive disease. *J Clin Oncol*, 5:125–131, 1987.

6. Thompson RA, Cambel EW, Kramer HC: Late invasive recurrence despite long-term surveillance for superficial bladder cancer. *J Urol*, 149:1010–5, 1993.

7. Herr HW, Wartinger DD: BCG therapy for superficial bladder cancer: A 10 years follow-up. *J Urol*, 149:40–5, 1992.

8. Parmar MKB, Freedman LS, Hargrave TB: Prognostic factors for recurrence and follow-up policies in the treatment of superficial bladder cancer. *J Urol* 142:284–9, 1989.

9. Allard P, Fradet Y, Tetu B, Bernard P: Tumor associated antigens as prognostic factors for recurrence in 382 primary transitional cell carcinoma of the bladder. *Clin Cancer Res*, 1:1195–1202, 1995.

10. Koch M, Hill GB, Mc Phee MS: Factors affecting recurrence rates in superficial bladder cancer. *JNCI*, 76:1025–31, 1986.

11. Kurth KH, Denis L, ten Kate JW, et al.: Prognostic factors in superficial bladder tumors. *Prob. Urol.* 6(3):339–51, 1992.

12. Bassi P, Piazza N, Abatangelo G, et al.: Unresponsive superficial bladder cancer, in Pagano F, Fair WR, Bassi P, (eds.): *Superficial bladder cancer*. Oxford, Isis Medical Media, 1997, pp. 158–68.

13. Frazier HA, Robertson J, Dodge RK, Paulson DF: The value of pathological factors in predicting cancer specific survival among patients treated with radical cystectomy for transitional cell carcinoma. *Cancer*, 71:3993–9, 1993.

14. Bassi P, Drago Ferrante GL, Piazza N, et al.: Prognostic factors of outcome after radical cystectomy for bladder cancer: A retrospective study of a homogeneous patient cohort. *J Urol* 161:1494–7, 1999.

15. Lerner SP, Skinner E, Skinner DG: Radical cystectomy in regionally advanced bladder cancer. *Urol Clin North Am* 19(4):713–22, 1992.

16. Pagano F, Bassi P, Prayer Galetti T, et al.: Results of contemporary radical cystectomy for invasive bladder cancer: A clinico-pathological study with an emphasis on the inadequacy of the tumor, nodes and metastases classification. *J Urol* 145:50–5, 1991.

17. Pollack A, Zagars GK, Cole JC, et al.: The relationship of local control to distant metastasis in muscle invasive bladder cancer. *J Urol* 154:2059–64, 1995.

18. Lerner SP, Skinner DG, Lieskowsky G, et al.: The rationale of "en bloc" pelvic node dissection for bladder cancer patients with nodal metastases: Long-term results. *J Urol* 149:758–64, 1993.

19. Robertson CG, Sagalowsky AI and Peters PC: Long-term patient survival after radical cystectomy for regional metastatic transitional cell carcinoma of the bladder. *J Urol* 146:36–9, 1991.

20. Vieweg J, Whitmore WF, Herr HW, et al.: The role of pelvic lymphadectomy and radical cystectomy for lymph node positive bladder cancer. *Cancer* 73:3020–6, 1994.

21. Vieweg J, Gschwend JE, Herr HW, Fair WR: The impact of primary stage on survival in patients with lymph node positive bladder cancer. *J Urol*, 161:72–6, 1999.

22. Vieweg J, Gschwend JE, Herr HW, Fair WR: Pelvic node dissection can be curative in patients with node positive bladder cancer. *J Urol* 161:449–54, 1999.

23. Leibovitch I, Ben-Chaim J, Ramon J, et al.: The significance of ureteral obstruction in invasive transitional cell carcinoma of the urinary bladder. *J Surg Oncol* 52:31–6, 1993.

24. Mostofi FK: *Histological typing of urinary bladder tumors*. Geneva, WHO, 1973.

25. Raghavan D, Shipley UW, Hall RR, Richie JP: Biology and management of invasive bladder cancer, in: Raghavan D, Scher HI, Leibel A, Lange PH, (eds.): *Principles and practice of genitourinary oncology*. Publishers, Philadelphia, Lippincott-Raven 1997, pp. 281–9.

26. Ghoneim MA, el Mekresh NM, el Baz MA, et al.: Radical cystectomy for carcinoma of the bladder: Critical evaluation of the results in 1026 cases. *J Urol* 158:393–9, 1997.

27. Lipponen PK, Eskelinen M, Jauhianinen K, et al.: Clinical prognostic factors in transitional cell cancer of the bladder. *Urol Int* 50:192–8, 1993.

28. Abel PD: Prognostic indices in transitional cell carcinoma of the bladder. *Brit J Urol* 62:103–11, 1998.

29. Angulo JC, Lopez JI, Flores N, Toledo JD: The value of tumor spread, grading and growth pattern as morphological predictive parameters in bladder carcinoma. A critical revision of the 1987 TNM classification. *J Cancer Res Clin Oncol* 119:578–84, 1993.

30. Lipponen PK: Review of cytometric methods in the assessment of prognosis in transitional cell bladder cancer. *Eur Urol* 21:177–83, 1992.

31. Borland RN, Partin AW, Epstein JI, Brendler CB: The use of nuclear morphometry in predicting recurrence of transitional cell carcinoma. *J Urol* 149:272–5, 1993.

32. Okamura K, Miyake K, Kosikawa T, Assai J: Growth fractions of transitional cell carcinomas of the bladder defined by the monoclonal antibody Ki-67. *J Urol* 144:875–8, 1990.

33. Lipponen PK, Eskelinen MJ: Cell proliferation of transitional cell bladder tumors determined by PCNA/cyclin immunostaining and its prognostic value. *Br J Cancer* 66:171–6, 1992.

34. Lipponen PK, Eskelinen MJ, Nordling S: Progression and survival in transitional cell bladder cancer: A comparison of established prognostic factors, S-phase fraction and ploidy. *Eur J Cancer* 27:877–81, 1991.

35. Logothetis C, Hu H-J, Ro J, et al.: Altered expression of the retinoblastoma protein and known prognostic variables in locally advanced bladder cancer. *J Natl Cancer Inst* 84:1256–61, 1992.

36. Cordon-Cardo C, Wartinger D, Petrylak D, et al.: Altered expression of the retinoblastoma gene product: Prognostic indicator in bladder cancer. *J Natl Cancer Inst* 84:1251, 1992.

37. Hollstein M, Sidransky D, Vogelstein B, Harris C: P53 mutations in human cancer. *Science* 253:49–54, 1991.

38. Dalbagni G, Cordon-Cardo C, Reuter V, Fair W: Tumor suppressor alterations in bladder cancer. *Surg Oncol Clin North Am* 4:231–8, 1995.

39. Esrig D, Elmajian D, Groshen S, et al.: Accumulation of nuclear p53 and tumor progression in bladder cancer. *N Engl J Med* 331:1259–66, 1994.

40. Lipponen P: Over-expression of the p53 nuclear oncoprotein in transitional cell carcinoma of the bladder and its prognostic value. *Int J Cancer* 53:365–70, 1993.

41. Sarkis A, Dalbagni B, Cordon-Cardo C, et al.: Nuclear over-expression of p53 protein in transitional cell carcinoma: A marker for disease progression. *J Nat Cancer Inst* 85:53–9, 1993.

42. Sarkis AS, Zhang Z-F, Cordon-Cardo C, et al.: p53 nuclear overexpression and disease progression in Ta. Bladder carcinoma. *Int J Oncol*, 3:355–60, 1993.

43. Sarkis AS, Dalbagni G, Cordon-Cardo C, et al.: Association of p53 nuclear over-expression and tumor progression in carcinoma in situ of the bladder. *J Urol* 152:388–94, 1994.

44. Lacombe L, Dalbagni G, Zhang Z-F, et al.: Overexpression p53 protein in a high-risk population of patients with superficial bladder cancer before and after bacillus Calmette-Guérin Therapy. Correlation to Clinical Outcome. *J Clin Oncol* 14(10):2646–52, 1996.

45. Pollack A, Zagars GK, Swanson DA: Muscle invasive bladder cancer treated with external beam radiotherapy: Prognostic factors. *Int Radiat Oncol Biol Phys* 30:267–77, 1994.

46. Sarkis AS, Bajorin DF, Reuter VE, et al.: Prognostic value of p53 nuclear overexpression in patients with invasive bladder cancer treated with neoadjuvant MVAC. *J Clin Oncol* 13:1384–90, 1995.

47. Cote RJ, Esrig D, Groshen S, et al.: p53 and treatment of bladder cancer. *Nature* 385:123–4, 1997.

48. Lianes P, Orlow I, Zhang Z-F, et al.: Altered patterns of MDM2 and TP53 expression in human bladder cancers. *J Nat Cancer Inst* 86:1325–30, 1994.

49. Habuschi T, Kinoshita H, Kakehi Y, et al.: Oncogene amplification in urothelial cancers with p53 gene mutation or MDM2 amplification. *J Nat Cancer Inst* 86:1131–5, 1994.

50. Stein JP, Ginsburg DA, Grossfeld GD, et al.: The effect of p21 expression on tumor progression in p53 altered bladder cancer. *J Urol* 155:628A, 1996.

51. Esrig D, Shi S-R, Bochner B, et al.: Prognostic importance of p53 and Rb alterations in transitional cell carcinoma of the bladder. *J Urol* 153:536A, 1995.

52. Grossman HB, Antelo M, Dinney CPN, et al.: p53 and Rb expression predict progression in T1 bladder cancer. *Proc AACR* 37:201, 1996.

53. Orlow I, Lacombe L, Hannan GJ, et al.: Deletion of the p16 and p15 genes in human bladder tumors. *J Nat Cancer Inst* 87:1524–9, 1995.

54. Folkman J: The role of angiogenesis in tumor growth. *Semin Cancer Biol* 3:65–71, 1992.

55. Jaeger TM, Weidner N, Chew K, et al.: Tumor angiogenesis correlates with lymph node metastasis in invasive bladder cancer. *J Urol* 154:69–71, 1995.

56. Dickinson AJ, Fox SB, Persad RA, et al.: Quantification of angiogenesis as an independent predictor of prognosis in invasive bladder cancer. Br. *J Urol* 74:762–6 1994.

57. Bochner BH, Cote RJ, Weidner N, et al.: Angiogenesis in bladder cancer: Relationship between microvessel density and tumor prognosis. *JNCI* 87(21):1603–12, 1995.

58. Babkowski RC, Zhang H-Z, Xia Y, et al.: Angiogenesis does not have prognostic value in T1 bladder cancer. *J Urol* 155:615A, 1996.

59. Fradet Y, Cordon-Cardo C: Critical appraisal of tumor markers in bladder cancer. *Semin Urol* 11:145–53, 1993.

60. Ravery V, Colombel M, Popov Z, et al.: Prognostic value of epidermal growth factor receptor, T138 and T43 expression in bladder cancer. *Br J Cancer* 71:196–200, 1995.

61. Aprikian AG, Sarkis AS, Reuter VE, et al.: Biological markers of prognosis in transitional cell carcinoma of the bladder: Current concepts. *Semin Urol* 11:137–44, 1993.

62. Goliganin D, Sherman Y, Shapiro A, Pode D: Detection of bladder tumors by immunostaining of the Lewis X antigen in cells from voided urine. *Urology* 46:173–7, l995.

63. Summers JL, Coon JS, Ward RM, et al.: Prognosis of carcinoma of the urinary bladder based on tissue blood group ABH and Thomsen-Friedenzeich antigen status and karyotype of the initial tumor. *Cancer Res* 43:934–9, 1983.

64. Shrahama T, Ikoma M, Muramatsu T, et al.: The binding site for fucose-binding proteins of Lotus tetragonolobus is a prognostic marker for transitional cell carcinoma of the human urinary bladder. *Cancer* 72:1329–34, 1993.

65. Shiozaki H, Tahara H, Oka H, et al.: Expression of immunoreactive E-cadherin adhesion molecules in human cancers. *Am J Pathol* 139:215–23, 1991.

66. Abou Farha KMM, Janknegt RA, Kester ADM, Arendt JW: Value of immunohistochemical laminin staining in transitional cell carcinoma of human bladder. *Urol Int* 50:133–40, 1993.

67. Abou Farha KMM, Menheere PPCA, Nieman FHM, et al.: Relation between basement membrane degradation and serum levels of laminin P1 in patients with transitional cell carcinoma of the bladder. *Urol Int* 50:13–6, 1993.

68. Fixen UH, Behrens J, Sachs M, et al.: E-cadherin-mediated cell–cell adhesion prevents invasiveness of human carcinoma cells. *J Cancer Res Clin Oncol* 121:303–8, 1995.

69. Bringuier PP, Umbas R, Schaafsma HE, et al.: Decreased E-cadherin immunoreactivity correlates with poor survival in patients with bladder tumors. *Cancer Res* 53:3241–5, 1993.

70. Otto T, Birchmeier W, Schmidt U, et al.: Inverse relation of E-cadherin and autocrine motility factor receptor expression as a prognostic factor in patients with bladder cancer. *Cancer Res* 54:3120–3, 1994.

71. Albeda SM: Biology of disease: Role of integrins and other cell adhesion molecules in tumor progression and metastasis. *Lab Invest* 68:4–17, 1993.

72. Liebert M, Wedemeyer G, Stein JA, et al.: The monoclonal antibody BQ16 identified the a6,B4 integrin in bladder cancers. *Hybridoma* 12:67–80, 1993.

73. Liebert M, Washtington R, Wedemeyer G, et al.: Loss of colocalization of $\alpha6\beta4$ integrin and collagen VII in bladder cancer. *Am J Pathol* 144:787–95, 1994.

74 Messing E: Clinical implications of the expression of epidermal growth factor receptors in human transitional cell carcinoma. *Cancer Res* 50:2530–7, 1990.

75. Liebert M: Growth factors in bladder cancer. *World J Urol* 13:349–55, 1995.

76. Berger MS, Greenfield C, Gullick WJ, et al.: Evaluation of epidermal growth factor receptors in bladder tumours. *Br J Urol* 56:533–7, 1987.

77. Gorgoulis VG, Barbatis C, Poulias I, Karameris AM: Molecular and immunohistochemical evaluation of epidermal growth factor receptor and c-erb-B2 gene product in transitional cell carcinomas of the urinary bladder: A study in Greek patients. *Mod Pathol* 8:758–64, 1995.

78. Sato K, Mariyama M, Morei S, et al.: An immunohistologic evaluation of c-erb-B2 gene products in patients with urinary bladder carcinoma. *Cancer*, 70:2493–8, 1992.

79. Moch H, Sauter G, Moore D, et al.: p53 and erbB-2 protein overexpression are associated with early invasion and metastasis in bladder cancer. *Virchows Arch Pathol Anat* 423:319–34, 1993.

80. Barritault D, Groux-Muscatelli B, Caruelle D, et al.: aFGF increases with malignancy in human chondrosarcoma and bladder cancer. *Ann NY Acad Sci* 638:387–93, 1991.

81. O'Brien TS, Smith K, Cranston D, et al.: Urinary basic fibroblast growth factor in patients with bladder cancer and benign prostatic hypertrophy. *Brit J Urol* 76:311–4, 1996.

82. Nguyen M, Watanabe H, Budson E, et al.: Elevated levels of angiogenic peptide basic fibroblast growth factor in urine of bladder cancer patients. *J Nat Cancer Inst* 85:241–2, 1993.

83. Chopin DK, Caruelle J-P, Colmbel M, et al.: Increased immunodetection of acidic fibroblast growth factor in bladder cancer, detectable in the urine. *J Urol* 150:1126–30, 1991.

84. Margulies IMK, Hoyhtya M, Evans C, et al.: Urinary type IV collagenase: Elevated levels are associated with bladder transitional cell carcinoma. *Cancer Epidemiol. Biomark Prev* 1:467–74, 1992.

85. Davis B, Waxman J, Wasan H, et al.: Levels of matrix metalloproteases in bladder cancer correlate with tumor grade and invasion. *Cancer Res* 53:5365–9, 1993.

86. Hasui Y, Marutsuka K, Suzumiya J, et al.: The content of urokinase-type plasminogen activator antigen as a prognostic factor in urinary bladder cancer. *Int J Cancer* 50:871–3, 1992.

87. Weiss RE, Liu BCS, Ahlering T, et al.: Mechanisms of human bladder tumor invasion: Role of protease cathepsin. *Brit J Urol* 144:798–804, 1990.

88. Dickinson AJ, Fox SB, Newcomb PV, et al.: An immunohistochemical and prognostic evaluation of cathepsin D expression in 105 bladder carcinomas. *J Urol* 154:237–41, 1995.

89. Zuk ERJ, Baithun SI, Martin JE, et al.: The immunocytochemical demonstration of basement membrane deposition in transitional cell carcinoma. *Virchows Arch Pathol Anat* 414:447–52, 1989.

90. Conn IG, Crocker J, Wallace DMA, et al.: Basement membranes in urothelial carcinoma. *Br J Urol* 60:536–42, 1987.

91. Daber N, Abourchild H, Bove N, et al.: Collagen IV staining pattern in bladder carcinomas: Relationship to prognosis. *Br J Cancer*, 55:665–71, 1987.

92. Liu L, Deapen D, Bernstein L, Ross R: Cancer incidence in Los Angeles County by race/ethnicity, 1988–1993. Los Angeles County Cancer Surveillance Program, University of South California, Los Angeles, in Petrovich Z, Baert L, Brady LW (eds.): *Carcinoma of the bladder.* Springer-Verlag, 1998, pp. 1–13.

93. Yu MC, Ross RK: Epidemiology of bladder cancer, in Petrovich Z, Baert L, Brady LW, (eds.): *Carcinoma of the bladder.* Berlin, Springer-Verlag, 1998, pp. 1–13.

94. Napalkov S, Maisonneuve P, Boyle P: Epidemiology of bladder cancer, in: Pagano F, Fair WR, Bassi P (eds.): *Superficial bladder cancer.* Oxford, Isis Medical Media, 1997, pp. 1–24.

95. Badawi AF, Mostafa MH, Probert A, O'Connor PJ: Role of schistomiasis in human bladder cancer: Evidence of association, etiological factors, basic mechanisms of carcinogenesis. *Eur J Cancer* 4:45–9, 1995.

96. Kiemeney LALM, Schoenberg M: Familial transitional cell carcinoma. *J Urol* 156:867–72, 1996.

97. Fleshner N, Garland JA, Moadel A, et al.: Influence of smoking status on the disease related outcome of patients with tobacco-associated superficial transitional cell carcinoma of the bladder. *Cancer* 86:2337–45, 1999.

98. Geller NL, Sternberg CN, Penenberg D: Prognostic factors for survival of patients with advanced urothelial tumors treated with MVAC chemotherapy. *Cancer* 67:1525–37, 1991.

99. Duncan W, Quilty PM: The results of a series of 936 patients with transitional cell carcinoma of the urinary bladder primarily treated by radical megavoltage x-ray therapy. *Radiother Oncol* 7:299–310, 1986.

100. Gospodarowicz MK, Hawkins NV, Rawlings GA, et al.: Radical radiotherapy for muscle invasive transitional cell carcinoma of the bladder: Failure analysis. *J Urol* 142:1448–53, 1989.

101. Greven KM, Solin LJ, Hanks GE: Prognostic factors in patients with bladder carcinoma treated with definitive irradiation. *Cancer*, 65:908–12, 1990.

OPHTHALMIC TUMORS

■■■■■■ CHAPTER 41

Intraocular Tumors

ARUN D. SINGH, CAROL L. SHIELDS, and JERRY A. SHIELDS

The eye structures are composed of a variety of tissue types derived from ectodermal and mesodermal germinal layers. Therefore, several kinds of benign and malignant tumors arise in and around the ocular structures. The two most common primary intraocular malignancies are melanoma of the uveal tract (iris, ciliary body, and choroid) and retinoblastoma. Uveal melanoma is usually seen in adults and retinoblastoma usually manifests in children less than 5 years of age. Although both arise primarily from the intraocular structures, each of these tumors is a distinct clinical entity with unique clinical features and systemic prognosis. In this chapter, prognostic factors that influence the survival in uveal melanoma and retinoblastoma are discussed.

PROGNOSTIC FACTORS IN UVEAL MELANOMA

Uveal melanoma is the most common primary intraocular malignant tumor with an annual incidence of approximately six cases per million per year.[1] The diagnosis of uveal melanoma is made by slit-lamp examination and indirect ophthalmoscopy, and ancillary studies such as fluorescein angiography and ultrasonography (Figure 41.1).[2] The traditional form of treatment, enucleation, has been challenged in recent years and alternative methods of treatment, including radiotherapy, local resection, and transpupillary thermotherapy, have been used more frequently.[2,3] Despite high accuracy of diagnosis,[2,4] the mortality due to uveal melanoma has remained unchanged.[1]

This investigation was supported by the Sarah B. Kant Fund, Philadelphia, PA (ADS), Macula Foundation, New York, NY (CLS), and the Paul Kayser Award of Merit in Retinal Research, Houston, TX (JAS).

Prognostic Factors in Cancer, 2nd edition, Edited by Mary K. Gospodarowicz.
ISBN 0-471-40633-3   Copyright © 2001 Wiley-Liss, Inc.

(a)

(b)

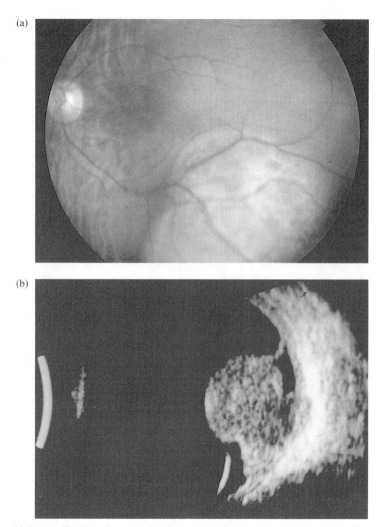

Figure 41.1 (a) Fundus photograph of the right eye showing a choroidal melanoma and (b) ultrasongraphy-B scan demonstrating a mushroom-shaped choroidal melanoma.

Approximately 40% of patients with posterior uveal melanoma who undergo enucleation develop metastatic melanoma to the liver within 10 years after initial diagnosis and treatment.[3] Clinically evident metastatic disease at the time of initial presentation is uncommon, however, indicating early subclinical metastasis in the majority of cases.[3] Using conventional methods such as serum liver enzymes and liver scans, metastatic disease can be detected in only 1–2% of patients at the time of presentation.[5] Systemic screening protocols using physical examinations, liver function tests, chest X rays, and liver imaging studies every 6 months to 1 year have been proposed but the effectiveness of the screening protocols remains to be established.[6]

To reduce uveal melanoma-specific mortality, there has been a recent trend in treatment of small choroidal melanocytic lesions that have a significant risk of growth, which strongly suggests transformation into melanoma.[7] Since 1995, with the availability of transpupillary thermotherapy, a noninvasive treatment modality, it has become possible to treat smaller tumors with fewer complications.[8,9] It is believed that treatment of small choroidal melanocytic lesions will translate into improved long-term survival, but the assumption remains to be proven.

The prognosis in uveal melanoma depends on both clinical and histopathologic features.

Clinical Prognostic Factors

Clinical prognostic factors that relate to prognosis include location, size, configuration of the tumor, and the method of treatment employed (Table 41.1).

Tumor Location   Uveal melanoma can arise either in the iris, ciliary body, or choroid. Iris melanomas (3% of cases) are mostly anterior and relatively small when diagnosed and treated.[10,11] Iris melanomas have the lowest mortality of about 3–5% in 10 years.[11,12] This may be due to the fact that these tumors are relatively small when diagnosed and hence have fewer malignant cell types as compared to posterior uveal melanoma.[13–15]

In 1958, Rones and Zimmerman reported a 10-year tumor-related mortality rate of 6% for iris melanoma.[12] Subsequently, in a larger series of 3432 cases of uveal melanoma reported from the same institution, McLean and associates reported 10 times lower mortality in iris melanoma as compared to ciliary body

TABLE 41.1   The Clinical Prognostic Factors in Uveal Melanoma

Category	Factor	Outcome	Result (%)	First Author	Year
Location	Iris	10-year mortality	6	Rones[12]	1958
		10-year mortality	5	Shields[11]	2000
	Ciliary body	5-year mortality	53	Seddon[17]	1983
		5-year mortality	22	Gunduz[18]	1999
	Choroidal	5-year mortality	14	Seddon[17]	1983
Size	Small	5-year mortality	16	Diener-West[22]	1992
		5-year mortality	3	Shields[7]	1995
		5-year mortality	1	COMS[a,24]	1997
	Medium	5-year mortality	32	Diener-West[22]	1992
	Large	5-year mortality	53	Diener-West[22]	1992
Configuration	Diffuse	5-year mortality	24	Shields[23]	1996
Treatment	Enucleation	8-year mortality	38	Augsburger[28]	1989
	Plaque	8-year mortality	24	Augsburger[28]	1989
	Plaque and helium ion	5-year mortality	24	Kroll[30]	1998
	Proton beam	5-year mortality	19	Seddon[29]	1990

[a]COMS: Collaborative Ocular Melanoma Study.

and choroidal melanoma.[16] More recently, Shields and coworkers identified risk factors for metastasis.[11] Using Kaplan-Meier life table analysis, metastasis was found in 3% at 5 years, 5% at 10 years, and 10% at 20 years. The statistically significant clinical factors predictive of subsequent metastasis from iris melanoma included increasing age at diagnosis, elevated intraocular pressure, extension of tumor posteriorly, extraocular extension, and prior surgical intervention.[11]

Ciliary body melanoma have a worse prognosis.[17] In a series of 267 patients with uveal melanoma treated by enucleation, the 5-year mortality for ciliary-body melanoma was 53% as compared to 14% for choroidal melanoma.[17] Of 136 patients with ciliary body melanoma treated with radioactive plaques, the Kaplan-Meier estimates showed 22% mortality rate at 5 years.[18] The median time to development of metastasis was 68 months (range 25–178 months). The only predictor of metastasis was tumor thickness greater than 7 mm. Patients with ciliary-body melanoma greater than 7 mm in thickness were 2.5 times more likely to develop metastasis than patients with thinner ciliary-body melanoma. Although ciliary-body melanomas tend to be larger at the time of diagnosis as compared to choroidal melanoma, it has been established by detailed statistical analysis that the poor prognosis with ciliary-body melanoma is independent of tumor size and cell type.[17,19]

Tumor Size   Various measurements have been used to represent the tumor size.[16–21] These include largest tumor dimension,[17] tumor volume,[19] and the area of the tumor base.[21] In a meta-analysis of eight published reports on mortality rates of uveal melanoma following enucleation, uveal melanomas were classified into three groups based upon the diameter and height.[22] The combined weighted estimates of 5-year mortality rates were 16% for small tumors, 32% for medium tumors, and 53% for large tumors.[22]

Small choroidal melanoma may be clinically indistinguishable from choroidal nevus. Therefore, management of small choroidal melanocytic tumors remains controversial. In a large retrospective study of 1329 small choroidal melanocytic lesions measuring less than 3 mm in thickness, 3% of the patients developed metastasis at 5 years.[23] The factors predictive of metastasis included tumor proximity to the optic disc, documented tumor growth, and greater tumor thickness. In a nonrandomized prospective study of 204 small choroidal melanomas, defined as choroidal melanocytic lesions with a height of 1–3 mm and diameter of 5–16 mm, 5-year melanoma-specific mortality was only 1%, indicating low rates of mortality in small choroidal melanoma.[24]

Tumor Configuration   The shape of uveal melanoma can vary from a relatively flat diffuse lesion to a dome-shaped tumor. Some tumors break through the Bruch's membrane and assume a mushroom shape. The presence of a break through Bruch's membrane is not a prognostic factor.[17,20] Diffuse choroidal melanomas have a poor prognosis.[23] In a study of 111 diffuse choroidal melanoma, 5-year mortality by Kaplan-Meier estimates was 24% at 5 years.[23] The clinical factors predictive of metastasis included diameter of 18 mm or more, optic nerve invasion, and poorly defined margins. The worse prognosis in diffuse choroidal melanoma may be attributed to a delay in correct diagnosis, greater proportion of epithelioid cells, and its tendency for extraocular extension.[23,25]

Method of Treatment   Zimmerman and associates in 1979 reported their observations on the rise of the mortality rate a few years after enucleation.[26,27] On the basis of 2300 case studies the postoperative mortality rate increased from the estimated preenucleation rate of 1% per year to a peak of 8% during the second year after enucleation, and then decreased. The authors postulated that the procedure of enucleation had a detrimental effect on the expected natural course of the disease.[26,27]

Based on retrospective studies, the mortality rates for uveal melanoma for comparable sized uveal melanoma treated by enucleation, plaque radiotherapy,[28] proton-beam radiotherapy,[29] and helium-ion therapy,[30] appear to be similar.

The Collaborative Ocular Melanoma Study (COMS) is an ongoing prospective study that is currently investigating the patient survival after treatment of choroidal melanoma.[31] The uveal melanomas have been classified into small, medium, and large categories. Tumors smaller than the dimension of a small choroidal melanoma were termed choroidal nevi. The COMS consists of (1) a randomized trial of patients with medium choroidal melanoma treated with enucleation versus iodine-125 plaque irradiation, (2) a randomized trial of patients with large choroidal melanoma treated with enucleation only versus preenucleation external-beam irradiation and enucleation,[32] and (3) a prospective observational study of patients with small choroidal melanoma.[24]

Histopathologic Prognostic Factors

Detailed histopathologic evaluation of the tumor in enucleated cases has led to identification of cell type, mitotic activity, microcirculation architecture, tumor infiltrating lymphocytes, and presence of extrascleral extension as significant predictors of survival (Table 41.2).

Cell Type   Callender in 1931 proposed a classification system for uveal melanoma based on the cell type.[33] The Callender classification was subsequently modified by McLean and associates with improved correlation between the cell type and the mortality.[34] Many of the spindle A cell tumors have been downgraded to benign tumors with no associated mortality. The spindle-cell uveal melanoma has the best prognosis, epithelioid-cell melanoma the worst, and the mixed-cell melanoma has an intermediate prognosis.[16] The 15-year tumor specific mortality of patients with mixed-cell-type melanoma was three times that of patients with spindle cell melanoma. The presence of epithelioid cells is associated with a poorer prognosis, and the tumors classified as mixed-cell type can vary in their content of the epithelioid cells.[34] The prognosis worsens with increasing number of epithelioid cells per high-power field (HPF) measured as an average of 40 HPF.[17]

TABLE 41.2   The Histopathologic Prognostic Factors in Uveal Melanoma

Category	Factor	Outcome	Result (%)	First Author	Year
Cell type	Spindle	15-year mortality	20	McLean[16]	1982
	Mixed	15-year mortality	60	McLean[16]	1982
	Epithelioid	15-year mortality	75	Shammas[20]	1977
Mitotic activity	Low	6-year mortality	15	McLean[19]	1977
	Medium	6-year mortality	43	McLean[19]	1977
	High	6-year mortality	56	McLean[19]	1977
Vascular networks	Absent	10-year mortality	10	Folberg[38]	1993
	Present	10-year mortality	50	Folberg[38]	1993
TIL[a]	Low	15-year mortality	30	de la Cruz[41]	1990
	High	15-year mortality	62	de la Cruz[41]	1990
Extrascleral extension	Absent	10-year mortality	37	Seddon[17]	1983
	Present	10-year mortality	75	Seddon[17]	1983

[a]TIL: Tumor-infiltrating lymphocytes.

Since characterization of cell type is subjective, morphometric criteria have been proposed.[35] The nucleolar area is greater and more pleomorphic in the more malignant variants of uveal melanoma. The standard deviation of the nucleolar area (SDNA), a measure of nucleolar pleomorphism, is prognostically significant.[36] However, measurement of SDNA requires specialized equipment and is time-consuming. The measurement of the mean of the diameters of the 10 largest nucleoli (MLN) is a simpler method and provides similar prognostic information.[35]

Mitotic Activity   Mitotic activity as measured by number of mitoses seen per HPF appears to be of prognostic value in some studies.[19] In one study, tumors with low mitotic activity (0–1 per HPF) had good prognosis, with 6-year mortality of 15% as compared with 56% mortality in tumors with high mitotic activity (9–48 per HPF).[19]

Microcirculation Architecture   Recent studies have suggested that the presence of microcirculation architecture (vascular patterns) is a strong prognosticator of metastatic death, even more significant than tumor size, cell type, and tumor location.[37,38] Nine types of microcirculation architecture are described, including normal, silent (absent), straight, parallel, arcs, loops, and networks.[38] The presence of vascular networks appears to be the most significant variable associated with tumor-specific mortality.[38]

Tumor-infiltrating Lymphocytes   About 5–12% of uveal melanoma show evidence of TILs.[39,40] Increased number of TILs per 20 HPF is significantly associated with decreased survival, even when controlled for other factors.[39–41]

Extrascleral Extension   The presence of extrascleral extension is observed in about 8% of eyes enucleated for uveal melanoma.[42] In such cases the 10-year mortality is doubled to about 75% as compared to those cases with no extrascleral extension.[17] Tumors arising from the ciliary body tend to be larger, and therefore are more likely to be associated with extraocular extension.[20]

Cytologic Prognostic Factors

Cell Proliferation   Various techniques have been used to assess the proliferative activity of uveal melanoma, including visualization of nucleolar organizer regions by silver staining, assessment of aneuploidy following labeling for DNA synthesis by flow cytometry, and immunohistochemical staining for Ki-67 and proliferating cell nuclear antigen (PCNA) (Table 41.3).

Nucleolar Organizer Regions   Nucleolar organizer regions are condensations of the nucleolar DNA seen as black dots when stained with silver staining (AgNOR).[43] Silver staining of nucleolar organizer regions is an objective method for evaluating the malignancy of a variety of tumors. The AgNOR count correlates with the tumor size and mitotic activity and can have prognostic value in uveal melanoma.[43]

Aneuploidy   Flow cytometry is a technique by which the DNA and RNA content of the cells can be assessed.[44] Normal cells show a diploid pattern with a single peak. Aneuploidy represents an abnormal amount of DNA, with multiple peaks representing either a hyperdiploid or hypodiploid pattern. The degree of DNA abnormality is expressed as a DNA index (DI). In a study of 79 patients with uveal melanoma, the clinical outcome was correlated with DNA content (ploidy).[44] The aneuploidy in uveal melanoma has been correlated with the presence of epithelioid cells.[45] Ploidy abnormalities probably reflect a genetically unstable population of cells that have greater ability to metastasize.[44,45] Ploidy abnormalities can be better prognostic indicators than conventional histopathologic parameters.[44,45]

TABLE 41.3   The Cytologic and Genetic Poor Prognostic Factors in Uveal Melanoma

Category	Factor	Author	Year
Cell proliferation			
Nucleolar organizer regions	High AgNOR count	Marcus[43]	1990
Aneuploidy (flow cytometry)	High DNA index	Meecham[44]	1986
Expression of Ki-67	High expression	Mooy[45]	1995
Expression of PCNA[a]	High expression	Seregard[49]	1996
Histocompatibility antigens	High expression of HLA-A	Jager[50]	1986
Cytogenetic	Monosomy 3	White[52]	1998
	Duplication 8q	White[52]	1998
Molecular genetic	c-myc expression	Mooy[45]	1995

[a]PCNA: proliferating cell nuclear antigen.

Expression of Ki-67 and PCNA   Uveal melanoma cells express a number of melanoma-associated antigens, which can be detected by immunohistochemical methods using monoclonal antibodies.[46] There are two antigens that are specific markers for cellular proliferation. Ki-67 and PCNA are expressed when cells are in the proliferative phase. The proliferative activity of uveal melanoma assessed by Ki-67[47] and PCNA[48] is reduced by irradiation of uveal melanoma. In one study, the cumulative 10-year survival proportion was 84% for the low positivity group and 40% for patients with highly positive tumors. Those with highly positive tumors had a 5.8 times greater risk of death from metastatic disease.[49] A similar prognostic value of Ki-67 antigen expression, measured as Mib-1 score, has been reported.[45]

Histocompatibility Antigens   Using immunohistochemical methods human leukocyte antigen (HLA) expression can be assessed.[50] One study suggested that micrometastasis of uveal melanoma cells with a low expression of HLA antigens into the systemic circulation facilitates their removal by natural killer cells and prevents the development of metastasis.[40]

Genetic Prognostic Factors

Cytogenetic   The cytogenetic investigations of choroidal and ciliary-body melanoma have demonstrated clonal abnormalities involving chromosomes 3, 6, and 8.[51,52] Abnormalities of chromosomes 3 and 8 usually coexist and are preferentially present in ciliary-body tumors. In contrast, abnormalities of chromosome 6 are more frequently associated with choroidal tumors.[53–55] In a study of 54 patients with uveal melanoma undergoing enucleation, the findings of monosomy 3 and duplication of 8q were associated with a survival rate of 40% at 3 years compared to 95% survival in the absence of these cytogenetic changes.[52] In addition, it has been observed that ciliary body and choroidal melanoma are cytogenetically distinct, with ciliary-body melanoma showing preferential monosomy of chromosome 3.[54] In a detailed cytogenetic study on uveal melanoma derived from 54 patients, 30 melanomas showed monosomy of chromosome 3. In 17 of these patients (57%) metastatic disease developed within 3 years. By contrast, of the 24 patients whose melanoma had a normal complement of chromosome 3, none developed metastatic disease.[54] The poor prognosis of ciliary-body melanoma can be partially explained on the basis of distinctive cytogenetic abnormalities.[52,54,55]

Molecular Genetics   The expression of c-myc, an oncogene involved in cellular proliferation, has been studied in detail because c-myc has been mapped to the 8q chromosomal region, the region observed to be commonly altered cytogenetically in uveal melanoma. In a immunohistochemical study of 24 uveal melanomas, c-myc expression in both nucleus and cytoplasm was observed in up to 85% of uveal melanoma.[56] c-myc expression correlated with the proliferative index, but not with the cell type.[56] In another study of 51 patients with uveal melanoma, multivariate analysis showed a prognostic significance of c-myc positive cells.[45] There seems to be an inverse correlation between expression of c-myc and HLA antigens, suggesting that c-myc down regulates HLA expression, thereby influencing immune response in uveal melanoma.[57]

The prognostic factors in uveal melanoma have been studied with the hope of detecting high-risk cases. These patients may be candidates for adjuvant systemic immune therapy or chemotherapy. At present, the role of these therapeutic methods is not clearly established.[58,59]

PROGNOSTIC FACTORS IN RETINOBLASTOMA

Retinoblastoma is the most common primary intraocular malignancy in children, with an incidence of 1 in 15,000 live births.[60] The average annual incidence of retinoblastoma in the United States has been estimated as 10.9 per million for children younger than 5 years and has remained stable from 1974 to 1985.[61] Most children present with a white pupillary reflex, or leukocoria (Figure 41.2). (see Reference 2, pp. 305–319). Ancillary studies such as ultrasonography, computed tomography, and magnetic resonance imaging can assist in confirming the diagnosis (see Reference 2, 363–376).

In recent years there has been a trend away from enucleation,[62] and the increased use of the alternative globe-conserving methods of treatment, including external-beam radiotherapy,[63] plaque radiotherapy,[64] laser photocoagulation,[65] cryotherapy,[66] and transpupillary thermotherapy.[67] Currently, chemotherapy is being increasingly used as chemoreduction, with other adjuvant therapy to avoid external-beam radiotherapy and enucleation.[68,69] Recent advances in the treatment of retinoblastoma have led to a reduced risk of metastasis and improved survival rates in the developed countries. The 5-year survival rates of 91, 93, and 88% have been reported from the United States,[61] Japan[70] and United Kingdom[62] respectively. However, in the underdeveloped countries retinoblastoma is still associated with high mortality.[71]

Retinoblastoma is a familial disorder with an autosomal dominant inheritance. Approximately 60% of the patients are considered sporadic and 40% are inheritable. Of the inheritable type of retinoblastoma 5–15% have an existing family history and the remaining 25% are due to new germline mutations.[72] The inheritable variant of retinoblastoma tends to be bilateral and present earlier with a mean age of 12 months. The sporadic type of retinoblastoma tends to be unilateral and presents later with a mean age of 24 months. All bilateral cases are considered inheritable and harbor germline mutation. In addition, about 15% of all unilateral cases are also inheritable. Patients with the inheritable variant of retinoblastoma are particularly susceptible to the development of pinealoblastoma and other second malignant neoplasms, particularly osteosarcoma.

Metastatic disease at the time of retinoblastoma diagnosis is very unlikely. Therefore, staging procedures such as bone scans, lumbar puncture, and bone marrow aspirations at initial presentation are not generally recommended.[73,74] The metastasis in retinoblastoma usually occurs within one year of diagnosis of retinoblastoma. If there is no metastatic disease within 5 years of retinoblastoma

(a)

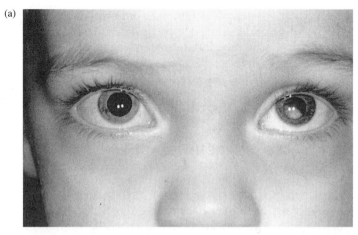

(b)

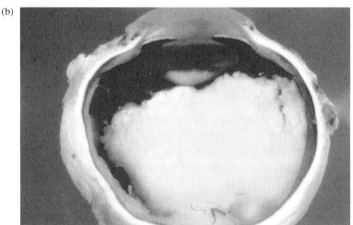

Figure 41.2   (a) External photograph of face showing leukocoria in the left eye, and (b) enucleated globe with a large retinoblastoma appearing as a white mass in the vitreous cavity.

diagnosis, the child is usually considered cured.[75] Involvement of the central nervous system and hematogenous spread are common. The survival with metastatic retinoblastoma is limited, with death occurring generally within 6 months.[75,76]

The prognosis for retinoblastoma can be related to the clinical factors and histopathologic factors (Table 41.4).

Clinical Prognostic Factors

Delay in Diagnosis   The commonest presentations of retinoblastoma include leukocoria and strabismus.[77] Children presenting with such symptoms or signs should be examined by an ophthalmologist to exclude retinoblastoma. In a study

TABLE 41.4 Adverse Prognostic Factors in Retinoblastoma

Clinical
  Delay in diagnosis (more than 6 months)
  Prior intraocular surgery
  Use of external beam radiotherapy
Histopathologic
  Choroidal invasion
  Optic nerve invasion
    Retrolaminar invasion
    Invasion up to the line of transection
  Orbital invasion

of 100 patients with retinoblastoma in the United Kingdom, a delay in diagnosis did not increase the likelihood of treatment by enucleation, but the risk of local tumor invasion was increased.[78] In another study from Brazil, the 3-year survival rate was 82% in the early-diagnosis group as compared with 44% in the late-diagnosis group. The worse prognosis in the late-diagnosis group correlated with the tendency of patients in this group to exhibit extraocular extension of the retinoblastoma.[79,80]

Prior Intraocular Surgery Extraocular spread of retinoblastoma is a poor prognostic factor. Intraocular surgical procedures such as pars plana vitrectomy inadvertently performed on patients with retinoblastoma, predisposes to orbital extension or metastasis of retinoblastoma. Stevenson and associates published three such cases, all of which developed orbital retinoblastoma following intraocular surgery.[81] Shields and coworkers reported 11 such patients all of whom received prompt enucleation and most received prophylactic orbital radiotherapy and chemotherapy with ultimate metastasis in only 1 case.[82]

Genetic Subtype The inheritable form of retinoblastoma has significant long-term prognostic implications. Second malignant neoplasms, which occur predominantly in the inheritable form of retinoblastoma, have now become significant contributors to overall mortality.[83] In a large study from the United Kingdom, the overall 3-year survival rate was 88%.[83] Patients with bilateral tumors had worse long-term survival rates because of later deaths from trilateral intracranial retinoblastoma or other second primary neoplasms.[62] Similar results were observed in a study from Japan.[70] The occurrence of a second neoplasm was the main cause of death in the hereditary cases 10 years after the diagnosis.[70]

Second Malignant Neoplasms It is now recognized that more children with retinoblastoma die from the second malignant neoplasms and trilateral retinoblastoma than from the retinoblastoma itself.[84] The incidence of second malignant neoplasm in the inheritable form of retinoblastoma has been reported to be between 5% and 90% in various reports due to differences in the methods of ascertainment of the cases and analysis of the data (Table 41.5).[84] In a study from the United Kingdom, Draper and associates reported a cumulative incidence rate of 8% after 18 years in 384 cases, with the inheritable form of retinoblastoma.[85] Roarty and associates calculated cumulative incidence using the life table method in 215 patients with bilateral retinoblastoma to be 18% at 20 years.[86] Mohney and associates estimated the incidence of second malignant neoplasm as 16% at 25 years and 30% at 40 years in 82 patients with heritable retinoblastoma using Kaplan-Meier analysis.[87] In a detailed study of 1604 patients with retinoblastoma, of which 961 patients had hereditary retinoblastoma, the cumulative incidence (Kaplan-Meier estimates) of second malignant neoplasms, 50 years after diagnosis of retinoblastoma, was ten times higher in hereditary cases versus nonhereditary cases (51% and 5%) (Figure 41.3).[88,89] It is estimated that the cumulative incidence rate of developing second malignant neoplasm in heritable retinoblastoma is about 1% per year.[89]

The second malignant neoplasms are of many types and at least 35 distinct types of neoplasms have been reported in association with retinoblastoma.[90] The majority of the neoplasms are osteosarcoma (37%) and other sarcomas (10%).[91] Cutaneous melanoma represents about 7% of all second malignant neoplasms.[91] The risk of developing bone tumors is increased about 400 times and that of connective and soft tissue tumors to about 100 times in heritable retinoblastoma as compared with the normal population.[89] The role of radiotherapy in the pathogenesis of second malignant neoplasm is discussed below.

Trilateral Retinoblastoma   The association between inheritable retinoblastoma and a primary intracranial malignancy, especially of the pineal gland, is

TABLE 41.5   Incidence of Second Malignant Neoplasms in Retinoblastoma

First Author	Year	Number[a]	Method	Outcome (Yr)	Result (%)
Draper[85]	1986	384	Cumulative incidence rate	18	8
Roarty[86]	1988	215	Cumulative incidence	10	4
			(Life table method)	20	18
				30	26
CNRR[70,b]	1992	409	Cumulative incidence rate	5	0
				10	5
				15	9
				20	16
Moll[91]	1997	87	Cumulative incidence	10	3
			(Kaplan-Meier)	20	11
Wong[89]	1997	961	Cumulative incidence	50	51
			(Kaplan-Meier)		
Mohney[87]	1998	82	Cumulative incidence	10	12
			(Kaplan-Meier)	25	16
				40	30

[a]Number: Includes only patients with inheritable retinoblastoma.
[b]CNRR: The Committee for the National Registry of Retinoblastoma, Japan.

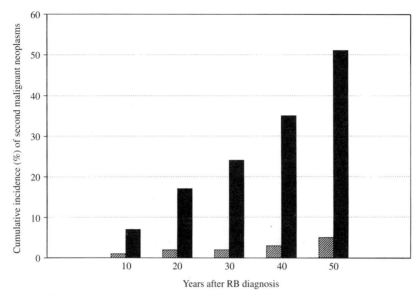

Figure 41.3   The cumulative incidence (Kaplan-Meier estimates) of second malignant neoplasms in hereditary cases (solid) and nonhereditary cases (shaded) of retinoblastoma. (Adapted from Reference 89.)

called "trilateral retinoblastoma."[92] In patients with bilateral retinoblastoma, the presence of an intracranial malignancy is now recognized to be the most frequent cause of death in the first decade of life, accounting for 50% of all deaths.[93]

Trilateral retinoblastoma occurs in about 8% of all inheritable retinoblastoma.[94] The primary intracranial malignant tumor can vary in its location and histopathologic features.[62] The majority of tumors are located in the pineal region, but the tumors can also occur in the suprasellar and parasellar regions.[95,96] The overall prognosis in the presence of trilateral retinoblastoma is poor.[97,98] The median survival time after diagnosis of trilateral retinoblastoma was 9 months.[98] It is hoped that earlier neuroimaging studies may detect the intracranial tumor and allow earlier treatment.

External-beam Radiotherapy   The relationship between radiation and second malignant neoplasms is complex.[84] At least two effects of external-beam radiotherapy in the pathogenesis of second malignant neoplasms in retinoblastoma patients have been identified. These include enhancement of the baseline risk and a localizing effect.[88] The effects of radiotherapy are influenced by the age of the recipient and are believed to be dose dependent.[88,89]

The previously mentioned risk of developing a second malignant neoplasms is doubled by the use of external-beam radiotherapy (Figure 41.4).[88,89] The influence of radiotherapy in causing second malignant neoplasm appears to be dependent upon the age of the child when radiotherapy is administered and the dose of radiation applied.[88,89] The cumulative incidence of a second

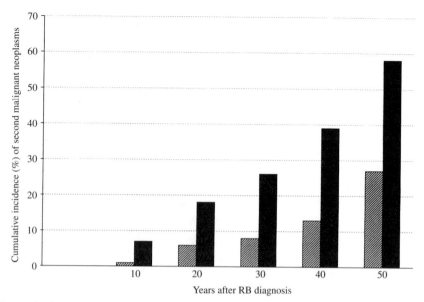

Figure 41.4 The cumulative incidence (Kaplan-Meier estimates) of second malignant neoplasms in hereditary cases of retinoblastoma treated with external-beam radiotherapy (solid) and without radiotherapy (shaded). (Adapted from Reference 89.)

malignant neoplasm is 9% at age 10 years and 34% at 30 years if the radiation is given to children who were less than 1 year of age as compared to 5% and 22%, respectively, for children who were older than 1 year when treated.[88] In addition, the effect of radiotherapy may be dose dependent, with elevated risk associated with doses higher than 50 Gy.[89] Currently with the megavoltage techniques, an average dose of 44 Gy is used to treat retinoblastoma, and the high-energy photon beams deliver a uniform dose to the bone and soft tissues.[63] With present techniques of external-beam radiotherapy for retinoblastoma, the enhancing influence of external-beam radiotherapy in the pathogenesis of second malignant neoplasm can be lower than the published data.

Use of Chemoreduction Chemoreduction involves the administration of chemotherapy for advanced intraocular retinoblastoma to achieve tumor reduction so that focal ophthalmic therapy can be applied to partially regressed tumors.[68,69] In a series of 160 children with intraocular retinoblastoma treated with chemoreduction none of the children developed trilateral retinoblastoma.[99] In the same cohort, 5–16 cases were expected to develop trilateral retinoblastoma. It is suspected that the chemoreduction might play a protective role against the development of the intracranial tumor.[99]

Histopathologic Prognostic Factors

Many studies have evaluated the histopathologic prognostic factors including tumor size, tumor growth pattern, tumor differentiation, extension into the choroid, optic nerve, anterior chamber, and extrascleral tissues.[75,80,100-104] Multivariate analysis, in which correction for confounding effects of multiple risk factors is made, is particularly helpful in identifying the influence of individual prognostic factor (Table 41.6).[75,80,100-102] Tumor parameters such as tumor size, tumor growth pattern (endophytic or exophytic),[104] and tumor differentiation[100] do not significantly influence the systemic prognosis.[105]

Choroidal Invasion   There are conflicting results as to whether extension of retinoblastoma into the choroid is believed to represent a poor prognostic factor.[75,106] In a histopathologic review of 74 retinoblastoma patients, choroidal invasion correlated with 100% survival provided that the sclera, iris, and optic nerve were not involved.[107] Studies using methods of multivariate analysis have supported the view that choroidal invasion by retinoblastoma increases the risk of metastatic disease.[80,101]

Optic-nerve Invasion   Optic-nerve invasion of retinoblastoma is a known poor prognostic factor for patients with retinoblastoma.[110] In fact, multivariate statistical analysis has indicated that histologic detection of optic-nerve invasion by retinoblastoma is one of the most highly predictive factors for death from retinoblastoma.[75] Since 1960, the frequency and severity of optic-nerve invasion has been less extensive due to the earlier diagnosis of retinoblastoma.[108]

TABLE 41.6   Histopathologic Poor Prognostic Factors in Retinoblastoma Identified by Multivariate Analysis

| First Author | Study Years | Number | Prognostic Factors | |
			Significant	Not Significant
Tosi[100]	1968–1985	54	Invasion of choroid/sclera	Differentiation AC extension ON invasion
Khelfaoui[101]	1977–1990	171	Extrascleral extension ON up to resection line Massive choroidal invasion Retrolaminar ON invasion	AC extension
Kopelman[75]	1922–1959	361	ON invasion Orbital extension	Tumor size Choroidal invasion
Messmer[80]	1956–1986	526	Late enucleation[a] Retrolaminar ON invasion ON up to resection line Choroidal invasion	Tumor size Secondary glaucoma Number of tumors AC extension
Magramm[102]	1922–1986	240	Age Extent of ON invasion Choroidal invasion	Scleral invasion Laterality

Abbreviations: ON: optic nerve; AC: anterior chamber.
[a]Late enucleation: More than 120 days after the initial presentation.

Optic-nerve invasion is present in about one-third of enucleated globes for retinoblastoma and correlates with the presence of choroidal or scleral extension.[102,107,109] Optic-nerve invasion is usually categorized as prelaminar, laminar, postlaminar, and up to the line of transection.[102] Prelaminar optic-nerve involvement is most common, representing about half of all cases of optic-nerve involvement.[109] The laminar and the retrolaminar involvement in equal portions accounts for the remaining half of the cases. In our experience, optic-nerve involvement up to the line of transection is very rare and was seen only in 2 out of 289 cases (1%).[109]

There is increasing mortality with increasing extent of optic-nerve involvement.[102] It is generally agreed, however, that prelaminar involvement of the optic nerve does not increase the risk of metastasis.[101,103,109,110] The impact of laminar involvement on metastasis is debated.[101,109,110] Retrolaminar involvement is a poor prognostic factor, and optic-nerve invasion by retinoblastoma up to the line of transection predicts the worst prognosis.[80,101,109]

Optic-nerve invasion can be predicted by the presence of a large exophytic retinoblastoma with secondary glaucoma and vitreous hemorrhage.[109] These findings should alert the clinician to suspect optic-nerve invasion. When enucleation is performed for retinoblastoma, an attempt should be made to salvage a long stump of optic nerve (about 10–15 mm long) so as to transect the optic nerve beyond the extent of involvement by retinoblastoma.[111]

Orbital Invasion Extrascleral or orbital extension of retinoblastoma is possibly the worst prognostic factor for death from retinoblastoma.[75] The presence of orbital invasion of retinoblastoma is associated with a 40% risk of metastasis as compared to 4% in cases with no orbital invasion.[101]

Prophylactic chemotherapy with adjuvant orbital radiotherapy has been advocated in retinoblastoma cases with prior prognostic indicators such as prior intraocular surgery, orbital extension of retinoblastoma, anterior chamber seeding, and in cases with extension of retinoblastoma, up to the line of optic-nerve transection.[101,110,111] The role of such prophylactic treatment in instances with isolated choroidal invasion and retrolaminar optic-nerve invasion remains controversial.[112,113]

SUMMARY

Various clinical and histopathologic prognostic factors have been identified in retinoblastoma. Early recognition of symptoms with a high index of suspicion and prompt referral to a specialized center will further improve survival in patients with retinoblastoma. Patients with germline mutations of retinoblastoma gene are at a risk for development of pinealoblastoma and other second malignant neoplasms. The use of external-beam radiotherapy enhances the risk for development of second malignant neoplasms. Uncontrolled clinical studies suggest that the use of prophylactic chemotherapy in high-risk retinoblastoma patients is effective in reducing the risk of metastasis. Due to the limited number of cases treated at a given center, there is a need for a collaborative prospective randomized clinical trial evaluating the efficacy of prophylactic chemotherapy in retinoblastoma patients with poor prognostic factors.

████████ **APPENDIX 41A.1**

Prognostic Factors in Uveal Melanoma

Prognostic Factors	Tumor Related	Host Related	Environment Related
Essential	Tumor location Tumor size		
Additional	Tumor configuration Tumor-cell type Microcirculation architecture TILs Extrascleral extension		
New and promising	Cell proliferation — Ki-67 Cytogenetic factors c-myc expression		

████████ **APPENDIX 41A.2**

Prognostic Factors in Retinoblastoma

Prognostic Factors	Tumor Related	Host Related	Environment Related
Essential	Tumor size	Familial retinoblastoma	Delay in diagnosis Prior intraocular surgery
Additional	Orbital invasion Optic-nerve invasion Choroidal invasion	Rb gene mutation	
New and promising	p53 CD44		

REFERENCES

1. Strickland D, Lee JA: Melanomas of eye: Stability of rates. *Am J Epidemiol* 113:700–2, 1981.

2. Shields JA, Shields CL: *Intraocular tumors, A text and atlas*. Philadelphia, Saunders, 1992, pp. 155–169.

3. Shields JA, Shields CL, Donoso LA: Management of posterior uveal melanoma. *Surv Ophthalmol* 36:161–95, 1991.

4. Shields JA, Augsburger JJ, Brown GC, Stephens RF: The differential diagnosis of posterior uveal melanoma. *Ophthalmology* 87:518–22, 1980.

5. Donoso LA, Folberg R, Naids R, et al.: Metastatic uveal melanoma. Hepatic metastasis identified by hybridoma-secreted monoclonal antibody Mab8-1H. *Arch Ophthalmol* 103:799–801, 1985.

6. Eskelin S, Pyrhonen S, Summanen P, et al.: Screening for metastatic malignant melanoma of the uvea revisited. *Cancer* 85:1151–9, 1999.

7. Shields CL, Shields JA, Kiratli H, et al.: Risk factors for growth and metastasis of small choroidal melanocytic lesions. *Ophthalmology* 102:1351–61, 1995.

8. Oosterhius J, Journee-de Korver HG, Kakebeeke-kemme HM, et al.: Transpupillary thermotherapy in choroidal melanomas. *Arch Ophthalmol* 113:315–21, 1995.

9. Shields CL, Shields JA, Cater J, et al.: Transpupillary thermotherapy for choroidal melanoma. Tumor control and visual results in 100 consecutive cases. *Ophthalmology* 105:581–90, 1998.

10. Jensen OA: Malignant melanomas of the human uvea. Recent follow up of cases in Denmark, 1943–1952. *Acta Ophthalmol* 48:1113–28, 1970.

11. Shields CL, Shields JA, Materin M, et al.: Iris melanoma: Risk factors in 169 consecutive cases. In press.

12. Rones B, Zimmerman LE: The prognosis of primary tumors of iris treated by iridectomy. *Arch Ophthalmol* 60:193–205, 1958.

13. Davidorf FH: The melanoma controversy. A comparison of choroidal, cutaneous, and iris melanomas. *Surv Ophthalmol* 25:373–7, 1981.

14. Arentsen JJ, Green WR: Melanoma of the iris: Report of 72 cases treated surgically. *Ophthalmic Surg* 6:23–7, 1975.

15. Jensen OA: Malignant melanoma of the iris. A 25-year analysis of Danish cases. *Eur J Ophthalmol* 3:181–8, 1993.

16. McLean IW, Foster WD, Zimmerman LE: Uveal melanoma: Location, size, cell type, and enucleation as risk factors in metastasis. *Hum Pathol* 13:123–32, 1982.

17. Seddon JM, Albert DM, Lavin PT, et al.: A prognostic factor study of disease-free interval and survival following enucleation for uveal melanoma. *Arch Ophthalmol* 101:1894–9, 1983.

18. Gunduz K, Shields CL, Shields JA, et al.: Plaque radiotherapy of uveal melanoma with predominant ciliary body involvement. *Arch Ophthalmol* 117:170–7, 1999.

19. McLean MJ, Foster WD, Zimmerman LE: Prognostic factors in small malignant melanomas of choroid and ciliary body. *Arch Ophthalmol* 95:48–58, 1977.

20. Shammas HF, Blodi FC: Prognostic factors in choroidal and ciliary body melanomas. *Arch Ophthalmol* 95:63–9, 1977.

21. Jensen OA: Malignant melanomas of the human uvea in Denmark, 1943–1952. *Acta Ophthalmol* 75:1–220, 1963.

22. Diener-West M, Hawkins BS, Markowitz JA, et al.: A review of mortality from choroidal melanoma. II. A meta-analysis of 5-year mortality rates following enucleation, 1966 through 1988. *Arch Ophthalmol* 110:245–50, 1992.

23. Shields CL, Shields JA, De Potter PV, et al.: Diffuse choroidal melanoma: Clinical features predictive of metastasis. *Arch Ophthalmol* 114:956–63, 1996.

24. Anonymous: Mortality in patients with small choroidal melanoma. COMS report no. 4. The Collaborative Ocular Melanoma Study Group. *Arch Ophthalmol* 115:886–93, 1997.

25. Font RL, Spaulding AG, Zimmerman LE: Diffuse malignant melanoma of the uveal tract: A clinicopathologic report of 54 cases. *Trans Am Acad Ophthalmol Otolaryngol* 72:877–95, 1968.

26. Zimmerman LE, McLean IW, Foster WD: Does enucleation of the eye containing a malignant melanoma prevent or accelerate the dissemination of tumour cells. *Br J Ophthalmol* 62:420–5, 1978.

27. Zimmerman LE, McLean IW: An evaluation of enucleation in the management of uveal melanomas. *Am J Ophthalmol* 87:741–60, 1979.

28. Augsburger JJ, Gamel JW, Shields JA: Cobalt plaque radiotherapy versus enucleation for posterior uveal melanoma: Comparison of survival by prognostic index groups. *Trans Am Ophthalmol Soc* 87:348–59, 1989.

29. Seddon JM, Gragoudas ES, Kathleen EM, et al.: Relative survival rates after alternative therapies for uveal melanoma. *Ophthalmology* 97:769–77, 1990.

30. Kroll S, Char DH, Quivey J, et al.: A comparison of cause-specific melanoma mortality and all-cause mortality in survival analyses after radiation treatment for uveal melanoma. *Ophthalmology* 105:2035–45, 1998.

31. Straatsma BR, Fine SL, Earle JD, et al.: Enucleation versus plaque irradiation for choroidal melanoma. *Ophthalmology* 95:1000–4, 1988.

32. Anonymous: The Collaborative Ocular Melanoma Study (COMS) randomized trial of pre-enucleation radiation of large choroidal melanoma II: Initial mortality findings. COMS report no. 10. *Am J Ophthalmol* 125:779–96, 1998.

33. Callender GR: Malignant melanotic tumors of the eye. A study of histologic types in 111 cases. *Trans Am Acad Ophthalmol Otolaryngol* 36:131–40, 1931.

34. McLean IW, Foster WD, Zimmerman LE, et al.: Modifications of Callender's classification of uveal melanoma at the Armed Forces Institute of Pathology. *Am J Ophthalmol* 96:502–9, 1983.

35. Gamel JW, McCurdy JB, McLean IW: A comparison of prognostic covariates for uveal melanoma. *Invest Ophthalmol and Vis Sci* 33:1919–22, 1992.

36. Seddon JM, Polivogianis L, Hsieh CC, et al.: Death from uveal melanoma. Number of epithelioid cells and inverse SD of nucleolar area as prognostic factors. *Arch Ophthalmol* 105:801–6, 1987.

37. Rummelt V, Folberg R, Woolson RF, et al.: Relation between the microcirculation architecture and the aggressive behavior of ciliary body melanomas. *Ophthalmology* 102:844–51, 1995.

38. Folberg R, Rummelt V, Parys-Van Ginderdeuren R, et al.: The prognostic value of tumor blood vessel morphology in primary uveal melanoma. *Ophthalmology* 100:1389–98, 1993.

39. Durie FH, Campbell AM, Lee WR, et al.: Analysis of lymphocytic infiltration in uveal melanoma. *Invest Ophthalmol Vis Sci* 31:2106–10, 1990.

40. de Waard-Siebinga I, Hilders CG, Hansen BE, et al.: HLA expression and tumor-infiltrating immune cells in uveal melanoma. *Graefe's Arch Clin Exp Ophthalmol* 234:34–42, 1996.

41. De la Cruz PO, Specht CS, McLean IW: Lymphocytic infiltration in uveal malignant melanoma. *Cancer* 65:112–5, 1990.

42. Anonymous: Histopathologic characteristics of uveal melanoma in eyes enucleated from the Collaborative Ocular Melanoma Study COMS report no. 6. *Am J Ophthalmol* 125:745–66, 1998.

43. Marcus DM, Minkovitz JB, Wardwell SD, et al.: The value of nucleolar organizer regions in uveal melanoma. The Collaborative Ocular Melanoma Study Group. *Am J Ophthalmol* 110:527–34, 1990.

44. Meecham WJ, Char DH: DNA content abnormalities and prognosis in uveal melanoma. *Arch Ophthalmol* 104:1626–9, 1986.

45. Mooy CM, Luyten GPM, Luider TM, et al.: An immunohistochemical and prognostic analysis of apoptosis and proliferation in uveal melanoma. *Am J Pathol* 147:1097–104, 1995.

46. Mooy CM, de Jong PTVM: Prognostic parameters in uveal melanoma: A review. *Surv Ophthalmol* 41:215–28, 1996.

47. Mooy CM, de Jong PTVM, van der Kwast TH, et al.: Ki-67 immunostaining in uveal melanoma; The effect of preenucleation radiotherapy. *Ophthalmology* 97:1275–80, 1990.

48. Pre'er J, Gnessin H, Shargal Y, Livni N: PC-10 immunostaining of proliferating cell nuclear antigen in posterior uveal melanoma. *Ophthalmology* 101:56–62, 1994.

49. Seregard S, Oskarsson M, Spanberg B: PC-10 as predictor of prognosis after antigen retrieval in posterior uveal melanoma. *Invest Ophthalmol Vis Sci* 37:1451–8, 1996.

50. Jager MJ, de Wolff-Rouendaal D, Breebaart AC, et al.: Expression of HLA antigens in paraffin sections of uveal melanomas. *Doc Ophthalmol* 64:69–76, 1986.

51. Singh AD, Bhogosian-Sell L, Wary KK, et al.: Cytogenetic findings in primary uveal melanoma. *Cancer Genet Cytogenet* 72:109–15, 1994.

52. White VA, Chambers JD, Courtright PD, et al.: Correlation of cytogenetic abnormalities with outcome of patients with uveal melanoma. *Cancer* 83:354–9, 1998.

53. Horsman DE, White VA: Cytogenetic analysis of uveal melanoma: Consistent occurrence of monosomy 3 and trisomy 8q. *Cancer* 71:811–9, 1993.

54. Prescher G, Bornfeld N, Hirche H, et al.: Prognostic implications of monosomy 3 in uveal melanoma. *Lancet* 347:1222–5, 1996.

55. Sisley K, Rennie IG, Parsons MA, et al.: Abnormalities of chromosomes 3 and 8 in posterior uveal melanoma correlate with prognosis. *Genes Chromosomes Cancer* 19:22–8, 1997.

56. Royds JA, Sharrad RM, Parsons MA, et al.: C-myc oncogene expression in ocular melanomas. *Graefe's Arch Clin Exp Ophthalmol* 230:366–71, 1992.

57. Blom DJ, Mooy CM, Luyten GP, et al.: Inverse correlation between expression of HLA-B and c-myc in uveal melanoma. *J Pathol* 181:75–9, 1997.

58. Shields JA: Management of uveal melanoma: A continuing dilemma. *Cancer* 72:2067–8, 1993.

59. McLean IW, Berd D, Mastrangelo MJ, et al.: A randomized study of methanol-extraction residue of bacille Calmette-Guerin as postsurgical adjuvant therapy of uveal melanoma. *Am J Ophthalmol* 110:522–6, 1990.

60. Bishop JO, Madsen EC: Retinoblastoma: Review of current status. *Surv Ophthalmol* 19:342–66, 1975.

61. Tamboli A, Podgor MJ, Horm JW: The incidence of retinoblastoma in the United States: 1974 through 1985. *Arch Ophthalmol* 108:128–32, 1990.

62. Shields CL, Shields JA: Recent developments in the management of retinoblastoma. *J Pediatr Ophthalmol Strabismus* 36:8–18, 1999.

63. Hernandez JC, Brady LW, Shields JA, et al.: External beam radiation for retinoblastoma: Results, patterns of failure and proposal for treatment guidelines. *Int J Rad Oncol Biol Phys* 35:125–32, 1996.

64. Shields JA, Shields CL, De Potter PV, et al.: Plaque radiotherapy for residual or recurrent retinoblastoma in 91 cases. *J Pediatr Ophthalmol Strabismus* 31:242–5, 1994.

65. Shields CL, Shields JA, Kiratli H, De Potter PV: Treatment of retinoblastoma with indirect ophthalmoscope laser photocoagulation. *J Pediatr Ophthalmol Strabismus* 32:317–22, 1995.

66. Shields JA, Parsons H, Shields CL, Giblin ME: The role of cryotherapy in the management of retinoblastoma. *Am J Ophthalmol* 108:260–4, 1989.

67. Shields CL, Santos MC, Diniz W, et al.: Thermotherapy for retinoblastoma. *Arch Ophthalmol* 117:885–93, 1999.

68. Ferris FL, Chew EY: A new era for the treatment of retinoblastoma. *Arch Ophthalmol* 114:1412, 1996.

69. Shields CL, Shields JA, Needle M, et al.: Combined chemoreduction and adjuvant treatment for intraocular retinoblastoma. *Ophthalmology* 104:2101–11, 1997.

70. Anonymous. Survival rate and risk factors for patients with retinoblastoma in Japan. The Committee for the National Registry of Retinoblastoma. *Jpn J Ophthalmol* 36:121–31, 1992.

71. Ajaiyeoba IA, Akang EE, Campbell OB, Olurin IO, Aghadiuno PU: Retinoblastomas in Ibadan: Treatment and prognosis. *West Afr J Med* 12:223–7, 1993.

72. Vogel F: Genetics of retinoblastoma. *Hum Genet* 52:1–54, 1979.

73. Pratt CB, Meyer D, Chenaille P, Crom DB: The use of bone marrow aspirations and lumbar punctures at the time of diagnosis of retinoblastoma. *J Clin Oncol* 7:140–3, 1989.

74. Mohney BG, Robertson DM: Ancillary testing for metastasis in patients with newly diagnosed retinoblastoma. *Am J Ophthalmol* 118:707–11, 1994.

75. Kopelman JE, McLean IW, Rosenberg SH: Multivariate analysis of risk factors for metastasis in retinoblastoma treated by enucleation. *Ophthalmology* 94:371–7, 1987.

76. McCay CJ, Abramson DH, Ellsworth RM: Metastatic patterns of retinoblastoma. *Arch Ophthalmol* 102:391–6, 1984.

77. Abramson DH, Frank CM, Susman L, et al.: Presenting signs of retinoblastoma. *J Pediatr* 25:210–1, 1998.

78. Goddard AG, Kingston JE, Hungerford JL: Delay in diagnosis of retinoblastoma: Risk factors and treatment outcomes. *Br J Ophthalmol* 83:1320–3, 1999.

79. Erwenne CM, Franco EL: Age and lateness of referral as determinants of extra-ocular retinoblastoma. *Ophthalmic Genet* 10:179–84, 1989.

80. Messmer EP, Fritze H, Mohr C, et al.: Long-term treatment effects in patients with bilateral retinoblastoma: Ocular and mid-facial findings. *Graefe's Arch Clin Exp Ophthalmol* 229:309–14, 1991.

81. Stevenson KE, Hungerford JL, Garner A: Local extraocular extension of retinoblastoma following intraocular surgery. *Br J Ophthalmol* 73:739–42, 1989.

82. Shields CL, Honavar S, Shields JA, et al.: Vitrectomy in eyes with unsuspected retinoblastoma. In Press.

83. Sanders BM, Draper GJ, Kingston JE. Retinoblastoma in Great Britain 1969–80: Incidence, treatment, and survival. *Br J Ophthalmol* 72:576–83, 1983.

84. Abramson DH: Second nonocular cancers in retinoblastoma: A unified hypothesis — The Franceschetti Lecture. *Ophthalmic Genet* 20:193–204, 1999.

85. Draper GJ, Sanders BM, Kingston JE: Second primary neoplasms in patients with retinoblastoma. *Br J Cancer* 53:661–71, 1986.

86. Roarty JD, McLean IW, Zimmerman LE: Incidence of second neoplasms in patients with bilateral retinoblastoma. *Ophthalmology* 95:1583–7, 1988.

87. Mohney BG, Robertson DM, Schomberg PJ, Hodge DO: Second nonocular tumors in survivors of heritable retinoblastoma and prior radiation therapy. *Am J Ophthalmol* 126:230–7, 1998.

88. Abramson DH, Frank CM: Second nonocular tumors in survivors of bilateral retinoblastoma: A possible age effect on radiation-related risk. *Ophthalmology* 105:573–9, 1998.

89. Wong FL, Boice JD, Abramson DH, et al.: Cancer incidence after retinoblastoma. Radiation dose and sarcoma risk. *J Am Med Assoc* 278:1262–7, 1997.

90. Dunkel IJ, Gerald WL, Rosenfield NS, et al.: Outcome of patients with a history of bilateral retinoblastoma treated for a second malignancy: The Memorial Sloan-Kettering experience. *Med Pediatr Oncol* 30:59–62, 1998.

91. Moll AC, Imhof SM, Bouter LM, Tan KEWP: Second primary tumors in patients with retinoblastoma. *Ophthalmic Genet* 18:27–34, 1997.

92. Singh AD, Shields CL, Shields JA: New insights into trilateral retinoblastoma. *Cancer* 86:3–5, 1999.

93. Blach LE, McCormick B, Abramson DH, Ellsworth RM: Trilateral retinoblastoma-incidence and outcome: A decade of experience. *Int J Rad Oncol Biol Phys* 29:729–33, 1994.

94. DePotter PV, Shields CL, Shields JA: Clinical variations of trilateral retinoblastoma: A report of 13 cases. *J Pediatr Ophthalmol Strabismus* 31:26–31, 1994.

95. Paulino AC: Trilateral retinoblastoma: Is the location of the intracranial tumor important? *Cancer* 86:135–41, 1999.

96. Becker LE, Hinton D: Primitive neuroectodermal tumors of the central nervous system. *Hum Pathol* 14:538–50, 1983.

97. Marcus DM, Brooks SE, Leff G, et al.: Trilateral retinoblastoma: Insights into histogenesis and management. *Surv Ophthalmol* 43:59–70, 1998.

98. Kivela T: Trilateral retinoblastoma: A meta-analysis of hereditary retinoblastoma associated with primary ectopic intracranial retinoblastoma. *J Clin Oncol* 17:1829–37, 1999.

99. Shields CL, Shields JA, Meadows AT: Chemoreduction for retinoblastoma may prevent trilateral retinoblastoma (Letter) *J Clin Oncol* 18:236–7, 2000.

100. Tosi P, Cintorino M, Toti P, et al.: Histopathological evaluation for the prognosis of retinoblastoma. *Ophthal Genet* 10:173–7, 1989.

101. Khelfaoui F, Validire P, Auperin A, et al.: Histopathologic risk factors in retinoblastoma: A retrospective study of 172 patients treated in a single institution. *Cancer* 77:1206–13, 1996.

102. Magramm I, Abramson DH, Ellsworth RM: Optic nerve involvement in retinoblastoma. *Ophthalmology* 96:217–22, 1989.

103. Shields CL, Shields JA, Baez KA, et al.: Choroidal invasion of retinoblastoma: Metastatic potential and clinical risk factors. *Br J Ophthalmol* 77:544–8, 1993.

104. Palazzi M, Abramson DH, Ellsworth RM: Endophytic vs. exophytic unilateral retinoblastoma: Is there any real difference? *J Pediatr Ophthalmol Strabismus* 27:255–8, 1990.

105. Ellsworth RM: Retinoblastoma: An overview, in Blodi FC (ed.): *Contemporary issues in ophthalmology: Retinoblastoma.* New York, NY, Churchill Livingston, 1985, pp. 1–10.

106. Wolter JR: Retinoblastoma extension into the choroid. Pathological study of the neoplastic process and thoughts about its prognostic significance. *Ophthal Genet* 8:151–7, 1987.

107. Stannard C, Lipper S, Sealy R, Sevel D: Retinoblastoma: Correlation of invasion of the optic nerve and choroid with prognosis and metastasis. *Br J Ophthalmol* 63:560–70, 1979.

108. Rootman J, Hofbauer J, Ellsworth RM, Kitchen D: Invasion of the optic nerve by retinoblastoma: A clinicopathological study. *Can J Ophthalmol* 11:106–14, 1976.

109. Shields CL, Shields JA, Baez K, et al.: Optic nerve invasion of retinoblastoma. Metastatic potential and clinical risk factors. *Cancer* 73:692–8, 1994.

110. Chantada GL, de Davila MT, Fandino A, et al.: Retinoblastoma with low risk for extraocular relapse. *Ophthal Genet* 20:133–40, 1999.

111. Shields JA, Shields CL, De Potter PV: Enucleation technique for children with retinoblastoma. *J Pediatr Ophthalmol Strabismus* 29:213–5, 1992.

112. White L: The role of chemotherapy in the treatment of retinoblastoma. *Retina* 3:194–9, 1983.

113. Honavar SG, Singh AD, Shields CL, et al.: Does post-enucleation prophylactic chemotherapy in high-risk retinoblastoma prevent metastasis? In press.

HEMATOLOGIC MALIGNANCIES

CHAPTER 42

Hodgkin's Disease

LENA SPECHT

The Ann Arbor staging classification[1] remains the basis for the evaluation of patients with Hodgkin's disease.[2] The Ann Arbor classification has been adopted by the American Joint Committee on Cancer (AJCC) and International Union Against Cancer (UICC) as the recommended staging classification for Hodgkin's disease (see Appendix 42A) It is evident, though, that this staging cannot be relied on as the only prognostic tool in Hodgkin's disease. A modification of the Ann Arbor system was proposed at the Cotswold meeting to incorporate a designation for number of sites and bulk.[3] These recommendations have not been universally adopted, however, and a multitude of other factors and combinations of factors are currently being employed worldwide. The anatomic extent of disease is the most important prognostic factor in Hodgkin's disease and forms the baseline for decision making regarding treatment. Because of this, the prognostic factors will be considered in the context of stage.

STAGE I AND II HODGKIN'S DISEASE

Clinical assessment of the anatomic extent of disease underestimates the degree of abdominal involvement, especially spleen involvement, which occurs in approximately 30% of patients with supradiaphragmatic clinical stage (CS) I–II Hodgkin's disease. Staging laparotomy with splenectomy was previously performed in many patients in CS I–II, yielding a more precise delineation of the extent of disease than clinical staging alone. However, because no survival benefit has been found in patients staged with laparotomy and treatment strategies have evolved to include chemotherapy for patients at high risk of relapse, the procedure has been largely abandoned.[4,5] Patients with early-stage Hodgkin's disease are routinely treated either with radiotherapy alone or combined modality treatment. A meta-analysis of all randomized trials comparing these two treatment

Prognostic Factors in Cancer, 2nd edition, Edited by Mary K. Gospodarowicz
ISBN 0-471-40633-3   Copyright © 2001 Wiley-Liss, Inc.

approaches showed that the addition of chemotherapy to radiotherapy prevents recurrence but does not improve the overall survival.[6] The size of the reduction in risk of failure with combined modality therapy in different prognostic subgroups was remarkably similar. Thus, there is no indication that the prognostic factors for patients who receive combined modality therapy are different from the factors for patients treated with radiotherapy alone when the overall survival is concerned.[7] Because fewer recurrences are seen with combined modality therapy, however, a larger number of patients need to be analyzed for a factor to show statistical significance for recurrence-free survival.

Tumor-related Factors

Anatomic Extent of Disease   The anatomic extent and volume of disease may vary considerably within early-stage disease. The number of involved regions has been shown to be prognostically important in many studies.[8–10] The volume of disease in individual regions, particularly in the mediastinum, has also been proven prognostically important.[8,11,12] An estimate of the total tumor burden, combining the number of involved regions with the tumor size in each region, has been shown to be the most important prognostic factor in early-stage disease.[13] Most centers will make decisions regarding intensity of treatment for early-stage disease based on some form of estimate of the extent of disease, often a combination of the number of involved regions and the presence of bulky disease (e.g., >10 cm in largest diameter or mediastinal mass >1/3 of chest diameter). There seems to be no evidence that particular localization (including localized extralymphatic) of disease affects prognosis when bulk of disease is taken into account.[7]

Systemic Symptoms   Systemic B symptoms (weight loss, unexplained fever, night sweats) have consistently been shown to influence prognosis in early-stage disease.[9,10] The presence of B symptoms is correlated with the amount of tumor, probably because the B symptoms are caused by aberrant production of endogenous cytokines, either by tumor cells or by reactive bystander cells.[14] The presence of B symptoms is thus a surrogate measure of the tumor burden and possibly the proliferative potential of the tumor.

Histologic Features   The prognostic importance of the Rye histopathologic classification of Hodgkin's disease[15] has decreased with the introduction of effective treatment. The overwhelming majority of early-stage patients have either the nodular-sclerosis (NS) or mixed-cellularity (MC) subtype, while histologic subtype usually does not provide prognostic information. In many series, NS constitutes up to 75% of all cases.[16] Attempts have been made to subdivide the NS type according to the cellular composition of the nodules of tumor tissue.[17] However, results have not been unequivocal and the issue is still unsettled.[7] The presence of mixed-cellularity Hodgkin's disease is associated with a higher risk of failure in patients treated with radiotherapy alone.[18] The International Lymphoma Study Group has proposed slight modifications of the Rye classification, the most important one being the recognition of lymphocyte predominance (LP) as a distinct entity.[19] LP early-stage disease has an excellent prognosis, and many centers will limit treatment for this type, often to involved field radiotherapy alone.[20] The lymphocyte depletion (LD) subtype is very rarely seen today in early-stage disease.

Biologic Parameters Several biologic parameters (hematologic, biochemical, or immunologic) have been shown to be prognostically significant. They provide an indirect indication of disease extent, and when staging is less accurate (e.g., without laparotomy) some biologic parameters offer independent prognostic information. This is particularly true of the erythrocyte sedimentation rate (ESR).[9,10,18,21] Anemia and a decreased serum albumin have also been shown prognostically significant.[10] A host of other biologic indicators have been shown to be correlated with disease activity, but their independent prognostic significance in early-stage disease has not been proved.

Host-related Factors

Age Older age has frequently been associated with a poorer prognosis in Hodgkin's disease, especially an increased risk of failure when treated with RT alone.[9,18] With adequate staging and treatment, however, older patients with early stage disease seem to have the same potential for cure as younger patients.[11,22] Nevertheless, underlying medical problems may preclude adequate staging and treatment in some older patients. Older age is also associated with a higher risk of occult abdominal disease.[23] Consequently, older age does adversely influence both disease-free survival and in particular overall survival, since relapse treatment seems to be less effective in older patients.

Gender and Race Male patients are more likely to have adverse prognostic factors.[16] Even when other prognostic factors are taken into account, males have a somewhat poorer prognosis.[9,10,21] Data on the prognostic influence of race are very sparse. When other prognostic factors are taken into account, prognosis seems the same irrespective of race.

Immune Status Patients with immune deficiencies, most commonly HIV-positive patients, usually present with advanced disease. Prognosis is distinctly poorer for these patients, more so the lower the CD4+ count.[24]

Environment-related Factors

Intensive, often complicated, and technically demanding treatment is a prerequisite for cure in Hodgkin's disease. Therefore, access to state-of-the-art treatment is important for prognosis.[25] Not surprisingly, a low socioeconomic status is associated with a poor prognosis, especially in Third World countries.[26,27]

STAGE III AND IV HODGKIN'S DISEASE

The distinction between early and advanced disease is not consistently applied. Most centers will include all stage III and IV patients in the advanced-disease category, and many will include stage IIB patients. Patients with advanced disease are treated with chemotherapy. Whether the addition of radiotherapy confers any advantage is at present unresolved.[28]

Tumor-related Factors

Extent of Disease   The anatomic extent and volume of disease are much more difficult to quantify in advanced disease than in early-stage disease. However, the number of involved areas,[29] the extent of infradiaphragmatic nodal disease,[30-32] the amount of tumor in the spleen,[30,31] and a very large mediastinal mass[32,33] have all been shown to be prognostically important. The presence of disseminated extranodal disease confers a poorer prognosis,[10] but it remains controversial whether any particular extranodal site carries a particularly bad prognosis within stage IV.[7] However, the number of involved extranodal sites have been shown to be independently prognostic.[34] These findings indicate that the total tumor burden also is important for prognosis in advanced disease.[13]

Systemic Symptoms   As in early-stage disease systemic B symptoms have been shown to influence prognosis and to be correlated with the amount of tumor and with biologic parameters that mirror both tumor burden and possibly the proliferative potential of the tumor (vide infra).[10]

Histologic Features   Histologic subtype plays a minor role as a prognostic factor in advanced Hodgkin's disease. Some studies show that MC or LD subtypes have a poorer prognosis,[10] but several others do not.[7,29,35] As in early stage disease, the LD subtype is rarely diagnosed today.[10]

Biologic Parameters   Several hematologic and biochemical parameters carry prognostic information in advanced disease. These include an elevated ESR, a decreased hemoglobin level, a decreased serum albumin, an elevated alkaline phosphatase, leukocytosis, and lymphocytopenia.[7,10,33,35] Different combinations of biologic parameters and other tumor-related and patient-related factors have been proposed as prognostic indices for advanced Hodgkin's disease.[32,33,36] None of these indices have gained general acceptance. The International Prognostic Factors Project on advanced Hodgkin's disease[35] has developed a prognostic score incorporating seven prognostic factors of approximately similar prognostic impact (see Appendix 42B.3). This International Prognostic Score is gaining international acceptance for reporting and comparing different data sets. It is, however, not capable of selecting out at diagnosis a sizable group of patients with a very poor prognosis for trials of high-dose therapy up front.

More specific immunologic indicators may possibly in the future provide better prognostic factors for patients with advanced Hodgkin's disease.[7] The neoplastic cells in Hodgkin's disease produce and express a number of cytokines and antigens. Increased levels of some cytokines and soluble forms of membrane-derived antigens can be detected in the serum of the majority of patients with untreated Hodgkin's disease. They are thought to correlate both with the number of tumor cells and with their proliferative activity. Of particular interest is the soluble form of the CD30 molecule.[37]

Host-related Factors

Age   Older age is a well-recognized adverse prognostic factor in advanced disease. This fact can be partly ascribed to greater natural mortality, more toxicity from treatment, and reduced disease control because of reduced, age-adapted treatment in older patients. Nevertheless, older age is also an independent adverse prognostic factor in age groups that may be assumed to have received standard treatment.[35] This may be related to adverse tumor biology in older patients, as unfavorable histologic subtypes have been shown to be more frequent with increasing age.[10]

Gender and Race   As in the case of early-stage disease, male patients have a somewhat poorer prognosis even when other prognostic factors are taken into account.[10,35,36] Data on the influence of race are very sparse, but the prognosis seems to be the same irrespective of race if socioeconomic factors are taken into account.[38]

Immune Status   Patients with immune deficiencies, most commonly HIV-positive patients, usually have widely disseminated disease at diagnosis. Their prognosis is much worse than that of immune-competent patients with advanced disease. A low number of CD4+ cells and prior AIDS diagnosis, reflecting the degree of immunosuppression, are associated with a particularly poor survival.[24]

Environment-related Factors

As in the case of early-stage disease, intensive and technically demanding treatment is a prerequisite for cure of advanced disease. Access to state-of-the-art treatment is important for prognosis and, hence, a low socioeconomic status is associated with a poor prognosis.

PROGNOSIS AFTER RELAPSE

Prognostic factors are considered at diagnosis to assist in decision making regarding management. However, prognostic factors may be defined for any scenario, such as relapse. Patients relapsing after initial treatment of Hodgkin's disease still have a reasonable chance of cure. In this scenario, a somewhat different set of prognostic factors comes into play. Relapses after initial treatment with radiotherapy alone are qualitatively different from relapses after initial chemotherapy with or without additional radiotherapy. Prognosis is considerably better for patients relapsing after radiotherapy alone.

RELAPSE AFTER INITIAL TREATMENT WITH RADIOTHERAPY ALONE

About 30% of early-stage patients treated with radiotherapy alone will relapse, but most of these can be successfully salvaged and durable remissions are obtained in about 60% of cases.

Tumor-related Factors

Extent of Disease   The extent of disease at relapse has consistently been shown to be important for prognosis. In studies where patients have been systematically restaged at relapse, the relapse stage was independently significant for prognosis.[39] Relapse site (nodal only vs. extranodal with or without nodal relapse) is correlated with relapse stage, and studies without systematic restaging at relapse show an adverse prognostic influence of extranodal relapse.[40]

Histologic Features   In contrast to the findings at initial treatment, the histologic subtype has been shown prognostically important after relapse.[39,40]

Host-related Factors

Age   Age consistently has been shown to be very important, the efficacy of salvage chemotherapy being much lower in older patients.[39,40]

RELAPSE AFTER INITIAL TREATMENT WITH CHEMOTHERAPY

Patients relapsing after initial treatment with chemotherapy or combined modality therapy, whether for early-stage or advanced disease, have a much poorer prognosis than patients relapsing after radiotherapy alone. With conventional second-line chemotherapy, durable remissions are achieved in only 10–30%. However, a subgroup of patients relapsing after chemotherapy have anatomically limited relapse in nodal sites alone, and for selected patients in this category, wide-field radiotherapy with or without additional chemotherapy offers a chance of durable disease control. Prognostic factor analyses indicate that patients suitable for this kind of relapse treatment are patients relapsing exclusively in supradiaphragmatic nodal sites, with no B symptoms, with favorable histology (LP or NS), and after a disease-free interval of more than a year.[41] For most patients, however, chemotherapy remains the only possible relapse treatment.

Tumor-related Factors

Extent and Durability of the First Remission   The most important prognostic factor for outcome after relapse in these patients is the extent and durability of the initial remission. Patients relapsing from complete remission lasting more than 1 year have a better prognosis than patients relapsing after a short first remission, and patients who do not even achieve a complete remission during primary treatment have the worst prognosis of all.[42]

Extent of Disease and Systemic Symptoms   The extent of disease at relapse is important here, too. Patients with advanced stage, extranodal disease, or more than three involved sites at relapse have a significantly poorer prognosis.[43] The presence of systemic B symptoms at relapse has also proved significant for prognosis.[43]

Histologic Features   Histologic subtype other than NS has been shown to be associated with a poorer prognosis after relapse.[43]

Host-related Factors

Age and Performance Status   Older age is associated with a poorer prognosis after relapse.[42] As opposed to the situation at primary treatment and relapse after radiotherapy alone, where patients rarely have a poor performance status except in relation to advanced age, in patients relapsing after initial chemotherapy a poor performance status has been shown to be prognostically important.[44]

PROGNOSTIC FACTORS FOR PATIENTS UNDERGOING HIGH-DOSE CHEMOTHERAPY AND STEM-CELL TRANSPLANTATION FOR RELAPSED OR REFRACTORY DISEASE

High-dose chemotherapy with stem-cell transplantation seems to improve the prognosis for patients failing after chemotherapy or combined modality therapy, although randomized evidence in support of this is at present sparse. Prognostic factors for outcome in this scenario have been analyzed in a number of series.

Tumor-related Factors

Chemosensitivity of the Disease   This factor is critical for outcome. Response to initial therapy, duration of initial remission, number of prior failed chemotherapy regimens, and response to conventional salvage therapy before transplant have all been shown to influence prognosis.[45,46]

Extent of Disease and Systemic Symptoms   The extent of disease before transplantation is also important for prognosis. Stage of disease, bulky disease, extranodal disease, and pleural involvement or multiple pulmonary nodules at transplantation have all been shown significant for prognosis, reflecting the tumor burden at the time of transplantation.[46,47] Systemic B symptoms at relapse have proved significant for prognosis after transplantation, indirectly reflecting the tumor burden at the time of transplantation.[48]

Biologic Parameters An elevated serum lactic dehydrogenase level has been shown to influence prognosis, possibly also indirectly reflecting the tumor burden at transplantation.[49]

Host-related Factors

As would be expected with this highly intensive treatment, a poor performance status is an important adverse prognostic factor.[46,49] Older patients have rarely undergone this treatment, and hence the prognostic significance of older age has not been examined. Pediatric patients have the same outcome as adults.[50]

Environment-related Factors

With complicated and intensive treatment like this, access to state-of-the-art treatment and, hence, socioeconomic status are extremely important for prognosis.

SUMMARY

Hodgkin's disease is a highly curable malignancy. Because of the success of treatment, prognostic factors are used to distinguishing between "good risk" patients, in whom treatment can be minimized, and "high risk" patients, who require treatment that is more aggressive. Currently prognostic factors in Hodgkin's disease are used to define the treatment options and to predict the success of therapeutic interventions not only in terms of survival but also in terms of recurrence.

████████ **APPENDIX 42A**

Ann Arbor Staging Classification Adopted by the UICC and AJCC

Clinical Stages

Stage I   Involvement of a single lymph node region (I), or localized involvement of a single extralymphatic organ or site (I_E)

Stage II   Involvement of two or more lymph-node regions on the same side of the diaphragm (II), or localized involvement of a single extralymphatic organ or site and its regional lymph node(s) with or without involvement of other lymph-node regions on the same side of the diaphragm (II_E)

[*Note*: The number of lymph-node regions involved may be indicated by a subscript (e.g., II_3)].

Stage III Involvement of lymph-node regions on both sides of the diaphragm (III), which may also be accompanied by localized involvement of an associated extralymphatic organ or site (III_E), or by involvement of the spleen (III_S), or both (III_{E+S})

Stage IV Disseminated (multifocal) involvement of one or more extralymphatic organs, with or without associated lymph-node involvement; or isolated extralymphatic organ involvement with distant (nonregional) nodal involvement

(*Note*: The site of Stage IV disease is identified further by specifying sites according to the following notation:

Pulmonary	PUL or L	Bone marrow	MAR or M
Osseous	OSS or O	Pleura	PLE or P
Hepatic	HEP or H	Peritoneum	PER
Brain	BRA	Adrenals	ADR
Skin	SKI or D	Others	OTH)

A and B Classification (Symptoms)

Each stage should be divided into A and B according to the absence or presence of defined general symptoms. These are:

1. Unexplained weight loss of more than 10% of the usual body weight in the 6 months prior to first attendance
2. Unexplained fever with temperature above 38°C
3. Night sweats

(*Note*: Pruritus alone does not qualify for B classification nor does a short, febrile illness associated with a known infection.)

Pathological Staging

The definitions of the four stages follow the same criteria as the clinical stages but with the additional information obtained following laparotomy. Splenectomy, liver biopsy, lymph-node biopsy, and marrow biopsy are mandatory for the establishment of pathological stages. The results of these biopsies are recorded as indicated earlier.

Source: Sobin LH, Wittekind Ch (eds.): *TNM classification of malignant tumors*, 5th ed. New York, Union Internationale Contre le Cancer Wiley-Liss, 1997.

━━━━ **APPENDIX 42B.1**

Prognostic Factors in Early-stage Disease

Prognostic Factors	Tumor Related	Host Related	Environment Related
Essential	Anatomic extent of disease, that is, number of involved regions, tumor bulk, tumor burden B symptoms Histologic type	Age Immune status	Access to state-of-the-art treatment Socioeconomic status
Additional	ESR, Hemoglobin, Serum albumin	Gender	

━━━━ **APPENDIX 42B.2**

Prognostic Factors in Advanced Disease

Prognostic Factors	Tumor Related	Host Related	Environment Related
Essential	Anatomic extent of disease B symptoms	Age Immune status	Access to state-of-the art treatment Socioeconomic status
Additional	Histologic features ESR, hemoglobin, serum albumin, serum alkaline phosphatase, leukocyte count, lymphocyte count	Gender	
New and promising	Serum cytokines and membrane-derived antigens (e.g., soluble CD30)		

■■■■■■ **APPENDIX 42B.3**

Adverse Prognostic Factors in the International Prognostic Factors Project Score for Advanced Hodgkin's Disease[35]

Age ≥45 years
Male gender
Stage IV disease
Hemoglobin <10.5 g/dL
Serum albumin <4.0 g/dL
Leukocytosis ≥15 × 10^9/L
Lymphocytopenia <0.6 × 10^9/L or <8% of white blood cell count

■■■■■■ **APPENDIX 42B.4**

Prognostic Factors after Relapse

Relapse after Initial Treatment with	Tumor Related	Host Related
Radiotherapy alone	Extent of disease at relapse (relapse stage, extranodal relapse) Histologic subtype	Age
Chemotherapy or combined modality therapy	Extent and duration of first remission Extent of disease at relapse (relapse stage, extranodal relapse, number of involved sites at relapse) B symptoms at relapse Histologic subtype	Age Performance status

■■■■■■ **APPENDIX 42B.5**

Prognostic Factors for Outcome after High-dose Chemotherapy and Stem-cell Transplantation

Prognostic Factors	Tumor Related	Host Related
Essential	Chemosensitivity of the disease (response to initial therapy, duration of initial remission, number of prior failed regimens, response to conventional salvage therapy)	Performance status
	Extent of disease before transplantation (stage, bulky disease, extranodal disease, pleural involvement or multiple pulmonary nodules) B symptoms	
Additional	Biologic parameters (elevated serum lactic dehydrogenase)	

REFERENCES

1. Carbone PP, Kaplan HS, Musshoff K, et al.: Report of the Committee on Hodgkin's Disease Staging Classification. *Cancer Res* 31:1860–1, 1971.

2. Sobin LH, Wittekind C (eds.): *TNM classification of malignant tumours*, 5th ed. New York, International Union Against Cancer Wiley-Liss, 1997.

3. Lister TA, Crowther D, Sutcliffe SB, et al.: Report of a committee convened to discuss the evaluation and staging of patients with Hodgkin's disease: Cotswolds meeting. *J Clin Oncol* 7:1630–6, 1989.

4. Bergsagel DE, Alison RE, Bean HA, et al.: Results of treating Hodgkin's disease without a policy of laparotomy staging. *Cancer Treat Rep* 66:717–31, 1982.

5. Carde P, Hagenbeek A, Hayat M, et al.: Clinical staging versus laparotomy and combined modality with MOPP versus ABVD in early-stage Hodgkin's disease: The H6 twin randomised trials from the European Organization for Research and Treatment of Cancer Lymphoma Cooperative Group. *J Clin Oncol* 11:2258–72, 1993.

6. Specht L, Gray RG, Clarke MJ, Peto R, for The International Hodgkin's Disease Collaborative Group: Influence of more extensive radiotherapy and adjuvant chemotherapy on long-term outcome of early-stage Hodgkin's disease: A meta-analysis of 23 randomized trials involving 3,888 patients. *J Clin Oncol* 16:830–43, 1998.

7. Specht L, Hasenclever D: Prognostic factors of Hodgkin's disease, in Mauch P, Armitage J, Diehl V, et al.: (eds.): *Hodgkin's disease*. Philadelphia, Lippincott Williams & Wilkins, 1999, pp. 295–325.

8. Mendenhall NP, Cantor AB, Barré DM, et al.: The role of prognostic factors in treatment selection for early-stage Hodgkin's disease. *Am J Clin Oncol (CCT)* 17:189–95, 1994.

9. Tubiana M, Henry-Amar M, Carde P, et al.: Toward comprehensive management tailored to prognostic factors of patients with clinical stages I and II in Hodgkin's disease. The EORTC Lymphoma Group controlled clinical trials: 1964–1987. *Blood* 73:47–56, 1989.

10. Henry-Amar M, Aeppli DM, Anderson J, et al.: Workshop statistical report, in Somers R, Henry-Amar M, Meerwaldt JK, Carde P (eds.): *Treatment strategy in Hodgkin's Disease. Colloque INSERM No. 196.* London, INSERM/John Libbey Eurotext, 1990, pp. 169–422.

11. Mauch P, Tarbell N, Weinstein H, et al.: Stage IA and IIA supradiaphragmatic Hodgkin's disease: Prognostic factors in surgically staged patients treated with mantle and paraaortic irradiation. *J Clin Oncol* 6:1576–83, 1988.

12. Longo DL, Glatstein E, Duffey PL, et al.: Alternating MOPP and ABVD chemotherapy plus mantle-field radiation therapy in patients with massive mediastinal Hodgkin's disease. *J Clin Oncol* 15:3338–46, 1997.

13. Specht L: Tumor burden as the main indicator of prognosis in Hodgkin's disease. *Eur J Cancer* 28A:1982–5, 1992.

14. Gorschlüter M, Bohlen H, Hasenclever D, et al.: Serum cytokine levels correlate with clinical parameters in Hodgkin's disease. *Ann Oncol* 6:477–82, 1995.

15. Lukes RJ, Craver LF, Hall TC, et al.: Report of the nomenclature committee. *Cancer Res* 26:1311, 1966.

16. Kaplan HS: *Hodgkin's disease*, 2nd ed. Cambridge, Mass, Harvard University Press, 1980.

17. MacLennan KA, Bennett MH, Tu A, et al.: Relationship of histopathologic features to survival and relapse in nodular sclerosing Hodgkin's disease. *Cancer* 64:1686–93, 1989.

18. Gospodarowicz MK, Sutcliffe SB, Clark RM, et al.: Analysis of supradiaphragmatic clinical stage I and II Hodgkin's disease treated with radiation alone. *Int J Radiat Oncol Biol Phys* 22:859–65, 1992.

19. Harris NL, Jaffe ES, Stein H, et al.: A revised European-American classification of lymphoid neoplasms: A proposal from the International Lymphoma Study Group. *Blood* 84:1361–92, 1994.

20. Diehl V, Sextro M, Franklin J, et al.: Clinical presentation, course, and prognostic factors in lymphocyte-predominant Hodgkin's disease: Report form the European Task Force on Lymphoma Project on Lymphocyte-predominant Hodgkin's Disease. *J Clin Oncol* 17:776–83, 1999.

21. Haybittle JL, Hayhoe FGJ, Easterling MJ, et al.: Review of British National Lymphoma Investigation studies of Hodgkin's disease and development of prognostic index. *Lancet* i:967–72, 1985.

22. Austin-Seymour MM, Hoppe RT, Cox RS, et al.: Hodgkin's disease in patients over sixty years old. *Ann Intern Med* 100:13–8, 1984.

23. Leibenhaut MH, Hoppe RT, Efron B, et al.: Prognostic indicators of laparotomy findings in clinical stage I-II supradiaphragmatic Hodgkin's disease. *J Clin Oncol* 7:81–91, 1989.

24. Tirelli U, Carbone A, Straus DJ: HIV-related Hodgkin's disease, in Mauch P, Armitage J, Diehl V, et al.: (eds.): *Hodgkin's disease*. Philadelphia, Lippincott Williams & Wilkins, 1999, pp. 701–11.

25. Smitt MC, Stouffer N, Owen JB, et al.: Results of the 1988–1989 Patterns of Care Study process survey for Hodgkin's disease. *Int J Radiat Oncol Biol Phys* 43:335–9, 1999.

26. Levy LM: Hodgkin's disease in black Zimbabweans. A study of epidemiologic, histologic, and clinical features. *Cancer* 61:189–94, 1988.

27. Glaser SL: Hodgkin's disease in black populations: A review of the epidemiologic literature. *Semin Oncol* 17:643–59, 1990.

28. Loeffler M, Brosteanu O, Hasenclever D, et al.: Meta-analysis of chemotherapy versus combined modality treatment trials in Hodgkin's disease. *J Clin Oncol* 16:818–29, 1998.

29. Somers R, Carde P, Henry-Amar M, et al.: A randomized study in Stage IIIB and IV Hodgkin's disease comparing eight courses of MOPP versus an alternation of MOPP with ABVD: A European Organization for Research and Treatment of Cancer Lymphoma Cooperative Group and Group Pierre-et-Marie-Curie controlled clinical trial. *J Clin Oncol* 12:279–87, 1994.

30. Mauch P, Goffman T, Rosenthal DS, et al.: Stage III Hodgkin's disease: Improved survival with combined modality therapy as compared with radiation therapy alone. *J Clin Oncol* 3:1166–73, 1985.

31. Hoppe RT, Cox RS, Rosenberg SA, Kaplan HS: Prognostic factors in pathologic stage III Hodgkin's disease. *Cancer Treat Rep* 66:743–9, 1982.

32. Straus DJ, Gaynor JJ, Myers J, et al.: Prognostic factors among 185 adults with newly diagnosed advanced Hodgkin's disease treated with alternating potentially noncross-resistant chemotherapy and intermediate-dose radiation therapy. *J Clin Oncol* 8:1173–86, 1990.

33. Proctor SJ, Taylor P, Mackie MJ, et al.: A numerical prognostic index for clinical use in identification of poor-risk patients with Hodgkin's disease at diagnosis. The Scotland and Newcastle Lymphoma Group (SNLG) Therapy Working Party. *Leuk Lymphoma* 7(Suppl. 7):17–20, 1992.

34. Fermé C, Bastion Y, Brice P, et al.: Prognosis of patients with advanced Hodgkin's disease: Evaluation of four prognostic models using 344 patients included in the Group d'Etudes des Lymphomes de l'Adulte Study. *Cancer* 80:1124–33, 1997.

35. Hasenclever D, Diehl V: A prognostic score for advanced Hodgkin's disease. International Prognostic Factors Project on advanced Hodgkin's disease. *N Engl J Med* 339:1506–14, 1998.

36. Gobbi PG, Cavalli C, Federico M, et al.: Hodgkin's disease prognosis: A directly predictive equation. *Lancet* i:675–9, 1988.

37. Gause A, Jung W, Keymis S, et al.: The clinical significance of cytokines and soluble forms of membrane-derived activation antigens in the serum of patients with Hodgkin's disease. *Leuk Lymphoma* 7:439–47, 1992.

38. Routh A, Hickman BT: Comparison of survival of black and white patients in each stage of Hodgkin's disease during 1970–1980. *Radiat Med* 7:28–31, 1989.

39. Roach M, Brophy N, Cox R, et al.: Prognostic factors for patients relapsing after radiotherapy for early-stage Hodgkin's disease. *J Clin Oncol* 8:623–9, 1990.

40. Horwich A, Specht L, Ashley S: Survival analysis of patients with clinical stages I or II Hodgkin's disease who have relapsed after initial treatment with radiotherapy alone. *Eur J Cancer* 33:848–53, 1997.

41. Wirth A, Corry J, Laidlaw C, et al.: Salvage radiotherapy for Hodgkin's disease following chemotherapy failure. *Int J Radiat Oncol Biol Phys* 39:599–607, 1997.

42. Longo DL, Duffey PL, Young RC, et al.: Conventional-dose salvage combination chemotherapy in patients relapsing with Hodgkin's disease after combination chemotherapy: The low probability for cure. *J Clin Oncol* 10:210–8, 1992.

43. Viviani S, Santoro A, Negretti E, et al.: Salvage chemotherapy in Hodgkin's disease. Results in patients relapsing more than twelve months after first complete remission. *Ann Oncol* 1:123–7, 1990.

44. Fermé C, Bastion Y, Lepage E, et al.: The MINE regimen as intensive salvage chemotherapy for relapsed and refractory Hodgkin's disease. *Ann Oncol* 6:543–9, 1995.

45. Bierman PJ, Anderson JR, Freeman MB, et al.: High-dose chemotherapy followed by autologous hematopoietic rescue for Hodgkin's disease patients following first relapse after chemotherapy. *Ann Oncol* 7:151–6, 1996.

46. Anderson JE, Litzow MR, Appelbaum FR, et al.: Allogeneic, syngeneic, and autologous marrow transplantation for Hodgkin's disease: The 21-year Seattle experience. *J Clin Oncol* 11:2342–50, 1993.

47. Poen JC, Hoppe RT, Horning SJ: High-dose therapy and autologous bone marrow transplantation for relapsed/refractory Hodgkin's disease: The impact of involved field radiotherapy on patterns of failure and survival. *Int J Radiat Oncol Biol Phys* 36:3–12, 1996.

48. Reece DE, Phillips GL: Intensive therapy and autologous stem cell transplantation for Hodgkin's disease in first relapse after combination chemotherapy. *Leuk Lymphoma* 21:245–53, 1996.

49. Lumley MA, Milligan DW, Knechtli CJ, et al.: High lactate dehydrogenase level is associated with an adverse outlook in autografting for Hodgkin's disease. *Bone Marrow Transplant* 17:383–8, 1996.

50. Williams CD, Goldstone AH, Pearce R, et al.: Autologous bone marrow transplantation for pediatric Hodgkin's disease: A case-matched comparison with adult patients by the European Bone Marrow Transplant Group Lymphoma Registry. *J Clin Oncol* 11:2243–9, 1993.

CHAPTER 43

Non-Hodgkin's Malignant Lymphoma

MICHAEL CRUMP and MARY GOSPODAROWICZ

The non-Hodgkin's lymphomas (NHLs) are a diverse group of diseases with large variation in tumor biology and course of disease. The 1980s and 1990s brought a great increase in our knowledge of the biology of the immune system. Insights into the immunology and molecular genetics of NHL have led to the recognition of a number of new pathological entities, with unique natural histories. In addition, the clinical approach to patients with NHL has relied increasingly on aggregate assessment of prognostic factors, rather than single attributes such as disease stage, presence of extranodal involvement, presence of constitutional symptoms, or specific biochemical abnormalities. Furthermore, it is increasingly recognized that these biological attributes are surrogate measures of a tumor's growth and invasion potential, the host's response to the tumor, and the host's ability to tolerate treatment. A better understanding of the significance of molecular and immunological attributes of lymphoma will hopefully replace these clinical surrogates in refining NHL's prognosis and therapy more precisely in the future.

TUMOR-RELATED PROGNOSTIC FACTORS

Histologic Type

The Revised European American Lymphoma (REAL) classification from the International Lymphoma Study Group was published in 1994, and has gained wide acceptance as the new standard lymphoma classification.[1] This classification emphasized that NHL is not a single disease but a group of diseases, each with distinctive features defined by a combination of morphologic, immunophenotypic, genetic, and clinical attributes. A number of new types of lymphoma were included. Among these were mantle cell lymphoma, marginal zone lymphoma, mucosa-associated lymphoid tissue (MALT) lymphoma, primary mediastinal

Prognostic Factors in Cancer, 2nd edition, Edited by Mary K. Gospodarowicz
ISBN 0-471-40633-3   Copyright © 2001 Wiley-Liss, Inc.

large B-cell lymphoma, and several T-cell lymphomas, including anaplastic large-cell lymphoma and T/NK-cell CD56 positive lymphoma. Clinical evaluation of this classification system was undertaken to determine the diagnostic accuracy of the criteria set forth in the REAL classification, and the degree of reproducibility of the diagnoses.[2] In a cohort of almost 1400 consecutive cases from nine centers in eight countries, the REAL classification was shown to be highly reproducible, particularly when accompanied by immunophenotyping. In that analysis, the histological types of lymphoma, as well as the clinical characteristics defined by the International Prognostic Index (IPI) (see below) predicted for failure-free and overall survival (Table 43.1). The new World Health Organization (WHO) classification is based on the principles of the REAL and includes the entities that were previously designated as provisional.[3] The WHO classification will represent the first true worldwide consensus on the classification of lymphoid neoplasms.[4]

Immunophenotype It is recognized that immunophenotype provides important prognostic information in NHL.[5]Although the majority of lymphomas are of B-cell origin, 15–30% of these tumors have a T-cell phenotype. Gisselbrecht et al.[6] showed that the outcome was significantly worse for patients with peripheral T-cell lymphoma compared to those with B-cell lymphoma treated with the same chemotherapy (the LNH-87 protocol).[7,8] Patients with T-cell lymphoma were more likely to present with Stage IV disease, B symptoms, bone marrow, and skin involvement, as well as elevated β_2 microglobulin, but less likely with bulky disease.[6] Remission rates (54% vs. 63%; $p = 0.004$) and overall survival (41% vs 53% OS at 5 years; $p = 0.0004$) were significantly inferior for patients with T-cell, compared to B-cell, NHL, with the possible exception of anaplastic

TABLE 43.1 Survival by Histologic Type and Number of Risk Factors According to International Prognostic Index

Consensus Diagnosis	% 5-yr OS		% 5-yr FFS	
	Index 0/1	Index 4/5	Index 0/1	Index 4/5
Follicular, all grades	84	17	55	6
Mantle cell	57	0	27	0
Marginal zone B cell, MALT	89	40	83	0
Marginal zone B cell, nodal	76	50	30	0
Small lymphocytic	75	38	35	13
Diffuse large B cell	73	22	63	19
Primary mediastinal large B cell	77	0	69	0
High-grade B cell, Burkitt-like	71	0	71	0
Precursor T lymphoblastic	29	40	29	40
Peripheral T cell, all types	36	15	27	10
Anaplastic large T/null-cell	81	83	49	83

Abbreviations: OS, overall survival; FFS, failure-free survival.

large-cell lymphoma. These observations were confirmed by a single institution series reported by Melnyk[9] and appeared to be true across all IPI categories (see below). Particular entities within the T/NK-cell category deserve mention. A small number of patients present with CD56+ T-cell lymphoma involving the nasopharynx and nasal cavity (referred to as angiocentric lymphoma in the REAL classification).[1] CD56+ lymphomas have also been described in other sites including skin, upper airway, digestive tract, and gastrointestinal tract. These tumors pursue an aggressive clinical course and generally have a poor outcome.[10,11] Both the nasal-type NK/T-cell lymphoma and aggressive NK-cell leukemia lymphoma have a strong association with Epstein-Barr virus (EBV).

In contrast, anaplastic large-cell lymphoma with a T-cell or null-cell phenotype, the second most common T-cell lymphoma in the REAL classification, has the best overall failure-free survival rate of any large-cell lymphoma.[12] Such patients generally present with low IPI scores, a young median age, and male predominance. These lymphomas are CD30+ and express the ALK protein because of a t(2;5)(p23;q35) chromosome translocation.[13]

Anatomic Extent of Disease

The Ann Arbor staging classification, developed for Hodgkin's disease, is the accepted staging classification for non-Hodgkin lymphomas and is included in the American Joint Committee on Cancer (AJCC) and the International Union Against Cancer (UICC) manuals.[14,15] Ann Arbor stage (see Appendix 43A) has been shown to be an independent prognostic factor in numerous studies of non-Hodgkin lymphomas.[16-20] In the Toronto experience with follicular lymphomas, the 10-year cause-specific survivals for patients with stage I, II, III, and IV were 68, 56, 42, and 18% respectively.[21] However, although stage is an important factor, considerable variation of outcomes exists within each stage. Therefore, further specification of tumor extent, such as tumor bulk, number of involved sites, or extranodal involvement, are indispensable in predicting outcome in patients with non-Hodgkin lymphomas.

Tumor bulk or burden has been found to be one of the most important prognostic factors in non-Hodgkin lymphomas, whether localized (stage I and II) or advanced (stage III and IV).[16,20-23] Tumor bulk predicts for relapse and survival in patients with localized disease treated with radiation alone and with combined chemotherapy and radiation. In patients treated with radiation therapy alone, tumor bulk >5 cm or >10 cm has been associated with a lower local control rate, higher risk of distant relapse, and lower survival, independent of other prognostic factors. In patients with stage IA and IIA intermediate and high-grade non-Hodgkin lymphomas treated with radiation alone, 39% of those with tumor bulk <5 cm relapsed, while 62% of those with tumor bulk >5 cm relapsed.[20] The impact of tumor bulk is greater in patients with intermediate and high-grade histology than in those with low-grade non-Hodgkin lymphomas. Other definitions of high tumor burden, which have been associated with poor outcome, include the presence of a large mediastinal mass (>1/3 of chest diameter), the presence of a palpable abdominal mass and a combination of para-aortic and pelvic-node involvement in stage III and IV disease.[16,19–22,24–27]

The number of sites of involvement, expressed either as the number of nodal regions involved in stage I and II disease, or the number of nodal and extranodal sites involved in stage III and IV disease, has been found to be an independent prognostic factor for disease-free and overall survival in patients treated with chemotherapy alone or combined modality therapy.[22,25,26,28] In a multivariate analysis of Vancouver patients with stage IIB-IV diffuse large-cell lymphoma treated with chemotherapy, involvement of >1 extranodal site carried a relative risk of death of 3.3, and involvement of >2 nodal sites, a relative risk of 3.7.[29]

Almost 50% of patients with stage I and II non-Hodgkin lymphomas present with disease in extranodal sites.[22,30,31] Extranodal involvement is also very common in stage III and IV disease. The gastrointestinal (GI) tract, in particular the stomach, is the commonest site of extranodal involvement. The GI tract has been identified as an adverse site of extranodal presentation in multivariate analysis of early-stage patients due to the impact of locally advanced, bulky, and unresectable disease not otherwise encountered in localized non-Hodgkin lymphomas.[16] Patients presenting with involvement of the Waldeyer's ring and those with resectable GI lymphoma have been found in multivariate analysis to have better survival than those presenting in other extranodal sites.[31,32] Sites of extranodal involvement associated with poor outcome include liver, Central nervous system (CNS), and extensive bone marrow involvement.[17,25,27] Primary brain non-Hodgkin's lymphoma is uncommon and is associated with a particularly poor outcome. The pattern of failure is mostly local and the main prognostic factors include degree of neurologic impairment and performance status.[33]

Symptoms

Systemic symptoms, including fever, night sweats, and weight loss (B-symptoms), are usually associated with stage III and IV disease, but their presence still has an independent prognostic effect after correction for Ann Arbor stage.[17,20,21,29,34,35] A large study of elderly patients with non-Hodgkin lymphomas identified B-symptoms as one of the most important prognostic factors.[36] In this study patients with B-symptoms had 2.2 times higher risk of dying than those without B-symptoms. The presence of B-symptoms is generally correlated with advanced stage, bulky disease, and elevated lactate dehydrogenase (LDH) levels, all indicators of high tumor burden.

Hematologic and Biochemical Factors

Elevated serum LDH is one of the more important adverse prognostic factors in patients with non-Hodgkin lymphoma,[37] and is thought to reflect tumor burden. While it correlates with stage and bulk, the serum LDH has been found to be one of the most important independent prognostic factors in both early-stage and stage III and IV lymphomas.[16,18,26–28,37–40] Elevated serum calcium has been found to be an independent prognostic factor in patients with T-cell lymphoma in Japan.[41] Other biochemical factors are important in special situations. For example, the level of the cerebrospinal fluid protein is an independent prognostic factor in patients with primary brain lymphomas.[42]

A high beta-2 microglobulin level was found to be an independent prognostic factor for complete response rate and time to treatment failure in all stages of patients with low-grade non-Hodgkin lymphomas.[43] In the analysis of the high-grade lymphomas (Kiel classification), the level of beta-2 microglobulin was one of the most important prognostic variables for response rate, disease-free, and the overall survival.[44] In this study of patients with high-grade non-Hodgkin lymphomas treated with chemotherapy, the 6-year survival for patients with high beta-2 microglobulin levels was 35%, while it was 70% for those with normal levels.[44] In an analysis of 220 patients with follicular lymphoma followed for a median of 9 years, beta-2-microglobulin at diagnosis was the only factor which predicted for transformation to a more aggressive histology.[45]

Cytogenetic and Molecular Markers

A large number of clonal cytogenetic abnormalities have been identified in patients with NHL, increasing our understanding of the pathogenesis and providing new insights into treatment and prognosis. Earlier reports suggested karyotypic abnormalities in general, and specific chromosomal abnormalities in particular, are associated with an adverse outcome in NHL.[46] Chromosomal translocations, such as the t(8;14) in Burkitt's lymphoma, or the t(14;18) in follicular lymphoma, not only help to define specific pathologic entities, but carry independent prognostic information.[47] The t(14;18) translocation is found in the majority of follicular lymphomas and in up to 30% of B-cell diffuse large cell lymphoma (DLCL).[48,49] Expression of bcl-2 protein in diffuse large cell NHL correlates with inferior disease-free survival and overall survival.[48,49] When both were assessed, there was almost no correlation between bcl-2 gene rearrangement and bcl-2 protein expression, and the prognostic significance of bcl-2 translocation (as distinct from increased bcl-2 protein expression) remains uncertain.

In contrast to diffuse large B-cell lymphoma, the complete response rate of patients with follicular lymphoma with no evidence of rearrangement bcl-2 gene was significantly lower than that in patients whose tumors exhibited rearrangement of the major breakpoint region (MBR) or the minor cluster region (mcr).[50] Patients germline for MBR or mcr tended to present more frequently with Stage IV disease and higher levels of β_2 microglobulin.[51] Patients with an mcr breakpoint may have more favorable failure-free survival compared to those with germline bcl-2 configuration.

Reciprocal rearrangements between the bcl-6 gene on chromosome 3q27 have been reported in 15–35% of B-cell DLCL. This rearrangement was shown by Offit et al.[52] to be associated with an improved prognosis; however, others have subsequently not been able to demonstrate this favorable effect.[53]

Cell-cycle Regulator Proteins Mutation of tumor suppressor gene p53 has been observed in a proportion of patients with aggressive histology NHL and has been associated with a lower complete response rate and shorter survival compared to patients with tumors containing wild-type p53.[54,55] In 102 patients with aggressive histology B-cell NHL, Ichikawa et al. reported that overall survival was significantly lower in patients with tumors that had a p53 mutation compared to those with wild-type p53 (16 vs. 64% at 5 years, $p < 0.001$).[56] p53 mutation was an independent marker in low-risk patients according to IPI criteria, but not in those with high-risk disease where the outcome was poor regardless of p53 status.[56] p53 overexpression is also frequently detected in de novo cases of diffuse large-cell lymphoma without evidence of mutations, suggesting up-regulation of the gene by another mechanism. p53 expression has also been associated with aggressive behavior in mantle-cell lymphoma.[55]

The antibody Ki67 (MIB1) detects a protein expressed during the G_1, S, G_2, and M phases of the cell cycle and is a widely accepted marker of cell proliferation. Increased expression of this protein was found associated with poor survival in small prospective[57] and retrospective[58] studies. The relationship is much less consistent between outcome and the expression of other cell-cycle regulatory proteins, such as MDM2, p21, and the retinoblastoma protein RB.[58] To date, studies on the contribution of expression of cell-cycle regulatory proteins to prognosis in NHL are intriguing, but should be considered preliminary.

Angiogenesis Vascular endothelial growth factor (VEGF) has an important role in the process of tumorigenesis and has been detected in lymphomas. In a retrospective analysis of patients with NHL of diverse histologies, Salven et al.[59] showed that higher than median serum VEGF levels were associated with poor performance status, high IPI, high LDH, and large cell histology. Patients with a lower than median VEGF at diagnosis had a superior survival rate compared to those with higher than median values ($p = 0.04$). In another study, event-free survival was significantly higher in patients with baseline VEGF and basic fibroblast growth factor (βFGF) below the median values.[60] Further prospective validation of these preliminary observations appears warranted.

Adhesion Molecule Expression The CD44 antigen facilitates the binding of lymphocytes to high endothelial venules and permits the extravasation of lymphocytes into nodal areas. A number of studies have shown that high levels of expression of CD44 correlate with advanced-stage disease presentation and shorter survival.[61,62] The expression of intercellular adhesion molecule 1 (ICAM-1) was similarly adversely associated with Stage IV disease, extranodal involvement, and bone marrow infiltration.[63] Patients with lymphoma expressing ICAM-1 had significantly higher overall survival, and in a multivariate analysis, ICAM-1 expression maintained its importance for predicting survival, along with histological type and IPI. Serum levels of soluble ICAM-1 are correlated with other adverse prognostic factors and were associated with worse disease-free and overall survival. Taken together, cell-surface or soluble adhesion molecule expression can carry independent prognostic information in patients with NHL. A variety of histologic subtypes were included in these studies,[63] however, and prospective evaluation of these markers in larger studies within individual disease entities is warranted.

HOST-RELATED PROGNOSTIC FACTORS

Age

Advanced age is an adverse prognostic factor in non-Hodgkin lymphomas regardless of stage and treatment. Patients over the age of 60 tend to have worse prognosis, as measured by overall survival and cause-specific survival. The main effect of age may be a reflection of a decreased tolerance to treatment beyond the age of 60. However, despite equivalent therapy, an increased risk of relapse has been noted in older patients treated with stage I and II disease.[17,18,20–23,26,29,32,64,65] A similar negative effect of age on outcome has been reported for stage III and IV follicular NHL[34,35] and diffuse large cell NHL.[37] In a series of patients with stage I and II intermediate-grade lymphoma treated with radiation alone, the 5-year survival and freedom from relapse were 97% and 58% for patients <60 years old and 51% and 27% for those >60 years old.[22]

Gender

Male gender has been found to correlate with other adverse prognostic factors, such as histology, stage, symptoms, and because of this correlation, in many series it was not considered to have an independent prognostic impact. However, male gender has been demonstrated to be an independently adverse prognostic factor in several reports of patients with low-grade non-Hodgkin lymphoma.[19,35,66]

Performance Status

Poor performance status has been shown to be an independent factor for adverse prognosis in patients with stage III and IV non-Hodgkin lymphomas.[17,19,32,37,38,41] It is, however, usually associated with other adverse factors such as advanced age and the extent of disease. The lack of influence of PS on outcome in large series of patients with advanced-stage follicular NHL may be related to the relatively low percentage of patients who present with poor performance status.[34,35] Performance status was an important prognostic factors in patients with primary brain lymphomas,[42] in aggressive histology in AIDS-related NHL,[67] and NHL in the elderly.[68]

Immunocompromised Host

HIV infection   NHL is the second most common malignancy associated with AIDS, with on incidence of approximately 3% across all HIV risk groups. Most NHL in AIDS patients is of aggressive histology.[69] Extranodal spread of disease is common, especially to CNS, GI tract, liver, and bone marrow. Outcome has been shown to be related to extent of underlying HIV or AIDS and is worse in patients with prior opportunistic infection, CD4 count <100/mL, KPS <70% LDH, and age.[67,70,71] Molecular characteristics (polyclonality, EBV negative),[72] may also influence outcome. The results of treatment and prognostic factors should be reported separately for HIV-related NHL.

Posttransplant Lymphoproliferative Disorder Posttransplant lymphoproliferative disorder (PTLD) is an EBV-associated disease[73], which should be considered distinct from NHL in immunocompetent individuals. Morphologic classification and use of molecular analysis to establish clonality have not been able to reliably predict clinical behavior in PTLD. A recently reported combined classification of PTLD into plasmacytic hyperplasia (polyclonal immunoglobulin (Ig) and EBV), polymorphic PTLD (mono/oligoclonal Ig or EBV), and NHL/multiple myeloma (monoclonal with altered N-ras, p53, or c-myc) may predict response to therapy.[74] Bcl-6 mutations may be more frequent in the latter two categories and were associated with failure of withdrawal of immunosuppression and shorter survival.

Other Host Factors

Recently, it has been shown that individuals with rare alleles of the H-RAS1 proto-oncogene may be more susceptible to developing non-Hodgkin's lymphoma.[75] Furthermore, patients with NHL of any histologic grade who harbored such germline changes were more likely to die of their disease. This is the first demonstration that a change in a patient's genome present before diagnosis can affect prognosis once NHL develops.

Prognostic Factor Models

Age and performance status were known as powerful prognostic factors in lymphoma, regardless of histologic type. In the 1990s, these host prognostic factors were integrated into prognostic factor models, together with anatomic extent of disease.[76] Recognizing the need for an improved ability to determine prognosis within the category of aggressive histology NHL, the IPI was developed.[37] The unfavorable factors included age >60 years, abnormal LDH, more than one site of extranodal disease, stage III or IV, and ECOG performance status ≤2. These factors also predicted for lower complete response rates, and higher relapse rates.[37] The IPI has been validated in other reports.[77,78] It has been shown to predict survival and relapse in patients with follicular lymphoma. The IPI appears to provide independent prognostic information across the majority of disease in REAL classification.

ENVIRONMENT-RELATED FACTORS

There is a paucity of studies dealing with the prognostic factors external to the tumor and patient. However, difficulties with pathologic diagnosis, and well-documented discrepancies in pathologic diagnosis, have potential to have an impact on therapy. Evidence from Mexico shows that malnourished patients treated with chemotherapy has a worse outcome than those with adequate nutrition.[79]

SUMMARY

Numerous prognostic factors have been identified in non-Hodgkin's lymphoma. These include factors related to tumor pathology and biology, anatomic tumor extent; symptoms associated with the disease and the host factors, such as age, performance status, and gender. The profound impact of these factors in outcome led to creation of the International Prognostic Index to help in evaluating treatment results in similar groups of patients. A summary of prognostic factors in current practice is presented in Appendix 43B. The currently used prognostic factors do not fully explain the variations in the outcome in lymphoma, and further search for molecular prognostic factors continues with some success.

■■■■■ **APPENDIX 43A.1**

Ann Arbor Staging Classification Adopted by the UICC and AJCC

Stage I   Involvement of a single lymph-node region (I), or localized involvement of a single extralymphatic organ or site (I_E)

Stage II   Involvement of two or more lymph-node regions on the same side of the diaphragm (II), or localized involvement of a single extralymphatic organ or site and its regional lymph node(s) with or without involvement of other lymph-node regions on the same side of the diaphragm (II_E)

[*Note:* The number of lymph-node regions involved may be indicated by a subscript (e.g. II_3)].

Stage III Involvement of lymph-node regions on both sides of the diaphragm (III), which may also be accompanied by localized involvement of an associated extralymphatic organ or site (III_E), or by involvement of the spleen (III_S), or both (III_{E+S})

Stage IV   Disseminated (multifocal) involvement of one or more extralymphatic organs, with or without associated lymph node involvement; or isolated extralymphatic organ involvement with distant (nonregional) nodal involvement

(*Note:* The site of Stage IV disease is identified further by specifying sites according to the notations listed earlier.)

A and B Classification (Symptoms)

Each stage should be divided into A and B according to the absence or presence of defined general symptoms. These are:

1.   Unexplained weight loss of more than 10% of the usual body weight in the 6 months prior to first attendance
2.   Unexplained fever with temperature above 38°C
3.   Night sweats

(*Note:* Pruritus alone does not qualify for B classification, nor does a short, febrile illness associated with a known infection.)

Pathological Staging

The definitions of the four stages follow the same criteria as the clinical stages, but with the additional information obtained following laparotomy. Splenectomy, liver biopsy, lymph-node biopsy, and marrow biopsy are mandatory for the establishment of pathological stages. The results of these biopsies are recorded as indicated earlier.

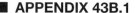 **APPENDIX 43B.1**

Prognostic Factors in non-Hodgkin's Lymphoma

Prognostic Factors	Tumor Related	Host Related	Environment Related
Essential	Histologic type Stage Presenting extranodal site	Age HIV status	
Additional	LDH Molecular/cytogenetics BCL-2 protein	IPI score	Malnutrition
New and Promising	CD44 Angiogenesis Proliferative index p53	H-*ras* mutations	

REFERENCES

1. Harris NL, Jaffe ES, Stein H, et al.: A Revised European-American Classification of Lymphoid Neoplasms: A Proposal From the International Lymphoma Study Group. *Blood* 84:1361–92, 1994.

2. The non-Hodgkin's Lymphoma Classification Project: A Clinical Evaluation of the International Lymphoma Study Group Classification of Non-Hodgkin's Lymphoma. *Blood* 89:3909–18, 1997.

3. Harris NL, Jaffe ES, Diebold J, et al: World Health Organization classification of neoplastic diseases of the hematopoietic and lymphoid tissues: Report of the Clinical Advisory Committee meeting-Airlie House, Virginia, November 1997. *J Clin Oncol* 17:3835–49, 1999.

4. Jaffe ES, Harris NL, Diebold J, Huller-Hermelink H-K: World Health Organization Classification of Neoplastic Diseases of the Hematopoietic and Lymphoid Tissues — A Progress Report. *Am J Clin Path* 111:S8–S12, 1999.

5. Lippman SM, Miller TP, Spier CM, et al.: The prognostic significance of the immunotype in diffuse large-cell lymphoma: A comparative study of the T-cell and B-cell phenotype. *Blood* 72:436–41, 1988.

6. Gisselbrecht C, Gaulard P, Lepage E, et al., for the Group d'Etudes des Lymphomes de l"Adulte (GELA): Prognostic significance of T-cell phenotype in aggressive non-Hodgkin's lymphomas. *Blood* 92:76–82, 1998.

7. Bosly A, Lepage E, Dupriez B, et al.: Alternance of chemotherapy does not improve results in aggressive non-Hodgkin's lymphoma: A prospective randomized study on 884 Patients LNH87 Protocol Group 3 (Abstr.): A GELA study. *Br J Haematol* 83:546, 1996.

8. Bastion Y, Blay JY, Divine M, et al.: Elderly patients with aggressive lymphoma survive longer if treated with a curative intent. A GELA study on 453 patients older than 69 years. *J Clin Oncol* 15:2945–53, 1997.

9. Melnyk A, Rodriguez A, Pugh W, Cabanillas F: Evaluation of the Revised European-American Lymphoma classification confirms the clinical relevance of immunophenotype in 560 cases of aggressive non-Hodgkin's lymphoma. *Blood* 89:4514–20, 1997.

10. Cheung MM, Chan JK, Lau WH, et al.: Primary non-Hodgkin's lymphoma of the nose and nasopharynx: Clinical features, tumor immunophenotype, and treatment outcome in 113 patients. *J Clin Oncol* 16:70–7, 1998.

11. Chan JK, Sin VC, Wong KF, et al.: Nonnasal lymphoma expressing the natural killer cell marker CD56: A clinicopathologic study of 49 cases of an uncommon aggressive neoplasm. *Blood* 89:4501–13, 1997.

12. Armitage JO, Weisenburger DD, for the non-Hodgkin's Lymphoma Classification Project. New approach to classifying non-Hodgkin's lymphomas: Clinical features of the major histologic subtypes. *J Clin Oncol* 16(8):2780–95, 1998.

13. Kinney MC, Kadin ME: The pathologic and clinical spectrum of anaplastic large cell lymphoma and correlation with ALK gene dysregulation. *Am J Clin Path* 111:S56–67, 1999.

14. Beahrs OH, Henson DE, Hutter RV, et al. (eds.): *American Joint Committee on Cancer. Manual for staging of cancer*, 4th ed. Philadelphia, Lippincott, 1992.

15. Hermanek P, Sobin L (eds.): *International Union Against Cancer. TNM classification of malignant tumors*, 4th ed., 2d rev. Germany, Springer-Verlag, 1992.

16. Mackintosh JF, Cowan RA, Jones M, et al.: Prognostic factors in Stage I and II high and intermediate grade non-Hodgkin's lymphoma. *Eur J Cancer Clin Oncol* 24(10):1617–22, 1988.

17. Hayward RL, Leonard RC, Prescott RJ: A critical analysis of prognostic factors for survival in intermediate and high grade non-Hodgkin's lymphoma. Scotland and Newcastle Lymphoma Group Therapy Working Party. *Br J Cancer* 63(6):945–52, 1991.

18. Lindh J, Lenner P, Osterman B, et al.: Prognostic significance of serum lactic dehydrogenase levels and fraction of S-phase cells in non-Hodgkin lymphomas. *Eur J Hematol* 50(5):258–63, 1993.

19. Steward WP, Crowther D, McWilliam LJ, et al.: Maintenance chlorambucil after CVP in the management of advanced stage, low-grade histologic type non-Hodgkin's lymphoma. A randomized prospective study with an assessment of prognostic factors. *Cancer* 61(3):441–7, 1988.

20. Sutcliffe SB, Gospodarowicz MK, Bush RS et al.: Role of radiation therapy in localized non-Hodgkin's lymphoma. *Radiother Oncol* 4:211–23, 1985.

21. Gospodarowicz MK, Bush RS, Brown TC, et al.: Prognostic factors in nodular lymphomas: A multivariate analysis based on the Princess Margaret experience. *Int J Radiat Oncol Biol Phys* 10:489–97, 1984.

22. Kaminski MS, Coleman CN, Colby TV, et al.: Factors predicting survival in adults with stage I and II large-cell lymphoma treated with primary radiation therapy. *Ann Intern Med* 104:747–56, 1986.

23. Velasquez WS, Fuller LM, Jagannath S, et al. Stages I and II diffuse large cell lymphomas: Prognostic factors and long-term results with CHOP-bleo and radiotherapy. *Blood* 77(5):942–7, 1991.

24. Prestidge BR, Horning SJ, Hoppe RT. Combined modality therapy for Stage I-II large cell lymphoma. *Int J Radiat Oncol Biol Phys* 15:633–9, 1988.

25. Romaguera JE, McLaughlin P, North L, et al.: Multivariate analysis of prognostic factors in Stage IV follicular low-grade lymphoma: A risk model. *J Clin Oncol* 9(5):762–9, 1991.

26. Velasquez WS, Jagannath S, Tucker SL, et al.: Risk classification as the basis for clinical staging of diffuse large-cell lymphoma derived from 10-year survival data. *Blood* 74(2):551–7, 1989.

27. Vitolo U, Bertini M, Brusamolino E, et al.: MACOP-B treatment in diffuse large cell lymphoma: Identification of prognostic groups in an Italian multicenter study. *J Clin Oncol* 10(2):219–27, 1992.

28. Bastion Y, Berger F, Bryon PA, et al.: Follicular lymphomas: Assessment of prognostic factors in 127 patients followed for 10 years. *Ann Oncol* 2(123):123–9, 1991.

29. Hoskins PJ, Ng V, Spinelli JJ, et al.: Prognostic variables in patients with diffuse large-cell lymphoma treated with MACOP-B. *J Clin Oncol* 9(2):220–6, 1991.

30. Bush RS, Gospodarowicz MK. The place of radiation therapy in the management of patients with localized non-Hodgkin's lymphoma, in Rosenberg SA, Kaplan HS (eds.): Malignant lymphomas: Etiology, immunology, pathology, treatment. Bristol Myers Cancer Symposia. New York, Academic Press, 1982, pp. 485–502.

31. Gospodarowicz MK, Sutcliffe SB, Brown TC, et al.: Patterns of disease in localized extranodal lymphomas. *J Clin Oncol* 5(6):875–80, 1987.

32. Shimoyama M, Ota K, Kikutchi M, et al.: Major prognostic factors of adult patients with advanced B-cell lymphoma treated with Vincristine, Cyclophosphamide, Prednisone and doxorubicin (VEPA) or VEPA plus Methotrexate (VEPA-M). *Jpn J Clin Oncol* 18:113–24, 1988.

33. Jellinger KA, Paulus W. Primary central nervous system lymphomas — An update [Editorial] [Review]. *J Cancer Res Clin Oncol* 119(1):7–27, 1992.

34. Decaudin D, Lepage E, Brousse N, et al.: Low-grade Stage III-IV follicular lymphoma: Multivariate analysis of prognostic factors in 484 patients — A study of the Group d'Etude des Lymphomes de l'Adulte. *J Clin Oncol* 17:2499, 1999.

35. Federico M, Vitolo U, Zinzani PL, et al., for the Intergruppo Italiano Linfomi. Prognosis of follicular lymphoma: A predictive model based on a retrospective analysis of 987 cases. *Blood* 95:783–9, 2000.

36. d'Amore F, Brincker H, Christensen BE, et al.: Non-Hodgkin's lymphoma in the elderly. A study of 602 patients aged 70 or older from a Danish population-based registry. The Danish LYEO-Study Group. *Ann Oncol* 3(5):379–86, 1992.

37. The International Non-Hodgkin's Lymphoma Prognostic Factors Project: A predictive model for aggressive Non-Hodgkin's lymphoma. *N Engl J Med* 329:987–94, 1993.

38. Kwak LW, Halpern J, Olshen RA, et al.: Prognostic significance of actual dose intensity in diffuse large-cell lymphoma: Results of a tree-structured survival analysis [see Comments]. *J Clin Oncol* 8(6):963–77, 1990.

39. Stein RS, Greer JP, Cousar JB, et al.: Malignant lymphomas of follicular centre cell origin in man. VII. Prognostic features in small cleaved cell lymphoma. *Hematol Oncol* 7(5):381–91, 1989.

40. Straus DJ, Wong G, Yahalom J, et al.: Diffuse large cell lymphoma. Prognostic factors with treatment. *Leukemia* 1(32):32–7, 1991.

41. Shimoyama M. Peripheral T-cell lymphoma in Japan: Recent progress. *Ann Oncol* 2(Suppl. 2):157–62, 1991.

42. Blay JY, Lasset C, Carrie C, et al.: Multivariate analysis of prognostic factors in patients with non HIV-related primary cerebral lymphoma. A proposal for a prognostic scoring. *Br J Cancer* 67(5):1136–41, 1993.

43. Litam P, Swan F, Cabanillas F, et al.: Prognostic value of serum beta-2 microglobulin in low-grade lymphoma. *Ann Intern Med* 114(10):855–60, 1991.

44. Slymen DJ, Miller TP, Lippman SM, et al.: Immunobiologic factors predictive of clinical outcome in diffuse large-cell lymphoma. *J Clin Oncol* 8(6):986–93, 1990.

45. Bastion Y, Sebban C, Berger F, et al.: Incidence, predictive factors, and outcome of lymphoma transformation in follicular lymphoma patients. *J Clin Oncol* 15:1587–94, 1997.

46. Ong ST, Le Beau MM. Chromosomal abnormalities and molecular genetics of non-Hodgkin's lymphoma. *Semin Oncol* 25:447–60, 1998.

47. Macpherson N, Lesack D, Klasa R, et al.: Small noncleaved, non-Burkitt's (Burkitt-like) lymphoma: Cytogenetics predict outcome and reflect clinical presentation. *J Clin Oncol* 17:1558–67, 1999.

48. Gascoyne RD, Adomat SA, Krajewski S, et al.: Prognostic significance of Bcl-2 protein expression and Bcl-2 gene rearrangement in diffuse aggressive Non-Hodgkin's lymphoma. *Blood* 90:244–51, 1997.

49. Hill ME, MacLennan KA, Cunningham DC, et al.: Prognostic significance of bcl-2 protein expression and bcl-2 major breakpoint region rearrangement in diffuse large cell Non-Hodgkin's lymphoma: A British National Lymphoma Investigation Study. *Blood* 88:1046–51, 1996.

50. Johnson A, Brun A, Dictor M, et al.: Incidence and prognostic significance of t(14;18) translocation in follicle center cell lymphoma of low and high grade. *Ann Oncol* 6:789, 1995.

51. Lopez-Guillermo A, Cabanillas F, McDonnell TI, et al.: Correlation of Bcl-2 rearrangement with clinical characteristics and outcome in indolent follicular lymphoma. *Blood* 93:3081–7, 1999.

52. Offit K, Lo CF, Louie DC, et al.: Rearrangement of the BCL-6 gene as a prognostic marker in diffuse large cell lymphoma. *N Engl J Med* 331:74–80, 1994.

53. Bastard C, Deweindt C, Kerckaert JP, et al.: LAZ3 rearrangements in Non-Hodgkin's lymphoma: Correlation with histology, immunophenotype, karyotype and clinical outcome in 217 patients. *Blood* 83:2423–7, 1994.

54. Moller MB, Gerdes AM, Skjodt K, et al.: Disrupted p53 function as predictor of treatment failure and poor prognosis in B- and T-Cell Non-Hodgkin's lymphoma. *Clin Cancer Res* 5:1085–91, 1999.

55. Zoldan MC, Inghirami G, Masuda Y, et al.: Large-cell variants of mantle cell lymphoma: Cytologic characteristics and p53 anomalies may predict poor outcome. *Br J Hematol* 93:475–86, 1996.

56. Ichikawa A, Kinoshita T, Watanabe T, et al.: Mutations of the p53 gene as a prognostic factor in aggressive b-cell lymphoma. *N Engl J Med* 337:529–35, 1997.

57. Miller TP, Grogan TM, Dahlberg S, et al.: Prognostic significance of the Ki-67-associated proliferative antigen in aggressive Non-Hodgkin's lymphomas: A prospective Southwest Oncology Group Trial. *Blood* 83:1460–6, 1994.

58. Sanchez E, Chacon I, Plaza MM, et al.: Clinical outcome in diffuse large B-cell lymphoma is dependent on the relationship between different cell-cycle regulator proteins. *J Clin Oncol* 16:1931–9, 1998.

59. Salven P, Teerenhovi L, Joensuu H: A high pretreatment serum vascular endothelial growth factor concentration is associated with poor outcome in Non-Hodgkin's lymphoma. *Blood* 90:3167–72, 1997.

60. Bertolini F, Paolucci M, Peccatori F, et al.: Angiogenic growth factors and endostatin in non-Hodgkin's lymphoma. *Br J Hematol* 106:504–9, 1999.

61. Jalkanen S, Joensuu H, Soderstrom KO, Klemi P: Lymphocyte homing and clinical behavior of non-Hodgkin's lymphomas. *J Clin Invest* 87:1835–40, 1991.

62. Drillenburg P, Wielenga VJ, Kramer MH, et al.: CD44 expression predicts disease outcome in localized large B-cell lymphoma. *Leukemia* 13:1448–1455, 1999.

63. Terol MJ, Lopez-Fuillermo A, Bosch F, et al.: Expression of the adhesion molecule icam-1 in Non-Hodgkin's lymphoma: Relationship with tumor dissemination and prognostic importance. *J Clin Oncol* 16:35–40, 1998.

64. O'Reilly SE, Hoskins P, Klimo P, et al.: MACOP-B and VACOP-B in diffuse large cell lymphomas and MOPP/ABV in Hodgkin's disease. *Ann Oncol* 1(17):17–23, 1991.

65. Soubeyran P, Eghbali H, Bonichon F, et al.: Localized follicular lymphomas: Prognosis and survival of stages I and II in a retrospective series of 103 patients. *Radiother Oncol* 13(2):91–8, 1988.

66. Dana BW, Dahlberg S, Nathwani BN, et al.: Long-term follow-up of patients with low-grade malignant lymphomas treated with doxorubicin-based chemotherapy or chemoimmunotherapy. *J Clin Oncol* 11(4):644–51, 1993.

67. Bermudez MA, Grant KM, Rodvien R, Mendes F: Non-Hodgkin's lymphoma in a population with or at risk for acquired immunodeficiency syndrome: Indications for intensive chemotherapy. *Am J Med* 86:71–6, 1989.

68. Zinzani PL, Storti S, Zaccaria A, et al.: Elderly aggressive-histology Non-Hodgkin's lymphoma: First-line VNCOP-B regimen experience on 350 patients. *Blood* 94:33–8, 1999.

69. Kaplan LD, Straus DJ, Testa MA: Low-dose compared with standard-dose m-BACOD chemotherapy for Non-Hodgkin's lymphoma associated with human immunodeficiency virus infection. *N Engl J Med* 336:1641–8, 1997.

70. Freter CE: Acquired immunodeficiency syndrome-associated lymphomas. *Monogr Natl Cancer Inst* 1990(10):45–54, 1990.

71. Vaccher E, Tirelli U, Spina M, et al.: Age and serum lactate dehydrogenase level are independent prognostic factors in human immunodeficiency virus-related Non-Hodgkin's lymphomas: A single-institute study of 96 patients. *J Clin Oncol* 14:2217–23, 1996.

72. Kaplan LD, Shiramizu B, Herndier B, et al. Influence of molecular characteristics on clinical outcome in human immunodeficiency virus-associated Non-Hodgkin's lymphoma: Identification of a subgroup with favorable clinical outcome. *Blood* 85:1727–35, 1995.

73. Lyons SF, Liebowitz DN: The roles of human viruses in the pathogenesis of lymphoma. *Semin Oncol* 25:461–75, 1998.

74. Cesarman E, Chadburn A, Liu Y-F, et al.: BCL-6 gene mutations in post-transplantation lymphoproliferative disorders predict response to therapy and clinical outcome. *Blood* 92:2294–302, 1998.

75. Calvo R, Pifarre A, Rosell R, et al.: H-RAS 1 minisatellite rare alleles: A genetic susceptibility and prognostic factor for non-Hodgkin's lymphoma. *J Nat Cancer Inst* 90:1095–8, 1998.

76. Coiffier B, Gisselbrecht C, Vose JM, et al.: Prognostic factors in aggressive malignant lymphomas: Description and validation of a prognostic index that could identify patients requiring a more aggressive therapy. *J Clin Oncol* 9:211, 1991.

77. Hermans J, Krol AD, van Groningen K, et al.: International prognostic index for aggressive non-Hodgkin's lymphoma is valid for all malignancy grades. *Blood* 86:1460–3, 1995.

78. Mounier N, Morel P, Haioun C, et al., for the Groupe d'Etudes des Lymphomes de l'Adulte. A multivariate analysis of the survival of patients with aggressive lymphoma. Cancer 82:1952–62, 1998.

79. Aviles A, Yanez J, Lopez T, et al.: Malnutrition as an adverse prognostic factor in patients with diffuse large cell lymphoma [see Comments]. *Arch Med Res* 26:31–4, 1995.

CHAPTER 44

Leukemia

MARK MINDEN

Leukemia, the malignant transformation of bone marrow blood-forming cells, is not a single entity. Prior to any form of therapy, which would include antibiotics and transfusion, the leukemias were classified as acute or chronic. The acute leukemias were rapidly fatal, with individuals dying in days to weeks from the time of diagnosis. In contrast, individuals with chronic leukemias could live for many years without any therapy. With the recognition of the stem-cell nature of blood formation and the identification of different lineages, it was possible to further subdivide the leukemias into those of the myeloid and lymphoid lineages; with the development of therapeutics, this distinction has proven to be important.

ACUTE LEUKEMIA

As just mentioned, without any treatment, individuals with acute leukemia will usually die of their disease in a very short period of time. In the acute leukemias there is overproduction of immature nonfunctional cells referred to as *blast cells*, and decreased production of the mature elements of the blood, such as red blood cells, neutrophils, and platelets. Death is due to leukostasis, anemia, infection, or bleeding. Some patients with acute leukemia present with low peripheral blood counts and relatively preserved production of red blood cells, neutrophils, and platelets. These individuals can live for several months, before succumbing to their disease.

With the development of effective chemotherapeutics and supportive care, the prognosis of patients has improved so that there are now long-term disease-free survivors. In contrast to other malignancies where local treatment modalities have produced cures, the leukemias are the first example of a malignant disease where systemic therapy successfully produced cures. Over the years, the overall prognosis of patients has improved. During this time it has become apparent from

Prognostic Factors in Cancer, 2nd edition, Edited by Mary K. Gospodarowicz
ISBN 0-471-40633-3   Copyright © 2001 Wiley-Liss, Inc.

a morphologic, cytogenetic, and biochemical point of view that the leukemias are a highly heterogeneous group of diseases. Dr. Renato Baserga, in discussing studies of cells in culture, makes three caveats: this is true for (1) these cells, (2) under these conditions, (3) at this time.[1] These caveats can be applied equally to patients with acute leukemia, paraphrased as: this is true for (1) these patients classified in this manner, (2) treated with this therapy, (3) given this support, at this time in medical history.

Classification of Acute Leukemias

The acute leukemias are classified by the French, American, British classification system into the acute myeloblastic leukemias (AML) and acute lymphoblastic leukemias (ALL).[2,3] These in turn are not single-disease entities, but rather represent broad groupings of leukemias classified according to morphology, cytochemical stains, and more recently,immunological markers. At this time cytogenetics has not been included in the classification; however, as will be evident below, with the increased knowledge that we now have, and the ready availability of testing, any new classification has to include this variable.

ACUTE MYELOBLASTIC LEUKEMIAS

The AMLs are classed as M0–M7, based upon the degree of differentiation.[2,3,] Using a standard chemotherapy such as daunorubicin intravenously for three days and cytosine arabinoside by continuous infusion for seven days, it is possible to assign a different prognosis to each of the groups.[4] For example in the M0, M6, and M7 groups, the response rate is low, and there are very few long-term survivors. In contrast, long-term survivors are found in the M2, M3, M4, and M5 groups. Even in these subgroups, there is heterogeneity in response to treatment and long-term survival. Some insight into this variability to response is provided by cytogenetic analysis.[5]

FAB-M2

The FAB-M2 phenotype is characterized by the presence of Auer rods and evidence of myeloid differentiation. At a cytogenetic and molecular level, a subset of these patients carries the t(8;21) chromosomal abnormality.[6] The molecular nature of this abnormality has been determined and is due to a chromosome translocation involving the AML-1 gene from chromosome 21 and the ETO gene on chromosome 8.[7] Within patients with FAB-M2, the t(8;21) is found in about 50% of patients.[8] This is likely an underestimate of the proportion of patients with FAB-M2 t(8;21), as molecular means will detect 10–20% more cases.[9] The t(8;21) is not restricted to the FAB-M2 group, nor is it the only abnormality found in patients with FAB-M2. Patients with FAB-M1 and M4 may also have a t(8;21).[10] Approximately 10% of patients with FAB-M2 have a tandem duplication of the MLL/ALL-1 gene at

11q23.[11] Patients with t(8;21) have a high complete remission rate and long-term survival.[12] The duration of remission is enhanced with high dose ara-C included in the induction or consolidation regimen.[12,13] In contrast to the patients with t(8;21), patients with a duplication of MLL/ALL-1 have a lower complete remission rate, and long-term remissions with chemotherapy alone are unusual.[11]

The preceding illustrates that even within a single FAB subtype, the disease is heterogeneous with regard to biology and response to therapy. Although FAB subtype is of prognostic value, the molecular characterization allows a more precise assignment of risk. It should also be noted that the risk is reduced by the addition of specific chemotherapy.

FAB-M3 (Acute Promyelocytic Leukemia)

Patients with FAB-M3 leukemia have increased numbers of blasts and promyelocytes in the bone marrow.[14] Due to the release of procoagulants by the leukemic cells, this group of patients has an ongoing disseminated intravascular coagulation (DIC) that is exacerbated by induction-style chemotherapy. When chemotherapy alone is used for treatment, there is a high induction mortality of approximately 20%, usually due to bleeding. The recognition of the DIC state with aggressive component replacement has resulted in a reduced mortality during the induction phase.[15] Chemotherapy alone achieves remission in 60–70% of patients. Long-term survival is approximately 20% with chemotherapy alone, with higher survival being correlated with higher doses of daunorubicin or idarubicin. The use of high-dose ara-C during induction therapy has been reported to have a negative impact on survival.[13]

Over the past 10 years, much has changed in the treatment of acute promyelocytic leukemia (APL). Based on in vitro studies demonstrating the induction of differentiation of HL-60 cells by all-*trans*-retinoic acid (ATRA),[16] a clinical trial was performed in which AML patients were treated with ATRA alone. No responses were seen in the non-M3 group of patients; however, the majority of cases of APL entered complete remission in 1–3 months. Unfortunately, most patients subsequently had a relapse of their disease.[17] Interestingly similar studies performed with 13-*cis*-retinoic acid did not result in any complete remissions. Since the initial observation, clinical trials have been conducted in which complete remission is achieved with ATRA, and then chemotherapy is given or ATRA and chemotherapy are given together.[18,19] With both of these approaches, complete remission rates of 80–90% have been achieved, and long-term remissions of 70% without bone marrow transplant are expected. ATRA has contributed to the improved survival in two major ways. First ATRA results in a rapid control of the DIC, reducing the early mortality in this disease. Second, the combination of ATRA with concomitant or sequential chemotherapy has produced a higher proportion of long-term survivors compared to chemotherapy alone. The mechanism for this is unknown, but likely relates to the ability of ATRA to enhance the degradation of the transforming protein responsible for the development of APL.

Cytogenetic analysis of APL indicates that approximately 70% of cases have t(15;17) using standard G-banding methodology. At about the same time that ATRA was being used to treat patients with APL, the t(15;17) breakpoint was cloned, identifying the formation of a fusion gene composed of the PML gene on chromosome 15 and the retinoic acid receptor (RAR) α gene on chromosome 17.[20,21] This fusion gene is referred to as PML–RAR. Further analysis indicated that the translocation can produce one of three distinct messages. Early studies suggested that the form of fusion message was of prognostic significance; however, more recent studies have not confirmed this. The presence of a fusion gene has made it possible to develop a highly specific molecular test for PML–RAR. Using this method, it was possible to show that 10–20% of cases of morphologically defined, but cytogenetically normal, APL did indeed contain the t(15;17).[22] Similar results have been obtained using fluorescent in situ hybridization probes that recognize the t(15;17) in metaphase and interphase cells. Most of the other cases of morphologic APL were found to have variant translocations of RARα involving chromosome 5 or 11.[23] In some cases of morphologic APL, it was not possible to find a rearrangement of RARα; this represents a small group of about 5%. The identification of t(15;17) is important, as cases lacking rearrangement of RARα or carrying the PLZF–RAR fusion product do not appear to benefit from the addition of ATRA. It is of note that current clinical trials in FAB-M3 leukemia require a molecular test to establish the presence of PML–RAR. Because response to ATRA and hence prognosis is dependent upon the presence of PML–RAR, it is likely that the naming of the disease should be changed to consider this.

The use of reverse-transcriptase and polymerase chain reaction (RT-PCR) to detect PML–RAR has also provided a very sensitive means of detecting the presence of cells that contain the fusion transcript.[24,25] Morphologic evaluation of bone marrow using a microscope is a poor way of assessing remission status, as up to 5% of the cells can have the morphologic character of blasts. In contrast, RT-PCR for PML–RAR is capable of detecting 1 in 1000 to 1 in 10,000 leukemic cells. This ability to detect minimal residual disease is of predictive value. Patients who are RT-PCR positive for PML–RAR at the end of induction and consolidation therapy have a very high risk of relapse.[26] Furthermore, reemergence of PML–RAR positivity in a patient whose bone marrow was previously negative also predicts for relapse.

Another feature that predicts for relapse in APL patients treated with ATRA and chemotherapy is a high white count >50,000 at presentation. Allogeneic or autologous bone marrow transplant may be of therapeutic value in patients who present with a high white count or are RT-PCR positive for PML–RAR at the end of therapy. Transplant for other patients is not necessary given the excellent results of treatment.

FAB-M4

This form of acute leukemia is characterized by the presence of markers of differentiation of both granulocytes and monocytes. At a cytogenetic and molecular level, it is a heterogeneous disease. For example, although t(8;21) is predominantly found in FAB-M2, some cases of FAB-M4 carry this abnormality. Trisomy 8, total loss or interstitial deletion of chromosomes 5 and 7 are also frequently found in leukemic cells with this morphology. The finding of one of these three abnormalities is a poor prognostic sign.[5,27] With standard chemotherapy the remission rate is 40–50% and long-term remissions are rare.

Chromosome translocations involving 11q23 are found in both ALL and AML FAB M4 and M5.[28,29] Over 15 different genes have been found to be involved in translocations targeted to 11q23. In both ALL and AML the partner gene at 11q23 is MLL or ALL-1. It appears that it is the partner gene that determines whether the translocation produces a lymphoid or myeloid type leukemia. In general the response rate to chemotherapy in such patients is 50–60%; however, the relapse rate is very high, with <10% long-term survivors.

FAB-M4 eo

A variant of FAB-M4 is FAB-M4 eo, in which there is an increased number of eosinophilic forms present in the peripheral blood and bone marrow. This form of leukemia is characterized by the presence of inv (16) or t(16;16).[30] Like the t(8;21) patients, these individuals have an improved prognosis when treated with a regimen that includes high-dose ara-C either in induction or consolidation therapy.[12]

FAB-M5

FAB-M5 differs from FAB-M4 in that the majority of blasts have a monocytic phenotype. Cytogenetic abnormalities such as trisomy 8, abnormalities of chromosome 5 and 7 and translocations involving 11q23 are also found in this form of AML. In contrast to other forms of AML, FAB-M5 leukemias tend to infiltrate normal tissues such as the gums. There is a high rate of CNS disease in these patients either at presentation or at relapse. The response to therapy is similar to that for patients with FAB-M4 leukemia and is predominantly affected by the cytogenetic abnormalities noted.[12]

FAB-M6

Blasts in FAB-M6 have features of erythroblasts. This is a relatively infrequent form of AML. Patients with this form of the disease have a low response rate, and short duration of remission, compared to other FAB types.[12]

FAB-M7

Blasts in FAB-M7 have the features of megakaryoblasts. Rearrangements in the region of the Evi-1 gene at 3q26 are often observed in this form of leukemia.[31] Patients with abnormalities of 3q26 or FAB-M7 have a low complete remission rate, and the duration of remission is frequently short.

Other Biologic Features

In addition to the FAB classification and attendant cytogenetic changes, other biologic features of AML blasts have prognostic significance; again the prognostic relevance is dependent upon the induction therapy used.

CD34 CD34 is a cell-surface marker expressed on immature normal blood progenitors. Patients with a high percentage of CD34 + ve blast cells have a worse prognosis than other groups. It is of interest that the in FAB-M3, blasts have relatively low CD34 expression, in keeping with the good prognosis seen in this group.[32,33]

Bcl-2 Bcl-2 is the founding member of a family of proteins involved in mediating cell survival and death. Patients whose blasts have high levels of Bcl-2 have a worse prognosis.[34,35]

P-glycoprotein P-Glycoprotein, or multidrug resistance gene 1, is expressed on early normal hematopoietic progenitor cells.[36,37] This cell-surface protein is involved in actively transporting xenobiotics and other molecules out of the cells. Included in the list of molecules transported out of the cell are anthracyclines such as daunorubicin and doxorubicin, and other chemotherapeutics such as etoposide, vincristine, vinblastine, and taxol. Patients who have a high level of expression of MDR-1 on the cell surface have a low response rate and short duration of remission. The use of agents that block drug efflux are being tested to see if they can overcome this form of resistance.

WT-1 The Wilm's tumor gene, WT-1, was first identified as a tumor suppressor gene in the pediatric kidney tumor.[38] In AML, however, it is likely that WT-1 is acting as an oncogene.[39,40] A high level of expression of the WT-1 transcription factor is associated with reduced rate of complete remission and shorter duration of remission. It is intriguing to note that the Bcl-2 promoter contains a WT-1 binding site, and that these two features cosegregate.

Minimal Residual Disease

The preceding factors relate to the endogenous biologic features of the leukemic cells. Minimal residual disease is a measure of the amount of leukemia present following completion of induction and consolidation therapy. Prior to molecular diagnostics, the level of detection was on the order of 5% leukemic cells, due to the presence of normal cells that have a blast-like appearance. With the development of probes that can detect specific chromosome translocations at a frequency of 1 in 10,000 to 1 in 100,000 cells, it is now possible to (1) identify the level of leukemic infiltration following treatment, and (2) determine the significance of residual disease. The best studied situations are PML–RAR arising from the t(15;17) and AML–ETO arising from t(8;21).[41,42] Interestingly the detection of PML–RAR at the completion of therapy is an excellent predictor of relapse,[24,43] while detection of AML–ETO is not of significance. The reason for these opposite findings is not known. Using more quantitative methods, it has been found that increasing levels of AML–ETO in postremission samples is a harbinger of disease relapse.

Host-related Factors

Age   Age is a significant risk factor in patients undergoing treatment for AML. Patients >55 years of age tend to have a lower complete remission rate and shorter remissions than younger patients do. This can be attributed to (1) greater incidence of poor risk cytogenetics; (2) more frequent history of antecedent hematologic abnormality; and (3) more frequent deaths during induction due to cardiac, neurologic and infectious complications.[4]

Antecedent Hematologic Abnormality   Patients who have an undefined hematologic abnormality for 3 months or more have a poorer response rate and duration of remission than patients who present with de novo disease. The longer period of abnormality also affects prognosis in a negative manner. The presence of an antecedent hematologic abnormality likely indicates the presence of an underlying myelodysplastic state. Poor risk cytogenetics such as trisomy 8, aberration of chromosome 5 and 7, and rearrangements of 3q26 are frequently associated with this condition.[44]

White Blood Count   Patients with a high white blood count at presentation are at greater risk of death during induction therapy due to (1) the development of leukostasis, and (2) the development of tumor lysis syndrome and subsequent renal and pulmonary failure. These patients are also at increased risk of relapse, often due to extramedullary and CNS disease.[44,45]

Secondary Leukemias   The secondary acute leukemias are those that develop following prior chemotherapy or radiotherapy for another malignancy or following a period of myelodysplasia, essential thrombocythemia, polycythemia vera, chronic myelogenous leukemia, or chronic myelomonocytic leukemia. Both of these conditions are associated with an increased frequency of poor-risk cytogenetics such as trisomy 8, aberration of chromosome 5 and 7, and rearrangements of 3q26. Patients with these abnormalities have a poor response remission rate and short remissions when treated with standard chemotherapy. Patients who lack these cytogenetic risk factors, or have good risk cytogenetic abnormalities respond in a manner similar to the respective cytogenetic group.[44,45]

Patients who develop leukemia following prior chemo- or radiotherapy have an increased risk of dying during induction therapy due to cardiac, pulmonary, and infectious complications, likely secondary to the effects of the previous treatment.

ACUTE LYMPHOBLASTIC LEUKEMIAS

Like AML, patients with ALL will die rapidly from their disease in the absence of any therapy. With supportive therapy such as transfusion and antibiotics, short-term survival of several months is possible. Chemotherapy has had a major impact on long-term survival of patients with this disease.

Tumor-related Factors

ALL is a heterogeneous collection of diseases; the disease is stratified in a number of different ways based either on size and morphology of the cells, cell-surface markers, or cytogenetics. As for AML there is an FAB classification consisting of L1, L2, and L3.[46] The L3 phenotype is similar to the morphology seen in patients with Burkitt's lymphoma. Using chemotherapy protocols that are generally successful in the treatment of pediatric ALL, L3 ALL has a low response rate and poor overall survival. However, when one employs a more aggressive, high-dose, short-course-type therapy, there is a complete remission rate in the order of 90% and long-term disease-free survival of 70% or more.[47]

By cell-surface markers it is possible to divide ALL into those of B-cell and T-cell lineage.[46,48] Based upon cell-surface expression of the antigen receptors and other markers, it is possible to further classify these leukemias into pre-pre, pre-, and mature cells of either the B or T lineage. Using chemotherapy regimens consisting predominantly of vincristine, prednisone, adriamycin, and methotrexate patients with T-cell-type ALL had a poor prognosis. However, with the development of risk adapted therapy and the addition of cyclophosphamide and high-dose ara-C to the treatment of patients with T-ALL, the complete remission rate and long-term survival is equal to that of patients with pre-pre-, and pre-B-cell ALL.[49,50] Patients with sIg-positive ALL, tend to do worse than sIg-negative patients.

Morphology and cell-surface markers indicate that ALL is a heterogeneous disease. This heterogeneity is most evident with regards to cytogenetics.[51] A variety of cytogenetic abnormalities have been noted in ALL, many of which are of prognostic significance. In infant ALL there is a very high incidence of chromosome translocation involving MLL/ALL-1 at 11q23.[29,52] These translocations are found in childhood and adult ALL, but at lower frequencies. Patients whose cells carry an 11q23 translocation have a relatively poor prognosis compared to patients with normal or hyperdiploid cytogenetics. In childhood ALL the most frequent abnormality found in patients with pre-B ALL is a t(12;21) involving the tel gene on chromosome 12 and the AML-1 gene on chromosome 21; approximately 25% of cases possess this abnormality.[53] By standard cytogenetics this is very difficult to see, and the usual means of identifying the abnormality is by RT–PCR for the fusion RNA. Patients with this abnormality treated with the Dana Farber Cancer Institute protocol have a very high complete remission rate, and relapses are rare.[54] Other groups have not presented the same favorable prognosis for this group of patients. This discrepancy may be explained by crucial differences in the treatment protocols.

Translocations of Tel-AML are found in only 3% of adult cases of ALL, and then predominantly in the younger adults. In contrast to t(12;21), the frequency of which decreases with age, the incidence of t(9;22) in patients with ALL increases with age.[55-57] In childhood ALL this abnormality, in which the bcr gene on chromosome 22 is linked to the abl gene on chromosome 9, is found in 5% of cases. In adults 20–30% of cases may contain the Philadelphia (Ph) chromosome. Despite a high initial response rate, in the absence of an allogeneic bone marrow transplant, all patients will eventually relapse and die of their disease.

Host-related Factors

Age   Age plays an important prognostic role in this disease.[58] Patients less than one year of age do not respond as well as older children.[49,59] The best response is in children 2–11 years of age. In this group long-term disease-free survival of >80% is expected. In the adult group, younger patients have a better response than older patients. It is fascinating that the different cytogenetic prognostic subgroups closely mirror the age-related prognostic groups.

White Blood Count   Patients with a high white blood count >50,000 have a worse prognosis compared to other patients. This does not hold for patients with T-ALL.

CHRONIC LEUKEMIAS

In acute leukemia the disease is characterized by the overproduction of nonfunctional blast cells and decreased production of normal cells. In the chronic leukemias, there is the overproduction of functional mature cells and at least in the early stages of the disease continued production of normal blood elements. Thus, unlike the acute leukemias, patients do not rapidly die of their disease. Similar to the acute leukemias, the chronic forms of the disease may exist as either a myeloid-or lymphoid-type disease. For the sake of brevity only the two most common forms of chronic leukemias, chronic myelogenous leukemia (CML) and chronic lymphocytic leukemia (CLL) are discussed.

Chronic Myelogenous Leukemia

CML represents 7–15% of adult leukemias and has a median onset of 50–60 years of age. CML is a progressive disease with three identifiable stages.[60] The first or chronic phase may last a few months to many years.During this time most patients are asymptomatic. Over time the disease evolves to an accelerated phase, in which there is the development of cytopenias and increased production of blast cells. After a variable period of time from weeks to months, this gives way to a myeloid or lymphoid blast crisis, which closely resembles the corresponding acute leukemia.

Over the years, with changes in therapy there has been an improvement in survival.[61,62] With hydroxyurea as the mainstay of therapy, patients with CML in the chronic phase can be divided into good, intermediate, and poor prognosis groups, with median survivals of 5.5, 3.5, and 2 years, respectively. For patients treated with interferon median survival is 9, 7.5, and 4.5 years for good, intermediate, and poor-risk patients. Features associated with poor prognosis are older age, symptoms at the time of diagnosis, splenomegaly, hepatomegaly, low performance status, anemia, thrombocytopenia or thrombocytosis, increased blasts and basophils in the peripheral blood or bone marrow, and cytogenetic clonal evolution. It is of interest to note that interferon has not changed the significance of these prognostic factors. The achievement of a major cytogenetic response, that is, a reduction of Philadelphia positive cells to <30%, predicts for progression-free survival of >8 years. Approximately 50% of patients with good-risk disease will have a major cytogenetic response, while about 20% of poor-risk patients will have a major cytogenetic response. A major cytogenetic response in a poor-risk patient produces the same 4-year survival as seen for interferon-responsive patients in the good and intermediate risk groups. Thus response to interferon is an independent prognostic factor.

Allogeneic bone marrow transplant has also significantly altered the prognosis of patients with chronic-phase CML. Long-term disease-free survival in patients treated with HLA identical-sibling bone marrow transplants is 50–70%.[63,64]

Once a patient has entered blast crisis, survival is short despite chemotherapy or bone marrow transplant. The recent introduction of the abl kinase inhibitor STI-571 holds promise for controlling this lethal complication of CML.

Chronic Lymphocytic Leukemia

CLL is a chronic disease characterized by the overproduction of mature B-cells.[65–67] Like CML, during the early phase of the disease there is maintenance of red cell, neutrophil, and platelet production. With the exception of the few patients who may be cured by allogeneic bone marrow transplantation, this is an indolent incurable disease. Two similar prognostic scales are commonly used by practitioners and clinical investigators treating this disease.[66,68] Both systems are based upon clinical and laboratory features, including lymphadenopathy, splenomegaly, anemia, and thrombocytopenia. The Rai classification has five levels, 0–IV. The median duration of survival in months is >150, 100, 70, and 20 for stages 0, I, II, and III and IV. The Binet has three levels, A, B, and C. Median survival in months for these three groups is >100, 80, and 20, respectively. Recently it has been found that the level of $\beta 2$ microglobulin and CD23 are of prognostic significance.[69]

SUMMARY

The leukemias are disseminated diseases from the onset. As such, early and long-term prognosis are dependent on two major factors: (1) chronic vs. acute disease, and (2) systemic therapy responsive vs. nonresponsive. Over time prognostic factors have changed, as more effective therapies have been identified. One of the best examples of this is acute promyelocytic leukemia in which the addition of all-*trans*-retinoic acid to chemotherapy has resulted in a significant improvement in long-term survival. In this case, a prognostic factor based on morphology was explained by a cytogenetic abnormality. Subsequently the presence of this abnormality was found to predict and explain response to a particular therapy. With our increasing understanding of the molecular basis of leukemias, it is likely that other "prognostic factors" will become the guideposts for successful therapies (see Appendix 44A).

■■■■■ APPENDIX 44A.1

Prognostic Factors in Acute Myeloblastic Leukemia

Prognostic Factors	Tumor Related	Host Related	Environment Related

Essential	Cytogenetics
	Cell-surface markers
	Expression of MDR-1
	WBC
		Age
		Cardiac disease
		Respiratory disease
		Availability of an
		  HLA-matched
		  individual
		Antecedent
		  hematologic
		  abnormality
			Secondary
			leukemia — treatment
			induced

Additional	Remission duration Response to initial therapy		

New and
  promising
	Identification of mutator
	  phenotype
	Identification of
	  aberrantly expressed
	  genes in the absence
	  of chromosomal
	  translocation
	VEGF levels
	Number of blood vessels
	  in bone marrow[70]		

Prognostic Factors in Acute Lymphoblastic Leukemia

Prognostic Factors	Tumor Related	Host Related	Environment Related
Essential	Cytogenetics Cell-surface markers WBC B vs. pre-B type Phenotype	Age	
Additional	Mutant p53 Response to primary therapy Early relapse		

New and
  promising
	Identification of
	  aberrantly
	  expressed genes		

Prognostic Factors in Chronic Myelogenous Leukemia

Prognostic Factors	Tumor Related	Host Related	Environment Related
Essential	Cytogenetics Splenomegaly Basophils	Age Ability to tolerate interferon Availability of an HLA-related individual	
Additional	Blast crisis Myelofibrosis Beta 2 microglobulin		

New and
  promising
	Deletions associated with
	  the development of
	  the Philadelphia
	  chromosome		

Prognostic Factors in Chronic Lymphocytic Leukemia

Prognostic Factors	Tumor Related	Host Related	Environment Related
Essential	Lymphocytosis Lymphadenopathy Splenomegaly Anemia Thrombocytopenia Cytogenetics	Age	
Additional	Beta 2 microglobulin Soluble CD23		
New and promising	VEGF levels		

REFERENCES

1. Baserga R: The cell cycle: Myths and realities. *Cancer Res* 50:6769–71, 1990.

2. Bennett JM, Catovsky D, Daniel MT, et al.: Proposed revised criteria for the classification of acute myeloid leukemia: A report of French-American-British cooperative group. *Ann Int Med* 103:620–4, 1985.

3. Bennett JM, Catovsky D, Daniel MT, et al.: Proposal for the recognition of minimally differentiated acute myeloid leukaemia (AML-MO). *Br J Haematol* 78:325–9, 1991.

4. Mayer RJ, Davis RB, Schiffer CA, et al.: Intensive postremission chemotherapy in adults with acute myeloblastic leukemia. *New Engl J Med* 331:896–903, 1994.

5. Mrozek K, Heinonen K, de la Chappelle A, Bloomfield CD: Clinical significance of cytogenetics in acute myeloid leukemia. *Semin Oncol* 24:17–31, 1997.

6. Byrd JC, Dodge RK, Carroll A, et al.: Patients with t(8;21)(q22;q22) and acute myeloid leukemia have superior failure-free and overall survival when repetitive cycles of high-dose cytarabine are administered. *J Clin Oncol* 17:3767–75, 1999.

7. Kozu T, Miyoshi H, Shimizu K, et al.: Junctions of the *AML1/MTG8(ETO)* fusion are constant in t(8;21) acute myeloid leukemia detected by reverse transcription polymerase chain reaction. *Blood* 82:1270–6, 1993.

8. Hagihara M, Kobayashi H, Miyachi H, Ogawa T: Clinical heterogeneity in acute myelogenous leukemia with the 8;21 translocation. *Keio J Med* 40:90–3, 1991.

9. Downing JR, Head DR, Curcio-Brint AM, et al.: An AML1/ETO fusion transcript is consistently detected by RNA-based polymerase chain reaction in acute myelogenous leukemia containing the (8;21)(q22;q22) translocation. *Blood* 81:2860, 1993.

10. Langabeer SE, Walker H, Rogers JR, et al.: Incidence of AML1/ETO fusion transcripts in patients entered into the MRC AML trials. MRC adult leukemia working party. *Br J Haematol* 99:925–8, 1997.

11. Caligiuri MA, Strout MP, Lawrence D, et al.: Rearrangement of ALL1 (MLL) in acute myeloid leukemia with normal cytogenetics. *Cancer Res* 58:55–9, 1998.

12. Bloomfield CD, Lawrence D, Byrd JC, et al.: Frequency of prolonged remission duration after high-dose cytarabine intensification in acute myeloid leukemia varies by cytogenetic subtype. *Cancer Res* 58:4173–9, 1998.

13. Head DR, Kopecky KJ, Willman C, Appelbaum FR: Treatment outcome with chemotherapy in acute promyelocytic leukemia: The Southwest Oncology Group (SWOG) experience. *Leukemia* 8 (Suppl. 2): S38–41, 1994.

14. Grignani F, Fagioli M, Alcalay M, et al.: Review: Acute promyelocytic leukemia: From genetics to treatment. *Blood* 83:10–25, 1994.

15. Tallman MS: The thrombophilic state in acute promyelocytic leukemia. *Semin Thromb Hemost* 25:209–15, 1999.

16. Collins SJ, Robertson KA, Mueller L: Retinoic acid-induced granulocytic differentiation of HL-60 myeloid leukemia cells is mediated directly through the retinoic acid receptor(RAR-alpha). *Mol Cell Biol* 10:2154–63, 1990.

17. Chen ZX, Xue YQ, Zhang R, et al.: A clinical and experimental study on all-trans retinoic acid-treated acute promyelocytic leukemia patients. *Blood* 78:1413–19, 1991.

18. Tallman MS, Andersen JW, Schiffer CA, et al. All-trans-retinoic acid in acute promyelocytic leukemia [see Comments] [Erratum appears in *N Engl J Med* 337(22):1639, 1997, *N Engl J Med* 337:1021–8, 1997.

19. Warrell RP Jr., Maslak P, Eardley A, et al.: Treatment of acute promyelocytic leukemia with all trans retinoic acid: An update of the New York experience. *Leukemia* 8:929–33, 1994.

20. Kakizuka A, Miller WH, Umesono K, et al.: Chromosomal translocation t(15;17) in human acute promyelocytic leukemia fuses RARalpha with a novel putative transcription factor PML. *Cell* 66:663–74, 1991.

21. de The H, Lavau C, Marchio A, et al.: The PML-RAR alpha fusion mRNA generated by the t(15;17) translocation in acute promyelocytic leukemia encodes a functionally altered RAR. *Cell* 66:675–84, 1991.

22. Allford S, Grimwade D, Langabeer S, et al.: Identification of the t(15;17) in AML FAB types other than M3: Evaluation of the role of molecular screening for the PML/RARalpha rearrangement in newly diagnosed AML. The Medical Research Council (MRC) Adult Leukaemia Working Party. *Br J Haematol* 105:198–207, 1999.

23. Hummel JL, Wells RA, Dube ID, et al.: Deregulation of NPM and PLZF in a variant t(5;17) case of acute promyelocytic leukemia. *Oncogene* 18:633–41, 1999.

24. Miller WH, Kakizuka A, Frankel SR, et al.: Reverse transcription polymerase chain reaction for the rearranged retinoic acid receptor α clarifies diagnosis and detects minimal residual disease in acute promyelocytic leukemia. *Proc Natl Acad Sci* USA 89:2694, 1992.

25. Muindi J, Frankel SR, Miller WH, et al.: Continuous treatment with all-trans retinoic acid causes a progressive reduction in plasma drug concentrations: Implications for relapse and retinoid "resistance" in patients with acute promyelocytic leukemia. *Blood* 79:299, 1992.

26. Miller WH, Jr., Levine K, DeBlasio A, et al.: Detection of minimal residual disease in acute promyelocytic leukemia by a reverse transcription polymerase chain reaction assay for the PML/RAR-α fusion mRNA. *Blood* 82:1689–94, 1993.

27. Bloomfield CD, de la Chappelle A: Chromosome abnormalities in acute nonlymphocytic leukemia: Clinical and biologic significance. *Semin Oncol* 14:372–83, 1987.

28. Downing JR, Look AT: MLL fusion genes in the 11q23 acute leukemias. *Cancer Treat Res* 84:73–92, 1996.

29. Rowley JD: The role of chromosome translocations in leukemogenesis. *Semin Hematol* 36:59–72, 1999.

30. Paietta E, Wiernik PH, Andersen J, et al.: Acute myeloid leukemia M4 with inv(16) (p13q22) exhibits a specific immunophenotype with CD2 expression. *Blood* 82:2595, 1993.

31. Testoni N, Borsaru G, Martinelli G, et al.: 3q21 and 3q26 cytogenetic abnormalities in acute myeloblastic leukemia: Biological and clinical features. *Haematologica* 84:690–4, 1999.

32. Leith CP, Kopecky KJ, Godwin J, et al.: Acute myeloid leukemia in the elderly: Assessment of multidrug resistance (MDR1) and cytogenetics distinguishes biologic subgroups with remarkably distinct responses to standard chemotherapy. A Southwest Oncology Group study. *Blood* 89:3323–9, 1997.

33. Sperling C, Buchner T, Creutzig U, et al.: Clinical, morphologic, cytogenetic and prognostic implications of CD34 expression in childhood and adult de novo AML. *Leuk Lymphoma* 17:417–26, 1995.

34. Pui CH, Evans WE: Genetic abnormalities and drug resistance in acute lymphoblastic leukemia. *Adv Exp Med Biol* 457:383–9, 1999.

35. Reed JC: Bcl-2 family proteins: Regulators of apoptosis and chemoresistance in hematologic malignancies. *Semin Hematol* 34:9–19, 1997.

36. Leith CP, Kopecky KJ, Chen IM, et al.: Frequency and clinical significance of the expression of the multidrug resistance proteins MDR1/P-glycoprotein, MRP1, and LRP in acute myeloid leukemia: A Southwest Oncology Group Study. *Blood* 94:1086–99, 1999.

37. Marie JP, Legrand O, Russo D, et al.: Multidrug resistance (MDR) gene expression in acute non lymphoblastic leukemia: sequential analysis. *Leuk Lymphoma* 8:261–5, 1992.

38. Call KM, Glaser T, Ito CY, et al.: Isolation and characteriztion of a zinc finger polypeptide gene at the human chromosome 11 Wilm's tumor locus. *Cell* 60:509–20, 1990.

39. Inoue K, Tamaki H, Ogawa H, et al.: Wilms' tumor gene (WT1) competes with differentiation-inducing signal in hematopoietic progenitor cells. *Blood* 91:2969–76, 1998.

40. Schmid D, Heinze G, Linnerth B, et al.: Prognostic significance of WT1 gene expression at diagnosis in adult de novo acute myeloid leukemia. *Leukemia* 11:639–43, 1997.

41. van Dongen JJ, Macintyre EA, Gabert JA, et al.: Standardized RT-PCR analysis of fusion gene transcripts from chromosome aberrations in acute leukemia for detection of minimal residual disease. Report of the BIOMED-1 Concerted Action: Investigation of minimal residual disease in acute leukemia. *Leukemia* 13:1901–28, 1999.

42. Jurlander J, Caligiuri MA, Ruutu T, et al.: Persistence of the AML1/ETO fusion transcript in patients treated with allogeneic bone marrow transplantation for t(8;21) leukemia [see Comments]. *Blood* 88:2183–91, 1996.

43. Rubnitz JE, Pui CH: Molecular diagnostics in the treatment of leukemia. *Curr Opin Hematol* 6:229–35, 1999.

44. Estey E: Prognostic factors in clinical cancer trials. *Clin Cancer Res* 3:2591–3, 1997.

45. Estey EH, Keating MJ, McCredie KB, et al.: Causes of initial remission induction failure in acute myelogenous leukemia. *Blood* 60:309–15, 1982.

46. Smith M, Arthur D, Camitta B, et al.: Uniform approach to risk classification and treatment assignment for children with acute lymphoblastic leukemia. *J Clin Oncol* 14:18–24, 1996.

47. Thomas DA, Cortes J, O'Brien S, et al.: Hyper-CVAD program in Burkitt's-type adult acute lymphoblastic leukemia. *J Clin Oncol* 17:2461–70, 1999.

48. Pui CH, Behm FG, Crist WM: Clinical and biologic relevance of immunologic marker studies in childhood acute lymphoblastic leukemia. *Blood* 82:343–62, 1993.

49. Rivera GK, Crist WM, Sallan SE: Biology and therapy of childhood acute lymphoblastic leukemia. *Rev Invest Clin Suppl* April; suppl. pm10 7886304 26–33, 1994.

50. Rubnitz JE, Pui CH: Recent advances in the biology and treatment of childhood acute lymphoblastic leukemia. *Curr Opin Hematol* 4:233–41, 1997.

51. Wetzler M, Dodge RK, Mrozek K, et al.: Prospective karyotype analysis in adult acute lymphoblastic leukemia: The cancer and leukemia Group B experience. *Blood* 93:3983–93, 1999.

52. Cimino G, Rapanotti MC, Sprovieri T, Elia L: ALL1 gene alterations in acute leukemia: Biological and clinical aspects. *Haematologica* 83:350–7, 1998.

53. Golub TR, Barker GF, Bohlander SK, et al.: Fusion of the TEL gene on 12p13 to the AML1 gene on 21q22 in acute lymphoblastic leukemia. *Proc Natl Acad Sci USA* 92:4917–21, 1995.

54. Loh ML, Silverman LB, Young ML, et al.: Incidence of TEL/AML1 fusion in children with relapsed acute lymphoblastic leukemia. *Blood* 92:4792–7, 1998.

55. Snyder DS, Nademanee AP, O'Donnell MR, et al.: Long-term follow-up of 23 patients with Philadelphia chromosome-positive acute lymphoblastic leukemia treated with allogeneic bone marrow transplant in first complete remission. *Leukemia* 13:2053–8, 1999.

56. Hoelzer D: Change in treatment strategies for adult acute lymphoblastic leukemia (ALL) according to prognostic factors and minimal residual disease. *Bone Marrow Transplant.* 6 (Suppl. 1):66–70, 1990.

57. Chao NJ, Blume KG, Forman SJ, Snyder DS: Long-term follow-up of allogeneic bone marrow recipients for Philadelphia chromosome-positive acute lymphoblastic leukemia [Letter]. *Blood* 85:3353–4, 1995.

58. Perentesis JP: Why is age such an important independent prognostic factor in acute lymphoblastic leukemia? *Leukemia* 11 (Suppl. 4): S4–7, 1997.

59. Silverman LB, Gelber RD, Young ML, et al.: Induction failure in acute lymphoblastic leukemia of childhood. *Cancer* 85:1395–1404, 1999.

60. Cortes J, Kantarjian HM, Giralt S, Talpaz M: Natural history and staging of chronic myelogenous leukaemia. *Baillieres Clin Haematol* 10:277–90, 1997.

61. Giralt S, Kantarjian H, Talpaz M: The natural history of chronic myelogenous leukemia in the interferon era. *Semin Hematol* 32:152–8, 1995.

62. Kantarjian HM, Smith TL, O'Brien S, et al.: Prolonged survival in chronic myelogenous leukemia after cytogenetic response to interferon-alpha therapy. The Leukemia Service. *Ann Intern Med* 122:254–61, 1995.

63. Cortes JE, Talpaz M, Kantarjian H: Chronic myelogenous leukemia: A review. *Am J Med* 100:555–70, 1996.

64. Messner HA, Fyles G, Meharchand J, et al.: Allogeneic bone marrow transplantation in chronic myeloid leukemia (CML). *New Strategies Bone Marrow Transplant* 145–154, 1991.

65. Cheson BD, Bennett JM, Grever M, et al.: National Cancer Institute-sponsored Working Group guidelines for chronic lymphocytic leukemia: Revised guidelines for diagnosis and treatment. *Blood* 87:4990–7, 1996.

66. Rai KR, Sawitsky A, Cronkite EP: Clinical staging of chronic lymphocytic leukemia. *Blood* 46:219–34, 1975.

67. Reed JC: Molecular biology of chronic lymphocytic leukemia: Implications for therapy. *Semin Hematol* 35:3–13, 1998.

68. Binet JL, Auquier A, Dighiero G, et al.: A new prognostic classification of chronic lymphocytic leukemia derived from a multivariate survival analysis. *Cancer* 48:198–206, 1981.

69. Molica S, Levato D, Cascavilla N, et al.: Clinico-prognostic implications of simultaneous increased serum levels of soluble CD23 and beta2-microglobulin in B-cell chronic lymphocytic leukemia. *Eur J Haematol* 62:117–22, 1999.

70. Aguayo A, Estey E, Kantarjian H, et al.: Cellular vascular endothelial growth factor is a predictor of outcome in patients with acute myeloid leukemia. *Blood* 94:3717–21, 1999.

BRAIN TUMORS

CHAPTER 45

Gliomas

HIROKO OHGAKI, GUIDO REIFENBERGER, KAZUHIRO NOMURA, and
PAUL KLEIHUES

Tumors of the nervous system amount to less than 2% of the total human cancer burden, the overall incidence being in the range of 7–9 new cases a year per 100,000 population. They affect all age groups and their etiology is largely unknown. More than 40 clinicopathological disease entities have been classified by the World Health Organization (WHO) and this makes the identification of factors with unequivocal prognostic value difficult.[1] Large, randomized therapy studies with long-term follow-up of a significant number of patients have concentrated on malignant gliomas of astrocytic and oligodendroglial origin.

During the past decade, numerous studies have been published that, in addition to conventional clinical and histopathological parameters, suggested certain genetic alterations as potential prognostic factors, but for tumors of the nervous system, few of these have been confirmed in subsequent reports. The establishment of reliable prognostic factors requires the critical, unbiased evaluation of large databases and often remains an elusive goal.

DIFFUSELY INFILTRATING ASTROCYTOMAS

Diffusely infiltrating astrocytomas are the most frequent intracranial neoplasms and account for more than 60% of all primary brain tumors. These gliomas share the following characteristics: (1) they can arise at any site in the central nervous system (CNS), mostly in the cerebral hemispheres, (2) they typically manifest in adults, (3) they have a wide range of histopathological features and biological behavior, (4) they diffusely infiltrate adjacent brain structures, and (5) they have an inherent tendency for malignant progression, with the glioblastoma as the most malignant phenotypic endpoint.[2] They must be strictly separated from the pilocytic astrocytoma of children and young adolescents, which is more

Prognostic Factors in Cancer, 2nd edition, Edited by Mary K. Gospodarowicz.
ISBN 0-471-40633-3   Copyright © 2001 Wiley-Liss, Inc.

confined, mostly affects the cerebellum and CNS midline structures, has a different biological basis, no tendency for malignant progression, and a more favorable clinical outcome (WHO, Grade I).

Diffusely infiltrating astrocytomas consist of three major entities, diffuse astrocytoma, anaplastic astrocytoma, and glioblastoma. The most frequently applied grading systems are those of WHO and St. Anne/Mayo (Table 45.1).

Diffuse Astrocytoma

The diffuse astrocytoma WHO Grade II is also referred to as low-grade diffuse astrocytoma or low-grade astrocytoma. This slowly growing astrocytic tumor typically affects young adults and is characterized by a high degree of cellular differentiation. Due to extensive infiltration of neighboring brain structures, diffuse astrocytomas usually recur, and this is often associated with progression to anaplastic astrocytoma or glioblastoma.[3]

Tumor-related Prognostic Factors

Several prognostic factors have been identified, but none of them allows a prediction of the clinical course in individual cases.

Histological Grading The mean survival time after surgical intervention is in the range of 6–8 years and thus is significantly longer than that of patients with anaplastic astrocytoma or glioblastoma (see below). Approximately 90% of patients with low-grade astrocytoma, but only 6% of patients with astrocytomas Grade III or IV, were found to survive more than 100 weeks.[4] The total length of disease ranges from less than 2 to more than 10 years and is mainly influenced by the dynamics of malignant progression to anaplastic astrocytoma or glioblastoma, which tends to occur after a mean time interval of 4–5 years.[5–8]

TABLE 45.1 Comparison of the World Health Organization and St. Anne/Mayo Grading System of Astrocytomas

WHO Grade	WHO Designation	St. Anne/Mayo Designation	St. Anne/Mayo Histological Criteria
I	Pilocytic astrocytoma		
II	Diffuse astrocytoma	Astrocytoma Grade 2	One criterion, usually nuclear atypia
III	Anaplastic astrocytoma	Astrocytoma Grade 3	Two criteria, usually nuclear atypia and mitotic activity
IV	Glioblastoma multiforme	Astrocytoma Grade 4	Three criteria: nuclear atypia, mitoses, endothelial proliferation and/or necrosis

Tumor Size The tumor size appeared to be an important predictive factor in a study of 379 gliomas (astrocytomas, oligodendrogliomas, and mixed oligoastrocytomas) in two multicentric randomized trials conducted by the European Organization for Research and Treatment of Cancer (EORTC).[9]

Histopathological Features It is generally acknowledged that low-grade astrocytomas with a significant fraction of *gemistocytes* tend to undergo malignant progression more rapidly than the ordinary fibrillary astrocytoma,[10–13] despite the fact that the majority of neoplastic gemistocytes are in a non-proliferative state (G_0 phase of the cell cycle) suggestive of terminal differentiation.[14]

The presence of numerous *microcysts* appears to be associated with a somewhat better prognosis.[13] Some studies indicate that *perivascular lymphocyte cuffing* is associated with a somewhat more favourable prognosis,[15,16] while others failed to note a correlation with patient survival.[17]

Microvessels Excessive angiogenesis (microvascular proliferation) is a hallmark of the glioblastoma, but incipient vessel proliferation and the secretion by glioma cells of vascular endothelial growth factor (VEGF) is already observed in some low-grade astrocytomas. The density of microvessels was predictive for a shorter survival for patients in retrospective series of 95 patients with low-grade astrocytomas, anaplastic astrocytomas, and glioblastomas. Patients carrying tumors with microvessel counts of 70 or more at × 200 magnification showed shorter survival (mean survival 51 weeks) compared to patients whose tumors had microvessel counts of less than 70 (mean survival of 106 weeks).[18] Similarly, patients with more microvessels in fibrillary low-grade astrocytoma had a significantly shorter survival time (mean 3.8 years) than those with fewer microvessels (mean survival 11.2 years).[19] Tumors with a higher density of microvessels also had a greater chance of undergoing malignant transformation. Similarly, significant staining for VEGF was correlated with shorter survival times and with more rapid malignant progression.[19]

Proliferation There is an overall correlation between the tumor growth fraction [as determined by the MIB-1 labeling index (LI)] and histological grade, with mean values of 3.8% for diffuse astrocytomas WHO Grade II, 18.4% for anaplastic astrocytomas WHO Grade III, and 31.6% for glioblastomas WHO Grade IV reported in one study.[20] Other authors have also found a correlation between LI and WHO Grade in astrocytic gliomas.[21,22] Accordingly, analyses of a wide range of astrocytic tumors showed a gross correlation of proliferation with clinical outcome.[23,24] A Ki67 LI >7.5% was associated with higher histological grade and poorer survival, and this value was a statistically more significant factor than histological grading.[25] In another study, a Ki67 LI of >5% was found to constitute a threshold value for predicting shorter survival.[4] Hsu et al.[22] suggested that a cutoff value of >1.5% MIB-1 LI was a significant independent predictor of shorter survival in patients with diffuse astrocytomas. Some studies suggest that in low-grade astrocytomas, the proliferative potential correlates inversely with survival and time to recurrence, but this finding is inconsistent and in individual cases, the size of the growth fraction as determined by the MIB-1 LI cannot be regarded as being prognostic.[13,17,25-27]

Genetic Alterations Neoplasms with *p53* mutations appear to progress more frequently, but the evidence for this correlation is still circumstantial.[28-30] The time interval until progression appears to be shorter in patients with low-grade astrocytomas carrying a *p53* mutation.[8] In the study by Chozick et al.,[31] immunoreactivity for p53 protein in diffuse astrocytomas was associated with shorter patient survival, but other studies showed that the presence of *p53* mutations or p53 accumulation had no effect on clinical outcome.[26,29,32,33] Even in the presence of a *p53* mutation in the first biopsy, long-term survival is possible in the absence of additional genetic alterations, for example, loss of heterozygosity (LOH) on chromosome 10 or chromosome arm 19q.[34]

Host-related Prognostic Factors

The only significant host-related factors appear to be the patients' age and the status of preoperative mental and neurological functions.

Age For the entire class of diffusely infiltrating astrocytomas, including diffuse astrocytomas WHO Grade II, manifestation at young age has been consistently predictive for a more favorable clinical course. Several studies showed that young age is clearly associated with a longer survival in low-grade astrocytomas.[35-37]

Preoperative Status Low-grade astrocytoma with epilepsy as the single symptom appears to have a better prognosis than if accompanied by other symptoms.[37] Conversely, presentation with a neurologic deficit is associated with a worse prognosis than presentation with seizures or pressure symptoms alone.[38]

Environment-related Prognostic Factors

Treatment-related Factors The discussion on prognostic factors in low-grade astrocytomas has largely concentrated on the extent of surgical resection and on whether or not adjuvant radio- or chemotherapy is advantageous.

Extent of Resection Survival rates at 1, 2, 3, and 4 years following surgery was 100%, 96%, 96%, and 96% for patients who underwent gross total resection, and 86%, 77%, 77%, and 64% for patients with subtotal resection of low-grade astrocytomas.[11] The cumulative recurrence or progression rates after 4 years were 26% after gross total resection and 80% after subtotal resection. In other studies the extent of surgery was highly significant ($P = 0.002$) on univariate analyses.[37,39] These reports suggest that an attempt to remove as many tumor cells as possible (cytoreductive surgery) is worth the effort. Other authors, however, maintain that at least for a subset of patients, diagnostic biopsy can be equally effective if followed by external radiation[40] or brachytherapy.[41]

Adjuvant Therapy The potential effect on patient survival of adjuvant radio- or chemotherapy has been discussed for many years and is still controversial.[40,42,43] Many oncology centers, particularly in North America, routinely apply adjuvant therapy,[44] while others, particularly in Europe, prefer a wait-and-see approach, recommending radiotherapy only after evidence for progression to anaplastic astrocytoma. The latter view is supported by a recent study showing no significant difference in survival between patients who did and those who did not receive radiotherapy for supratentorial fibrillary astrocytomas.[26] Survival was similar for 13 patients with supratentrial low-grade astrocytomas treated immediately after diagnosis and for 17 patients initially followed up and treated only after clinical or radiological progression (63% survival rate after 5 years).[37]

Anaplastic Astrocytoma

This lesion is histologically defined as diffusely infiltrating astrocytoma with focal or dispersed anaplasia and marked proliferative potential (Table 45.1). Anaplastic astrocytoma corresponds to WHO Grade III.[45] Anaplastic astrocytomas typically develop from low-grade diffuse astrocytoma WHO Grade II, but are also diagnosed at first biopsy.

Predictive Factors The progression of anaplastic astrocytoma to glioblastoma is a key prognostic factor. The time interval (time till progression) varies considerably, with a mean of 2 years[8] and a total length of disease of 3 years.[46] Factors predicting the clinical outcome have often been analyzed in conjunction with those for glioblastoma patients (see below) and showed increased survival associated with young age at onset, high preoperative Karnofsky score, and extent of surgical resection.[38] As for other gliomas with predominant astrocytic phenotype, the presence of an oligodendroglial component is associated with a significant increase in survival.[46]

Glioblastoma

This most malignant astrocytic tumor is composed of poorly differentiated neoplastic astrocytes and corresponds to WHO Grade IV. Histopathological features include cellular polymorphism, nuclear atypia, brisk mitotic activity, vascular thrombosis, microvascular proliferation, and necrosis (Table 45.1). Glioblastomas are preferentially located in the cerebral hemispheres and typically manifest in adults. They may develop from low-grade diffuse or anaplastic astrocytomas ("secondary glioblastoma"), but more frequently, they manifest after a short clinical history *de novo*, with no evidence of a less malignant precursor lesion ("primary glioblastoma").[47,48] It is still a matter of controversy, whether the prognosis of patients with secondary glioblastoma is better than,[49] or similar to,[50] that of patients with primary (*de novo*) lesions.

Numerous clinical trials have been conducted to determine prognostic factors for patients with glioblastoma, but to date, individual prediction of clinical outcome has remained an elusive goal. These attempts should be judged in view of the fact that glioblastomas are among the most malignant human neoplasm, patients with primary glioblastoma having a mean total length of disease of less than one year. A recent population-based study showed that after exclusion of glioblastomas with a significant oligodendroglial component, only 5 out of 279 patients (<2%) survived more than 3 years, irrespective of aggressive radio- and chemotherapy.[51]

Tumor-related Prognostic Factors

Histological Grading   The chance of a long, recurrence-free survival is closely associated with the intrinsic biology of the neoplasm as reflected in its histopathological features. Significant indicators of anaplasia include nuclear atypia, mitotic activity, cellularity, vascular proliferation, and necrosis. Historically, grading according to the four-tiered Kernohan system[52] prevailed, but today, the malignancy scale of the WHO classification is widely accepted.[1] For diffusely infiltrating astrocytomas, the St Anne/Mayo grading system has proved to be both reproducible and predictive of patient survival.[53,54] The grading schemes clearly distinguish glioblastomas from anaplastic astrocytomas. A decisive criterion for the diagnosis of glioblastoma is the presence of microvascular proliferation and/or necrosis. Barker et al.[55] carried out a multivariate analysis of postoperative survival in 275 glioblastoma patients and observed that the difference in survival between patients with necrosis-containing glioblastomas and patients with necrosis-free glioblastomas was only 2 months and the observed median survival was only 10.5 months, still significantly shorter than the survival of patients with anaplastic astrocytoma (3.5 years).

Necrosis   Several studies suggest that the presence and extent of necrosis in glioblastomas correlates with poor clinical outcome.[55–58] The area of necrosis was usually smaller in young adults, reflecting their overall more favorable prognosis (see below).

Proliferation   While some studies suggest that glioblastomas can be subdivided on the basis of their proliferative activity,[20,59,60] others have failed to detect significant differences.[61–64] There is general consensus that the MIB-1 LI and related proliferation markers do not allow a prognosis in individual patients. A hypertriploid DNA profile appears to correlate with prolonged survival,[65] and this correlates with the observation that the presence of multinucleated giant cells in glioblastomas is associated with a slightly better outcome.[56]

Genetic Alterations   Primary and secondary glioblastomas develop through different genetic pathways.[48] Amplification and/or overexpression of the *EGF* receptor *(EGFR)* gene is a hallmark of the primary *(de novo)* glioblastoma. Some studies have reported that amplification and overexpression of the *EGFR* gene in anaplastic astrocytomas and glioblastomas is associated with poor prognosis.[60,66–68] However, other investigators have not confirmed this finding.[62,69–71]

Mutation of the p53 tumor suppressor gene is the earliest genetic alteration in diffuse astrocytomas that progress to secondary glioblastoma. The presence of this mutation however, does not correlate with survival of glioblastoma patients.[70] Similarly, nuclear accumulation of the p53 protein in glioblastoma cells showed no prognostic significance.[38,62] Kaplan-Meier survival estimation demonstrated that *MDM2* overexpression in patients with anaplastic astrocytoma or with glioblastoma was associated with a shorter survival time,[70] but the Cox proportional hazards model did not confirm this tendency.[70] The presence of a *PTEN* mutation was not associated with survival,[72] but in one study, high levels of expression of *PTEN/MMAC1*[73] were found to be associated with longer survival. Low p16 expression was associated with poor survival in astrocytomas.[74] c-Met overexpression detected by immunohistochemistry was independent from MIB-1 LI, and patients with high-grade astrocytomas with c-Met overexpression showed a significant shorter survival $(P < 0.05)$.[75] There was no significant difference in postoperative survival between patients whose tumors expressed either c-myc or L-myc.[76]

Combinations of Genetic Alterations   Significant differences in patient survival were observed for glioblastomas with a *p53* mutation only (mean survival 13 months) and those with *p53* mutations and complete LOH on chromosome 10 (survival 5.2 months, $P = 0.0058$), and between patients with *p53* mutations only and those with complete LOH on chromosome 10 and *EGFR* amplification (mean survival 4 months, $P = 0.0033$).[77] The age-corrected survival time for patients with complete LOH on chromosome 10 and *EGFR* amplification was significantly shorter than that for patients with *p53* mutations only.[77] Newcomb et al.[78] examined the survival of 80 adult glioblastoma patients stratified by age to determine whether genetic alterations were associated with different survival outcomes. Survival testing using Kaplan-Meier plots for glioblastoma patients with or without altered expression of p16, p53, EGFR, MDM2, or Bcl-2 showed no significant differences by age group or by gene expression, indicating a lack of prognostic value for glioblastomas. Similarly, Galanis et al.[79] analyzed amplification of the *EGFR, CDK4, MDM2, N-MYC, CYCD1, PDGFR-α, MET, c-MYC* genes by Southern blot in 186 high-grade malignant gliomas and found no apparent correlation between the occurrence of gene amplification and patient survival.

Host-related Prognostic Factors

Age   Virtually every therapy trial has shown that young patients (below 45 years) have a considerably better prognosis than the elderly.[56,62,65,76,80,81] This can be explained, in part, by the higher frequency of secondary glioblastomas in younger patients,[56,82] but most data suggest an intrinsically more rapid malignant progression in elderly patients.[35] In a recent study, long-term glioblastoma survivors had a mean age of 45 years, and thus were significantly younger than all glioblastoma patients combined.[51]

Preoperative Status   A high score (≥ 70) in the preoperative Karnofsky Performance Status (KPS) has been shown to be associated with longer survival.[83,84]

Environment-related Prognostic Factors

Treatment-related Prognostic Factors

Extent of resection   Evaluation of the extent of resection as prognostic factor has been controversial, but there is some evidence that complete resection favors longer survival.[49,85–87] In one study using magnetic resonance imaging, individuals with malignant gliomas for which residual tumor visualized postoperatively, had a significantly higher (6.6-fold) risk of death (shorter survival time) than those in whom all of the contrast-enhancing tumor had been removed.[85] Not all studies show a significant survival difference for lesions with a greater extent of resection.[70,88] Bouvier-Labit et al.[62] reported that total or subtotal surgical excision were associated with a longer survival ($P < 0.05$) in a retrospective series of 63 glioblastomas. Similarly, Keles et al.[89] found that percent of resection related positively and volume of residual disease related negatively to patient survival.

Adjuvant Therapy   It is generally acknowledged that postoperative radiotherapy increases the mean survival of glioblastoma patients by 3–4 months.[70] However, doses of ≥ 60 gray (Gy) appear to be necessary. There is a large body of literature on various radiation sources, fractionation schemes as well as on external radiation versus implanted radioactive sources and intraoperative brachytherapy. Additional chemotherapy can increase the mean survival. In a meta-analysis the estimated increase in survival for patients treated with combination radiation and chemotherapy was 10.1% at 1 year and 8.6% at 2 years.[90] Another meta-analysis confirmed an effect of chemotherapy on patients' survival, nitrosoureas and platinums being most effective.[91] However, there are no unequivocal criteria that predict response to adjuvant therapy.

OLIGODENDROGLIOMAS

Oligodendroglioma (WHO Grade II) is a well-differentiated, slowly growing diffusely infiltrating tumor of adults typically located in the cerebral hemispheres and composed predominantly of cells morphologically resembling oligoden-droglia. Anaplastic oligodendroglioma (WHO Grade III) is an oligodendroglioma with focal or diffuse histological features of malignancy and a less favorable prognosis.[92]

Tumor-related Prognostic Factors

Tumor Size   The size of oligodendroglioma does not appear to be correlated with either survival or histologic grade.[93]

Location of Tumors   Location in the frontal lobe was found to carry a more favorable prognosis.[93–95]

Neuroimaging   Lack of contrast enhancement on neuroimaging is associated with better prognosis.[96]

Histological Grading   The WHO grading system recognizes two malignancy grades for oligodendroglial tumors: WHO Grade II for well-differentiated and WHO Grade III for anaplastic oligodendrogliomas. Grading according to WHO has been shown to be significantly predictive of survival.[97,98] Histological features typical for anaplastic oligodendroglioma (necrosis, high mitotic activity, increased cellularity, nuclear atypia, cellular pleomorphism, and microvascular proliferation) have been shown to be associated with worse prognosis.[99–104] The 5-years survival for oligodendroglioma of Grade II was 46% and for Grade III 10%.[105]

The four-tiered Kernohan and the St. Anne/Mayo grading system have also been applied to oligodendrogliomas and oligoastrocytomas. Tumor grade, as determined by these systems, was strongly associated with survival of *oligodendroglioma* patients.[103] Patients with Grade 1 or 2 tumors by either grading method had a median survival time of 9.8 years and 5- and 10-year survival rates of 75%, and 46%, respectively, compared to 3.9 years, 41%, and 20% for Grade 3 or 4 tumors.[103] Similarly, in a study of 71 patients with supratentorial *mixed oligoastrocytomas*, histological grade according to the Kernohan system was strongly associated with survival.[106]

Proliferation and Apoptosis   Numerous studies have focused on the prognostic significance of the growth fraction (Ki-67/MIB-1 LI) for patients with oligodendroglial tumors.[93,94,100,107,108] In a study of 89 oligodendroglioma patients, the 5-year survival rate was 83% for patients whose oligodendrogliomas had a MIB-1 LI of less than 5%, but only 24% for patients with tumors displaying more than 5% MIB-1 positive cells.[100] Similar data were reported by Coons et al.[107] Kros et al.[94] found the Ki-67 LI was of prognostic significance independent of patient age, tumor site, and histological grade. Other studies showed no correlation with survival[98] or response to chemotherapy.[109] In a study of 85 cases, 31% of tumors were diploid, 39% were tetraploid, and 31% were aneuploid, but there was no correlation with survival.[110] Determination of the apoptotic index is not of prognostic relevance in oligodendrogliomas.[98,118]

Genetic Alterations Patients whose anaplastic oligodendrogliomas have LOH on chromosome arm 1p or combined LOH on chromosome arms 1p and 19q have substantially prolonged survival (mean, approximately 10 years) compared with those patients whose tumors lack these genetic changes (mean survival of about 2 years).[109] A more recent study of 162 diffuse gliomas has confirmed the prognostic significance of combined LOH on 1p and 19q for oligodendroglioma patients, but not for patients with an astrocytoma or a mixed oligoastrocytoma.[111] Homozygous deletions of the *CDKN2A* gene were primarily detected in those anaplastic oligodendrogliomas that lacked 1p and 19q losses.[109] Patients whose tumors had *CDKN2A* deletions generally had shorter survivals.[109] Expression of *p16*, which is encoded by the *CDKN2A* locus, was frequently decreased in oligodendrogliomas and anaplastic oligodendrogliomas, and lack of *p16* expression predicted poor survival.[74] In one study,[112] there was no significant correlation between p53 protein accumulation or *EGFR* overexpression and prognosis of patients with oligodendrogliomas. In contrast, two other studies suggested that immunoreactivity for p53 in tumor cell nuclei correlates with reduced patient survival.[113,114]

Host-related Factors

Overall, up to three-quarters of patients with oligodendrogliomas survive 5 years from the time of diagnosis, with a median survival reported to be in the range of 6–10 years. For those with anaplastic oligodendrogliomas, median survival is in the range of 3–4 years (see review in Reference 115).

Age In a study of 208 patients with histologically confirmed oligodendrogliomas, the patients' age at diagnosis was 47 years, with a range of 3–76 years, and 6% of the oligodendrogliomas occurred in children.[101] Younger age at surgery is associated with longer survival.[93–95,103,106,116] One study reported a median survival of 17.5 years for the group of patients younger than 20 years and 13 months for the group of patients older than 60 years.[105] In a study of 19 children with oligodendrogliomas and mixed oligoastrocytomas, the 5-year survival was 65%, and younger children (<12 years) had a better prognosis than older children (12–18 years).[117]

Performance Score High postoperative Karnofsky score (>90) was associated with longer survival.[95] In addition, oligodendroglioma patients without neurological deficits had a 5-year survival rate of 43%, while those with neurological deficits had a 5-year survival rate of only 5%.[95]

Environment-related Prognostic Factors

Treatment-related Factors

Extent of Resection   In most studies, an association was found between the extent of resection and prolonged survival, in both oligodendroglioma and oligoastrocytoma.[95,100,101,103] In the study by Shaw et al.,[103] 19 patients who underwent gross total resection of their tumor had a median survival time of 12.6 years and 5- and 10-year survival rates of 74% and 59%, respectively, as compared to 4.9 years, 46%, and 23%, respectively, for 63 patients who had subtotal resection.

Genetic Alterations   The presence of ring enhancement on initial neuroimaging has been reported to correlate with a lack of response to PCV treatment and poor prognosis.[109] In addition, there is recent evidence that molecular genetic analysis may provide a more powerful means of separating anaplastic oligodendrogliomas into therapeutically and prognostically significant subgroups. Those anaplastic oligodendrogliomas that have allelic loss on the short arm of chromosome 1, or combined allelic losses on 1p and 19q, are typically sensitive to procarbazine, CCNU and vincristine (PCV) chemotherapy, with about half of such tumors showing complete neuroradiological responses to PCV.[109] On the other hand, only 25% of tumors that lack these genetic changes respond to PCV, with only rare complete responses. Thus, there appear to be at least two biologically distinct types of anaplastic oligodendrogliomas with markedly different clinical behavior. Whether such powerful molecular predictors of chemosensitivity apply also to low-grade oligodendrogliomas and mixed oligoastrocytomas remains to be shown.

SUMMARY

Primary glial brain tumors are a challenge to both physicians and patients. The examination of prognostic factors is difficult. There is no clinically useful staging classification for brain tumors. However, tumor size is an important prognostic factor. The histologic type and grade are essential factors, but of equal importance are patients' age, performance status, and degree of neurologic deficit (see Appendix 45A). Newer genetic alterations hold promise in predicting the outcome, but few are used in clinical practice today.

Prognostic factors in Brain Tumors

	Prognostic factors	Tumor Related	Host Related	Treatment Related
Diffuse low-grade astrocytoma	Essential[a]	Small tumor size	Young age No neurologic deficit	Gross total resection
	Additional[b]	Low proliferation rate (MIB-1 index) Lack of VEGF expression Absence of *p53* mutation		Radiotherapy Chemotherapy
Glioblastoma	Essential	Less extensive necrosis	Young age High preoperative performance status	Radiotherapy
	Additional	No *EGFR* overexpression		Gross total resection Adjuvant chemotherapy
Oligodendrogliomas	Essential	WHO grade II Frontal location Absence of contrast enhancement (MRI) LOH on 1p & 19q	Young age High preoperative performance status No neurologic deficit	Gross total resection Chemotherapy (tumor with LOH on 1p & 19q)
	Additional	No *p53* accumulation		

[a]Consistent finding in several independent studies.
[b]Predictive value controversial or borderline.

REFERENCES

1. Kleihues P, Cavenee WK (eds.): *Pathology and genetics of tumors of the nervous system*, Lyon, IARC Press, 2000.
2. Cavenee WK, Furnari FB, Nagane M, et al.: Diffusely infiltrating astrocytomas, in Kleihues P, Cavenee WK (eds.): *Pathology and genetics of tumors of the nervous system*. Lyon, IARC Press, 2000, pp. 10–21.

3. Kleihues P, Davis RL, Ohgaki H, et al.: Diffuse astrocytoma, in Kleihues P, Cavenee WK (eds.): *Pathology and genetics of tumors of the nervous system*. Lyon, IARC Press, 2000, pp. 22–6.

4. Jaros E, Perry RH, Adam L, et al.: Prognostic implications of p53 protein, epidermal growth factor receptor, and Ki-67 labelling in brain tumors. *Br J Cancer* 66:373–85, 1992.

5. McCormack BM, Miller DC, Budzilovich GN, et al.: Treatment and survival of low-grade astrocytoma in adults — 1977–1988. *Neurosurgery* 31:636–42, 1992.

6. Roelcke U, von Ammon K, Hausmann O, et al.: Operated low grade astrocytomas: A long term PET study on the effect of radiotherapy. *J Neurol Neurosurg Psychiatry* 66:644–7, 1999.

7. Vertosick FT, Jr., Selker RG, Arena VC: Survival of patients with well-differentiated astrocytomas diagnosed in the era of computed tomography. *Neurosurgery* 28:496–501, 1991.

8. Watanabe K, Sato K, Biernat W, et al.: Incidence and timing of *p53* mutations during astrocytoma progression in patients with multiple biopsies. *Clin Cancer Res* 3:523–30, 1997.

9. Karim AB, Maat B, Hatlevoll R, et al.: A randomized trial on dose-response in radiation therapy of low-grade cerebral glioma: European Organization for Research and Treatment of Cancer (EORTC) Study 22844. *Int J Radiat Oncol Biol Phys* 36:549–56, 1996.

10. Krouwer HG, Davis RL, Silver P, Prados M: Gemistocytic astrocytomas: A reappraisal. *J Neurosurg* 74:399–406, 1991.

11. Peraud A, Ansari H, Bise K, Reulen HJ: Clinical outcome of supratentorial astrocytoma WHO Grade II. *Acta Neurochir (Wien)* 140:1213–22, 1998.

12. Russell DS, Rubinstein LJ (eds.): *Pathology of tumors of the nervous system*, London, Arnold, 1989.

13. Schiffer D, Chio A, Giordana MT, et al.: Prognostic value of histologic factors in adult cerebral astrocytoma. *Cancer* 61:1386–93, 1988.

14. Watanabe K, Tachibana O, Yonekawa Y, et al.: Role of gemistocytes in astrocytoma progression. Lab Invest 76:277–84, 1997.

15. Brooks WH, Markesbery WR, Gupta GD, Roszman TL: Relationship of lymphocyte invasion and survival of brain tumor patients. *Ann Neurol* 4:219–24, 1978.

16. Palma L, Di Lorenzo N, Guidetti B: Lymphocytic infiltrates in primary glioblastomas and recidivous gliomas: Incidence, fate, and relevance to prognosis in 228 operated cases. *J Neurosurg* 49:854–61, 1978.

17. Ito S, Chandler KL, Prados MD, et al.: Proliferative potential and prognostic evaluation of low-grade astrocytomas. *J Neurooncol* 19:1–9, 1994.

18. Leon SP, Folkerth RD, Black PM: Microvessel density is a prognostic indicator for patients with astroglial brain tumors. *Cancer* 77:362–72, 1996.

19. Abdulrauf SI, Edvardsen K, Ho KL, et al.: Vascular endothelial growth factor expression and vascular density as prognostic markers of survival in patients with low-grade astrocytoma. *J Neurosurg* 88:513–20, 1998.

20. Wakimoto H, Aoyagi M, Nakayama T, et al.: Prognostic significance of Ki-67 labeling indices obtained using MIB-1 monoclonal antibody in patients with supratentorial astrocytomas. *Cancer* 77:373–80, 1996.

21. Ellison DW, Steart PV, Bateman AC, et al.: Prognostic indicators in a range of astrocytic tumors: An immunohistochemical study with Ki-67 and p53 antibodies. *J Neurol Neurosurg Psychiatry* 59:413–9, 1995.

22. Hsu DW, Louis DN, Efird JT, Hedley-Whyte ET: Use of MIB-1 (Ki-67) immunoreactivity in differentiating grade II and grade III gliomas. *J Neuropathol Exp Neurol* 56:857–65, 1997.

23. Hoshino T, Ahn D, Prados MD, et al.: Prognostic significance of the proliferative potential of intracranial gliomas measured by bromodeoxyuridine labeling. *Int J Cancer* 53:550–5, 1993.

24. Prados MD, Krouwer HG, Edwards MS, et al.: Proliferative potential and outcome in pediatric astrocytic tumors. *J Neurooncol* 13:277–82, 1992.

25. Montine TJ, Vandersteenhoven JJ, Aguzzi A, et al.: Prognostic significance of Ki-67 proliferation index in supratentorial fibrillary astrocytic neoplasms. *Neurosurgery* 34:674–8, 1994.

26. Hilton DA, Love S, Barber R, et al.: Accumulation of p53 and Ki67 expression do not predict survival in patients with fibrillary astrocytomas or the response of these tumors to radiotherapy. *Neurosurgery* 42:724–9, 1998.

27. Hoshino T, Rodriguez LA, Cho KG, et al.: Prognostic implications of the proliferative potential of low-grade astrocytomas. *J Neurosurg* 69:839–42, 1988.

28. Iuzzolino P, Ghimenton C, Nicolato A, et al.: p53 protein in low-grade astrocytomas: A study with long-term follow-up. *Br J Cancer* 69:586–91, 1994.

29. Kraus JA, Bolln C, Wolf HK, et al.: TP53 alterations and clinical outcome in low grade astrocytomas. *Genes Chromosomes Cancer* 10:143–9, 1994.

30. Rasheed BK, McLendon RE, Herndon JE et al.: Alterations of the *TP53* gene in human gliomas. *Cancer Res* 54:1324–30, 1994.

31. Chozick BS, Pezzullo JC, Epstein MH, Finch PW: Prognostic implications of p53 overexpression in supratentorial astrocytic tumors. *Neurosurgery* 35:831–7, 1994.

32. al Sarraj S, Bridges LR: p53 immunoreactivity in astrocytomas and its relationship to survival. *Br J Neurosurg* 9:143–9, 1995.

33. Schlegel U: [p53: An important or most overvalued tumor gene?] *Laryngol Rhinol Otol* 73:651–3, 1994.

34. Ohgaki H, Watanabe K, Peraud A, et al.: A case history of glioma progression. *Acta Neuropathol* 97:525–35, 1999.

35. Shafqat S, Hedley Whyte ET, Henson JW: Age-dependent rate of anaplastic transformation in low-grade astrocytoma. *Neurology* 52:867–9, 1999.

36. Shinoda J, Sakai N, Nakatani K, Funakoshi T: Prognostic factors in supratentorial WHO Grade II astrocytoma in adults. *Br J Neurosurg* 12:318–24, 1998.

37. van Veelen ML, Avezaat CJ, Kros JM, et al.: Supratentorial low grade astrocytoma: Prognostic factors, dedifferentiation, and the issue of early versus late surgery. *J Neurol Neurosurg Psychiatry* 64:581–7, 1998.

38. Danks RA, Chopra G, Gonzales MF, et al.: Aberrant p53 expression does not correlate with the prognosis in anaplastic astrocytoma. *Neurosurgery* 37:246–54, 1995.

39. Iwabuchi S, Bishara S, Herbison P, et al.: Prognostic factors for supratentorial low grade astrocytomas in adults. *Neurol Med Chir Tokyo* 39:273–9, 1999.

40. Lunsford LD, Somaza S, Kondziolka D, Flickinger JC: Brain astrocytomas: Biopsy, then irradiation. *Clin Neurosurg* 42:464–79, 1995.

41. Kreth FW, Faist M, Rossner R, et al.: Supratentorial World Health Organization Grade 2 astrocytomas and oligoastrocytomas. A new pattern of prognostic factors. *Cancer* 79:370–9, 1997.

42. Loiseau H, Dartigues JF, Cohadon F: Low-grade astrocytomas: Prognosis factors and elements of management. *Surg Neurol* 44:224–7, 1995.

43. Trautmann TG, Shaw EG: Supratentorial low-grade glioma: Is there a role for radiation therapy? *Ann Acad Med Singapore* 25:392–6, 1996.

44. Shaw EG: The low-grade glioma debate: Evidence defending the position of early radiation therapy. *Clin Neurosurg* 42:488–94, 1995.

45. Kleihues P, Davis RL, Coons SW, Burger PC: Anaplastic astrocytoma, in Kleihues P, Cavenee WK (eds.): *Pathology and genetics of tumors of the nervous system.* Lyon, IARC Press, 2000, pp. 27–8.

46. Donahue B, Scott CB, Nelson JS, et al.: Influence of an oligodendroglial component on the survival of patients with anaplastic astrocytomas: A report of Radiation Therapy Oncology Group 83–02. *Int J Radiat Oncol Biol Phys* 38:911–4, 1997.

47. Kleihues P, Burger PC, Collins VP, et al.: Glioblastoma, in Kleihues P, Cavenee WK (eds.): *Pathology and genetics of tumors of the nervous system.* Lyon, IARC Press, pp. 29–39, 2000.

48. Kleihues P, Ohgaki H: Primary and secondary glioblastomas: From concept to clinical diagnosis. *Neuro-Oncology* 1:44–51, 1999.

49. Winger MJ, Macdonald DR, Cairncross JG: Supratentorial anaplastic gliomas in adults. The prognostic importance of extent of resection and prior low-grade glioma. *J Neurosurg* 71:487–93, 1989.

50. Dropcho EJ, Soong SJ: The prognostic impact of prior low grade histology in patients with anaplastic gliomas: A case-control study. *Neurology* 47:684–90, 1996.

51. Scott JN, Rewcastle NB, Brasher PM, et al.: Long-term glioblastoma multiforme survivors: A population-based study. *Can J Neurol Sci* 25:197–201, 1998.

52. Kernohan JW, Mabon RF, Svien HJ, Adson AW: A simplified classification of gliomas. *Proc Staff Meet Mayo Clin* 24:71–5, 1949.

53. Daumas-Duport C, Scheithauer B, O'Fallon J, Kelly P: Grading of astrocytomas. A simple and reproducible method. *Cancer* 62:2152–65, 1988.

54. Kim TS, Halliday AL, Hedley Whyte ET, Convery K: Correlates of survival and the Daumas-Duport grading system for astrocytomas. *J Neurosurg* 74:27–37, 1991.

55. Barker FG, Davis RL, Chang SM, Prados MD: Necrosis as a prognostic factor in glioblastoma multiforme. *Cancer* 77:1161–6, 1996.

56. Burger PC, Green SB: Patient age, histologic features, and length of survival in patients with glioblastoma multiforme. *Cancer* 59:1617–25, 1987.

57. Nelson JS, Tsukada Y, Schoenfeld D, et al.: Necrosis as a prognostic criterion in malignant supratentorial, astrocytic gliomas. *Cancer* 52:550–4, 1983.

58. Pierallini A, Bonamini M, Pantano P, et al.: Radiological assessment of necrosis in glioblastoma: Variability and prognostic value. *Neuroradiology* 40:150–3, 1998.

59. Haapasalo HK, Sallinen PK, Helen PT, et al.: Comparison of three quantitation methods for PCNA immunostaining: Applicability and relation to survival in 83 astrocytic neoplasms. *J Pathol* 171:207–14, 1993.

60. Torp SH, Helseth E, Dalen A, Unsgaard G: Relationships between Ki-67 labelling index, amplification of the epidermal growth factor receptor gene, and prognosis in human glioblastomas. *Acta Neurochir (Wien)* 117:182–6, 1992.

61. Barker FG, Prados MD, Chang SM, et al.: Bromodeoxyuridine labeling index in glioblastoma multiforme: Relation to radiation response, age, and survival. *Int J Radiat Oncol Biol Phys* 34:803–8, 1996.

62. Bouvier-Labit C, Chinot O, Ochi C, et al.: Prognostic significance of Ki67, p53 and epidermal growth factor receptor immunostaining in human glioblastomas. *Neuropathol Appl Neurobiol* 24:381–8, 1998.

63. Pigott TJ, Lowe JS, Palmer J: Statistical modelling in analysis of prognosis in glioblastoma multiforme: A study of clinical variables and Ki-67 index. *Br J Neurosurg* 5:61–6, 1991.

64. Scott CB, Nelson JS, Farnan NC, et al.: Central pathology review in clinical trials for patients with malignant glioma. A Report of Radiation Therapy Oncology Group 83–02. *Cancer* 76:307–13, 1995.

65. Salmon I, Dewitte O, Pasteels JL, et al.: Prognostic scoring in adult astrocytic tumors using patient age, histopathological grade, and DNA histogram type. *J Neurosurg* 80:877–83, 1994.

66. Eppenberger U, Mueller H: Growth factor receptors and their ligands. *J Neurooncol* 22:249–54, 1994.

67. Hiesiger EM, Hayes RL, Pierz DM, Budzilovich GN: Prognostic relevance of epidermal growth factor receptor (EGF-R) and c-neu/erbB2 expression in glioblastomas (GBMs). *J Neurooncol* 16:93–104, 1993.

68. Hurtt MR, Moossy J, Donovan Peluso M, Locker J: Amplification of epidermal growth factor receptor gene in gliomas: Histopathology and prognosis. *J Neuropathol Exp Neurol* 51:84–90, 1992.

69. Bigner SH, Burger PC, Wong AJ, et al.: Gene amplification in malignant human gliomas: Clinical and histopathologic aspects. *J Neuropathol Exp Neurol* 47:191–205, 1988.

70. Rainov NG, Dobberstein KU, Bahn H, et al.: Prognostic factors in malignant glioma: Influence of the overexpression of oncogene and tumor-suppressor gene products on survival. *J Neurooncol* 35:13–28, 1997.

71. Waha A, Baumann A, Wolf HK, et al.: Lack of prognostic relevance of alterations in the epidermal growth factor receptor-transforming growth factor-α pathway in human astrocytic gliomas. *J Neurosurg* 85:634–41, 1996.

72. Zhou XP, Li YJ, Hoang-Xuan K, et al.: Mutational analysis of the *PTEN* gene in gliomas: Molecular and pathological correlations. *Int J Cancer* 84:150–4, 1999.

73. Sano T, Lin H, Chen X, Langford LA, et al.: Differential expression of *MMAC/PTEN* in glioblastoma multiforme: Relationship to localization and prognosis. *Cancer Res* 59:1820–4, 1999.

74. Miettinen H, Kononen J, Sallinen P, et al.: CDKN2/p16 predicts survival in oligodendrogliomas: Comparison with astrocytomas. *J Neurooncol* 41:205–11, 1999.

75. Hirose Y, Kojima M, Sagoh M, et al.: Clinical importance of c-Met protein expression in high grade astrocytic tumors. *Neurol Med Chir Tokyo* 38:851–9, 1998.

76. Herms JW, von Loewenich FD, Behnke J, et al.: c-myc oncogene family expression in glioblastoma and survival. *Surg Neurol* 51:536–42, 1999.

77. Leenstra S, Oskam NT, Bijleveld EH, et al.: Genetic sub-types of human malignant astrocytoma correlate with survival. *Int J Cancer* 79:159–65, 1998.

78. Newcomb EW, Cohen H, Lee SR, et al.: Survival of patients with glioblastoma multiforme is not influenced by altered expression of p16, p53, EGFR, MDM2 or Bcl-2 genes. *Brain Pathol* 8:655–67, 1998.

79. Galanis E, Buckner J, Kimmel D, et al.: Gene amplification as a prognostic factor in primary and secondary high-grade malignant gliomas. *Int J Oncol* 13:717–24, 1998.

80. Korkolopoulou P, Christodoulou P, Lekka-Katsouli I, et al.: Prognostic significance of proliferating cell nuclear antigen (PCNA) expression in gliomas. *Histopathology* 25:349–55, 1994.

81. Sneed PK, Prados MD, McDermott MW, et al.: Large effect of age on the survival of patients with glioblastoma treated with radiotherapy and brachytherapy boost. *Neurosurgery* 36:898–904, 1995.

82. Watanabe K, Tachibana O, Sato K, et al.: (1996) Overexpression of the EGF receptor and *p53* mutations are mutually exclusive in the evolution of primary and secondary glioblastomas. *Brain Pathol* 6:217–224

83. Ampil FL, Nanda A, Willis BK, Apple S: Treatment in patients with glioblastoma multiforme and poor performance status: Is it worthwhile? *Radiat Med* 16:109–12, 1998.

84. Barker FG2, Chang SM, Gutin PH, et al.: Survival and functional status after resection of recurrent glioblastoma multiforme. *Neurosurgery* 42:709–20, 1998.

85. Albert FK, Forsting M, Sartor K, et al.: Early postoperative magnetic resonance imaging after resection of malignant glioma: Objective evaluation of residual tumor and its influence on regrowth and prognosis. *Neurosurgery* 34:45–60, 1994.

86. Devaux BC, O'Fallon JR, Kelly PJ: Resection, biopsy, and survival in malignant glial neoplasms. A retrospective study of clinical parameters, therapy, and outcome. *J Neurosurg* 78:767–75, 1993.

87. Wood JR, Green SB, Shapiro WR: The prognostic importance of tumor size in malignant gliomas: A computed tomographic scan study by the Brain Tumor Cooperative Group. *J Clin Oncol* 6:338–43, 1988.

88. Kreth FW, Warnke PC, Scheremet R, Ostertag CB: Surgical resection and radiation therapy versus biopsy and radiation therapy in the treatment of glioblastoma multiforme. *J Neurosurg* 78:762–6, 1993.

89. Keles GE, Anderson B, Berger MS: The effect of extent of resection on time to tumor progression and survival in patients with glioblastoma multiforme of the cerebral hemisphere. *Surg Neurol* 52:371–9, 1999.

90. Fine HA, Dear KB, Loeffler JS, et al.: Meta-analysis of radiation therapy with and without adjuvant chemotherapy for malignant gliomas in adults. *Cancer* 71:2585–97, 1993.

91. Huncharek M, Muscat J: Treatment of recurrent high grade astrocytoma: Results of a systematic review of 1,415 patients. *Anticancer Res* 18(2B):1303–11, 1998.

92. Reifenberger G, Kros JM, Burger PC, et al.: Oligodendroglioma, in Kleihues P, Cavenee WK (eds.): *Pathology and genetics of tumors of the nervous system.* Lyon, IARC Press, 2000, pp. 56–61.

93. Kros JM, Pieterman H, Van Eden CG, Avezaat CJ: Oligodendroglioma: The Rotterdam-Dijkzigt experience. *Neurosurgery* 34:959–66, 1994.

94. Kros JM, Hop WC, Godschalk JJ, Krishnadath KK: Prognostic value of the proliferation-related antigen Ki-67 in oligodendrogliomas. *Cancer* 78:1107–13, 1996.

95. Schiffer D, Dutto A, Cavalla P, et al.: Prognostic factors in oligodendroglioma. *Can J Neurol Sci* 24:313–9, 1997.

96. Daumas-Duport C, Tucker ML, Kolles H, et al.: Oligodendrogliomas. Part II: A new grading system based on morphological and imaging criteria. *J Neurooncol* 34:61–78, 1997.

97. Hagel C, Krog B, Laas R, Stavrou DK: Prognostic relevance of TP53 mutations, p53 protein, Ki-67 index and conventional histological grading in oligodendrogliomas. *J Exp Clin Cancer Res* 18:305–9, 1999.

98. Wharton SB, Hamilton FA, Chan WK, et al.: Proliferation and cell death in oligo-dendrogliomas. *Neuropathol Appl Neurobiol* 24:21–8, 1998.

99. Burger PC, Rawlings CE, Cox EB, et al.: Clinicopathologic correlations in the oligodendroglioma. *Cancer* 59:1345–52, 1987.

100. Dehghani F, Schachenmayr W, Laun A, Korf HW: Prognostic implication of histopathological, immunohistochemical and clinical features of oligodendrogliomas: A study of 89 cases. *Acta Neuropathol* 95:493–504, 1998.

101. Mork SJ, Lindegaard KF, Halvorsen TB, et al.: Oligodendroglioma: Incidence and biological behavior in a defined population. *J Neurosurg* 63:881–9, 1985.

102. Mork SJ, Halvorsen TB, Lindegaard KF, Eide GE: Oligodendroglioma. Histologic evaluation and prognosis. *J Neuropathol Exp Neurol* 45:65–78, 1986.

103. Shaw EG, Scheithauer BW, O'Fallon JR, et al.: Oligodendrogliomas: The Mayo Clinic experience. *J Neurosurg* 76:428–34, 1992.

104. Smith MT, Ludwig CL, Godfrey AD, Armbrustmacher VW: Grading of oligoden-drogliomas. *Cancer* 52:2107–14, 1983.

105. Westergaard L, Gjerris F, Klinken L: Prognostic factors in oligodendrogliomas. *Acta Neurochir (Wien)* 139:600–5, 1997.

106. Shaw EG, Scheithauer BW, O'Fallon JR, Davis DH: Mixed oligoastrocytomas: A survival and prognostic factor analysis. *Neurosurgery* 34:577–82, 1994.

107. Coons SW, Johnson PC, Pearl DK: The prognostic significance of Ki-67 labeling indices for oligodendrogliomas. *Neurosurgery* 41:878–84, 1997.

108. Heegaard S, Sommer HM, Broholm H, Broendstrup O: Proliferating cell nuclear antigen and Ki-67 immunohistochemistry of oligodendrogliomas with special reference to prognosis. *Cancer* 76:1809–13, 1995.

109. Cairncross JG, Ueki K, Zlatescu MC, et al.: Specific genetic predictors of chemotherapeutic response and survival in patients with anaplastic oligoden-drogliomas. *J Natl Cancer Inst* 90:1473–9, 1998.

110. Kros JM, Van Eden CG, Vissers CJ, et al.: Prognostic relevance of DNA flow cytometry in oligodendroglioma. *Cancer* 69:1791–8, 1992.

111. Smith JS, Perry A, Borell TJ, et al.: Alterations of chromosome arms 1p and 19q as predictors of survival in oligodendrogliomas, astrocytomas, and mixed oligoastrocytomas. *J Clin Oncol* 18:636–45, 2000.

112. Broholm H, Bols B, Heegaard S, Braendstrup O: Immunohistochemical investi-gation of p53 and EGFR expression of oligodendrogliomas. *Clin Neuropathol* 18:176–80, 1999.

113. Kros JM, Godschalk JJ, Krishnadath KK, van Eden CG: Expression of p53 in oligodendrogliomas. *J Pathol* 171:285–90, 1993.

114. Pavelic J, Hlavka V, Poljak M, et al.: p53 immunoreactivity in oligodendrogliomas. *J Neurooncol* 22:1–6, 1994.

115. Peterson K, Cairncross JG: Oligodendroglioma. *Cancer Invest* 14:243–51, 1996.

116. Shimizu KT, Tran LM, Mark RJ, Selch MT: Management of oligodendrogliomas. *Radiology* 186:569–72, 1993.

117. Razack N, Baumgartner J, Bruner J: Pediatric oligodendrogliomas. *Pediatr Neurosurg* 28:121–9, 1998.

118. Schiffer D, Dutto A, Cavalla P, Chio A, Migheli A, Piva R (1997b) Role of apoptosis in the prognosis of oligodendrogliomas. Neurochem Int 31:245–250.

PEDIATRIC TUMORS

CHAPTER 46

Pediatric Cancers

KAREN J. MARCUS and DAVID HODGSON

Pediatric cancers include a broad spectrum of diseases. Cancer is diagnosed in only 8400 children in the United States less than 15 years of age annually, although death from cancer is the second major cause of mortality in developed countries. Childhood cancers differ from adult cancers in their origins and histologic subtypes, their etiologies, their response to treatment, and the outcomes. In the adult population, epithelial cancers are most common and many are related to environmental carcinogens. In contrast, pediatric malignancies more commonly arise in hematopoietic tissue or in the central nervous system (CNS).

The most common pediatric malignancies are acute leukemia, non-Hodgkin's lymphoma, Hodgkin's disease, and primary CNS tumors. Neuroblastoma, Wilms' tumor, rhabdomyosarcoma, and retinoblastomas are the most common solid tumors occurring in children. The etiology of most childhood malignancies is unknown, although some solid tumors do occur in association with recognized genetic defects. Bilateral retinoblastoma, for instance, occurs in children with mutations in the retinoblastoma tumor suppressor gene *RB1*.[1] Wilms' tumor occurs in association with mutations in the *WT1* gene in the Denys-Drash Syndrome. Rhabdomyosarcomas are seen in children with the LiFraumeni syndrome with *p53* gene mutations.[2,3]

Major advances in cancer genetics and the molecular biology of cancer have been gained through research in pediatric malignancies. Despite its rarity in comparison to adult malignancies, many of the most important discoveries about cancer biology and cancer genetics have come from research in pediatric cancers. In addition, the role of prognostic factors in determining treatment for an individual patient is best exemplified by neuroblastoma which is discussed in this chapter. At the present time, only a limited number of cancers in children have prognostic factors that have been prospectively evaluated and confirmed. In this chapter, we review those pediatric cancers that have clearly defined

Prognostic Factors in Cancer, *2nd edition*, Edited by Mary K. Gospodarowicz.
ISBN 0-471-40633-3 Copyright © 2001 Wiley-Liss, Inc.

prognostic factors. The understanding of cancer genetics gained from the study of pediatric cancers, the identification of prognostic factors, their confirmation in clinical trials, and their widespread acceptance can be viewed as a paradigm for prognostic factors in cancer patient management.

NEUROBLASTOMA

Neuroblastoma (NBL), the fourth most common pediatric malignancy, representing 8–10% of cancers in children under 15 years of age, is a tumor for which prognostic factors, tumor and host-related, have been established and are used in not only assessing prognosis but in determining therapy. Neuroblastoma originates from the autonomic nervous system and can occur anywhere this tissue is found. The most common sites are the abdomen (with an adrenal primary), the spinal ganglia, the thoracic ganglia, or the pelvis (primary in the organ of Zuckercandl). Presentation of patients varies depending on the primary site and extent of disease. The median age at diagnosis is 2 years; however, half of all malignancies are diagnosed in the first month of life, and one-third of all malignancies diagnosed in the first year of life are NBL.

Neuroblastoma is unique among human cancers in its ability to undergo spontaneous differentiation and regression. Disseminated NBL in a subset of infants with metastatic disease involving the liver, skin, and limited infiltration of the bone marrow can spontaneously regress. Residual microscopic disease following a resected localized NBL rarely results in recurrence of disease. The unique clinical behavior has been known for several years; however, recent research in the molecular biology of NBL has led to advances in the treatment of the disease.

Prognostic factors that are used to stratify patients into risk groups include those that are tumor related and those that are host related. The tumor-related factors are the stage of disease, *MYCN* gene amplification, Shimada histopathology, DNA ploidy, deletions of chromosome 1, gains of chromosome 17, and nerve growth-factor receptor (TRK-A) expression. The latter factor is being confirmed in clinical trials, whereas the others are currently accepted as prognostic factors.

The staging system now recommended for NBL is known as the International Staging System (INSS). Developed by an international conference the INSS was presented for discussion at the Fourth International Research Symposium on Advances in Neuroblastoma Research held in Philadelphia in May 1987 (Table 46.1). In addition to the newly agreed-upon staging system, criteria for the diagnosis of NBL and strict definitions of response were established.[4] Patients with Stage 1–2A disease are considered to have low stage, those with Stage 2B–3 are considered to have intermediate stage, and those with Stage 4 disease are considered advanced.

The other tumor-related factors have shown clinical significance in patients with NBL. Amplification of *MYCN* was found in approximately 25% of primary tumors and was strongly correlated with advanced disease.[5,6] Independent of age

TABLE 46.1   International Neuroblastoma Staging System

Stage	
1	Localized tumor with complete gross excision, with or without microscopic residual disease; representative ipsilateral lymph nodes negative for tumor microscopically (lymph nodes adherent to and removed with primary may be positive)
2A	Localized tumor with incomplete gross excision; representative ipsilateral nonadherent lymph nodes negative for tumor microscopically
2B	Localized tumor with or without complete gross excision, with ipsilateral nonadherent lymph nodes positive for tumor; enlarged contralateral lymph nodes must be negative microscopically
3	Unresectable unilateral tumor infiltrating across the midline, with or without regional lymph-node involvement; or localized unilateral tumor with contralateral regional lymph-node involvement; or midline tumor with bilateral extension by infiltration (unresectable) or by lymph-node involvement
4	Any primary tumor with dissemination to distant lymph nodes, bone, bone marrow, liver, skin, and/or other organs (except as defined for stage 4S)
4S	Limited to infants under 1 yr of age and localized primary tumor (as defined for stage 1, 2A, or 2B) with dissemination limited to skin, liver, and/or bone marrow (bone marrow involvement must be less than 10% of total nucleated cells identified as malignant on bone marrow biopsy or aspirate; more extensive bone marrow involvement is considered Stage 4.

and stage of the patients, however, *MYCN* amplification was associated with rapid tumor progression and poor clinical outcome.[5,6] These studies suggest that *MYCN* amplification is a marker of aggressive tumor biology in some patients. Loss of heterozygosity of chromosome 1p is strongly associated with *MYCN* amplification, and both of these markers are associated with poor outcome of patients; however, it is not known whether these two markers are independent prognostic variables.[7,8] Gain of chromosome 17 is now a negative prognostic factor in NBL.[9]

Although the pathogenesis of NBL is unknown, the tumor is believed to originate the sympathoadrenal cells of the neural crest. Studies of neurotrophic factors and their tyrosine kinase receptors in NBL have shown a correlation between the expression of the nerve growth-factor receptor TRK-A and clinical outcome.[10] TRK-A expression showed a strong correlation with survival; the 5-year survival of patients with high expression was 86% compared to 14% survival in the patients with low TRK-A expression ($p < 0.001$). Although the biologic role of nerve growth factor and TRK-A in NBL is unknown, some theorize that the expression of these factors reflect the propensity of NBL to regress or differentiate.

The principal host-related factor in NBL is the age of the patient. Children under one year have a significantly improved outcome than those over one year. This is true independent of stage. Neuroblastomas can be divided into genetically distinct groups based on biological properties. When these biologic characteristics are combined with clinical properties, patients can be stratified into risk groups and therapy can be tailored based on these clinical and biological groupings.

WILMS' TUMOR

Wilms' tumor is the most common primary malignant renal tumor of childhood. Several prognostic factors have been identified through the National Wilms' Tumor Study Group (NWTS) trials, which are used to determine treatment for patients with Wilms' tumor. The tumor-related factors include histology, stage of disease, vascular invasion capsular invasion, presence of lymph-node metastases, and tumor size. As treatments have improved, some factors have diminished significance. The staging system for Wilms' tumor is a surgical staging system that includes such factors as margin status, invasion of the renal sinus, integrity of the renal capsule, tumor spill, prior biopsy, and lymph-node status, but does not take into account the size of the tumor or histology (Table 46.2).

TABLE 46.2   Staging System for Wilms' Tumor from National Wilms' Tumor Study Group

STAGE I	Tumor limited to the kidney, completely excised. Renal capsule has an intact outer surface. Tumor not ruptured or sampled for biopsy prior to removal (fine needle aspiration excluded). Vessels of renal sinus are not involved. No evidence of tumor at or beyond the margins of resection.
STAGE II	Tumor extended beyond kidney but was completely excised. Regional extension such as penetration of renal capsule or extensive invasion of renal sinus; blood vessels outside renal parenchyma including vessels of renal sinus, may contain tumor.; biopsy performed prior to resection, excluding fine needle aspiration; spillage before or during surgery that was confined to the flank and did not involve the peritoneal surface. No evidence of tumor at or beyond the margins of resection.
STAGE III	Residual nonhematogenous tumor is present, confined to the abdomen. Any of the following: a) lymph nodes within the abdomen or pelvis involved by tumor; intrathoracic or other extra-abdominal lymph nodes are considered Stage IV b) tumor penetrated peritoneal surface c) tumor implants found on peritoneal surface d) gross or microscopic tumor remains post-operatively e) tumor not completely resectable because of local infiltration into vital structures f) tumor spillage not confined to the flank before or during surgery
STAGE IV	Hematogenous metastases (lung, liver, bone, brain, etc) or lymph node metastases outside the abdominopelvic region.
STAGE V	Bilateral renal involvement is present at diagnosis. Each side should be staged individually.

Histology is the most important prognostic determinant. Wilms' tumor pathology is classified as favorable histology, favorable histology with focal anaplasia, and unfavorable histology or diffuse anaplasia. Wilms' tumor is classically composed of three cell types: blastemal, stromal, and epithelial. Anaplastic tumors contain cells with giant polypoid nuclei. Tumors are considered focally anaplastic if the anaplastic features are confined to a single focus within the tumor; tumors with more extensive anaplasia are considered to be diffusely anaplastic. Patients with diffuse anaplasia have a worse prognosis than those whose tumors contain no anaplasia or only focal anaplasia. The 4-year relapse-free survival rate for children with diffuse anaplastic Wilms' tumor treated on the NWTS-IV study was 54.8% for those patients who received cyclophosphamide in their treatment regimen and 27.2% for those who did not.[11]

There are two other categories of Wilms' tumor pathology, which also arise in the kidney in children and have been included on the NWTS trials. Clear-cell sarcoma of the kidney is associated with a higher relapse rate and lower survival rate than favorable histology Wilms' tumor. Clear-cell sarcoma is also known to metastasize to bone, and lung and its propensity to go to bone is much higher than favorable histology Wilms' tumor.[12,13] Rhabdoid tumor of the kidney is not related to classic Wilms' tumor. The cell of origin is unknown. This tumor is also associated with separate primary neuroectodermal tumors of the brain. This histologic subtype is also associated with a worse outcome than favorable histology Wilms' tumor.

The principal host-related factor of clear prognostic significance is the age of the patient. Children less than 2 years of age had a significantly better prognosis than those over 2, as reported on NWTS-I.[14] Children with genitourinary abnormalities, as well as those with hemihypertrohpy, and other genetic syndromes, such as Beckwith-Wiedemann, Denys-Drash, and WAGR syndrome, are at increased risk of developing a Wilms' tumor and are also at increased risk for developing bilateral Wilms' tumor.[15-17] Precursor lesions to Wilms' tumor, nephrogenic rests, are found in the normal kidney of 30% of patients with Wilms' tumor. Children with nephrogenic rests are also at increased risk of developing a Wilms' tumor.[18] However, the presence of these factors does not alter the prognosis once a Wilms' tumor is diagnosed.

Prospective randomized trials by the NWTS have contributed greatly not only to the best clinical management but to the understanding of the pathogenesis of Wilms' tumor. Children with favorable histology Wilms' tumor Stages I–III have 4-year overall survival of over 90%, and those with favorable histology and Stage IV disease have 4-year survival of approximately 80%. Those with unfavorable histology Stages I–III have survival close to 70%, while survival for those with Stage IV disease and unfavorable histology is 50%. Children with the clear-cell variant have an expected 4-year survival of approximately 75%, while those patients with the rhabdoid variant have an expected it year survival of only 25%.

One of the objectives of the current Wilms' tumor study is to determine the prognostic significance of various biologic markers. These include chromosomal abnormalities such as the loss of heterozygosity of chromosome 16q, loss of heterozygosity of chromosome 1p, and DNA content of the tumor cells. These represent new and potentially promising prognostic factors.

ACUTE LYMPHOBLASTIC LEUKEMIA

Acute leukemia represents over one-third of malignancies in children.[19] The majority of these leukemias are lymphoblastic. A uniform approach to prognostic factors for risk classification and treatment has been developed.[20] Several essential tumor-related factors have been identified for childhood ALL. The presenting white blood cell count (WBC) has powerful prognostic significance for B-precursor ALL. A WBC of less than 50,000 is considered standard risk, with higher counts indicating high-risk disease. The immunophenotyping considers tumors with B-precursor phenotype to be standard risk, while most groups consider those with T-cell immunophenotype high risk. Tumor cytogenetics is a second tumor-related factor, with the specific chromosomal abnormalities t(9;22), t(4;11), t(1;19) having adverse prognostic significance.[21,22] By contrast, the TEL-AML1 translocation is a cytogenetic abnormality that appears to carry a favorable prognosis.[23-25] CNS involvement is considered an adverse prognostic factor. Children who present with CNS blasts are considered high risk.[26] Additional tumor factors in ALL have been identified. The DNA index as determined by flow cytometry has been shown to be an important prognostic factor, with hyperdiploid tumor cells (DI >1.6) considered favorable. Early response to therapy is recognized as a critical prognostic factor.[20] For several groups this is determined by the day-14 bone marrow; that is, the bone marrow obtained after 14 days of induction chemotherapy.[27] (BFM) studies use an 8-day corticosteroid response in the peripheral blood to assign patients to risk strata.[28] The uniformly agreed-upon host-related factor in childhood ALL is the age at diagnosis. Children under one year or over 9 years are considered high risk. Infants and adolescents have a poorer prognosis.

RHABDOMYOSARCOMA

Rhabdomyosarcoma (RMS), a tumor of skeletal muscle derivation, is the most common soft tissue tumor of childhood and represents 5% to 8% of all cancers in children. The clinical grouping is a surgicopathologic system that was developed by the Intergroup Rhabdomyosarcoma Study (IRS) (Table 46.3). The IRS stage is determined principally by the site of the primary, size of the tumor, presence of involved lymph nodes, and presence of metastatic disease (Table 46.4). Prognostic factors in children with RMS have been identified and are used to determine treatment. The essential tumor-related factors in RMS are the clinical group, the stage, and histology.[29,30] Additional tumor factors include extensive bony erosion for paramenigeal tumors, DNA ploidy, and tumor response to therapy.

The IRS grouping and staging systems are predictive of survival and are used to determine risk-based therapy. The two main histologic subtypes of

TABLE 46.3   Clinical Grouping Used in IRS I–III

Clinical Group	Extent of Disease and Surgical Result
I	A. Localized tumor, confined to site of origin completely resected
	B. Localized tumor, infiltrating beyond site of origin, completely resected
II	A. Localized tumor, gross total resection, microscopic residual disease
	B. Locally extensive tumor (spread to regional lymph nodes), completely resected
	C. Extensive tumor (spread to nodes) gross total resection, microscopic residual
III	A. Localized or locally extensive tumor, gross residual after biopsy
	B. Localized or locally extensive tumor, gross residual after major resection (>50% debulking)
IV	Any size tumor with or without nodal involvement with distant mets

TABLE 46.4   TNM Staging of Rhabdomyosarcoma

Stage	Site	T Invasiveness	T Size	N	M
1	Orbit	T1 or T2	a or b	N0, N1, Nx	M0
	H/N — nonparameningeal				
	GU — nonbladder/prostate				
2	Bladder/prostate	T1 or T2	a	N0 or Nx	M0
	Extremity				
	Parameningeal				
	Retroper, trunk				
3	Bladder/prostate	T1 or T2	a	N1	M0
	Extremity	T1 or T2	b	N0, N1, Nx	M0
	Parameningeal				
	Retroper, trunk				
4	All	T1 or T2	a or b	N0 or N1	M1

Abbreviations: T1: confined to anatomic site of origin; T2: extension; T2a: <5 cm in diameter; T2b: >5 cm in diameter; N0: nodes not clinically involved; N1: nodes clinically involved; Nx: clinical status of nodes unknown; M1: distant mets present.

RMS are embryonal and alveolar. Each subtype has characteristic clinical and pathologic features. Embryonal RMS typically occurs in younger children and most often presents in the head/neck, genitourinary tract, and orbit, and has a favorable prognosis. Alveolar RMS often occurs in older children and adolescents, presenting in the trunk or extremities. Over 70% of alveolar RMS have a characteristic chromosomal translocation, the t(2;13)(q35;q14).[31] This translocation involves the juxtaposition of the PAX3 gene and the FKHR gene. The PAX3 gene is believed to regulate transcription during neuromuscular development, and the FKHR gene is a member of the forkhead family of transcription factors. Approximately 10–15% of alveolar RMS will have a t(1;13)(p36;q14) translocation.[31,32] The different fusions may have prognostic significance, which is a being studied.[32] Embryonal RMS demonstrates a variety of chromosomal abnormalities, including deletions of chromosome 1p with hyperdiploidy, trisomy 2, and ring chromosome 13.[31] Embryonal RMS tumors can also show loss of heterozygosity at the 11p15 locus. No tumor-specific translocations in embryonal RMS have been identified, and the prognostic significance of the chromosomal abnormalities seen in some tumors is uncertain.

Children with stage 1 RMS, Clinical Groups I, II, and III, and embryonal histology have a 3 year event-free survival of 90% based on IRS studies.[29] Children with stage 2 or 3 (RMS), Groups I–II embryonal histology also have a 3 year event-free-survival of over 80%, based on IRS studies. These subgroups are considered "low risk" RMS. Children with stage 2–3, Group III RMS of embryonal histology or all sites, Group I–III with alveolar histology have an intermediate prognosis with a 5-year event-free survival of 55%. Children with stage 4 (also considered Clinical Group IV) are considered high risk with a poor prognosis, with the exception of younger children as discussed below.

The principal host-related factor in RMS is the age of the patient, particularly for the embryonal histology. Patients less than 10 years of age have a better prognosis than those over 10.[33] Included in this intermediate-risk group are children less than 10 years of age who have metastatic disease (considered stage 4 or Clinical Group IV) and whose tumors are embryonal in histologic subtype. Children with stage 4 (or Group IV, as both indicate metastatic disease), with alveolar histology and of any age, or with embryonal histology and over 10 years of age have a 5-year survival of 30%. Future potential prognostic factors in RMS will focus on the chromosomal translocations as indicators of tumor biology and tumor response to specific agents or combinations of agents.

EWING'S SARCOMA

The Ewing family of tumors includes Ewing's sarcoma (ES) and primitive neuroectodermal tumor (PNET). These tumors are the second most common malignant bone tumor of childhood. The annual incidence of this tumor is approximately 2.1 cases per million children throughout the world, except among Blacks and Asians, among whom the incidence is much lower.[34,35] Most ES and PNET have a clonal translocation in the malignant cells. The most frequent translocation is between the long arms of chromosomes 11 and 22.[36] The break point of this translocation has been cloned and shown to occur within the EWS gene on chromosome 22 and the FLI-1 gene on chromosome 11. Although the t(11;22) translocation is the most common translocation in ES, others seen are t(21;22) and rarely t(7;22).[37]

Ewing's sarcoma can present in almost any bone in the body. The pelvic bones, extremities, and axial skeleton are most after the primary itself. The soft tissue PNET often occurs near bones. Approximately 25% of patients will present with metastatic disease, involving the lung (approximately 50% of metastases), bone (approximately 25% of metastases), and bone marrow (approximately 20% of metastases). The chief essential tumor-related prognostic factor for ES/PNET is the extent of disease (localized vs. metastatic). Additional factors are the size of the primary tumor (over 8 cm being a poor prognostic factor), site of the primary tumors site of metastasis (lung metastases alone convey a better prognosis than the presence of metastases to the bone or bone marrow), tumor response (both radiologically and pathologically) to therapy, and serum LDH at diagnosis. The site of the primary is considered by many to have prognostic significance, with the pelvic primary considered a poor prognostic factor. This may be due to the size of the tumor at the time of diagnosis, as pelvic tumors tend to be larger at presentation, so poorer outcome may be due to large size rather than site. A large European trial did not find site to be prognostic on multivariate analysis.[38] The host-related factors for ES/PNET are those of age, with younger children having a better prognosis than older adolescents. The promising factors in ES/PNET focus on the biological differences among the translocations described earlier.

MEDULLOBLASTOMA

Medulloblastoma is the most common brain tumor of childhood. Numerous multi-institutional trials have been performed to investigate the optimal treatment for pediatric medulloblastoma, and current information about prognosis is largely based on subset analyses of these studies.

The extent of disease is the most reliable indicator of progression-free and overall survival following treatment for medulloblastoma. The Chang staging system classifies both the local extent of the primary tumor and also metastatic spread. (Table 46.5) Multiple studies have demonstrated that the presence of metastatic disease is associated with poor prognosis.[39-41] In a trial involving 233 patients, Evans et al. found that patients with M0 disease had 59% 5-year event-free survival, in contrast to 36% for those with M1–M3 disease.[42] The presence of M+ disease was also associated with worse event-free survival in the International Society of Pediatric Oncology (SIOP) II study.[43] The significance of tumor cells in the cerebral spinal fluid (CSF) without gross

TABLE 46.5   Chang Staging System for Medulloblastoma

T1	Tumor <3 cm in diameter	M0	No evidence of subarachnoid or hematogenous metastases
T2	Tumor ≥3 cm in diameter	M1	Tumor cells found in CSF
T3a	Tumor >3 cm in diameter with extension	M2	Intracranial tumor beyond primary site
T3b	Tumor >3 cm in diameter with brainstem invasion	M3	Gross nodular seeding in spinal subarachnoid space
T4	Tumor >3 cm in diameter, with invasion beyond aqueduct of Sylvius and/or beyond foramen magnum	M4	Metastases outside cerebrospinal axis

Source: Reference 56.

metastatic disease (M1) remains controversial. In a Children's Cancer Group (CCG) trial of 203 patients, increasing M stage (M0 vs. M1 vs. M2+) was associated with decreasing progression-free survival. Patients with M1 disease had 57% 5-year progression free survival compared to 70% for those with M0 disease.[39] However, an analysis of patients with metastatic disease treated with the "eight drugs in one day" protocol revealed that M1 patients had an overall survival rate comparable to published survival rates seen in patients with M0 disease, although there were no M0 patients in the study itself.[44]

The local extent of disease and its resectability appear to be closely related. Chang classification of local tumor extent may be difficult to reproduce,[43] and its use in describing the prognosis associated with local tumor extent has largely been replaced by postoperative assessments of the completeness of resection. Complete resection is a favorable prognostic factor in many studies, but not all. Zeltzer et al. reported that for the subset of patients with M0 disease, those with >1.5 cm^2 of residual tumor on postoperative imaging had significantly worse 5-year progression-free survival than those with ≤ 1.5 cm^2 (54% versus 78%).[39] A large CCG study found a trend of borderline statistical significance toward improving 5-year event-free survival, comparing partial resection, subtotal resection, and complete resection.[42] After controlling for T- and M-stage, however, complete resection was not associated with outcome. Also, there was no clear trend for worse outcome with increasing Chang T-stage.[42] These results probably indicate that stage and resectability are closely related and provide overlapping information with respect to prognosis. Not all studies find an association between completeness of resection and outcome, however. In a randomized POG study of 78 patients, the extent of surgery was not related to 5-year overall survival,[45] and in a report of the French M7 protocol, 7-year disease-free survival was not significantly different for those with total versus subtotal resection.[46]

Young age is associated with worse outcome in numerous studies. In a multi-institutional trial of 233 patients, children less than 4 years age had significantly worse 5-year event-free survival (32%) than older children (53% for those older than 14 years),[42] and on multivariable analysis of prognostic factors, only age was significant. The CCG 921 study also reported worse 5-year progression-free survival for children 1.5–3 years old compared to those >3 years old.[39] The SIOP I study also found a small, though not statistically significant effect of age, with patients less than 2 having 5-year overall survival of 38.5% versus 47% for those age greater than 10 years.[47] The neurocognitive side effects of treatment are more severe in younger children, frequently leading to less aggressive therapy in these patients. This may in part contribute to their poorer survival. Even so, clinical decisions regarding the management of young children with brain tumors should not be based only on expected relapse rates, but also quality of life for those who are long-term survivors.

In several studies, girls have better survival rates following treatment for medulloblastoma than boys.[45,47–48] In a study of 109 patients, Weil et al. found that after controlling for the presence of metastases and the extent of surgical resection, the hazard of death in males was roughly twice that for females. Similar findings have been reported in other multi-institutional trials,[45,47] although other studies have not found this relationship.[39,42]

Preliminary studies indicate that biological markers may soon provide additional prognostic information for patients with medulloblastoma. Tumor-cell DNA ploidy has been associated with prognosis in medulloblastoma. Patients with hyperdiploid tumors had a significantly longer estimated 5-year survival rate (89%) than those with diploid tumors (48%) in a series reported by Gajjar et al.[49] Similar results have been reported elsewhere,[50] although in a series reported by Zerbini et al., patients with aneuploid tumors had worse prognosis than those with diploid/tetraploid tumors.[51] High levels of expression of the mRNA for trkC, the receptor for neurotrophin 3, have been associated with better progression-free survival in a small series reported by Segal et al.[52] Also, the chromosomal deletion of 17p has been associated with worse survival in some studies,[53,54] but not in others.[55]

ASTROCYTIC TUMORS

For children with astrocytomas, histologic grade is a significant prognostic factor for progression-free and overall survival. There are several different grading systems for astrocytic tumors, but the relative merits of each is beyond the scope of this review.[57] The revised World Health Organization (WHO) classification recognizes four categories and appears to correlate with survival[58] Using the WHO classification, Finlay et al. reported 3-year progression-free survival for anaplastic astrocytoma (AA) was approximately 10% higher than for glioblastoma multiforme (GBM).[59] Marchese and Chang found that 5-year overall survival was 4% in children with GBM versus 36% in those AA.[60] Also, patients with pilocytic astrocytomas have better survival rates than those with higher-grade astrocytomas.[61] In adult patients, mixed astrocytoma with oligodendroglial components has associated with longer survival than pure astrocytoma, though it is uncertain if this is also true in the pediatric population.[62]

The extent of resection is a significant prognostic factor, with the persistence of gross disease following surgery associated with poor survival. In a CCG study of 172 patients, patients with AA and >90% resection had a median time to progression of 31 months, compared to 12 months for those with ≤90% resection.[59] In a series of 41 patients treated at St. Jude Children's Research Hospital, 3-year progression-free survival for patients who underwent Gross Total Resection (GTR) was 60%, compared to 4% for those who underwent subtotal resection (STR) or biopsy. The impact of resection was found to be independent of tumor location.[63] Other studies have also documented the negative impact of subtotal resection on survival.

Location appears to be associated with prognosis in so far as it relates histologic grade, bulk of disease, neurologic compromise, and resectability. Brainstem gliomas, for example, which are both unresectable and often anaplastic, have poor outcomes. Short duration of symptoms prior to diagnosis appears to be a major adverse prognostic factor in brainstem gliomas.[64] Other midline tumors have also been associated with poor outcome, though it can be difficult to distinguish the impact of location independent of resectability.[60] Certain clinical/anatomic entities, such as cervicomedullary tumors, tectal gliomas, and dorsal exophytic astrocytomas, are associated with prolonged survival, in some cases even after incomplete resection see References,[65,66] and articles referred to therein).

Proliferation index has shown promise as a prognostic factor for children with malignant gliomas. In a study of 101 children with nonpilocytic astrocytoma, Ho et al. found that higher MIB-1 labeling index was associated with higher grade.[67] In the subgroup of patients with anaplastic astrocytoma, those with high MIB-1 index had survival rates comparable to the group with GBM, whereas AA patients with low MIB-1 index had a survival rate similar to those with low grade astrocytoma.[67] Similar findings have been reported by other groups.[68–70] Increasing S-phase fraction has also been associated with shorter survival in adult patients.[71]

EPENDYMOMA

Ependymomas are the third most common brain tumor of childhood. Data regarding prognostic factors in pediatric ependymoma come most commonly from retrospective analyses of single-institution series. Typically, the number of patients in these series is less than 100, with even fewer events (relapses or deaths) providing the basis for analysis. Consequently, while some factors emerge in several series as having prognostic value, few are unanimously identified in all series.

The histologic typing and grading of ependymoma remains controversial. The 1993 WHO classification recognizes four types: subependymoma and myxopapillary ependymoma (Grade I), ependymoma (Grade II), and anaplastic ependymoma (Grade III).[58] Marked variability in the proportion of anaplastic cases reported in different series indicates the uncertain consistency with which this system is applied in practice.

Some studies report worse overall survival among patients with anaplastic tumors (5-yr survival 10–55% worse than for those with Grade II ependymoma),[72–74] although some studies have not found this difference.[75,76] In addition to the problem of small sample sizes just noted, the assessment of grade as a prognostic factor can be hampered by treatment selection bias, in which patients with anaplastic tumors receive more aggressive treatment, thereby diluting the association between high-grade and worse outcome.

In multiple series, complete resection is associated with better progression-free and overall survival.[77–79] Five-year progression-free survival is typically 80% for patients with radiologically confirmed complete resection and 25% for those with residual disease following surgery. In two series with long-term follow-up, 71–75% of patients were alive 10 years after complete resection, whereas no patients were alive and free of disease 10 years after subtotal resection.[79,80]

Young age has been reported to be associated with worse progression-free and overall survival in several series, although "young" is variably defined.[72,79,81,82] Frequently, however, younger patients are more likely to have anaplastic tumors, which may confound the assessment of the impact of age. Also, younger patients may receive less aggressive treatment than older patients, because of concerns regarding toxicity. In analyses controlling for potential cofounders of age, conflicting results have been reported so it remains uncertain whether age provides additional prognostic information.

Tumor location appears to have prognostic significance in univariate tests in some series. Epenymomas of the spine and cauda equina, which are more often Grade I or II, have been associated with 5-year survival rates >90%.[73,83] Some studies report that patients with supratentorial tumors have better survival rates than those with infrantentorial tumors,[72,77,81,82] though other studies do not support this finding.[75,79,83] Tumor location is associated with other prognostic factors (e.g., grade and resectability), making it difficult to assess the independent effect of location on prognosis in small series.

There are relatively few series examining the prognostic value of molecular markers in ependymoma. MIB-1 labeling index >20% was associated with worse survival in one series.[84] The small number of patients in single-institution series has made the recognition of biological prognostic factors more difficult for ependymoma than for other pediatric tumors.

SUMMARY

The summary table (Appendix 46A) lists the prognostic factors in childhood cancers that we have just discussed. The improvement in the outcome of many childhood cancers is due in large part to the enrollment of children in Cooperative Group randomized trials. Through these trials, prognostic factors can be identified to stratify patients and guide therapy to improve outcomes and minimize late effects.

███████ **APPENDIX 46A**

Prognostic Factors in Pediatric Cancer

Prognostic Factors	Tumor Related	Host Related	Environment Related
Neuroblastoma			

Essential	INSS stage
	MYCN amplification
	Shimada
	  (histopathology)
	DNA ploidy (children
	  <2)
		Age
		  (<1 yr is
		  favorable)
			Treatment by multidisciplinary
			  team with experience in
			  pediatric oncology

Additional			
New and promising	Gain of chromosome 17 LOH chromosome 1p TRK A expression		
Wilms' Tumor			

Essential	Histology
	  Stage
		Age
		  (<2 yr is
		  favorable)
			Treatment by multidisciplinary
			  team with experience in
			  pediatric oncology

Additional	Size
	Capsular invasion
	Lymphatic vessel
	  invasion
		GU abnor-
		  malities
		Nephrogenic
		  rests
		Beckwith-
		  Wiedemann
		Denys-
		Drash
		  syndrome
		
		WAGR
		  syndrome	

New and promising			
Acute Leukemia			

Essential	WBC at dx (< 50 K is
	  favorable)
	Immunophenotype (pre-
	  B-cell is favorable)
	Tumor cytogenetics
	CNS (+) is unfavorable
		Age (1–9
		  yrs is
		  favorable)
			Treatment by multidisciplinary
			  team with experience in
			  pediatric oncology

Additional	DNA index Early response to therapy		

New and
  promising
	TEL-AML1 translocation
	  is favorable		

Prognostic Factors	Tumor Related	Host Related	Environment Related
Rhabdomyosarcoma			
Essential	Histology Stage Clinical group	Age	Treatment by multidisciplinary team with experience in pediatric oncology Surgeon experience/expertise
Additional			
New and promising	t(2;13) and t(1;13)		
Ewing's Sarcoma			
Essential	Stage Size Site Tumor response to therapy	Age	Treatment by multidisciplinary team with experience in pediatric oncology
Additional			
New and promising	Differences in translocations		
Medulloblastoma			
Essential	Metastasis (stage) Resectability		Treatment by multidisciplinary team with experience in pediatric oncology Surgeon experience Radiation oncologist experience
Additional		Age (young unfavorable) Sex (male unfavorable)	
New and promising	DNA ploidy TrkC expression Chromosome 17p deletion		
Astrocytoma			
Essential	Grade/classification Extent of resection Tumor location (e.g., infiltrating brainstem glioma)		
Additional			
New and promising	Proliferation index (MIB-1, S-phase fraction)		

Prognostic Factors	Tumor Related	Host Related	Environment Related
		Ependymoma	
Essential	Local extent/resectability Grade/classification		
Additional	Tumor location	Age (young unfavorable)	
New and promising	Proliferation index (MIB-1)		

REFERENCES

1. Yandell DW, Campbell TA, Dayton SH, et al.: Oncogenic point mutations in the human retinoblastoma gene: Their application to genetic counseling. *N Engl J Med* 321:1689–95, 1989.

2. Li FP, Fraumeni JF Jr., Mulvihill JJ, et al.: A cancer family syndrome in twenty-four kindreds. *Cancer Res* 48:5358–62, 1988.

3. Santibanez-Koref MF, Birch JM, Hartley AL, et al.: p53 germline mutations in Li-Fraumeni syndrome. *Lancet* 338:1490–1, 1991.

4. Brodeur GM, Seeger RC, Barrett A, et al.: International criteria for diagnosis, staging, and response to treatment in patients with neuroblastoma. *J Clin Oncol* 6:1874–81, 1988.

5. Brodeur GM, Seeger RC, Schwab M, et al.: Amplification of N-myc in untreated human neuroblastomas correlates with advanced disease stage. *Science* 224:1121–4, 1984.

6. Seeger RC, Brodeur GM, Sather H, et al.: Association of multiple copies of the N-myc oncogene with rapid progression of neuroblastomas. *N Engl J Med* 313:1111–6, 1985.

7. Fong CT, Dracopoli NC, White PS, et al.: Loss of heterozygosity for chromosome 1p in human neuroblastomas: Correlation with N-myc amplification. *Proc Natl Acad Sci USA* 86:3753–7, 1989.

8. Hayashi Y, Kanda N, Inaba T, et al.: Cytogenetic findings and prognosis in neuroblastoma with emphasis on marker chromosome 1. *Cancer* 63;126–32, 1989.

9. Brown N, Cotterill S, Lastowska M, et al.: Gain of chromosome arm 17q and adverse outcome in patients with neuroblastoma. *N Engl J Med* 340:1954–61, 1999.

10. Nakagawara A, Arima M, Azar CG, et al.: Inverse relationship between trk expression and N-myc amplification in human neuroblastomas. *Cancer Res* 52f:1364–8, 1992.

11. Green DM, Beckwith JB, Breslow NE, et al.: Treatment of children with stages II-IV anaplastic Wilms' tumor: A report from the National Wilms' Tumor study group. *J Clin Oncol* 12:2126–31, 1994.

12. Beckwith JB, Palmer NF: Histopathology and prognosis of Wilms tumor. Results of the National Wilms Tumor Study. *Cancer* 41:1937–48, 1978.

13. Marsden HB, Lawler W, Kumar PM: Bone metastasizing renal tumor of childhood. *Cancer* 42:1922–8, 1978.

14. Breslow NE, Palmer NF, Hill LR, et al.: Wilms' tumor: Prognostic factors for patients without metastases at diagnosis. *Cancer* 41:1577–89, 1978.

15. Miller RW, Fraumeni JF, Manning MD: Association of Wilms' tumor with aniridia, hemihypertrophy and other congenital malformations. *N Engl J Med* 270:922–7, 1964.

16. Drash A, Sherman F, Hartmann Wh, Blizzard RM: A syndrome pseudohemaphroditism, Wilms' tumor, hypertension and degenerative renal disease. *J Pediatr* 76:585–9, 1970.

17. Coppes MJ, Huff V, Pelletier J: Denys-Drash syndrome: Relating a clinical disorder to genetic alteration in the tumor suppressor gene WT1. *J Pediatr* 123:673–8, 1993.

18. Beckwith JB, Kiviat NB, Bonadio J: Nephrogenic rests, nephroblastomatosis and the pathogenesis of Wilms' tumor. *Pediatr Pathol* 10:1–36, 1990.

19. Liner MS, Ries LAG, Smith MA, et al.: Cancer surveillance series: Recent trends in childhood cancer incidence and mortality in the United States. *Journal of the National Cancer Institute (JNCl)* 91:1051–8, 1999.

20. Smith MA, Arthur D, Camitta B, et al.: Uniform approach to risk classification and treatment assignment for children with acute lymphoblastic leukemia. *J Clin Oncol* 14:18–24, 1996.

21. Pui C-H, Frankel L, Carroll A, et al.: Clinical characteristics and treatment outcome of childhood acute lymphoblastic leukemia with the t(4;11)(q21;q23): A collaborative study of 40 cases. *Blood* 77:440–7, 1991.

22. Fletcher J, Lynch E, Kimball V, et al.: Translocation (9;22) is associated with extremely poor prognosis in intensively treated children with acute lymphoblastic leukemia. *Blood* 77:435–9, 1991.

23. McLean TW, Ringold S, Neuberg D, et al.: TEL-AML1 dimerizes and is associated with a favorable outcome in childhood acute lymphoblastic leukemia. *Blood* 88:4252–8, 1996.

24. Rubnitz JE, Downing JR, Pui CH, et al.: TEL gene rearrangement in acute lymphoblastic leukemia: A new genetic marker with prognostic significance. *J Clin Oncol* 15:1150–57, 1997.

25. Borowitz MJ, Rubnitz J, Nash M, et al.: Surface antigen phenotype can predict TEL-AML1 rearrangement in childhood B-precursor ALL: A Pediatric Oncology Group study. *Leukemia* 12:1764–70, 1998.

26. Mahmoud H, Reivera G, Hancock M, et al.: Low leukocyte counts with blasts in cerebrospinal fluid of children with newly diagnosed acute lymphoblastic leukemia. *N Eng J Med* 329:314–9, 1993.

27. Miller D, Coccia P, Bleyer W, et al.: Early response to induction therapy as a predictor of disease-free-survival and ate recurrence of childhood acute lymphoblastic leukemia: A report from the Children's Cancer Study Group. *J Clin Oncol* 7:1807–15, 1989.

28. Reiter A, Schrappe M, Ludwig W-D, et al.: Chemotherapy in 998 unselected childhood acute lymphoblastic leukemia patients. Results and conclusions of the multicenter trial ALL-BFM 86. *Blood* 84:3122–33, 1994.

29. Crist W, Gehan EA, Ragab AH, et al.: The third Intergroup Rhabdomyosaroma Study. *J Clin Oncol* 13:610–30, 1995.

30. Rodary C, Gehan EA, Flamant F, et al.: Prognostic factors in 951 non-metastatic rhabdomyosarcoma in children: A report from the International Rhabdomyosarcoma Workshop. *Med Pediatr Oncol* 19:89–95, 1991.

31. Whang-Peng J, Knutsen T, Theil K, et al.: Cytogenetic studies in subgroups of rhabdomyosarcoma. *Genes Chromosomes Cancer* 5:299–310, 1992.

32. Kelly KM, Womer RB, Sorensen PH, et al.: Common and variant gene fusions predict distinct clinical phenotypes in rhabdomyosarcoma. *J Clin Oncol* 15:1831–6, 1997.

33. Anderson JR, Link M, Qualman S, et al.: Improved outcome for patients with embryonal histology but not alveolar histology rhabdomyosarcoma: Results from Intergroup Rhabdomyosarcoma Study-IV. American Society of Clinical Oncology (ASCO), Los Angeles, CA, May 16–19, 1998.

34. Fraumeni JF, Glass AG: Rarity of Ewing's sarcoma among US negro children. *Lancet* 1:366, 1981.

35. Li FP, Tu J-T, Liu F-S, et al.: Rarity of Ewing's sarcoma in China. *Lancet* 1:1255, 1980.

36. Delattre O, Zucman J, Melot T, et al.: The Ewing family of tumors: A subgroup of small-round-cell tumors defined by specific chimeric transcripts. *N Engl J Med* 331:294–9, 1994.

37. Sorensen PH, Lessnick Sl, Lopez-Terrada D, et al.: A second Ewing's sarcoma translocation, t(21;22), fuses the EWS gene to another ETS-family transcription factor, ERG. *Nat Genet* 6:146–51, 1994.

38. Sauer R, Jurgens H, Burger JMV, et al.: Prognostic factors in the treatment of Ewing's sarcoma. *Radiother Oncol* 10:101–10, 1987.

39. Zeltzer PM, Boyett JM, Finaly JL, et al.: Metastasis stage, adjuvant treatment and residual tumor are prognostic factors for medulloblastoma in children: Conclusions form the Children's Cancer Group 921 randomized phase III study. *J Clin Oncol* 17(3):832–45, 1999.

40. Yao MS, Mehta MP, Boyett JM, et al.: The effect of M-stage on patterns of failure in posterior fossa primitive neuroectodermal tumors treated on CCG-921: A phase III study in a high risk population. *Int J Radiat Oncol Biol Phys* 38(3):469–76, 1997.

41. Merchant TE, Wang MH, Haida T, et al.: Medulloblastoma: Long term results of patients treated with definitive radiation therapy during the computed tomography era. *Int J Radiat Oncol Biol Phys* 36(1):29–35, 1996.

42. Evans AE, Jenkin RD, Sposto R, et al.: The treatment of medulloblastoma: Results of a prospective randomized trial of radiation therapy with and without CCNU, vincristine and prednisone. *J Neurosurg* 72(4):572–82, 1990.

43. Bailey CC, Gnekow A, Wellek S, et al.: Prospective randomized trial of chemotherapy given before radiotherapy in childhood medulloblastoma. International Society of Pediatric Oncology (SIOP) and the (German) Society of Pediatric Oncology (GPO): SIOP II. *Med Pediatr Oncol* 25:166–78, 1995.

44. Bouffet E, Gentet JC, Doz F, et al.: Metastatic medulloblastoma: The experience of the French cooperative M7 group. *Eur J Cancer* 30A(10):1478–83, 1994.

45. Krischer JP: Abdelsalem RH, Kun L, et al.: Nitrogen mustard, vincristine, procarbazine, and prednisone as adjuvant chemotherapy in the treatment of medulloblastoma. A Pediatric Oncology Group Study. *J Neurosurg* 74:905–9, 1991.

46. Gentet JC, Bouffet MD, Doz F, et al.: Preirradiation chemotherapy including "eight drugs in 1 day" regimen and high-dose methotrexate in childhood medulloblastoma: results of the M7 French Cooperative Study. *J Neurosurg* 82:608–14, 1995.

47. Tait DM, Thornton-Jones H, Bloom HJG, et al.: Adjuvant chemotherapy for medulloblastoma: The first multi-centre controlled trail of the International Society of Paediatric Oncology (SIOP I). *Eur J Cancer* 26(8):464–9, 1990.

48. Weil MD, Lamborn K, Edwards MS, Wara WM: Influence of a child's sex on medulloblastoma outcome. *JAMA* 279:1474–6, 1998.

49. Gajjar AJ, Heideman RL, Douglass EC, et al.: Relation of tumor-cell ploidy to survival in children with medulloblastoma. *J Clin Oncol* 11(11):2211–7, 1993.

50. Yasue M, Tomita T, Engelhard H, et al.: Prognostic importance of DNA-ploidy in medulloblastoma of childhood. *J Neurosurg* 70:385–91, 1989.

51. Zerbini C, Gelber RD, Weinberg D, et al.: Prognostic factors in medulloblastoma including DNA ploidy. *J Clin Oncol* 11:616–22, 1993.

52. Segal RA, Goumnerova LC, Kwon YK, et al.: Expression of the neurotrophin receptor TrkC is linked to a favorable outcome in medulloblastoma. *Proc Natl Acad Sci USA* 91:12867–71, 1997.

53. Batra SK, McLendon RE, Koo JS, et al.: Prognostic implications of chromosome 17p deletions in human medulloblastomas. *J Neurooncol* 24:39–45, 1995.

54. Cogen PH, McDonald JD.: Tumor suppressor genes and medulloblastoma. *J Neurooncol* 29:103–12, 1996.

55. Beigel JA, Janss AJ, Raffel C, et al.: Prognostic significance of chromosome 17p deletions in childhood primitive neuroectodermal tumors (medulloblastomas) of the central nervous system. *Clin Cancer Res* 3:473–8, 1997.

56. Fuchs H, Friedman HS, Halperin EC: Medulloblastomas, in Black PMcL, Loeffler JS (eds.): *Cancer of the nervous system.* Oxford, Blackwell, 1997, pp. 567–75.

57. Nicholas MK, Prados MD, Larson DA, Gutin PH: Malignant astrocytomas, in Black PMcL, Loeffler JS (eds.): *Cancer of the nervous system.* Oxford, Blackwell, 1997, pp. 464–91.

58. Kleihues P, Burger PC, Scheithauer BW: The WHO classification f brain tumors. *Brain Pathol* 3:255–68, 1993.

59. Finlay JL, Boyett JM, Yates AJ, et al.: Randomized phase III trial in high grade childhood astrocytoma comparing vincristine, lomustine and prednisone with the eight-drugs-in-one day regimen. Children's Cancer Group. *J Clin Oncol* 13(1):112–23, 1995.

60. Marchese MJ, Chang CH: Malignant astrocytic gliomas in children. *CANCER* 65(12):2771–8, 1990.

61. Pollack IF, Claassen D, al-Shboul Q, et al.: Low grade gliomas in the cerebral hemispheres of children: An analysis of 71 cases. *J Neurosurg* 82(4):536–47, 1995.

62. Donahue B, Scott CB, Nelson JS, et al.: Influence of an oligodendroglial component on the survival of patients with anaplastic astrocytomas: A report of radiation therapy oncology group 83–02. *Int J Radiat Oncol Biol Phys* 38(5):911–4, 1997.

63. Heideman RL, Kuttesch J Jr, Gajjar AJ, et al.: Supratentorial malignant gliomas in childhood: A single institution perspective. *Cancer* 80(3):497–504, 1997.

64. Kaplan AM, Albright AL, Zimmerman RA, et al.: Brainstem gliomas in children: A Children's Cancer Group Review of 119 cases. *Pediatr Neurosurg* 24:185–92, 1996.

65. Pollack IF, Hoffman HJ, Humphries RP, Becker L: The long term outcome after surgical treatment of dorsally exophytic brain stem gliomas. *J Neurosurg* 78(6):859–63, 1993.

66. Epstein F, Wisoff J: Intra-axial tumors of the cervicomedullary junction. *J Neurosurg* 67:483–7, 1987.

67. Ho DM, Wong TT, Hsu CY: MIB-1 labelling index in non-pilocytic astrocytoma of childhood: A study of 101 cases. *Cancer* 82(12):2459–66, 1998.

68. Pollack IF, Cambell JW, Hamilton RL, et al.: Proliferation index as a predictor of prognosis in malignant gliomas of childhood. *Cancer* 79(4):849–56, 1997.

69. Schiffer D, Cavalla P, Chio A, et al.: Proliferative activity and prognosis of low grade astrocytomas. *J Neurooncol* 34(1):31–5, 1997.

70. McKeever PE, Strawderman MS, Yamini B, et al.: MIB-1 proliferation index predicts survival among patients with grade II astrocytoma. *J Neuropath Exp Neurol* 57(10):931–6, 1997.

71. Coons SW, Johnson PC, Pearl DK: Prognostic significance of flow cytometry deoxyribonicleic acid analysis of human astrocytomas. *Neurosurgery* 35(1):119–25, 1994.

72. Chiu JK, Woo SY, Ater J, et al.: Intracranial ependymoma in children: Analysis of prognostic factors. *J Neurooncol* 13(3):283–90, 1992.

73. Schild SE, Nisi K, Scheithauer BW, et al.: The results of radiotherapy for ependymomas: The Mayo Clinic experience. *Int J Radiat Oncol Biol Phys* 42(5):953–8, 1998.

74. Ernestus RI, Schroder R, Stutzer H, Klug N: The clinical and prognostic relevance of grading in intracranial ependymomas. *Br J Neurosurg* 11(5):421–8, 1997.

75. Goldwein JW, Leahy JM, Packer RJ, et al.: Intracranial ependymomas in children. *Int J Radiat Oncol Biol Phys* 19:1497–502, 1990.

76. Gerszten PC, Pollack IF, Matinez AJ, et al.: Intracranial ependymomas of childhood. Lack of correlation of histopathology and outcome. *Pathol Res Pract* 192(6):515–22, 1996.

77. Perilongo G, Massimo M, Sotti G, et al.: Analyses of prognostic factors in a retrospective review of 92 children with ependymoma: Italian Pediatric Neuro-oncology Group. *Med Pediatr Oncol* 29(2):79–85, 1997.

78. Roberston PL, Zelter PM, Boett JM et al.: Survival and prognostic factors following radiation therapy and chemotherapy for ependymomas in children: A report of the Children's Cancer Group. *J Neurosurg* 88(4):695–703, 1998.

79. Healey EA, Barnes PD, Kupsky WJ, et al.: The prognostic significance of postoperative residual tumor in ependymoma. *Neurosurgery* 28(5):666–71, 1991.

80. Pollack IF, Gertzen PC, Martinez, AJ et al.: Intracranial ependymomas in childhood: Long term outcome and prognostic factors. *Neurosurgery* 37:655–67, 1995.

81. Sak F, Talacchi A, Mazzo C, et al.: Prognostic factors in childhood intracranial ependymomas: The role of age and tumor location. *Pediatr Neurosurg* 28(3):135–42, 1998.

82. Nazar GB, Hoffman HJ, Becker LE, et al.: Infratentorial ependymomas in childhood: Prognostic factors and treatment. *J Neurosurg* 72(3):408–17, 1990.

83. Marks JE, Adler SJ: A comparative study of ependymoma by site of origin. *Int J Radiat Oncol Biol Phys* 8:37–43, 1982.

84. Ritter AM, Hess KR, McLendon RE, Langford LA: Ependymomas: MIB-1 proliferation index and survival. *J Neurooncol* 40(1):51–7, 1998.

The process of rendering prognosis is an essential part of the practice of medicine, and it is especially important in cancer, a disease associated with an overwhelming fear of death. With the progress in treatment of cancer, attention has shifted away from prognosis to diagnosis and treatment. Indeed, none of the major cancer textbooks devote space to the formal consideration of the study of prognosis. This book has been written to fill the gap in this area and to place some order on the field of prognosis in cancer.

The First Edition of *Prognostic Factors in Cancer*[1] presented a compilation of prognostic factors that influence the outcome in cancer patients without an attempt to put them in the context of rendering the prognosis. This edition provides a framework for considering prognostic factors as an activity of medical practice, within the concept of a management scenario. Part A considers the principles for studying prognosis, and for reflecting upon and deliberating about prognostic factors in cancer. Just as the TNM classification allows an orderly consideration and coding of the anatomic extent of disease, the prognostic factor classification provides a similar framework for prognostic factors. The management scenario, which includes the tumor, host, and environment prognostic factors at a specific point, is used to project outcome in the context of a planned intervention. Several concepts and classifications are introduced. The subject-based classification of prognostic factors (tumor, host, environment) allows for the inclusion of all attributes, while the relevance-based classification (essential, additional, new and promising) focuses the reader's attention on the current use of prognostic factor information. The former provides the capacity for including all the important factors needed to estimate outcome, while the latter focuses on the application of prognostic factors in everyday practice.

While we do not expect the subject-based classification to change with time, it is expected that the relevance-based classification will change with the introduction of new treatments and with the discovery of new factors. Progress in technology has fuelled a veritable "prognostic factor industry" that is expected to fill the literature with the flurry of new attributes.[2] The literature is crowded with studies of prognostic factors in cancer that suffer from methodological weaknesses. The most common problems include failure to formulate hypotheses, failure to provide adequate sample size or adequate follow-up with a sufficient number of events, inappropriate multiple significance testing, overfitting the model, and failure to verify prognostic factors with an independent data set. Here we highlight the importance of

769

proper methodology of studying prognostic factors while also introducing the concept of artificial neural networks as a means of studying prognosis. In view of the importance of prognosis in the practice of oncology, we consider it relevant to describe the issues surrounding the measurement of the accuracy of prognosis.

To write Part II of the book, "Prognostic Factors in Selected Cancers," we invited an international group of experts to outline the prognostic factors for specific cancers using the classifications and format described in Chapter 2. The authors make up a diverse group of experts representing many countries, and many professional disciplines dealing with cancer patients, including diagnostic radiologists, pathologists, surgeons, radiation, and medical oncologists from different countries. This diversity is by design and reflects the international mandate of the UICC. A considerable heterogeneity in the approach to prognostic factors for the specific cancers contained in Part B can be considered to reflect the state of the art in this area. Most authors of disease-specific chapters concentrated on factors that have an effect on prognosis in the newly diagnosed cancer patient. However, the proposed framework for prognostic factors viewed in the context of a management scenario does not have to be restricted to only initial presentation. It can be applied equally at the time of recurrence, or at any time in the course of the disease. The authors also focused on prognostic factors for overall survival. The proposed framework, however, is applicable to any management scenario with any endpoint, as long as both are defined. The authors give most attention to *tumor*-related factors, as they are most commonly studied and described in the literature. The *host*- and *environment*-related factors are much less frequently considered and only limited data are available to substantiate their importance. In spite of this, environmental factors have a profound impact on the outcome of cancer patients. Furthermore, in many instances, no new knowledge is required to influence these factors and improve the results of cancer.

Progress in cancer biology, biochemistry, and genetics opened the door to the study of new targets for prognostic factor study. Although thousands of papers are published each year dealing with the immunohistochemical factors, proliferation markers, apoptosis, and other factors, the clinical relevance of the newer prognostic factors still awaits confirmation. While there is now more information about the molecular prognostic factors, few of them were assigned to the essential category. In fact, the time-honored and well-tested factors such as anatomic extent of disease, tumor type, and application of appropriate treatment intervention are consistently considered essential in today's clinical practice.

What is the future of prognostic factor study and its application in clinical practice? With the advent of the DNA microarray methodology, many new molecular prognostic factors are expected to be found during the next few years. New and improved computational and statistical methods are required to handle the enormous amount of information and to test the clinical relevance of these putative prognostic factors. With progress in computer science, handling of large amounts of data is already possible. Besides the progress in computing and data analysis, standardization of terminology is urgently needed. The field of medical informatics deals with data recording, storage retrieval, and analysis. Further development of a medical lexicon is needed to formalize a uniform and unambiguous use of terms coming into use and represents one of the challenges faced by the discipline of medical informatics.[3] Implementation of better standards for the presentation of the results of prognostic factors research in peer-reviewed journals would assist in improving the understanding of the subject. A more difficult venture is the development of the standards for application of prognostic factors to clinical practice, cancer research, and cancer control programs.

REFERENCES

1. Hermanek P, Gospodarowicz M, Henson D, et al.: *Prognostic factors in cancer*, UICC (ed.): Heidelberg, Springer-Verlag, 1995.
2. Hall PA, Going JJ: Predicting the future: A critical appraisal of cancer prognosis studies. *Histopathology* **35**:489–94, 1999.
3. Coiera E: Medical informatics. *BMJ* **310**:1381–7, 1995.

Accuracy The closeness of a measurement or judgment to the true value of the quantity of interest.

Additional prognostic factor Attributes that allow refinements in predicting outcome, although they are not currently used in the decision-making process, for example, do not alter treatment.

Adjuvant therapy Treatment given following the primary treatment to enhance the effectiveness of the primary treatment. Adjuvant therapy may be chemotherapy, radiation therapy, or hormone therapy.

Ageism Prejudice or discrimination against a particular age group and especially the elderly.

Biomarkers Substances sometimes found in an increased amount in the blood, other body fluids, or tissues, and that may suggest the presence of some types of cancer. Biomarkers include CA 125 (ovarian cancer), CA 15-3 (breast cancer), CEA (ovarian, lung, breast, pancreas, and GI tract cancers), and PSA (prostate cancer). Also called *tumor markers*.

Calibration Determination, by measurement or comparison with a standard, of the correct value of each scale reading on a meter or other measuring instrument; or determination of the settings of a control device that correspond to particular values of voltage, current, frequency, or other output.

Clinical decision making The process of making a selective intellectual judgment when presented with several complex alternatives consisting of several variables, and usually defining a course of action or an idea.

Clinical practice guidelines Systematically developed statements designed to help practitioners and patients make decisions about appropriate health care for specific circumstances.

Combined modality therapy Two or more types of treatment used to supplement each other. For instance, surgery, radiation, chemotherapy, hormonal, or immunotherapy may be used alternatively or together for maximum effectiveness.

Cox's model A regression-based technique for estimating how survival depends on a set of independent variables.

Discrimination The extent to which a test or judgment distinguishes between two states or items.

DNA arrays Matrix of a large number of known DNA molecules (or parts of molecules) attached to an inert substrate. Such matrices can be hybridized with unknown mixtures of mRNAs or DNAs to identify which genes are being expressed or are the subject of genomic imbalance in the cells from which the mixtures were derived.

Ellipsis Omission; a figure of syntax, by which one or more words, which are obviously understood, are omitted.

Endpoint A category of data used to compare the outcome in different arms of a clinical trial. Common endpoints are severe toxicity, disease progression, or fall in such surrogate markers as PSA level, or death.

Environment The aggregate of social and cultural conditions that influence the life of an individual or community; the sum of all external conditions affecting the life, development, and survival of an organism.

Environment-related prognostic factor Factors that operate external to the patient and affect the prognosis; examples include socioeconomic status, treatment, quality of care, health care system.

Error The difference between the approximate result and the true result; used particularly in the rule of double position.

Error analysis The study of the observed discrepancies between the data and the values predicted by a model, often aimed at checking assumptions and diagnosing faults in the model.

Errors of measurement The part of the variation in the distribution of items that is due to faulty measurement instruments, observation errors, and other human factors.

Essential prognostic factors Factors that are fundamental to decisions about the goals and choice of treatment, including details of selection of treatment modality and specific interventions for example, anatomic extent of tumor.

Event Something that happens; an occurrence.

Evidence-based practice The conscientious, explicit, and judicious use of current best evidence in making decisions about the care of individual patients.

Frequency Number of occurrences in a given class, for example, percentage of cancers that are lymphomas.

Health services accessibility The degree to which individuals are inhibited or facilitated in their ability to gain entry to and to receive care and services from the health care system. Factors influencing this ability include geographic location, architectural, transportational, and final considerations, among others.

Health services research The integration of epidemiologic, sociological, economic, and other analytic sciences in the study of health services. Health services research is usually concerned with relationships between need, demand, supply, use, and outcome of health services. The aim of the research is evaluation, particularly in terms of structure, process, output, and outcome.

Host-related prognostic factor Inherent characteristics, such as age, gender, and racial origin, and other factors, such as performance status, comorbid conditions, and immune status, that affect the prognosis, but are not related to the presence of tumor.

Incidence   Rate, range, or amount of occurrence or influence; for example, number of new cases of cancer occurring in 100,000 people of a defined population per year.

Independent prognostic factors   Not dependent upon another quantity in respect to value or rate of variation; said of quantities or functions. See **statistical independence**.

Independent variable   The terms *dependent* and *independent* variable apply mostly to experimental research where some variables are manipulated, and in this sense they are "independent" from the initial reaction patterns, features, intentions, and so forth, of the subjects.

Management scenario   Is the setting for the host with a set of prognostic attributes existing at the time, in a given environment. The prognosis associated with a scenario is influenced by the history of prior events, the choice of planned intervention, and the outcome of interest. A scenario is a chapter in the history of the disease. It is characterized by the date of diagnosis of the disease for the first time or the date of a recurrence for a subsequent scenario and ends with elimination of disease for an appropriate period of time for that disease or until last follow-up. A new scenario normally exists when disease recurrence manifests, but, in contrast, persisting disease at the same site would be continuation of the same scenario.

Meta-analysis   A quantitative method of combining the results of independent studies (usually drawn from the published literature), and synthesizing summaries and conclusions that may be used to evaluate therapeutic effectiveness or to plan new studies.

Milieu   The physical or social setting in which something occurs or develops.

Molecular prognostic factors   Substances, usually proteins, that control tumor growth and spread, and can predict for the presence of occult metastatic spread, virulence of the cancer, or the response to specific therapies, for example, Ki 67. Molecular factors can also be themselves the targets for newer forms of therapy.

Multiple regression   A method, the general purpose of which is to analyze the relationship between several independent variables and a dependent variable.

Multivariate analysis   A statistical method that allows analysis of the influence of several factors on prognosis or outcome after treatment to determine which factors may be independently predictive of that outcome.

Natural history of disease   The course and features of a disease, particularly in the absence of treatment.

Neural network   A computational network, often for pattern recognition, composed of mathematically defined elements that are thought to approximate the working of biological neurons; often composed of a layer that receives and organizes inputs, a hidden layer, and an output layer in which individual "neurons" identify particular patterns.

New and promising prognostic factor   Factors that shed new light about the biology of disease, but for which currently there is, at best, incomplete evidence of an independent effect on outcome or prognosis.

Oncogene   Mutated and/or overexpressed version of a normal gene of animal cells (the proto-oncogene) that in a dominant fashion can release the cell from normal restraints on growth, and thus alone or in concert with other changes, convert a cell into a tumor cell.

Outcome   Evaluation procedure that focuses on the status (*outcome assessment*) of the patient at the end of an episode of care — presence of symptoms, level of activity, and mortality; and the process (process assessment); what is done for the patient diagnostically and therapeutically.

Outcome assessment   Research aimed at assessing the quality and effectiveness of health care as measured by the attainment of a specified end result or outcome. Measures include parameters such as improved health, lowered morbidity or mortality, and improvement of abnormal states.

p53   A gene that encodes a protein that regulates cell growth and is able to cause potentially cancerous cells to destroy themselves.

p-value   In testing, the probability of observing a value of the test as discrepant from the null hypothesis as the one actually observed. Small *p*-values are taken to be evidence that the null hypothesis should be rejected.

Palliative therapy   Treatment given to relieve symptoms caused by advanced cancer. Palliative therapy does not alter the course of a disease, but improves the quality of life.

Physician Data Query (PDQ)   A comprehensive database produced by the National Cancer Institute that provides up-to-date cancer information. PDQ contains peer-reviewed information summaries on screening, prevention, supportive care, genetics, and treatment of cancer. These summaries are provided in two versions: one written in technical language for health care professionals, and a second written in nontechnical language. Editorial boards comprising cancer experts review the current medical literature to develop and update the content of PDQ each month. PDQ also contains a registry of approximately 1800 cancer clinical trials that are open to patients worldwide; and directories of physicians, genetics professionals, and organizations that provide cancer care.

Power   The probability that a clinical trial will be able to detect a real difference between two treatments. The power of a study depends strongly on its sample size.

Practice guidelines   Directions or principles presenting current or future rules of policy for the health care practitioner to assist him or her in patient care decisions regarding diagnosis, therapy, or related clinical circumstances. The guidelines may be developed by government agencies at any level, institutions, professional societies, governing boards, or by the convening of expert panels.

The guidelines form a basis for the evaluation of all aspects of health care and delivery.

Precision   The extent to which a measurement is free of random error. Precision reflects the ability to reach the same value each time one measures the same object. It is the reciprocal of variability.

Prediction   Any declaration or estimate regarding the future.

Predictive factor = prognostic factor   In some instances used only for factors that predict response to treatment, but such a distinction is arbitrary.

Probability   The measure of the uncertainty associated with events of unknown outcome. Interpretations of probability include physical properties of phenomena, subjective states of uncertainty, and logical relations between sentences.

Prognosis   The act or art of foretelling the course of a disease; a forecast as to the probable outcome of an attack or disease; the prospect as to recovery from a disease as indicated by the nature and symptoms of the case.

Prognostic factor   (1) That which prognosticates; a sign by which a future event may be known or foretold; an indication, a sign or omen; hence, a foretelling; a prediction. (2) A detectable feature of a cancer or patient that can be used to predict the likely outcome of treatment of the cancer.

Prognostic index   A value reflecting the combined effect of multiple *prognostic factors* for an individual patient.

Quality assurance (health care)   Activities and programs intended to assure or improve the quality of care in either a defined medical setting or a program. The concept includes the assessment or evaluation of the quality of care; identification of problems or shortcomings in the delivery of care; designing activities to overcome these deficiencies; and follow-up monitoring to ensure effectiveness of corrective steps.

Quality of health care   The levels of excellence that characterize the health service or health care provided based on accepted standards of quality.

Quality of life   A generic concept reflecting concern with the modification and enhancement of life attributes, for example, physical, political, moral, and social environment.

Random error   A random variable included in a variety of statistical models to summarize discrepancies between the data and the model that are due to unpredictable sources or to sampling variation.

Randomized clinical trial   A study in which participants are assigned by chance to separate groups that compare different treatments. Neither the researcher nor the participant can choose the group. Using chance to assign people means that the groups will be similar and the treatments they receive can be compared. At the time of the trial, there is no way for the researchers to know which of the treatments is best or who may be in control groups.

Rb   Tumor suppressor gene encoding a nuclear protein that, if inactivated, enormously raises the chances of development of cancer, classically retinoblastoma, but also other sarcomas and carcinomas.

Receiver-operating-characteristics (ROC) curve A technique for assessing the efficacy of a diagnostic test based on knowledge of the true-positive and false-positive rates for the test in question.

Recurrence The point when cancer cells from the primary tumor are detected following the primary treatment for the cancer.

Relative risk The proportion of diseased people among those exposed to the relevant risk factor divided by the proportion of diseased people among those not exposed to the risk factor. This process should be used in those cohort studies where those with and without disease are followed to observe which individuals become diseased.

Resection margins The edges delineating the resected and the remaining tissues following biopsy or surgical excision of a lesion. Normally these are described in relation to whether tumor extends to the resection margin or whether there is a definite layer of normal tissue separating the resection margin from the edge of the tumor within the resected specimen.

Response to treatment The regression of cancer following treatment, or spontaneously. Usually categorized as *complete response* or *partial response*.

Complete response The disappearance of all clinical evidence of disease. This does not necessarily mean cure, as microscopic metastases may remain undetected, are likely to regrow and become resistant to treatment.

Partial response A decrease of at least 50% in the sum of the measurements of all evaluable target lesions or tumors seen in a study.

Risk The probability that an event will occur. It encompasses a variety of measures of the probability of a generally unfavorable outcome.

Risk factor A clearly defined occurrence or characteristic that has been associated with the increased rate of a subsequently occurring disease.

ROC curve See **Receiver-operating-characteristics (ROC) curve**.

Scenario See **management scenario**.

Sensitivity The probability that a diagnostic test will identify those patients who have a given disease or attribute.

Shared decision making Two-way exchange of information, with decisions shared between by the doctor and the patient, not only about risks and benefits but also patient-specific characteristics and values.

Significant In statistics: probably resulting from something other than chance; probably having a systematic cause.

Specificity The probability that a negative diagnostic test will correctly identify those patients who do not have a given disease or attribute.

Stage The extent to which cancer has spread from its original site. Usually denoted by a number from Stage I (least severe), for example, small and organ confined, to Stage IV (most advanced), that is distant metastasis.

Staging In cancer: the *grouping* of cases with similar features of anatomic spread and similar prognosis. The *TNM* system classifies the tumor by its size, site, and spread. The numbers I, II, III, and IV are used to denote the grouping of Ts, Ns, and Ms into stages, and each number refers to a possible combination of TNM factors. For example, a Stage I cancer can include both *T1, N0, M0*, where T1 — tumor is small; N0 — no regional lymph-node metastasis, M0 — no distant metastasis and T2, N0, M0 (a larger localized primary tumor) if their prognoses are similar. It is important to separate the concepts of "staging" as an activity involving investigations and procedures to define the extent of disease versus "staging" as a process to classify and permanently record the stage using the TNM nomenclature.

Statistical independence   The case in which the occurrence of one event does not affect, nor is affected by, the occurrence of another event.

Statistical significance (*p*-level)   The statistical significance of a result is an estimated measure of the degree to which it is "true" (in the sense of "representative of the population"). The higher the *p*-level, the less we can believe that the observed relation between variables in the sample is a reliable indicator of the relation between the respective variables in the population. Specifically, the *p*-level represents the probability of error that is involved in accepting the observed result as valid, that is, as "representative of the population." For example, the *p*-level of .05 (i.e.,1/20) indicates that there is a 5% probability that the relation between the variables found in the sample is due to chance alone, just a coincidence, a "fluke." In many areas of research, the *p*-level of .05 is customarily treated as a "borderline acceptable" error level.

Supportive care   Treatment given to prevent, control, or relieve complications and side effects and to improve the patient's comfort and quality of life.

Surrogate marker   A measurement that indirectly indicates the effect of treatment on disease state; a *prognostic factor* that indirectly reflects another prognostic factor, for example, mitotic activity may be a surrogate marker for proliferation as measured by the Ki-67 index.

Systematic error   A sampling error that causes the resulting measurement to be incorrect in a systematic way.

TNM   A system that classifies the anatomic extent of cancer. T refers to the size or extent of spread of the primary tumor; N refers to the presence or absence of tumor in regional lymph nodes, and M to the presence or absence of distant metastases.

Treatment intervention   Planned action in the management of the disease; may involve observation, surgery, chemotherapy, radiation therapy, or a combination of any of these.

Tumor marker   A substance detected (usually in excess) in the body, that indicates the presence of cancer. These markers can be specific for certain types of cancer and are usually detected in tumor tissue or in the blood. Tumor markers include CA 125 (ovarian cancer), CA 15-3 (breast cancer), CEA (ovarian, lung, breast, pancreas, and GI tract cancers), and PSA (prostate cancer).

Tumor prognostic factors   The characteristics of the tumor, or the effects of the tumor on the host, that affect the *prognosis*, for example, extent of tumor (*TNM*) and histologic grade.

Tumor registry   A site in which data on cancer patients is recorded.

Tumor suppressor gene   A gene that encodes a product that normally negatively regulates the cell cycle and that must be mutated or otherwise inactivated before a cell can proceed to rapid division.

Univariate analysis   The study of the distribution of a single random variable.

Variable   Items that are measured, controlled, or manipulated, particularly in research.

■■■■■ ■ INDEX